Intra-abdominal Infections

José M. Tellado
Nicolas V. Christou

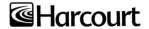

Madrid - Barcelona - Boston - Filadelfia
Londres - Orlando - Sidney - Tokio - Toronto

Es una publicación

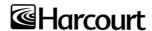

© 2000 Ediciones Harcourt, S.A.
Velázquez, 24-5.º Dcha
28001 - Madrid, España

Ediciones Harcourt, S.A.
Harcourt International
División Iberoamericana

ISBN: 84-8174-506-5
Depósito legal: M-29249-2000
Impreso en España por: Gráficas Marte, S.A.

Consulte el catálogo de publicaciones on-line
Internet: www.harcourt.es

Contributors

Frederico Aun MD PhD FACS
Department of Surgery
University of Sao Paulo
Sao Paulo, Brazil

José L. Balibrea MD PhD FACS (Hon.)
Chairman, Department of Surgery
Complutense University
H.C.U. San Carlos
Madrid, Spain

Henri Bismuth MD
Professor and Chair
Hepato-Biliary Surgery and Liver Transplant
Research Center
C.H.U. Paul Brousse
Villejuif, France

Félix Broche Valle MD
Research Fellow
Surgical Infection Unit
Department of Surgery
H.G.U. "Gregorio Marañón"
Madrid, Spain

Michael Budd, B.S
Surgical Research Associate
Department of Surgery
UCI Medical Center
Orange CA, USA

Emilia Cercenado Pharm.D.
Associate Professor of Microbiology
Complutense University
Division of Clinical Microbiology
H.G.U. "Gregorio Marañón"
Madrid, Spain

Nicolas V. Christou MD PhD FRCS (C) FACS
Professor of Surgery
Head, Division General Surgery and SICU
McGill University Health Centre
Montreal, PQ, Canada

Ricardo E. Cohen MD Ph.D.FACS
Department of Surgery
University of Sao Paulo
Sao Paulo, Brazil

John Miriam Davis MD FACS
Program Director of Surgery
Jersey Shore Medical Center
Neptune NJ, USA

Jesús Esquivel, M.D.
Chief Resident in Surgery
Jersey Shore Medical Center
Neptune NJ, USA

Eduard H. Farhmann MD
Professor and Chairman
Department of Surgery
Universität Freiburg
Freiburg, Germany

Frazier W. Frantz MD
Resident in Pediatric Surgery
Division of Pediatric Surgery
Children's Hospital Medical Center
Cincinnati, OH, USA

Fernando García-Garrote Sc.D. Ph.D
Resident in Microbiology
Division of Clinical Microbiology
H.G.U. "Gregorio Marañón"
Madrid, Spain

Harry van Goor MD PhD
Department of Surgery
Academisch Ziekenhuis Nijmegen
Nijmegen, The Netherlands

Jan Goris MD
Chairman, Departmen of Surgery
Academisch Ziekenhuis Nijmegen
Nijmegen, The Netherlands

Rudolf Häring MD
Chirurgische Universitätsklinik Freiburg
Universität Freiburg
Freiburg, Germany

Randeep S. Jawa MD
Clinical and Research Fellow
Division of Surgical Infectious Diseases
Department of Surgery
University of Cincinnati Medical Center
Cincinnati OH, USA

Fernando E. Kafie, M.D
Surgeical Research Fellow
Department of Surgery
UCI Medical Center
Orange CA, USA

Jina Krissat MD
Hepato-Biliary Surgery and Liver Transplant
Research Center
C.H.U. Paul Brousse
Villejuif, France

William J. Ledger MD
Professor and Chair
Department of Obstetrics and Gynaecology
New York Hospital-Cornell Medical Center
New York NY, USA

John Marshall MD FRCS (C) FACS
Associate Professor of Surgery,
Toronto General Hospital
Toronto, ON, Canada

Miguel Navasa Anadón MD
Liver Unit
Institut de Malalties Digestives
Hospital Clinic
Barcelona, Spain

Juan C. Puyana MD FACS
Chairman, Trauma and Critical Care Center
Brighan's and Women's Hospital
Boston MA, USA

Faouzi Saliba MD
Hepato-Biliary Surgery and Liver Transplant
Research Center
C.H.U. Paul Brousse
Villejuif, France

Ulrich Schöffel MD PhD
Chirurgische Universitätsklinik Freiburg
Department of Surgery
Freiburg, Germany

Joseph S. Solomkin MD
Chief, Division of Surgical Infectious Diseases
Department of Surgery
University of Cincinnati Medical Center
Cincinnati OH, USA

Daniel E. Swartz MD
Clinical and Research Fellow
Royal Victoria Hospital
McGill University Health Centre
Montreal PQ, Canada

José M. Tellado MD FACS
Surgical Infection Unit
Department of Surgery
H.G.U. "Gregorio Marañón"
Madrid, Spain

Daniel Vega MD
Chief Resident in Surgery
Department of Surgery
H.G.U. "Gregorio Marañón"
Madrid, Spain

Russell A. Williams MD
Professor of Surgery
Department of Surgery
UCI Medical Center
Orange CA, USA

Dietmar H. Wittman MD
Professor of Surgery
Venice, Fl USA

Moritz M. Ziegler MD
Director, Division of Pediatric Surgery
Children's Hospital Medical Center
Cincinnati, OH, USA

*To our fathers Alberto Tellado Rey
(1920 -1999) and Venizelos
Christou (1921-1992).
To our families (Carmen, Alberto
Scott, Sara and Katina, Velos, John)
for being understanding,
supportive and tolerant in many
illuminating ways.*

Preface

To Lloyd D. McLean MD FRCS (C) FACS
Former Chairman, Department of Surgery,
McGill. University at Montreal, and
ex-President of the American College of Surgeons

When setting out this project, our spirit and mode were in Ithaca, with the universal Greek poet Konstantinos Kavafis (1863-1933) who once remarked, "...for Ithaca has given you the lovely trip, without her you would not have set your course...". Even today this assertion is still a true leitmotif. Indeed, contemporary medicine flourishes in apparently contrasting lands, inasmuch as it has many undiscovered new worlds existing side by side with ancient Ithacas to go over again. Without reservation, intra-abdominal infections are one of those Ithacas and a recurrent theme in surgical infectious diseases. Here is an area in which much understanding has been accomplished, yet much remains to be done.

There have been sound advances in the care of intra-abdominal infections, from diagnosis to rational antimicrobial use. Nevertheless, new groups of patients and technology not seen before have emerged into the clinical scenario of intra-abdominal infections which deserve particular attention and a review is timely. The high prevalence of chronic viral infections and the long-term survival rate of transplant recipients under active immune suppression are clear examples of this new frontier. Parasitic endemic diseases are no longer confined outside western society boundaries. Innovative radical surgery, in many occasions under clinical trial itself, has been central to cancer cure or palliation, but when unsuccessful, becomes a true challenge for every surgeon in the pursuance of an effective surgical source control. Consequently, these high risk patients have pushed to the limit our current standardisation of clinical trials and the preventive measures to control hospital-acquired bacterial ecology ultimately, yielding new entities such as tertiary peritonitis and multiple organ dysfunction. These problems and developments in our field of surgical infectious diseases are considered in this edition, which has intended to take into account, both the expansion of knowledge and the change in scope yet retained the primary emphasis on the application and practical value.

However, in the modern global village encompassed by scientific information, medicine progresses by assembling fresh evidence and by creating new paradigms, rather than by individual experience as was the vogue of the ancient traveller. To ensure fairness we

asked each author to verity the forner approach based upon scientific evidence using their distinctive and unquestionable expertise. We were fortunate to gather around this monograph a worldwide faculty from the surgical and non-surgical international community. We thank all the authors for their scholarly contributions and we hope that this collective venture does indeed prove to be invaluable to the Medical community.
As our venerable pilgrims, we were ".... enriched by all you gained upon the way, and not expecting Ithaca to give you further wealth... ". In a project such as this, many colleagues provided helpful suggestions and certainly enlightened our view with their constructive critiques, particularly Roberto Urbez who was certainly the spine and by no means less substantial, the financial bauber until the end. We are greatly indebted to the Editorial Assistance of Mrs. Amor Tripiana for her persistence and good-humoured, in spite of continuous delays. We were also most grateful for the hard work, intellectual input and help provided by our Chief Residents Jose A. Alcazar MD PhD, Jose Rueda MD, Jose A. Lopez-Baena MD, Daniel Vega MD (at the H.G.U. Gregorio Marañon in Madrid) which certainly palliated our daily clinical duties. Finally, no portion of this monograph deals specifically with abscess formation or organ dysfunction, because outstanding monographs have already been published.

José M. Tellado MD FACS
Surgical Infection Unit
Department of Surgery
H.G.U. Gregorio Marañon
Madrid

Nicolas V. Christou MD PhD FRCS(C) FACS
Professor of Surgery
Head, Division of General Surgery
McGill University Health Centre and McGill
University
Montreal

Contents

Pág.

Host Defense Mechanisms of the Peritoneal Cavity 1
J.M. Tellado, F. Broche, D. Vega, J.L. Balibrea

The Microbial Ecology of the Gastrointestinal Flora 13
J.C. Marshall

Diagnosis and Minimally Invasive Treatment
of Occult Intra-abdominal Infections 31
J.C. Puyana

Monitoring Intra-abdominal Infection 45
H. van Goor, R.J.A. Goris

Issues in the Desing of Clinical Trials
of Anti-Infectives for Intra-abdominal Infections 65
J.S. Solomkim, R.S. Jawa

Primary Peritonitis 77
M. Navasa

Secondary Peritonitis 97
D.E. Swartz, N.V. Christou

Intra-abdominal Infections: Antibiotics in Secondary Peritonitis 119
J. Esquivel, J. Mihran Davis, R. Wook

Tertiary Peritonitis 143
D.H. Wittmann

Newer Methods of Operative Therapy for Peritonitis 153
D.H. Wittmann

Therapeutics Challenges of Tertiary Peritonitis 179
E. Cercenado, F. García-Garrote

Intra-abdominal Infections Originated in Solid Organs 193
E.H. Farthmann, R. Häring, U. Schöffel

Specific Approaches to Intra-abdominal Infections
in Liver Transplant Recipients 247
F. Saliba, J. Krissat, H. Bismuth

Common Intra-abdominal Infections in Aids Patients 259
F.E. Kafie, M. Budd, R. Williams

Pediatric Intra-abdominal Infections 283
F.W. Frantz, M.M. Ziegler

Pelvic Inflammatory Disease 341
W.J. Ledger

Intra-abdominal Infections Originated from Tropical Surgical Diseases 365
R.V. Cohen, F. Aun

Host Defense Mechanisms of the Peritoneal Cavity

José M. Tellado, MD FACS, Félix Broche Valle, MD,
Daniel Vega MD, José L. Balibrea MD FACS

The peritoneum belongs to a distinct family of body tissues known as the serosa which share the same cellular composition and exhibit identical histoarchitecture. It is traditionally accepted that the peritoneal surface area is approximately the same as the surface area of the skin, although a more accurate measurement indicates an average of 177 cm^2/Kg body weight [1]. This large compartment, the peritoneal cavity, was imagined to confront bacterial invasion in three ways by bacterial clearance via the diaphragmatic stomata, by cellular exudation and phagocytosis and throughout bacteria sequestration and abscess formation. Beneath this paradigm was a vaguely defined role of the peritoneum as a simple boundary structure [2]. In contradistinction to earlier concepts, the peritoneal cavity is no longer viewed as a mere leaky linning of mesothelial cells but a complex dynamic scenario where a variety of activities occur even in the steady-state, such as bacterial and viral sensing, visceral lubrication, particle absorption and non-self rejection. The exposure of the peritoneum to bacteria prompts the response of the peritoneal defense systems, both innate and adaptative, in a sequential and coordinated set of interactions by immune and non-immune mesenchymal cells.

1. RESIDENT CELLS WITHIN THE PERITONEAL CAVITY

1.1. Human Peritoneal Macrophages (HPMØ)

The mononuclear phagocyte is the predominal cell type found in peritoneal fluid from healthy animals, in peritoneal dialysate from uninfected patients undergoing acute or chronic peritoneal dialysis and in peritoneal fluid from normal and infertile woman. Extensive morphological and cytochemical studies (non-specific stearate, myeloperoxidase, acid phosphatase, leucine-amino peptidase) in animal models and humans have shown that peritoneal fluid contains macrophages on different activation states, ranging from resident macrophages in the unstimulated peritoneal cavity to elicit-macrophages in the peritoneal dialysate from CAPD patients and healthy women.

The uninfected peritoneal cavity (steady-state condition) contains in general, a small resident population of HPMØ ($\sim 10^3$-10^4), although the individual variability from subject-to-subject can be greater (3-74%) [3]. Labelling studies in animal models performed under steady-state conditions show that the kinetics of HPMØ replacement either from monocyte influx or from local production occurs at the rate of 7 x 10^3/ hr [4]. Under chronic inflammatory stimuli, such as peritoneal dialysis, the phenotype of HPMØ migrating into the peritoneum (elicit-macrophages) becomes increasingly immature with time, presumably as a result of continuous loss during effluent drainage. This reduction in maturity is accompanied by an increased ability to synthesize inflammatory cytokines *in vitro*, suggesting that increasing immaturity is associated with a deregulation in the control of the synthesis of pro-inflammatory cytokines. Under acute inflammatory conditions, the kinetics of HPMØ infiltration and accumulation in the peritoneal cavity appears to peak 24 hours after the onset of neutrophil influx.

HPMØ secrete at least 80 different products, including coagulation factors, complement cascade components, enzymes, cytokines, growth factors, eicosanoids and prostanoids, reactive oxygen species and extracellular matrix proteins, among others [5]. In the steady state, HPMØ release both cyclooxygenase and lipoxygenase products of arachidonic acid metabolism, TXB_2 and PGE_2 being the major cyclooxygenase products. HPMØ isolated during episodes of peritonitis appear to behave as elicited or primed cells rather than as a resident macrophage population, producing pro-inflammatory cytokines ($IL-1_\beta$, TNFα), and down-regulating PGE_2 production in an enhanced manner [6].

1.2. Human Peritoneal Mesothelial Cells (HPMC)

For its anatomical location, the mesothelial barrier is the interface between the blood and the serous cavity. Mesothelial cell shape, microvilli and pinocytic vesicles clearly change in number upon stimulation with a variety of chemical agents [7] whereas physical movements (systole/diastole and lung inflation receptively) affect the mesothelium lining in the human atria and pleura. The abundance of microvilli on the apical surface increases notably the functional surface of the peritoneum, thus enhancing its transport functions and exudative avility [8].

Human peritoneal mesothelial cells (HPMC) can be differentiated from endothelial cells and tissue-macrophages by morphology and by membrane-receptor expression (Table I). Resting mesothelial cells express ICAM-1 and V-CAM and the surface expression is increased by exposure to TNFα and IFNγ. Unlike endothelial cells, mesothelial cells did not express ICAM-2 and E-selectin [9]. HPMC synthesise *in vitro* pro-inflammatory cytokines (G-CSF, GM-CSF, M-CSF, IL-1α, IL-1β, IL-6, IL-8) and growth factors (TGFβ, IGF-II) [10] in a constitutive manner, increasing the rate of production after inflammatory and infectious stimuli. Whereas IL-1 and IL-6 are constantly expressed, GM-CSF and G-CSF are increasingly released with ageing. Several proliferative signals have been described for mesothelial cells such as $IL-1_\beta$ TNFα, IL-13 and EGF [11]. In the presence of macrophage-derived cytokines (IL-1β, TNFα), mesothelial cells produce bioactive $IL-1_\alpha$ and $IL-1_\beta$ [12], IL-6 [13], IL-8 [14] as well as other chemokines, monocyte chemotactic protein-1 (MCP-1), macrophage inflammatory protein-1 (MIP-1α) and RANTES (Regulated on Activation Normal T cell Expressed and Secreted), but not T-cell derived cytokines (IL-2 to IL-7) [15]. This secretion (up to five to twelve fold increase above background levels) is stimuli-specific and dose-dependent and requires *de novo* synthesis,

Table 1
Mesothelial cell markers

	HPMC	ENDOTHELIUM	HPMØ
MICROFILAMENTS			
Cytokeratin 8	+	−	−
Cytokeratin 18	+	−	−
Vimentin	+	+	−
PRO-COAGULANT ANTIGENS			
Factor VIII	−	+	−
ADHESION RECEPTORS			
ICAM-1/CD54	+	+	+
ICAM-2/CD102	−	+	+
V-CAM/CD106	+	+	−
E-Selectin	−	+	−
β_1 integrins	+		+
β_2 integrins	−		+
β_3 integrins	+		
LEUKOCYTE MARKERS			
CD16	−		+
HLA-DA	−		+

being the time-frame variable (three to 24 hours).

HPMC express receptors for IGF-I and IGF-II, as well as for insulin. In addition, they express RNA transcripts for IGF-II, suggesting that IGF-II may function as autocrine or paracrine growth factor to modulate the growth of these cells *in vivo*. In the presence of growth factors, they are capable of synthesizing a variety of interstitial and basement membrane proteoglycans (dermatan and several heparan sulphate proteoglycans) [16, 17]. Other human mesothelial cells (pleura cavity) possess receptors for several growth factors (PDGF, TGFβ, FGF and EGF), express mRNA for TGFβ and secrete TGFβ. Finally, tumour-derived mesothelial cell lines (mesothelioma cell lines) express higher levels of mRNAs for $PDGF_\alpha$ and $PDGF_\beta$ [18].

1.3. Peritoneal-associated Lymphoid Tissue (PALT)

The PALT includes the omental milky spots, the lymphocytes within the peritoneal fluid and the draining lymph nodes [19]. It has been suggested that the peritoneum might provide a micro environment that favours the expansion, accumulation or both, of a particular T cell repertoire or might even serve as a site for thymus-independent T cell differentiation. In fact, the peritoneal fluid contains a heterogeneous population of cells with the capability of viral and bacterial sensing. The phenotypical characterisation of the peritoneal cell yield shows a 2% CD22+ B-lymphocytes. Functionally distinct subsets of B cells bearing a CD5+ phenotype are rare in blood or lymph nodes but are common in the peritoneum, particularly in the human fetal

omentum [20]. Up the 65% of the peritoneal B cells express surface antigen CD5,
which can repopulate the intestinal lamina
propia with IgA producing cells as well as
contribute to the majority of serum IgM
[21] and among their functions is the response to T-independent lipopolysacchari-
des (for example, capsulated *M.meningiti-
dis*, *H.influenza* and *S. pneumoniae*).
Moreover, 7-8% of the peritoneal lymphocyte population are natural killer cells
(CD3- CD7+ CD16+ CD56+) although the
highest proportion are CD2+ T lymphocytes
(42%). The majority of peritoneal lymphocytes are single-positive (CD3+ CD4+,
CD3+) and the peritoneal CD4/CD8 ratio is
inverted, which may suggest a preferential
accumulation of the cytotoxic or suppres-
sor lymphocytes in the peritoneal cavity
(Figure 1). All CD3+ peritoneal lymphocytes express high levels of CD11a, CD18,
CD49d, CD44s and CD w60.

In areas where macrophages accumulate in
large numbers the omentum appears grossly
to contain "milky spots" (MS). Free tissue
macrophages originate in the milky spots
from precursors and migrate into the peritoneal cavity. Several features characterize these highly capillarized omental structures, as
to their position directly under the mesothelium lining and their glomerular-like form (sinusoids) surrounded by lymphatic cells and
infiltrated by non-myelinated nerve fibers.
Moreover, lymphatic drainage from omental
milky spots follows a separate circuit, which
is not connected with the main intestinal
lymphatic drainage system via the thoracic
duct [22]. During peritoneal inflammation,
MS seems to be the major route through
which leukocytes (PMNs. HPMØ) migrate
into the peritoneal cavity [23].

The thoracic duct is part of the normal circuit of recirculation of certain subpopula-

Figure 1

**The mayorly of peritoneal lymphocites are single-positive (CD3+ CD4+; CD3+ CD8+)
and the peritoneal CD4/CD8 ratio is inverted**

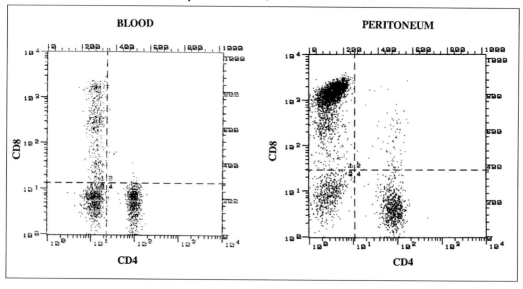

tions of lymphocytes and thoracic duct lymph contains enormous amounts of these cells, which, in addition, may be redistributed to the intestinal lymphatic tissue. The lymphatic peritoneal drainage, as opposed to portal blood, bypasses the reticulo-endothelial filter of the liver. Only two studies have attempted to investigate the GALT /PALT during SIRS indirectly by evaluating their connection to the systemic circulation through the thoracic duct [24, 25]. The markedly elevated percentage of T lymphocytes in thoracic duct lymph expressing CD45RA+ CD45RO+ and the gut homing receptor α4β7 on CD4+ and CD8+ T only certify the peritoneal origin of these cells.

2. EARLY PERITONEAL INFLAMMATORY RESPONSE TO INFECTION

The model proposed by Nicholas Topley [26] put into perspective the increasing evidence that the HPMC via their interactions with HPMØ play a central role in the initial response of the peritoneum to infection (*initiation phase*), during the *amplification phase* to control the recruitment of leukocytes and during the early stages of the resolution of inflammation (*healing phase*).

Although the evidence of the prime role of mesothelium in initiating and amplifying the peritoneal response to invading microorganisms is indirect, nevertheless the amount of mesothelial cells outnumber HPMØ by a factor of 10 [6]. Any contaminant in the peritoneal cavity is immediately in contact with mesothelial cells from the visceral, parietal peritoneum or both. Gram positive cocci can attach and be ingested by and activate cultured mesothelial cells, which result in the activation of mesothelial cell IL-8 secretion. On the other hand,

HPMØ synthesize and release IL-1β and TNFα in the presence of bacteria or bacterial products which in turn affect cytokine and eicosanoids release into the peritoneal cavity by HPMC. The close contact among the parietal, visceral and omental peritoneal membranes, resulting from breathing and bowel peristalsis facilitate the intercommunication among peritoneal cells (HPMØ, HPMC, mast cells, PALT) [27].

After intra-abdominal inoculation, fluid is both filtered and absorbed from the peritoneal space through the peritoneum. The absorption rate is dependent upon the size of the material absorbed. Particles and cells (up to 1 μm diameter) are removed through stomata within minutes and then through the lymphatic channels of the diaphragm into the thoracic duct and into the blood stream within 12 minutes with each diaphragmatic excursion [28]. The action of the diaphragm generates a cephalad flow of peritoneal fluid and in radiolabeled studies with E. Coli, few (less than 3%) free bacteria may be present in the peritoneal cavity after two hours [29]. The presence of large fibrin plugs result in the saturation of the stomata, decreasing the trans-diaphragmatic absorption. In addition, other factors may greatly influence the ability of the abdominal cavity to absorb large quantities of bacterial and fibrinopurulent debris, such as the ratio between the intrathoracic (decreasing efferent lymph flow) and the intra-abdominal pressure (increasing absorption and lymph flow), the presence of ascites, ileus or even, the patient's posture [30].

The sequential polarised release of chemokines by HPMC into the basal membrane and into the submesothelial interstitium submits signals for endothelial and mast, cell activation. Stimulation with macrophages-derived cytokines (IL-1β, TNFα), bacterial LPS, T-cell derived IFN-γ, heat-killed bacteria or a combination of these inflammatory stimuli results in substantial induction of mRNA synthesis and chemokines expression by HPMC in a quite specific time frame [31, 32]. IL-8 is a potent neutrophil chemoattractant and is one of the first chemokine (24 hours) to be associated with heparin-like surface structures on basal HPMC membrane. MCP-1 and MIP-1α are released later into the apical membrane of HPMC and are major monocyte chemoattractants, driving the later monocyte infiltration (> 24 hours) into the peritoneal cavity.

The passage of proteins across the peritoneal membrane during bacterial peritonitis is directly related to prostaglandin content in the peritoneal fluid. Macrophages-derived cytokines (IL-1β, TNFα) increase the expression of both cyclooxygenase forms (Cox-1 and Cox-2 mRNA) in HPMC, triggering the production of 6-keto-PGF$_1$ and PGE$_2$ [33]. In contrast, HPMØ stimulated with bacteria increase the release of lypoxigenase-dependent leukotriene generation (LTB$_4$, a major neutrophil chemoattractant) with concomitant dose-dependent decrease of PGE$_2$). Therefore, during peritonitis, locally produced vasodilatory prostaglandins contribute to hyperemia (increasing pre-capillary flow) and protein exudation (albumin, fibrin) by increasing post-capillary permeability. The exact nature of this process is unknown, although resident peritoneal mast cells may add complexity with mast cell-derived inflammatory mediators and chemoattractants. For example, histamine produces cytoskeleton changes in HPMC, modifying mesothelial cell shape and permeability, therefore, facilitating neutrophil trans-mesothelial migration [35].

Central to the process of inflammation is a dramatic increase in endothelial [36] and mesothelial-cell [37] surface expression of molecules that support the adhesion and migration of blood leukocytes. HPMC constitutively express high levels of adhesion receptor of the immunoglobulin super family ICAM/CD54 and VCAM/CD106 which are the ligands for the counter-receptors of the integrin family on leukocytes CD11a/CD18 (lymphocytes) and CD11b/CD18 (neutrophils and macrophages), α4β1 (VLA-4 in basophils and monocytes) and α4β7, respectively. Proinflammatory cytokines TNFα and IFN-γ alone or in combination up-regulate or induce the synthesis of ICAM-1 and VCAM-1 during peritonitis. In addition, HPMC also express PECAM-1/CD31, which is concentrated in the lateral borders of mesothelial cells. PECAM-1 is essential for neutrophils to cross the endothelium toward the extracellular matrix and from the submesothilium space into the peritoneal cavity through the intercellular mesothelial junctions.

During the amplification of the early inflammatory peritoneal response to bacterial invasion, fibrinogen-rich fluid exudate passes into the abdominal cavity producing third-space fluid shifts [38]. The presence of fibrinous exudate is essential for bacterial sequestration, initially by deposition of fribinous peel layering the visceral and parietal peritoneum and then, through organised adhesions and abscesses sealed by and around the omentum and the intestinal loops. The formation of fibrin is due in part to the inactivation of fibrinolysis during peritonitis. Several peritoneal cells, mainly HPMC and HPMØ, express tissue factor (TF) and procoagulant activity due to cell damage and bacteria stimuli, respectively [39]. During the exudative wave of blood borne cells and proteins into the peritoneal cavity, primed neutrophils interact with activated HPMC releasing proteases and oxidative oxygen species which are thought to be responsible for the acute alterations observed in peritoneal membrane function [40]. Whereas LPS predominantly promote plasminogen-dependent fibrinolysis *in vitro* by HPMØ, TNFα modifies cell shape and fibrinolytic activity of HPMC. On stimulation with inflammatory mediators, HPMC decrease the antigen tissue-type plasminogen activator (tPA) with a concomitant increase of type 1 and 2 plasminogen activator inhibitor (PAI-1 and PAI-2) [41]. A marked decrease of peritoneal fibrinolytic activity has been demonstrated in animal models with peritonitis [42] as well as in human appendicitis and in human secon-

dary peritonitis [43]. Nevertheless, the net balance between pro-coagulant and fibrinolytic responses to bacterial peritonitis is still largely unknown, particularly the time frame and signals switching on/off both cellular activities.

3. LATE PERITONEAL RESPONSE TO INFECTION

Neutrophil influx into the peritoneal cavity is followed by an increase in the number of monocytes, which rapidly differentiate into macrophages. This influx of monocytes is greater than local macrophage production

Figure 2.

Early healing phase with the dominancy of peritoneal remesothelialization and the restoration of fibrinolytic activity

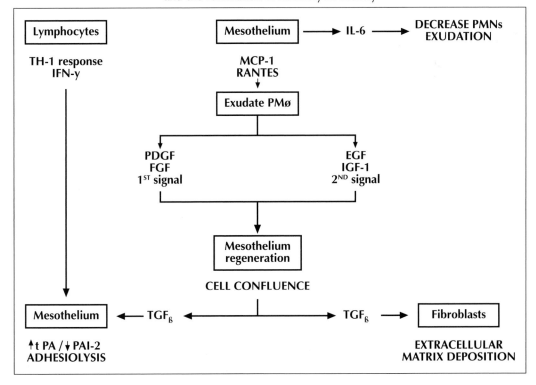

over the first 6 to 48 hours depending upon the stimulus employed. After post-operative day 5, the predominant cells in the peritoneal fluid are macrophages, which are critical to the resolution of surgical injury and to the peritoneal healing process. At this stage, macrophages-derived growth factors such as Platelet-derived growth factor (PDGF), Fibroblast growth factor (FGF), Epidermal growth factor (EGF) and Insulin-like growth factor (IGF-1) stimulate the proliferation and expression of differentiated functions on a variety of cell types, particularly fibroblasts and mesothelial cells. EGF and FGF are involved in the transition of HPMC from G_0 to S phase, whereas IGF-I stimulates the proliferation by affecting the transition from S phase to the M phase [44]. Interestingly, cell confluence and contact seems, at least *in vitro*, to be the pivotal signal to drive the peritoneal re-epithelization and tissue repair process toward extracellular matrix remodelling (Figure 2).

In this new context, mesothelium-derived transforming growth factor β (TGF-β) provides a powerful chemotactic signal for fibroblasts as well as induces a profound effect on dermatan sulphate proteoglycan production. Additionally, HPMC are also target cells for TGF-β, which potentiate the recovery of the fibrinolytic activity and the accumulation of PAI-1 [45]. Peritoneal fibrinolysis is essential in the prevention of fibrous adhesions and in the resolution of fibrous exudates. Several factors potentiate adhesion formation during intra-abdominal infections, such as bleeding, certain surgical procedures on solid organs (pancreas and liver), extensive surgery and severe and recurrent serous injury such as in peritonitis. If injury is continuously present, fibrinolytic activity is suppressed; fibrin clots achieve complete organisation, including neo-angiogenesis and firm collagen deposition.

Still, it is certainly obscure the stimuli perpetuating and triggering the morphogenesis of adhesion formation (pathological response) and the dominant regulator(s) of peritoneal remesothelialization (physiological response) remain unclear. To date, no single therapeutic approach has proven universally effective in preventing formation of post-operative intraperitoneal adhesions.

Abscess formation is a later pathological phase in the evolution of intra abdominal infections. Abscesses contain a polymicrobic flora consisting of both obligate anaerobes and facultative species and can be experimentally reproduced with capsular polysaccharide of *Bacteroides fragilis* [46]. It was also shown that the protection against abscess development relies on T cell dependent immunity, with the antigen surface profile of $CD8^+$ lymphocytes. Immunochemical characterisation of the capsular polysaccharide of *B.fragilis* revealed two components, termed polysaccharide A (PSA) and polysaccharide B (PSB) essential for preventing and provoking abscess formation [47]. Both polysaccharides induce IL-1β and TNFα production by HPMC, IL-8 released by polymorphonuclear leukocytes and IL-10 by HPMØ and peritoneal lymphocytes. IL-10 is a potent immunoregulator and a Th2-type cytokine, which regulates the humoral immune response and appears to be more effective in providing help for primary immunoglobulin secretion. The highly unusual nature of this response in the peritoneal compartment is not clear, since Th2-type $CD8^+$ lymphocytes have been associated with impaired immunity [48].

4. SUMMARY

The peritoneal cavity is a peculiar compartment which possesses matchless structures such as the omental milky spots and the subdiaragmatic lymphatic drainage system and contains a heterogeneous population of cells, some unique or rare in other lymphoid tissues such as CD5[+] B lymphocytes and CD34[+] dendritic cell precursors. Whether the peritoneal cavity functions as an "intestinal thymus", or is part of the gut-associated lymphoid tissue (GALT), only seems to indicate the undisputed primacy of the peritoneal defence system in intra-abdominal infections. However, the intricate immune mechanisms that contribute to deal with bacterial invasion during peritonitis have been frequently overlooked if not ignored. A clear understanding of the molecular and cellular events underlying peritoneal functions will aid future treatment of peritonitis, particularly several poorly understood clinical disorders such as abscess and adhesion formation, primary and tertiary peritonitis and the role of lymphatic peritoneal drainage as a trigger mechanism for septic shock.

REFERENCES

1. Esperanca MJ, Collins DL. Peritoneal dialysis efficiency in relation to body weight. J Ped Surg 1966; 1:162-169.

2. Dobbie JW. New concepts in molecular biology and ultrastructural pathology of the peritoneum: their significance for peritoneal dialysis. Am J Kidney Dis 1990; 15:97-109.

3. Kubicka U, Olszewski WL, Maldyk J, Wierzbicki Z, Orkiszewska A. Normal human immune peritoneal cells: phenotypic characteristics. Immunobiol 1989; 180: 80-92.

4. van Furth R. Phagocytic cells: developmenty and distribution of mononuclear phagocytes in normal steady-state and inflammation. In: Gallin JL, Goldstein IM, Synderman E (Eds.): Inflammation: basic principles and clinical correlates. Raven Press, New York, pp. 2 81-295.

5. Zerbala M, Arherson GL. Human Monocytes; Academic Press, London 1989.

6. Stylianou E, Mackenzie R, Davies M, Coles GA, Williams JD. The interaction of organism, phagocyte and mesothelial cell. In: Coles GA, Davies M, Williams JD (Eds.): CAPD, Host defense, Nutrition and ultrafiltration. Contrib Nephrol Basel, Karger 1990, 85: 30-38.

7. NW Thomas. Embryology and structure of the mesothilium. In J.S.P. Jones (Ed.): Pathology of the mesothelium. Springer-Verlag, Berlin 1987, pp. 1-13.

8. diZerega GS, Rodgers KE. The peritoneum. Springer-Verlag, New York, 1992.

9. Jonjic N, Peri G, Bernasconi S, Sciacca FL, Colotta F, Pelicci P, Lanfrancone L, Mantovani A. Expression of adhesion molecules and chemotactic cytokines in cultured human mesothelial cells. J Exp Med 1992, 176: 1165-1174.

10. Rutten AA; Bermudez E; Stewart W; Everitt JI; Walker CL. Expression of insulin-like growth factor II in spontaneously immortalized rat mesothelial and spontaneous mesothelioma cells: a potential autocrine role of insulin-like growth factor II. Cancer Res 1995 15; 55: 3634-3639.

11. Sironi M, Sciacca FL, Matteucci C, Conni M, Vecchi A, Bernasconi S, Minty A, Caput D, Ferrara P, Colotta F, Mantovani A. Regulation of endothelial and mesothelial cell function by interleukin-13: selective induction of vascular cell adhesion molecule-1 and amplification of interleukin-6 production. Blood 1994, 84: 1913-1921.

12. Douvdevani A, Rapoport J, Konforty A, Argov S, Ovnat A, Chaimovitz C. Human peritoneal mesothelial cells synthesize IL-1 and. Kidney Int 1994, 46: 993-1001.

13. Topley N, Jorres A, Luttmann W, Petersen MM, Lang MJ, Thierauch KH, Muller C, Co-

les GA, Davis M, Willians JD. Human peritoneal mesothelial cells synthesize interleukin-6: induction by IL-1 and TNF. Kidney Int. 1993, 43: 226-233.

14. Goodman RB, Wood RG, Martin TR, Hanson-Painton O, Kinasewitz GT. Cytokine-stimulated human mesothelial cells produce chemotactic activity for neutrophils including NAP/IL-8. J Immunol 1992, 148: 457-465.

15. Lanfrancone L, Boraschi D, Ghiara B, Falini B, Grignani F, Peri G, Mantovani A, Pelicci A. Human peritoneal mesothelial cells produce many cytokines (granulocyte colony-stimulating factor CSF, granulocyte-monocyte-CSF, macrophage-CSF, interleukin-1 IL-1 and IL-6) and are activated and stimulated to grow by IL-1. Blood 1992, 80: 2835-2842.

16. Milligan SA; Owens MW; Henderson RJ Jr; Grimes SR Jr. Characterization of proteoglycans produced by rat pleural mesothelial cells in vitro. Exp Lung Res 1995; 21: 559-575.

17. Yung S; Thomas GJ; Stylianou E; Williams JD; Coles GA; Davies M. Source of peritoneal proteoglycans. Human peritoneal mesothelial cells synthesize and secrete mainly small dermatan sulfate proteoglycans. Am J Pathol 1995 ;146: 520-529.

18. Asplund T, Versnel MA, Laurent TC, Heldin P. Human mesothelioma cells produce factors that stimulate the production of hyaluranate by mesothelial cells and fibroblasts. Cancer Res 1993, 53: 388-392.

19. Hall JC, Heel KA, Papadimitriou JM, Platell C. The pathobiology of peritonitis. Gastroenterology 1998; 114: 185-196.

20. Solvason N, Kearney JF. The human fetal omentum: a site of B cell generation. J.Exp. Med. 1992; 175: 397-404.

21. Donze HH, Lue C, Julian BA, Kutteh WH, Kantele A, Mestecky J. Human peritoneal B1 cells and the influence of continuos ambulatory peritoneal dialysis on peritoneal and peripheral blood mononuclear cell (PBMC)

composition and immunoglobulin levels. Clin Exp Immunol 1997; 109: 356-361.

22. Koten JW, Otter WD. Are omental milky spots an intestinal thymus? Lancet 1991, 338: 1189-1190.

23. Doherty NS, Griffiths RJ, Hakkinen JP, Scampoli DN, Milici AJ. Post-capillary venules in the "milky spots" of the greater omentum are the major site of plasma protein and leukocyte extravasation in rodent models of peritonitis. Inflamm Res 1995; 44: 169-177.

24. Lemaire LC, van Deventer SJ, van Lanschot JJ, Meenan J, Gouma DJ. Phenotypical characterization of cells in the thoracic duct of patients with and without systemic inflammatory response syndrome and multiple organ failure. Scand J Immunol 1998; 47: 69-75.

25. Sánchez García M, Prieto A, Tejedor A, Martín-Duce A, Fernández Sánchez FJ, Granell J, Álvarez-Mon M. Characteristics of thoracic duct lymph in multiple organ dysfunction syndrome. Arch Surg 1997; 132: 13-18.

26. Davenport A; Li FK ; Robson R; Wilkinson TS; McLoughlin R; Topley R. Early peritoneal responses to bacterial invasion: Cellular exudation. Sepsis 1999; 3: 303-309.

27. Kinnaert P; De Wilde JP; Bournonvillie B, Husson C; Salmon I. Direct activation of human peritoneal mesothelial cells by heat-killed micro-organisms. Ann Surg 1996; 224: 749-755.

28. van Goor H: Fibrinolytic therapy in generalized peritonitis to prevent intra-abdominal abscess formation. An experimental and clinical study. PhD Thesis, Nijmagen 1996.

29. Dunn DL, Barke RA, Ewald DC, Simmons RL. Macrophages and translymphatic absorption represent the first line of host defense on the peritoneal cavity. Arch Surg 1987, 122:105-110.

30. Fry DE. Peritonitis. Futura Publishing Co., Mount Kisco, New York. 1993.

31. Li FK, Davenport A, Robson RL, Loetscher P, Rothlein R, Williams JD, Topley N. Leukocyte migration across human peritoneal mesothelial cells is dependent on directed chemokine secretion and ICAM-1 expression. Kidney Int 1998; 54: 2170-2183.

32. Topley N, Brown Z, Jorres A, Westwick J, Davies M, Coles GA, Williams JD. Human peritoneal mesothelial cells synthesize interleukin-8. Synergistic induction by interleukin-1 (and tumor necrosis factor-β). Am J Pathol 1993; 142: 1876-1886.

33. Topley N; Petersen MM,Mackenzie R, Neubauer A, Stylianou E, Kaever V, Davies M, Coles GA, Jorres A, Williams JD. Human peritoneal mesothelial cell prostaglandin synthesis: induction of cyclooxygenase mRNA by peritoneal macrophage-derived cytokines. Kidney Int. 1994; 46: 900-909.

34. Davenport A; in FK; Robson R; Wilkinson TS, McLoughilin R; Topley N. Early Peritoneal Responses to Bacterial Invasion: Cellular Exudation Sepsis 1999; 3:303-309.

35. Bird SD, Walker RJ. Mast cell histamine-induced calcium transients in cultured human peritoneal mesothelial cells. Perit Dial Int 1998; 18: 626-636.

36. Tellado JM, Feijoo E. Anti-adhesion oriented therapies. in Tellado JM, Forse RA, Solomkin JS (Eds.): Modulation of the inflammatory response in severe sepsis. Prog.Surg. Basel, Karger, 1995; 20:91-102.

37. Garlanda C, Mantovani A. Cytokines and adhesion molecules in mesothelial cell pathophysiology. Sepsis 1999; 3:271-283.

38. Ahrenholz DH, Simmons RL. Fibrin in peritonitis. I. Beneficial and adverse effects of fibrin in experimental E.coli peritonitis. Surgery 1980; 88: 41-47.

39. Rosenthal GA, Levy G, Rotstein OD. Induction of macrophage procoagulant activity by Bacteroides Fragilis Infect Immun 1989, 57: 338-343.

40. Andreoli SP. Mallet C, Williams K, McAteer JA, Rothlein R, Doerschuk CM. Mechanisms of polymorphonuclear leukocyte mediated peritoneal mesothelial cell injury. Kidney Int 1994; 46: 1100-1109.

41. van Hinsbergh VW, Kooistra T, Scheffer MA, Hajo van Bockel J, van Muijen GN. Characterization and fibrinolytic properties of human omental tissue mesothelial cells. Comparison with endothelial cells. Blood 1990; 75: 1490-1497.

42. Hau T, Payne WD, Simmons RL. Fibrinolytic activity of the peritoneum during experimental peritonitis. Surg Gynecol Obstet 1979; 148: 415-418.

43. van Goor H, Bom VJJ, van der Meer J, Sluiter WJ, Bleichrodt RP. Coagulation and fibrinolytic responses in human peritoneal fluid and plasma to bacterial peritonitis. Br J Surg 1996; 83: 1133-1135.

44. Pledger WJ, Stiles CD, Antoniades HN, Scher CD. An ordered sequence of events is required before BALB/c-3T3 cells have become committed to DNA synthesis. Proc Natl Acad Sci 1978; 74: 2839-2848.

45. Tietze L, Elbrecht A, Schauerte C, Klosterhalfen B, Amo-Takyi B, Gehlen J, Winketau G, Mittermayer C, Handt S. Modulation of pro- and antifibrinolytic properties of human peritoneal mesothelial cells by transforming growth factor beta 1 (TGF-beta 1), tumor necrosis factor alpha (TNF-alpha) and interleukin 1 beta (IL-1 beta). Tromb Haemost 1998; 79: 362-370.

46. Joiner KA, Gelfand JA, Onderdonk AB, Bartlett JG, Gorbach SL. Host factors in the formation of abscesses. J Infect Dis 1980; 142: 40-49.

47. Tzianabos AO, Onderdonk AB, Rosner B, Cisneros RL, Kasper DL. Structural features of polysaccharides that induce intra-abdominal abscesses. Science 1993; 262: 416-419.

48. Birkhofer A, Rehbock J, Fricke H. T lymphocytes from the normal human peritoneum contain high frequencies of Th2-type CD8+ T cells. Eur J Immunol 1996; 26: 957-960.

The Microbial Ecology of the Gastrointestinal Flora

John C. Marshall, MD, FRCSC

"The adult human organism is said to be composed of approximately 10^{13} eukaryotic animal cells. That statement is only an expression of a particular point of view. The various body surfaces and the gastrointestinal canals of humans may be colonized by as many as 10^{14} indigenous prokaryotic and eukaryotic microbial cells. These microbes profoundly influence some of the physiological processes of their animal host. From another point of view, therefore, the normal human organism can be said to be composed of over 10^{14} cells, of which only about 10% are animal cells."

- Savage, 1977 [1]

1. INTRODUCTION

The normal gastrointestinal tract harbours more than 400 separate species of bacteria [2] in intimate proximity to a complex network of immunologic tissues. It is not surprising, therefore, that the GI tract in health serves as an important organ of immune homeostasis. Conversely, alterations in the normal indigenous flora have been implicated in the pathogenesis of a diverse group of disorders characterized by alterations in systemic immune homeostasis and inclu-

ding cirrhosis [3], autoimmune thyroiditis [4] and arthritis [5,6].

2. NORMAL FLORA OF THE GI TRACT

The microbial flora of the gastrointestinal tract increases in both numbers and diversity from proximal to distal. Patterns of colonization at differing anatomic sites vary widely [7]. Gram positive organisms and anaerobes predominate in the oral cavity, while the stomach and proximal small bowel are relatively sterile. Numbers of Gram negatives increase in the more distal small bowel and anaerobes appear in large numbers in the colon. The composition of the indigenous flora, although variable from one individual to another, is remarkably constant in a given individual over time [8].

2.1. Terminology and Methodological Considerations

Dubos and co-workers suggested that the gastrointestinal flora comprises three related microbial populations [9]. The *autochthonous flora* consists of those organisms which are present during the evolution of the animal, while the *normal microbiota* consists of a group of organisms which are ubiquitous in the natural environment of the animal and which thus establish residence in all members of the species. These two groups of organisms make up the *indigenous flora* of the animal and are distinguished from *pathogens* which are acquired from the environment and are capable of establishing residence within the gut of the host and of inducing systemic alterations of disease.

Accurate qualitative and quantitative characterization of the normal indigenous gastrointestinal flora has proved difficult [10], and variable findings from one study to another frequently reflect differences in study methodology. An appreciation of the limitations of methodology is critical to an understanding of the true complexity of the normal gastrointestinal flora.

2.1.1. Mucosal and Luminal Flora

The indigenous flora consists of at least two separate compartments- organisms which are intimately associated with the epithelial cell layer of the gut and its mucous blanket and those which reside within the intestinal lumen. The mucosal-associated flora has been best characterized in non-primates, although it is generally accepted that a similar flora is present in humans [11-14].

Bacterial colonization of the mucosal surface is further compartmentalized: some organisms attach to epithelial cells of the gut mucosa, while others survive in suspension in the blanket of mucus overlying the epithelium [15]. Variations in the composition of this flora reflect the complexity of the host-microbial interactions which maintain the biologic stability of the indigenous flora. *Lac-*

tobacilli, for example, colonize the stomach by attachment of one pole of the bacterial cell to the gastric epithelium. This attachment is highly specific: certain strains of *Lactobacilli* attach only to rat epithelial cells, while others associate exclusively with chicken cells [16]. Organisms colonizing the mucous blanket of the small bowel and colon generally display a spiral morphology and it is thought that their shape and motility favour their persistence in an anatomic site of rapid cell turnover [14]. Symbiosis between the colonizing organism and the local microenvironment assures the stability of the flora over time and serves to inhibit mucosal colonization by potentially pathogenic micro-organisms, a phenomenon known as "colonization resistance" [17] (vide infra).

Organisms free within the gut lumen are more accessible to sampling but less representative of the stable component of the indigenous flora. The luminal flora consists of a mixture of organisms shed from the mucosa and swallowed organisms; this component of the indigenous flora is by far the larger, with microbial cells making up 40% of the mass of normal feces [1].

2.1.2. Limitations of Sampling Techniques

Bacteriological studies of gut flora employ one of three techniques- culture of the mucosal surface of accessible portions of the GI tract (the oropharynx and rectum), culture of fluid or stool expelled from the gut, or sampling of intestinal contents obtained via indwelling sampling devices. Each technique has methodological limitations which potentially influence the results obtained.

Swabs of the mucosal surface can only be obtained from accessible portions of the GI tract- the oropharynx and rectum. Although these may reflect the dominant colonizing species, they are not quantitative and only sample that flora which exists in loose association with the mucosal surface: strongly adherent species and luminal organisms will not be represented.

Culture of expelled gut contents permits a highly detailed examination of the luminal flora and fecal cultures have been the basis for the characterization of the rich diversity of the normal flora [2]. This flora may, however, differ both quantitatively and qualitatively from the mucosal flora and patterns of growth or death of organisms in formed feces may not reflect relative concentrations higher in the GI tract where conditions such as pH, redox potential and water content are different [10].

Various forms of indwelling tubes have been used to sample the flora of the stomach and small bowel. While such techniques provide direct access to portions of the GI tract which are otherwise inaccessible for study, the insertion of the tube may result in contamination of the area of study by organisms from the nose or oropharynx and the very presence of the tube may later local peristalsis or other factors important in the regulation of microbial populations [18]. Gorbach and co-workers compared the results of samples obtained via indwelling tubes with those obtained directly at laparotomy in a group of dogs and showed that although direct sampling yielded higher concentrations of bacteria, the indwelling tube accurately reflected both the composition of the flora and the relative numbers of each isolate [19]. Drasar and Shiner have used a swallowed capsule, positioned fluoroscopically in the bowel segment of interest to circumvent the potential problems arising from contamination of the specimen

by secretions from higher in the GI tract [20].

Direct sampling of fluid from normally inaccessible portions of the gut may be possible under certain circumstances. Culture of ileostomy or colostomy effluent provides information on the resident flora of these sites, although the effects both of the prior surgery and the underlying disease process may alter the results [21]. Samples obtained at laparotomy are subject to similar influences [22] and may be further affected by the administration of systemic antibiotics or by the effects of prolonged hospitalization. Samples obtained from previously healthy trauma victims undergoing laparotomy for abdominal injury may be most representative of the normal flora [23].

Characterization of the normal flora may also be affected by specimen handling and culture techniques. Organisms present in low concentrations are particularly difficult to isolate and inappropriate handling may result in an underestimation of the numbers and types of anaerobes present [18].

However, these considerations notwithstanding, it has been possible to derive a comprehensive picture of patterns of GI colonization in the normal healthy individual, as well as beingable to characterize the alterations which occur in association with a variety of disease states.

2.2. Oropharyngeal Flora

The normal oropharyngeal flora consists predominantly of *Streptococci, Actinomyces*, and anaerobes [24]. Gram negative organisms are found in only 6% of healthy individuals but in up to 75% of critically ill hospitalized patients [25]; such colonization is a significant risk factor for the subsequent development of nosocomial respiratory tract infection [26].

2.3. Gastric Flora

The normal stomach is sterile or sparsely populated with organisms such as *Streptococci*, lactobacilli and anaerobic cocci [19,27,28]; mean numbers rarely exceed 10^3 CFU/mL. *Candida* is found in approximately 30% of normal individuals [27,29] and in a similar proportion of patients with gastric ulcers [30]. *Helicobacter pylori*, has recently been identified as a prominent component of the mucosal flora of the stomach in normal individuals and appears to play a role in the pathogenesis of gastritis, peptic ulceration, and possibly, malignancies of the stomach [31].

The stomach can be exposed to rapid changes in bacterial numbers through eating or swallowing secretions from the oropharynx. In health, normal gastric acidity is the predominant factor responsible for maintaining a state of relative sterility in the stomach. Although gastric acid is the most important factor controlling patterns of colonization, the influence of other as yet undefined factors is suggested by the fact that at a given pH, preprandial gastric juice demonstrates more potent antibacterial activity than postprandial gastric juice [32].

2.4. Small Intestinal Flora

The microbial flora of the small intestine increases both qualitatively and quantitatively from proximal to distal; duodenal bacteriology is similar to that of the stomach, while the flora of the terminal ileum is essentially the same as that of the cecum. Both Gram negative organisms and anaerobes become more numerous in the distal small bowel [18].

Like the stomach, the jejunum is sparsely populated with bacteria. Approximately one third of specimens obtained from the jejunum using an indwelling tube [33] and up to 80% of jejunal specimens obtained directly at the time of laparotomy [22,23] are sterile, while *Streptococci* and facultative anaerobes are present in colonized patients; mean bacterial counts are low, averaging fewer than 100 CFU/mL [19]. Normal gastric acidity contributes to the relative sterility of the jejunum and the upper GI tract of the achlorhydric patient is more heavily colonized [34]. Numbers of Gram negatives and obligate anaerobes increase along the ileum, reaching concentrations of 10^5 to 10^8CFU/mL in the terminal ileum [19].

Candida can be cultured from the small bowel fluid of approximately 50% of normal individuals [29]; viruses, on the other hand, are not found [33].

2.5. Colonic Flora

The normal colonic flora is a complex mixture of as many as 400 different microbial species [2], with anaerobes outnumbering aerobes by a factor of 1,000 to 1 [1. Although stool cultures have been the source of what is known about the **diversity** of the colonic flora, because of the capacity of the colon to absorb water they provide a poor reflection of the **concentration** of organisms present. While concentrations of bacteria in the feces may exceed 10^{10} CFU/mL [1], specimens obtained by aspiration of colonic contents at the time of laparotomy yield numbers of bacteria which are two to three logarithmic units lower [35]. *Candida* is slightly more common in the feces than in the small bowel and can be isolated from 65% of specimens [29].

The mucosal flora of the colon, like that of the small bowel, is not truly reflected by cultures of luminal contents. The mucosal flora of the colon comprises spiral organisms whose predominance appears to be favoured by their motility and by local differences in oxygen tension and the acidity of mucin [14].

2.6. Establishment and Persistence of the Indigenous Flora

The gastrointestinal tract of the fetus is sterile. Acquisition of the indigenous flora begins at birth and continues over the first two years of life; normal adult patterns of colonization are generally established by the age of two [36].

The temporal sequence of normal colonization has been best characterized in the mouse [37]. Animals delivered by Cesarean section are germfree. *Lactobacilli* and *Flavobacteria* are present throughout the gut by two days. The former increase in numbers over the ensuing four weeks while the latter decline in numbers and disappear by the end of the second week. Enterococci are present in the colon by the second day of life; their numbers increase progressively over the next two weeks. Coliforms are first evident at 10 days post partum, while *Bacteroides* and other anaerobes do not appear until more than two weeks after birth when the animal has begun to eat solid food [37].

Studies of the fecal flora of human neonates demonstrate a similar pattern. *Streptococci* and *E. coli* appear during the first few days of life; their numbers are particularly high in infants fed formula. Anaerobes such as *Bifidobacterium*, *Clostridium*, and *Bacteroides* become evident by one week. *Streptococci*, *Bifidobacteria*, and *E. coli* are the dominant organisms by two weeks. Concentrations of anaerobic Gram positive cocci, *Bacteroides* and *Clostridia* increase over the ensuing two years and the fecal composition becomes similar to that of the adult [36,38].

While the microbial ecology of the environment exerts an influence on the acquisition of the indigenous flora as evidenced, for example, by transient differences in the flora between breast-fed and formula-fed infants [36], local factors in the gut microenvironment seem to play the most important role in establishing a flora that is remarkably similar amongst members of a given species. When germfree animals are fed pure cultures of a single organism, predictable patterns of colonization develop: *Lactobacilli* and anaerobic *Streptococci* associate closely with the mucosal surface throughout the GI tract, while *Bacteroides* becomes established only in the colon [39].

Studies of the longterm stability of the GI flora in a given individual are not available, although serial studies do show that the composition of the fecal flora remains relatively constant over a period of half a year [2,8].

3. REGULATION OF NORMAL MICROBIAL ECOLOGY

The stability of the normal gastrointestinal flora is maintained by physiological, microbiologic, and immunological mechanisms working in concert; disruption of these, in turn, can induce abnormal patterns of gut colonization.

3.1. Gastric Acidity

Gastric acidity is the dominant influence responsible for the relative sterility of the stomach and upper GI tract [34,40,41]. Gram negative organisms are most susceptible to the bactericidal effects of gastric acidity. Complete eradication of the organism occurs within one hour, following oral administration of as much as 10^9 Serratia [28]. Conversely, hypochlorhydria as a consequence of medical [42-44], or surgical [45,46] vagotomy or in conjunction with pernicious anemia [28] is associated with significant overgrowth by Gram negative organisms. Susceptibility to gastric acidity appears to be greatest for Gram negative organisms; the effects of pH on Gram positive organisms and yeasts is not well-defined.

By reducing the numbers of organisms reaching the duodenum and jejunum, gastric acid also regulates the microbial flora of the small bowel [19,47], although it is evident from studies in IgA-deficient subjects that gastric achlorhydria alone is not sufficient to permit uncontrolled small bowel bacterial proliferation [48].

3.2. Bile Acids

Intestinal microorganisms play a significant role in normal bile acid metabolism, converting primary bile acids to secondary bile acids and deconjugating bile acids within the intestinal lumen [49,50]. Bile acids, in turn, appear to exert an influence on patterns of colonization of the small bowel, although the extent of this influence in vivo is undefined. Simple bile acids- cholic and deoxycholic acid- inhibit the growth of enterococci, *Bacteroides* and lactobacilli in vitro, whereas conjugated bile acids lack this inhibitory activity [51,52]. The human

small bowel, however, rarely contains significant concentrations of unconjugated bile acids I[1], and feeding exogenous conjugated bile acids has little effect on small bowel bacteriology [53]. On the other hand, germfree animals acquire resistance to colonization with *Shigella* only after they have been colonized with indigenous organisms capable of deconjugating bile acids and only in association with the presence of the metabolite 7-ketodeoxycholic acid in the intestinal contents [54]. Similarly, reduction of luminal bile salt concentrations by bile duct ligation results in significantly greater numbers of *E. coli* in the cecal contents of experimental animals compared to their sham-operated controls [55].

The role of bile in normal gut microbial ecology, therefore, remains uncertain although it has been suggested that the most important influence of bile acids is the prevention of colonization by organisms not normally found within the GI tract [1]. Since certain strains of organisms, notably *S. fecalis*, are capable of deconjugating bile acids, the indigenous flora itself may play a permissive role in maximizing the contribution of bile acids to normal colonization resistance [52].

3.3. Intestinal Motility

The rapid transit time of the stomach and small bowel influences not only the numbers of organisms present but also their composition. Stasis is associated with increased concentrations of anaerobes, while certain spiral organisms which constitute a major component of the mucosal flora of the small bowel appear to be selectively favoured by their rapid motility [14]. Intestinal obstruction results in significant increases in the density of the flora of the stomach and small bowel [56]. Impaired motility may be the explanation for bacterial overgrowth in the presence of duodenal [57] or jejunal [58] diverticula.

The microbial flora of the intestine, in turn, influences intestinal motility. Abrams and Bishop showed that animals with an intact and normal flora display enhanced gastric emptying and increased transit through the small and large intestine in comparison to germ-free animals [59]; the mechanism of this effect is unknown.

3.4. Microbial factors

The indigenous flora itself may well be the predominant factor responsible for the stability of patterns of gut colonization over time and for the resistance of the GI tract to colonization with exogenous species [60-62]. The mechanisms by which the autochthonous flora regulates patterns of GI colonization are complex and incompletely defined, yet critical to an understanding of the factors which promote pathologic colonization and its consequences.

3.4.1. The Concept of Colonization Resistance

Investigations by van der Waaij and co-workers into the pathogenesis of radiation injury demonstrated that mortality following lethal irradiation was a consequence of systemic infection by bacteria from the GI tract and could be minimized by pretreatment with oral non-absorbed antibiotics. The effect of antibiotics, however, was variable: if given in conjunction with oral administration of antibiotic-resistant organisms, antibiotics actually increased mortality for treated animals. Mortality co-

rrelated with fecal concentrations of Gram negative organisms and it became apparent that the discrepant results of antibiotic administration were a consequence of their variable effects on patterns of gut colonization [63]. These investigations established a role for certain components of the normal flora in resisting colonization by exogenous microbial species, a phenomenon which was termed "colonization resistance" [17].

Colonization resistance describes the inhibitory influence exerted by the indigenous flora on colonization by non-indigenous organisms. It has been defined quantitatively as the number of organisms required to establish fecal colonization at a level of more than 10^3 CFU/mL in 50% of treated animals [63], or the number of facultative anaerobes such as *E. coli* present at a given site in the gut [14] and qualitatively as the biological mechanism responsible for prevention of abnormal gut colonization by potentially pathogenic micro-organisms. Bacteriologic studies of the effects of antibiotics on colonization resistance indicated that the indigenous Gram positive anaerobes were the dominant species responsible for colonization resistance [61].

3.4.2. Consequences of Antibiotic Administration

The most compelling data demonstrating the central role of the indigenous flora in stabilizing the microbial ecology of the gut comes from studies in which the normal flora has been disrupted by the administration of antibiotics. This subject has been extensively documented elsewhere [61,64,65], and has significant clinical consequences, for example, *C. difficile* colitis and the promotion of the growth of resistant microbial strains are well-recognized. The role of antibiotics in promoting gut colonization with pathogens of importance in ICU-acquired infections is considered below.

3.4.3. Competition for Nutrients and Binding Sites

It is generally believed that competition for specific nutrients and/or binding sites within the GI tract is the major factor regulating microbial populations within the gut lumen [14,66].

Competition for nutrient substrate, although intuitively attractive as a mechanism for the regulation of bacterial populations, has been difficult to characterize because of the complexity of the normal flora and the large numbers of potential nutrients present. Moreover, the food sources used by the indigenous flora are not primarily ingested food but desquamated epithelial cells, mucus and the products of metabolism of other bacteria [14,67]. In vitro studies show that cecal contents do not support the growth of *E. coli* in the absence of exogenous substrate [68]. The low oxygen tension of the gut lumen favours the growth of anaerobic bacteria in the colon, whereas aerobic bacteria preferentially colonize the mucosa where they are able to derive oxygen from adjacent epithelial cells [1]. The growth of certain strains of *E. coli* associated with the cecal mucosa is dependent on their ability to metabolize mucus as an energy source [69]. Similarly, *Bacteroides fragilis* is able to use mucin as its sole carbohydrate energy source [70].

Competition for binding sites is an additional factor influencing patterns of colonization. Studies in the germfree animal show that twice as many *Candida* cells can adhere to oral epithelium in the absence of a normal colonizing flora [71]. Microbial attachment to epithelial surfaces occurs through the interaction of specific bacterial adhesins or lectins with complementary receptors on the epithelial cell. These receptors vary in the structure of their carbohydrate chain and this biochemical diversity is likely responsible for the development of discrete and distinctive patterns of colonization at different anatomic sites of the GI tract [72]. In the oropharynx, for example, normal colonization with *Streptococci* is not homogeneous but rather different species selectively localize to discrete anatomical niches [73] and differing strains of the organism demonstrate differential adhesion to cultured epithelial cells [74]. Similarly in the rat stomach, *Lactobacilli* and *S. epidermidis* are capable of adhering to gastric epithelial cells, while *S. fecalis*, *E. coli* and *Bacteroides* are unable to do so [75].

The mucus blanket of the gut epithelium plays a significant role in the regulation of normal gut colonization through the inhibition of bacterial binding to the underlying epithelial cells [76], an effect which is augmented in the presence of a specific IgA antimicrobial response [77].

Both bacterial and host factors contribute to the preferential association of certain species with distinct sites. Gut colonization by pathogens is favoured by the presence of colonization factors [78] or flagella [79] on the surface of the organism, as well as by the ability of the organism to grow in colonies [80]. Both the presence of pili on the bacterium [81] and the intrinsic hydrophobicity of Gram negative bacteria [82] favour binding of organisms to epithelial cell glycoproteins. Piliation appears to be an important factor in the development of pathologic colonization in critical illness [83]. IgA functions to prevent adhesion and there is evidence that certain bacterial strains such as *Pseudomonas* [84] and *Neisseria* [85] elaborate proteases capable of degrading IgA and thereby facilitating adherence. Host factors regulating microbial adhesion to epithelial surfaces include pH [86], surface charge [87] and the presence of fibronectin [88], as well as IgA, discussed in greater detail below.

3.4.4. Production of Antimicrobial Factors by the Indigenous Flora

Products of bacterial metabolism can both inhibit and promote the growth of other organisms. Volatile fatty acids produced by anaerobic bacteria, particularly butyric acid, inhibit the growth of facultative anaerobes and appear to play a role in regulating numbers of *E. coli* [89], as well as in preventing establishment of exogenous pathogens such as *Shigella* [90]. Both acetic and butyric acid, present in feces or in anaerobic culture supernatants suppress the growth of *Pseudomonas* in vitro [91]. A reduction in volatile fatty acid concentrations in the cecum resulting from dietary manipulation [92] or cecectomy [93] is associated with reduced colonization resistance to both exogenous organisms and endogenous facultative anaerobes. Others have questioned the importance of volatile fatty acids in vivo since there is no correlation between their levels and numbers of *E. coli* in mice in whom colonization has become established [94]; in this study, an inverse relationship between numbers of *E. coli* and cecal concentrations of propionic acid was documented, suggesting that this fatty acid may be important in regulating the density of colonization with *E. coli*. In addition to their biological contribution to the regulation of the normal gut flora, volatile fatty acids are an important source of energy for the colo-

nocyte [95]. Work by Freter et al in an in vitro system suggests that hydrogen sulfide may also inhibit the growth of *E. coli* [66].

A wide variety of Gram positive and Gram negative bacteria produce antibiotic substances known as bacteriocins which inhibit the growth of other bacterial strains [96]. Colicins elaborated by *E. coli* are among the best characterized bacteriocins and are known to inhibit the growth of other gram negative organisms in vitro. There is little evidence, however, that colicin production contributes significantly to the regulation of gut bacterial populations in vivo [97,98]. Bacteriocins produced by *S. mutans* appear to play an important role in the establishment of this species in dental plaque and there is some evidence that a class of low molecular weight bacteriocins known as microcins may play a role in the establishment of colonization resistance in humans [96]. Bacteriocins produced by *viridans Streptococci* of the oropharynx are believed to be an important barrier, preventing pathologic colonization by Gram negative bacteria and Group A *Streptococci* [72,99]. Enocin, an antibiotic substance produced by *S. salivarius*, inhibits the growth of Group A *Streptococci* by interfering with normal utilization of pantothenate [100].

A dialysable factor produced by certain strains of *E. coli* inhibits the growth of *Candida* in vitro and in vivo. Germfree mice monoassociated with *Candida* demonstrate significantly lower levels of fungal gut colonization when the inhibitory strain is administered than when a non-inhibitory strain of *E. coli* is given [101].

Lactobacilli exert an inhibitory influence on the growth of a number of bacterial species including *S. aureus*, *E. coli*, *Salmonella* and *Clostridia* [102]. *Lactobacilli* release natural antibiotics such as acidophilin and bulgari-can [103], as well as hydrogen peroxide which inhibits the growth of *S. aureus* [104] and *Pseudomonas* [105]. Moreover, they al-so stimulate the production of specific IgA antibody to potential gut pathogens such as *S. typhi* [106].

3.5. Immunologic Regulation of the Indigenous Flora

Although the gastrointestinal tract is richly endowed with lymphatic tissue, the eviden-ce that specific immunological factors play an important role in the regulation of nor-mal GI colonization is scant. On the other hand, the indigenous flora exerts a signifi-cant influence on systemic immune home-ostasis.

3.5.1. Immunoglobulin A

IgA is secreted by plasma cells of the mu-cosal lymphoid tissues as a dimer with an additional polypeptide chain- the J chain. Dimeric IgA binds to the secretory compo-nent, a product of epithelial cells, and the complex, known as secretory IgA (sIgA) is transported across the epithelial cell and re-leased into the intestinal lumen [107]. Alt-hough B cells of the gut-associated lymp-hoid tissues are the major site of synthesis of secretory IgA in the gut lumen, the liver of the rodent also synthesizes both IgA [108-110] and the secretory component [111]. Hepatic production of IgA has been demonstrated in humans [112], however the contribution of the liver to the IgA pool of the gut appears to be minimal. Secretory IgA concentrations are higher in portal ve-nous blood than in systemic blood, sugges-ting that tissues drained by the portal vein are the major site of IgA synthesis [113].

IgA-producing plasma cells decrease in number from the duodenum to the colon [114]. Micro-organisms within the gut are a potent stimulus for the proliferation of IgA-producing plasma cells and the release of IgA. The intestinal mucosa of the germfree animal contains few plasma cells [114,115] while bacterial overgrowth induces an in-crease in the luminal release of IgA specific for the colonizing species [116] and intesti-nal pathogens such as *Shigella* induce a lo-cal specific IgA response [117]. Local IgA release is regulated by non-microbial fac-tors as well, increasing in response to cho-lecystokinin and secretin [118] and decrea-sing in response to atropine [119].

The primary biological function of IgA is the prevention of bacterial adhesion to epithe-lial cells [120]. IgA in sputum, for example, inhibits the binding of *Pseudomonas* to tra-cheal epithelial cells [121], while urinary IgA exerts a similar inhibitory effect on the binding of *E. coli* to epithelial cells of the bladder [122].

IgA deficiency, a relatively common immu-ne disorder with a prevalence of approxi-mately 3 cases per thousand in the general population, is not associated with significant alterations in the microbial flora of the pro-ximal GI tract [48,123], presumably becau-se of a compensatory increase in the release of IgM linked to the secretory component [107]. On the other hand, IgA deficiency in association with vagotomy and ablation of the pylorus results in significantly greater proximal gut colonization than vagotomy and drainage alone [48]. A single case of isolated secretory component deficiency has been reported: interestingly, the affected individual presented with diarrhea and in-testinal Candidiasis, with small bowel fun-gal overgrowth but apparently minimal evi-dence of bacterial overgrowth [124].

3.5.2. Cell-mediated Immunity

Cell-mediated immunity appears to have relatively little influence on patterns of gut colonization. Homozygous athymic nude mice have a flora which is similar to that of their heterozygous littermates [125] and similar cecal concentrations of bacteria following monoassociation with antibiotic-resistant *E. coli* in association with orally administered antibiotics [126].

3.5.3. Other Immune Mechanisms

Paneth cells found in the crypts of Lieberkuhn of the small intestine appear to play a significant role in the antibacterial defenses of the small bowel. They release IgA [127] and lysozyme [128] and bacterial debris has been identified within their phagolysozomes [129]. Paneth cells contain mRNA for tumour necrosis factor [130] and have been shown to secrete cryptdins, two closely related defensins which demonstrate potent broad spectrum antibacterial activity [131,132]. Another antibacterial peptide known as cecropin has been isolated from pig intestine [133].

4. THE GUT FLORA AND INTRA-ABDOMINAL INFECTION

Primary peritonitis arises by one of two routes- ascending spread from the genital tract of women and translocation across an intact gut mucosa in the cirrhotic [134]. In the latter case, changes in the composition of the flora of the proximal gut [135] likely play a role in predisposing the cirrhotic to translocation. Microbial translocation is also important in the colonization and infection of peripancreatic necrotic tissue in pancreatic infections [136]. Secondary peritonitis typically results from a mechanical breach of the integrity of the gut wall, exposing the peritoneal cavity to the entire spectrum of organisms resident in the gastrointestinal tract [137].

Tertiary peritonitis, defined as the persistence or recurrence of peritonitis after the apparently adequate management of primary or secondary peritonitis [138], is associated with a strikingly different microbial flora from that of secondary peritonitis. The most common infecting species are coagulase-negative *Staphylococci*, *Candida*, *Enterococci* and *Pseudomonas* [139-141], the same species that are the most common organisms colonizing the proximal GI tract in critical illness [142]. Thus, like primary peritonitis in the cirrhotic, tertiary peritonitis appears to be caused by the translocation of an altered flora across the gastrointestinal tract.

5. CONCLUSIONS

The ecology of the normal microbial flora is enormously complex and the organisms resident in the gut influence systemic homeostasis in multiple ways. The complexity of the flora accounts for the microbial complexity of intra-abdominal infection. Perhaps more importantly, however, interactions between the flora and the gut associated lymphoid tissues regulate normal immunologic homeostasis and changes in these normal interactions may contribute to the broad spectrum of systemic manifestations that evolve in the critically ill patient with peritonitis [143,144].

REFERENCES

1. Savage DC: Microbial ecology of the gastrointestinal tract. Ann Rev Microbiol 31:107-133, 1977.

2. Moore WEC, Holdeman LV: Human fecal flora: The normal flora of 20 Japanese-Hawaiians. Appl Microbiol 27:961-979, 1974.

3. Rutenburg AM, Sonnenblick E, Koven I, Aprahamian HA, Reiner L, Fine J: The role of intestinal bacteria in the development of dietary cirrhosis in rats. J Exp Med 106:1-14, 1957.

4. Penhale WJ, Young PR: The influence of the normal microbial flora on the susceptibility of rats to experimental autoimmune thyroiditis. Clin Exp Immunol 72:288-292, 1988.

5. Midtvedt T: Intestinal bacteria and rheumatic disease. Scand J Rheumatol 64 (Suppl):49-54, 1987.

6. Eerola E, Mottonen T, Hannonen P, Luukainen R, Kantola I, Vuori K, Tuominen J, Toivanen P: Intestinal flora in early rheumatoid arthritis. Br. J. Rheumatol. 33:1030-1038, 1994.

7. Lee A: Neglected niches. The microbial ecology of the gastrointestinal tract. Adv Microb Ecol 8:115-162, 1985.

8. Gorbach SL, Nahas L, Lerner PI, Weinstein L: Studies of intestinal microflora. I. Effects of diet, age and periodic sampling on numbers of fecal organisms in man. Gastroenterology 53:845-855, 1967.

9. Dubos R, Schaedler RW, Costello R, Hoet P: Indigenous, normal and autochthonous flora of the gastrointestinal tract. J Exp Med 122:67-76, 1965.

10. Donaldson RM: Normal bacterial populations of the intestine and their relation to intestinal function. N Engl J Med 270:938-945, 1964.

11. Nelson DP, Mata LJ: Bacterial flora associated with the human gastrointestinal mucosa. Gastroenterology 58:56-61, 1970.

12. Takeuchi A, Jervis HR, Nakagawa H, Robison DM: Spiral-shaped organisms on the surface colonic epithelium of the monkey and man. Am J Clin Nutr 27:1287-1296, 1974.

13. Savage DC: Associations of indigenous microorganisms with gastrointestinal epithelial surfaces. pp55-78 in Hentges DJ (ED) Human Intestinal Microflora in Health and Disease. Academic Press New York, 1983.

14. Lee A: Neglected niches. The microbial ecology of the gastrointestinal tract. Adv Microb Ecol 8:115-162, 1985.

15. Rozee KR, Cooper D, Lam K, Costerton JW: Microbial flora of the mouse ileum mucous layer and epithelial surface. Appl Environ Microbiol 43:1451-1463, 1982.

16. Suegara N, Morotomi M, Watanabe T, Kawai Y, Matai M: Behaviour of microflora in the rat stomach: Adhesion of lactobacilli to the keratinized epithelial cells of the rat stomach in vitro. Infect Immun 12:173-179, 1975.

17. van der Waaij D, Berghuis-de Vries JM, Lekkerkerk-van der Wees JEC: Colonization resistance of the digestive tract in conventional and antibiotic-treated mice. J Hyg 69:405-411, 1971.

18. Finegold SM, Sutter VL, Mathisen GE: Normal indigenous intestinal flora. pp3-31 in Hentges DJ (ED) Human Intestinal Microflora in Health and Disease. Academic Press New York, 1983.

19. Gorbach SL, Plaut AG, Nahas L, Weinstein L, Spanknebel G, Levitan R: Studies of intestinal microflora. II. Microorganisms of the small intestine and their relations to oral and fecal flora. Gastroenterology 53:856-867, 1967.

20. Drasar BS, Shiner M: Studies on the intestinal flora. II. Bacterial flora of the small intestine in patients with gastrointestinal disorders. Gut 10:812-819, 1969.

21. Finegold SM, Sutter VL, Boyle JD, Shimada K: The normal flora of ileostomy and transverse colostomy effluents. J Infect Dis 122:376-381, 1970.

22. Corrodi P, Wideman PA, Sutter VL, Drenick EJ, Passaro E, Finegold SM: Bacterial flora of the small bowel before and after bypass pro-

cedure for morbid obesity. J Infect Dis 137:1-6, 1978.

23. Thadepalli H, Lou MA, Bach VT, Matsui TK, Mandal AK: Microflora of the human small intestine. Am J Surg 138:845-850, 1979.

24. Palmer LB: Bacterial colonization: Pathogenesis and clinical significance. Clin Chest Med 8:455-466, 1987.

25. Johanson WG, Pierce AK, Sanford JP: Changing pharyngeal flora of hospitalized patients. Emergence of gram negative bacilli. N Engl J Med 281:1137-1140, 1969.

26. Johanson WG, Pierce AK, Sanford JP, Thomas GD: Nosocomial respiratory infections with Gram-negative bacilli. The significance of colonization of the respiratory tract. Ann Intern Med 77:701-706, 1972.

27. Franklin MA, Skoryna SC: Studies on natural gastric flora: I. Bacterial flora of fasting human subjects. CMAJ 95:1349-1355, 1966.

28. Gianella RA, Broitman SA, Zamcheck N: Gastric acid barrier to ingested micro-organisms in man: studies in vivo and in vitro. Gut 13:251-256, 1972.

29. Cohen R, Roth FJ, Delgado E, Ahearn DG, Kalser MHi: Fungal flora of the normal human small and large intestine. N Engl J Med 280:638-641, 1969.

30. Gotlieb-Jensen K, Andersen J: Occurrence of *Candida* in gastric ulcers. Significance for the healing process. Gastroenterology 85:535-537, 1983.

31. Parsonnet J, Hansen S, Rodriguez L, Gelb AB, Warnke RA, Jellum E, Orentreich N, Vogelman JH, Friedman GD: *Helicobacter pylori* infection and gastric lymphoma. N. Engl. J. Med 330:1267-1271, 1994.

32. Peterson WL, Mackowiak PA, Barnett CC, Marling-Cason M, Haley ML: The human gastric bactericidal barrier: Mechanisms of action, relative antibacterial activity and dietary influences. J Infect Dis 159:979-983, 1989.

33. Kalser MH, Cohen R, Arteaga I, Yawn E, Mayoral L, Hoffert WR, Frazier D: Normal viral

and bacterial flora of the human small and large intestine. N Engl J Med 274:500-505, 1966.

34. Drasar BS, Shiner M, McLeod GM: Studies on the intestinal flora. I. The bacterial flora of the gastrointestinal tract in healthy and achlorhydric persons. Gastroenterology 56:71-79, 1969.

35. Bentley DW, Nichols RL, Condon RE, Gorbach SL: The microflora of the human ileum and intraabdominal colon: Results of direct needle aspiration at surgery and evaluation of the technique. J Lab Clin Med 79:421-429, 1972.

36. Stark PL, Lee A: The microbial ecology of the large bowel of breast-fed and formula-fed infants during the first year of life. J Med Microbiol 15:189-203, 1982.

37. Schaedler RW, Dubos R, Costello R: The development of the bacterial flora in the gastrointestinal tract of mice. J Exp Med 122:59-66, 1965.

38. Cooperstock MS, Zedd AJ: Intestinal flora of infants. pp79-99 in Hentges DJ (ED) *Human Intestinal Microflora in Health and Disease.* Academic Press New York, 1983.

39. Schaedler RW, Dubos R, Costello R: Association of germfree mice with bacteria isolated from normal mice. J Exp Med 122:77-82, 1965.

40. Shiner M, Waters TE, Gray JDA: Culture studies of the gastrointestinal tract with a newly devised capsule. Gastroenterology 45:625-632, 1963.

41. Howden CW, Hunt RH: Relationship between gastric secretion and infection. Gut 28:96-107, 1987.

42. Ruddell WSJ, Axon ATR, Findlay JM, Bartholomew BA, Hill MJ: Effect of cimetidine on the gastric bacterial flora. Lancet 1:672-674, 1980.

43. Stockbrugger RW, Cotton PB, Eugenides N, Bartholomew BA, Hill MJ, Walters CL: Intragastric nitrates, nitrosamines and bacterial overgrowth during cimetidine treatment. Gut 23:1048-1054, 1982.

44. Mehta S, Archer JF, Mills J: pH-dependent bactericidal barrier to gram-negative aerobes: its relevance to airway colonisation and prophylaxis of acid aspiration and stress ulcer syndromes- study in vitro. Intensive Care Med 12:134-136, 1986.

45. Greenlee HB, Vivit R, Paez J, Dietz A: Bacterial flora of the jejunum following peptic ulcer surgery. Arch Surg 102:260-265, 1971.

46. Broido PN, Gorbach SL,Condon RE, Nyhus LM: Upper intestinal microfloral control. Effects of gastric and vagal denervation on bacterial concentrations. Arch Surg 106:90-93, 1973.

47. Gray JDA, Shiner M: Influence of gastric pH on gastric and jejunal flora. Gut 8:574-581, 1967.

48. McLoughlin GA, Hede JE, Temple JG, Bradley J, Chapman DM, McFarland J: The role of IgA in the prevention of bacterial colonization of the jejunum in the vagotomized subject. Br J Surg 65:435-437, 1978.

49. Hentges DJ: Role of the intestinal microflora in host defense against infection. pp 311-331 in Hentges DJ (Ed) *Human Intestinal Microflora in Health and Disease.* Academic Press New York, 1983.

50. Hylemon PB, Glass TL: Biotransformation of bile acids and cholesterol by the intestinal microflora. pp 189-213, in Hentges DJ (Ed) *Human Intestinal Microflora in Health and Disease.* Academic Press New York, 1983.

51. Floch MH, Gershengoren W, Elliot S, Spiro HM: Bile acid inhibition of the intestinal microflora- a function of simple bile acids? Gastroenterology 61:228-233, 1971.

52. Floch MH, Binder HJ, Filburn B, Gershengoren W: The effect of bile acids on intestinal microflora. Am J Clin Nutr 25:1418-1426, 1972.

53. Williams RC, Showalter R, Kern F: In vivo effect of bile salts and cholestyramine on intestinal anaerobic bacteria. Gastroenterology 69:483-491, 1975.

54. Tazume S, Hashimoto K, Sasaki S: Intestinal flora and bile acids metabolism: Influence of bile acids on rejection of *Shigella flexneri* 2a from the intestine. Nippon Saikingaku Zasshi 34:745-754, 1979.

55. Deitch EA, Sittig K, Li M, Berg R, Specian RD: Obstructive jaundice promotes bacterial translocation from the gut. Am J Surg 159:79-84, 1990.

56. Bishop RF, Anderson CM: Bacterial flora of stomach and small intestine in children with intestinal obstruction. Arch Dis Childhood 35:487-491, 1960.

57. Skar V, Skar AG, Osnes M: The duodenal bacterial flora in the region of papilla of Vater in patients with and without duodenal diverticula. Scand J Gastroenterol 24:649-656, 1989.

58. King CE, Toskes PP: Small intestine bacterial overgrowth. Gastroenterology 76:1035-1055, 1979.

59. Abrams GD, Bishop JE: Effect of the normal microbial flora on gastrointestinal motility. Proc Soc Exp Biol Med 126:301-304, 1967.

60. Sprunt K, Redman R: Evidence suggesting importance of role of interbacterial inhibition in maintaining balance of normal flora. Ann Intern Med 68:579-590, 1968.

61. van der Waaij D: The ecology of the human intestine and its consequences for overgrowth by pathogens such as *Clostridium difficile.* Annu Rev Microbiol 43:69-87, 1989.

62. Salminen S, Isolauri E, Onnela T: Gut flora in normal and siordered states. Chemotherapy 14 (Suppl) 1:5-15, 1995.

63. van der Waaij D, Berghuis-de Vries JM: Determination of the colonization resistance of the digestive tract of individual mice. J Hyg 72:379-387, 1973.

64. Finegold SM, Mathisen GE, George WL: Changes in human intestinal flora related to the administration of antimicrobial agents. pp 355-446 in Hentges DJ (ED) *Human In-*

testinal Microflora in Health and Disease. Academic Press New York, 1983.

65. Hooker KD, DiPiro JT: Effect of antimicrobial therapy on bowel flora. Clin Pharm 7:878-888, 1988.

66. Freter R, Brickner H, Botney M, Cleven D, Aranki A: Mechanisms which control bacterial populations in continuous flow culture models of mouse large intestinal flora. Infect Immun 39:676-685, 1983.

67. Hoskins LC, Boulding ET: Mucin degradation in the human colon ecosystems. Evidence for the existence and role of bacterial subpopulations producing glycosidases as extracellular enzymes. J Clin Invest 67:163-172, 1981.

68. Guiot HFL: Role of competition for substrate in bacterial antagonism in the gut. Infect Immun 38:887-892, 1982.

69. Waldowski EA, Laux DC, Cohen PS: Colonization of the streptomycin-treated mouse large intestine by a human fecal *Escherichia coli* strain: Role of growth in mucus. Infect Immun 56:1030-1035, 1988.

70. Roberton AM, Stanley RA: In vitro utilization of mucin by *Bacteroides fragilis*. Appl Environ Microbiol 43:325-330, 1982.

71. Liljemark WF, Gibbons RJ: Suppression of *Candida albicans* by human oral streptococci in gnotobiotic mice. Infect Immun 8:846-849, 1973.

72. Mackowiak PA: The normal microbial flora. N Engl J Med 307:83-93, 1982.

73. Gibbons RJ, van Houte J: Selective bacterial adherence to oral epithelial surfaces and its role as an ecological determinant. Infect Immun 3:567, 1971.

74. Valentin-Weigand P, Chhatwal GS, Blobel H: A simple method for quantitative determination of bacterial adherence to human and animal epithelial cells. Microbiol Immunol 31:1017-1023, 1987.

75. Kawai Y, Suegara N: Specific adhesion of lactobacilli to keratinized epithelial cells of the rat stomach in vitro. Am J Clin Nutr 30:1777-1780, 1977.

76. McNabb PC, Tomasi TB: Host defense mechanisms at mucosal surfaces. Ann Rev Microbiol 35:477-496, 1981.

77. Walker RI, Owen RL: Intestinal barriers to bacteria and their toxins. Annu Rev Med 41:393-400, 1990.

78. Neeser J-R, Chambaz A, Golliard M, Link-Amster H, Fryder V, Kolodziejczyk E: Adhesion of colonization factor antigen II-positive enterotoxigenic *Escherichia coli* strains to human enterocytelike differentiated HT-29 cells: a basis for host-pathogen interactions in the gut. Infect Immun 57:3727-3734, 1989.

79. Pavlovskis OR, Rollins DM, Haberberger RL, Green AE, Habash L, Strocko S, Walker RI: Significance of flagella in colonization resistance of rabbits immunized with *Campylobacter* spp. Infect Immun 59:2259-2264, 1991.

80. Cohen PS, Kjelleberg S, Laux DC, Conway PL: *Escherichia coli* F-18 makes a streptomycin-treated mouse large intestine colonization factor when grown in nutrient broth containing glucose. Infect Immun 58:1471-1472, 1990.

81. Knutton S, Lloyd DR, Candy DCA, McNeish AS: Adhesion of enterotoxigenic *Escherichia coli* to human small intestinal enterocytes. Infect Immun 48:824-831, 1985.

82. Drumm B, Neumann AW, Policova Z, Sherman PM: Bacterial cell surface hydrophobicity properties in the mediation of in vitro adhesion by the rabbit enteric pathogen *Escherichia coli* strain RDEC-1. J Clin Invest 84:1588-1594, 1989.

83. Donaldson SG, Azizi SQ, Dal Nogare AR: Characteristics of aerobic Gram-negative bacteria colonizing critically ill patients. Am Rev Respir Dis 144:202-207, 1991.

84. Milazzo FH, Delisle GJ: Immunoglobulin A proteases in gram-negative bacteria isolated from human urinary tract infections. Infect Immun 43:11-13, 1984.

85. Mulks MH, Plaut AG: IgA protease production as a characteristic distinguishing pathogenic from harmless neisseriaceae. N Engl J Med 299:973-976, 1978.

86. Palmer LB, Merrill WW, Niederman MS, Ferranti RD, Reynolds HY: Bacterial adherence to respiratory tract cells. Relationships between in vivo and in vitro pH and bacterial attachment. Am Rev Respir Dis 133:784-788, 1986.

87. Ayars GH, Altman LC, Fretwell MD: Effect of decreased salivation and pH on the adherence of Klebsiella species to human buccal epithelial cells. Infect Immun 38:179-182, 1982.

88. Woods DE, Straus DC, Johanson WG, Bass JA: Role of salivary proteases activity in adherence of gram-negative bacilli to mammalian buccal epithelial cells in vivo. J Clin Invest 68:1435-1440, 1981.

89. Lee A, Gemmell E: Changes in the mouse intestinal microflora during weaning: Role of volatile fatty acids. Infect Immun 5:1-7, 1972.

90. Maier BR, Hentges DJ: Experimental *Shigella* infections in laboratory animals. I. Antagonism by normal flora components in gnotobiotic mice. Infect Immun 6:168-173, 1972.

91. Levison ME: Effect of colon flora and short-chain fatty acids on growth in vitro of *Pseudomonas* and Enterobacteriaceae. Infect Immun 8:30-35, 1973.

92. Brockett M, Tannock GW: Dietary influence on microbial activities in the cecum of mice. Can J Microbiol 28:493-499, 1982.

93. Voravuthikunchai SP, Lee A: Cecectomy causes long-term reduction of colonization resistance in the mouse gastrointestinal tract. Infect Immun 55:995-999, 1987.

94. Koopman JP, Welling GW, Huybregts AWM, Mullink JWMA, Prins RA: Association of germ-free mice with intestinal floras. Z Verstuchstierkd 23:145-154, 1981.

95. Rolandelli RH, Koruda MJ, Settle RG, Rombeau JL: Effect of intraluminal short chain fatty acids on healing of colonic anastamosis in the rat. Surgery 100:198-1986.

96. Govan JRW: In vivo significance of bacteriocins and bacteriocin receptors. Scand J Infect Dis Suppl 49:31-37, 1986.

97. Ikari NS, Kenton DM, Young VM: Interaction in the germfree mouse intestine of colicinogenic and colicin-sensitive microorganisms. Proc Soc Exp Biol Med 130:1280-1284, 1969.

98. Mason TG, Richardson G: A review of *Escherichia coli* and the human gut: Some ecological considerations. J Appl Bacteriol 1:1-6, 1981.

99. Crowe CC, Sanders WE, Longley S: Bacterial interference. II. Role of the normal throat flora in prevention of colonization by Group A *Streptococcus*. J Infect Dis 128:527-532, 1973.

100. Sanders CC, Sanders WE: Enocin: An antibiotic produced by *Streptococcus salivarius* that may contribute to protection against infections due to Group A Streptococci. J Infect Dis 146:683-690, 1982.

101. Hummel RP, Oestreicher EJ, Maley MP, MaMillan BG: Inhibition of *Candida albicans* by *Escherichia coli* in vitro and in the germfree mouse. J Surg Res 15:53-58, 1973.

102. Shahani KM, Ayebo AD: Role of dietary lactobacilli in gastrointestinal microecology. Am J Clin Nutr 33:2448-2457, 1980.

103. Shahani KM, Vakil JR, Kilara A: Natural antibiotic activity of Lactobacillus acidophilus and bulgaricus. II. Isolation of acidophilin from L. acidophilus. Cult Dairy Prod J 12:8, 1977.

104. Collins EB, Aramaki K: Production of hydrogen peroxide by Lactobacillus acidophilus. J Dairy Sci 63:353-357, 1980.

105. Price RJ, Lee JS: Inhibition of *Pseudomonas* species by hydrogen peroxide producing

lactobacilli. J Milk Food Technol 33:13-18, 1970.

106. Link-Amster H, Rochat F, Saudan KY, Mignot O, Aeschlimann JM: Modulation of a specific humoral immune response and changes in intestinal flora mediated through fermented milk intake. FEMS Immunol. Med. Microbiol. 10:55-63, 1994.

107. Bienenstock J, Befus AD: Mucosal immunology. Immunology 41:249-270, 1980.

108. Manning RJ, Walker PG, Carter L, Barrington PJ, Jackson GDF: Studies on the origins of biliary immunoglobulins in rats. Gastroenterology 87:173-179, 1984.

109. Alverdy J, Chi HS, Sheldon GF: The effect of parenteral nutrition on gastrointestinal immunity. The importance of enteral stimulation. Ann Surg 202:681-684, 1985.

110. Altorfer J, Hardesty SJ, Scott JH, Jones AL: Specific antibody synthesis and biliary secretion by the rat liver after intestinal immunization with cholera toxin. Gastroenterology 93:539-549, 1987.

111. Vaerman JP, Buts JP, Lescoat G: Ontogeny of secretory component in rat liver. Immunology 68:295-299, 1989.

112. Nagura H, Smith PD, Nakane PK, Brown WR: IgA in human bile and liver. J Immunol 126:587-595, 1981.

113. Challacombe SJ, Greenall C, Stoker TAM: A comparison of IgA in portal and peripheral venous blood. Immunology 60:111-116, 1987.

114. Crabbe PA, Bazin H, Eyssen H, Heremans JF: The normal microbial flora as a major stimulus for plasma cells synthesizing IgA in the gut. Ant Arch Allergy 34:362-375, 1968.

115. Kenworthy R, Allen WD: Influence of diet and bacteria on small intestinal morphology, with special reference to early weaning and *Escherichia coli*. Studies with germfree and gnotobiotic pigs. J Comp Path 76:291-296, 1966.

116. Lichtman S, Sherman P, Forstner G: Production of secretory immunoglobulin A in rat self-filling blind loops. Local secretory immunoglobulin A immune response to luminal bacterial flora. Gastroenterology 91:1495-1502, 1986.

117. Keren DF, McDonald RA, Scott PJ, Rosner AM, Strubel E: Effect of antigen form on local immunoglobulin A memory response of intestinal secretions to *Shigella flexneri*. Infect Immun 47:123-128, 1985.

118. Shah PC, Freier S, Park BH, Lee PC, Lebenthal E: Pancreozymin and secretin enhance duodenal fluid antibody levels to cow's milk proteins. Gastroenterology 83:881-888, 1982.

119. Freier S, Eran M, Faber J: Effect of cholecysotkinin and of its antagonist, of atropine and of food on the release of immunoglobulin A and immunoglobulin G specific antibodies in the rat intestine. Gastroenterology 93:1242-1246, 1987.

120. Williams RC, Gibbons RJ: Inhibition of bacterial adherence by secretory immunoglobulin A: a mechanism of antigen disposal. Science 177:697-699, 1972.

121. Niederman MS, Merrill WW, Polomski LM, Reynolds HY. Gee JBL: Influence of sputum IgA and elastase on tracheal cell bacterial adherence. Am Rev Respir Dis 133:255-260, 1986.

122. Svanborg-Eden C, Svennerholm AM: Secretory immunoglobulin A and G antibodies prevent adhesion of *Escherichia coli* to human urinary tract epithelial cells. Infect Immun 22:790-797, 1978.

123. Brown WR, Savage DC, Dubois RS, Alp MH, Mallory A, Kern F: Intestinal microflora of immunoglobulin-deficient and normal human subjects. Gastroenterology 62:1143-1152, 1972.

124. Strober W, Krakauer R, Klaeveman HL, Reynolds HY, Nelson DL: Secretory component deficiency. A disorder of the IgA immune system. N Engl J Med 294:351-356, 1976.

125. Brown JF, Balish E: Gastrointestinal micro-ecology of BALB/c nude mice. Appl Environ Micobiol 36:144-159, 1978.

126. Maddaus M, Wells C, Platt JL, Condie MS, Simmons RL: Effect of T cell modulation on the translocation of bacteria from the gut and mesenteric lymph node. Ann Surg 207:387-398, 1988.

127. Erlandsen SL, Rodning CB, Montero C, Parsons JA, Lewis EA, Wilson ID: Immunocytochemical identification and localization of immunoglobulin A within Paneth cells of the rat small intestine. J Histochem Cytochem 24:1085-1092, 1976.

128. Deckx RJ, Vantrappen GR, Parein MM: Localization of lysozyme activity in a Paneth cell granule fraction. Biochim Biophys Acta 139:204-209, 1967.

129. Erlandsen SL: Paneth cell function: ultrastructural evidence for the absorption of bacterial debris from the lumen of the intestinal crypt. J Cell Biol 47:57a, 1970.

130. Keshav S, Dawson L, Chung P, Stein M, Perry VH, Gordon S: Tumor necrosis factor mRNA localized to Paneth cells of normal murine intestinal epithelium by in situ hybridization. J Exp Med 171:327-332, 1990.

131. Ouellette AJ, Greco RM, James M, Frederick D, Naftilan J, Fallon JT: Developmental regulation of cryptdin, a corticostatin/defensin precursor mRNA in mouse small intestinal crypt epithelium. J Cell Biol 108:1687-1695, 1989.

132. Eisenhauer PB, Harwig SSL, Lehrer RI: Cryptdins: Antimicrobial defensins of the murine small intestine. Infect Immun 60:3556-3565, 1992.

133. Lee J-Y, Boman A, Chuanxin S, Andersson M, Jornvall H, Mutt V, Boman HG: Antibacterial peptides from the pig intestine: isolation of a mammalian cecropin. Proc Natl Acad Sci USA 86:9159-9162, 1989.

134. Crossley IR, Williams R: Spontaneous bacterial peritonitis. Gut 26:325-31, 1985.

135. Martini GA, Phear EA, Ruebner B, Sherlock S: The bacterial content of the small intestine in normal and cirrhotic subjects: relation to methionine toxicity. Clin Sci 16:35-51, 1956.

136. Gianotti L, Munda R, Alexander JW: Pancreatitis induced microbial translocation: a study of the mechanisms. Research in Surgery 4:87-91, 1992.

137. Wittmann DH, Schein M, Condon RE: Management of secondary peritonitis. Ann Surg 224:10-8, 1996.

138. Rotstein OD, Meakins JL: Diagnostic and therapeutic challenges of intraabdominal infections. World J Surg 1990; 14:159-66.

139. Rotstein OD, Pruett TL, Simmons RL: Microbiologic features and treatment of persistent peritonitis in patients in the intensive care unit. Can J Surg 29:247-50, 1986.

140. Sawyer RG, Rosenlof LK, Adams RB, May AK, Spengler MD, Pruett TL: Peritonitis into the 1990's: changing pathogens and changing strategies in the critically ill. Am Surg 58:82-7, 1992.

141. Nathens AB, Rotstein OD, Marshall JC: Tertiary peritonitis: Clinical features of a complex nosocomial infetion. World J Surg (In Press).

142. Marshall JC, Christou NV, Meakins JL: The gastrointestinal tract. The "undrained abscess" of multiple organ failure. Ann Surg 218:111-9, 1993.

143. Carrico CJ, Meakins JL, Marshall JC, Fry D, Maier RV: Multiple organ failure syndrome. The gastrointestinal tract: The 'motor' of MOF. Arch Surg 121:196-208, 1986.

144. Reemst PH, van Goor H, Goris RJ: SIRS, MODS, and tertiary peritonitis. Eur J Surg 576 Suppl:47-8, 1997.

Diagnosis and Minimally Invasive Treatment of Occult Intra-abdominal Infections

Juan Carlos Puyana, MD

1. INTRODUCTION

The diagnosis of intra-abdominal infection in the ICU is a challenging endeavor, as the patient usually presents with a conglomerate of events that make the clinical assessment rather limited [1,2,3]. Regardless of the primary pathology that prompts admission to the ICU, there are a number of risk factors common to the critically ill condition(s) that renders the patient extremely vulnerable for the development of intra-abdominal septic complications. These factors include hemodynamic instability, hypoxemia, systemic hypoperfusion, overwhelming infection, bacterial and/or fungal colonization and chronic disruption of mucosal barriers.

The patient may present severely ill and unstable as a result of an acute intra-abdominal process with peritonitis from a hollow viscus perforation (diverticulitis, gastric or duodenal ulcers, appendicitis) or with a severe intra-abdominal inflammatory focus such as, acute pancreatitis or severe retroperitoneal infection's (perinephric and psoas abscesses).

Conversely, the patient may manifest intra-abdominal sepsis as a secondary event added to the primary condition. Usually this septic pattern appears later in the course and may be protracted and difficult to identify. The most common culprits in this case include acalculous cholecystitis, perforation and peritonitis occurring after ischemia of the small or large bowel due to shock or secondary to severe constipation and paralytic ileus of the colon with subsequent ischemia and perforation. In addition, patients that have undergone intra-abdominal surgery may manifest intra-abdominal septic complications directly related to their primary operation such as, anastomotic leak, intracavitary abscesses, etc.

The patient is usually obtunded, on mechanical ventilation requiring intravenous sedatives and paralyzing agents. The clinical evaluation is usually difficult, however, it is of primordial importance to perform a thorough physical examination to rule out non-intra-abdominal sources of systemic infection that can be easily identified. The detection of severe sinusitis, a perirectal abscess, infected decubiti, superficial or deep phlebitis, will prompt early intervention avoiding expensive and strenuous diagnostic algorithms for intra-abdominal infection [2].

If the initial evaluation points to a possible intraabdominal source, a systematic approach should be used in order to achieve the best possible result with the most adequate utilization of resources, time and personnel. The decision to obtain an abdominal CT for example, should weigh the risks and benefits related to transporting an unstable patient to the radiology suite versus the yield for positive results. Anticipation of these results can be best accomplished by a thorough understanding of the possible causes and precipitating factors that prompted the patient into "SIRS and sepsis" in the first place [4,5].

Perhaps our own limitations in predicting or anticipating the events that trigger intra-abdominal catastrophes in the ICU translated into an aggressive approach based on exploratory laparotomy as a diagnostic intervention in the search of "occult" intra-abdominal infection [5,6,7]. This approach has not withstood the test of time. The *unaffordable* price of non-therapeutic laparotomies continue to be reported [8]. Such interventions have been associated with high mortality and morbidity, prolonged length of stay and consequently increased cost of health care [9]. Therefore, there is an imperative need to develop practical, safe and inexpensive interventions to diagnostic accuracy for the ICU patient with suspected intraabdominal foci as a source of SIRS/Sepsis.

2. CLASSICAL APPROACH COMPUTED TOMOGRAPHY (CT) AND OTHER ALTERNATIVES

The introduction of intensive care units and the progression of improved organ support

over the last 30 years has resulted in more severe patients rendered vulnerable to severe septic complications in the ICU. The abdominal cavity, bearing organs with a large bacterial burden, has long been recognized as a potential source of severe infection. The technological advances witnessed in the ICU have been paralleled with those in the area of imaging. The resolution, feasibility, speed and experience in computerized tomography, ultrasound, digital subtraction angiograms and nuclear medicine have significantly improved our ability to diagnose many conditions in the critically ill patient. However, there is a subgroup of ICU patients whose overall clinical condition and underlying pathology preclude the practical and safe application of some of these diagnostic tools. Furthermore, certain diagnoses, such as bowel ischemia, may not be easily identified with standard radiologic techniques, especially in patients with severe low flow status. Acalculous cholecystitis may be identified by ultrasound, however, this diagnostic modality is operator dependent and some of the classic changes described to establish the presence of inflammation may be prevalent in a significant number of patients resulting in a high incidence of false positive examinations [10,11,12].

Data on the outcome of ICU patients submitted to laparotomy for abdominal sepsis offers an additional insight to the magnitude of this problem.

A review of 100 laparotomies performed in 71 ICU patients was published in 1984 [3]. The objective of this study was to define preoperative criteria for and improve specificity of, laparotomy. Infection or ischemic process were identified in 81 explorations. 19 were negative. Preoperative features associated with a positive laparotomy included: 1) objective evidence of intra-abdominal sepsis by physical examination, CT or Ultrasound; 2) septic shock; 3) positive blood culture. Septic shock or bacteremia had a 90% mortality regardless of finding at exploration. The best accuracy (89%) and survival (51%) were achieved with directed exploration before septic shock or bacteremia. The authors conclude that early use of sensitive detection techniques will improve survival. Furthermore, these data strongly suggest that prompt diagnosis will translate in a lower rate of non-therapeutic laparotomy and will permit early and more effective intervention before the patient reaches irreversible "sepsis induced mediator disease."

If the original condition that brought the patient to the ICU is the result of an abdominal catastrophe, the outlook for non-directed relaparotomy as a mean of identifying intraabdominal sepsis is worse. In 192 patients who underwent relaparotomy for complications of primary laparotomy mortality ranged from 12.8% to 82.6%. Only 13% (2/15) non-directed laparotomies in patients with multiple organ dysfunction syndrome yielded positive results [5].

3. TO THE TOP OF THE COLUMN

The reintroduction of laparoscopy in the surgical armamentarium offers a diagnostic alternative for severely ill patients. There are several series in the literature describing high risk patients suspected to have severe intra-abdominal conditions who are taken to the operating room for diagnostic laparoscopy [13]. The learning curve has evolved quickly and most newer series report that bedside laparoscopy can be performed safely with similar diagnostic accuracy and comparable side effects [14]. Ideally, the bedside technique could further be impro-

ved to make the intervention less cumbersome by maximizing portability without sacrificing quality imaging, cost efficiency and maintaining the same safety standards. It is possible that in the near future smaller cameras and trocars as well as portable laparoscopy kits will be easily utilized to perform a laparoscopy as simply as inserting a Swan Ganz catheter. If such an ideal situation could be introduced, the true role of laparoscopy in the ICU will be better established. Unfortunately, most reports are limited to a small number of patients without specific prospective protocols. Such studies will be required to define clearly the high risk patients most likely to benefit of early laparoscopy as well as the best time for such interventions in relation to multiple clinical conditions.

3.1. Diagnostic peritoneal lavage

Diagnostic peritoneal lavage has been used extensively in trauma and there is a large body of data indicating the sensitivity and specificity for intra-abdominal bleeding in both blunt and penetrating trauma [13]. Unfortunately, there is no such evidence available for the role of DPL to evaluate acute inflammatory intra-abdominal disease. Bailey et al described 26 patients who underwent DPL for evaluation of acute intra-abdominal process [15]. DPL indicated the presence of sepsis in 10 patients. Sepsis was confirmed in 7/10 by laparotomy or postmortem examination. One patient was considered to have a false positive DPL. Sixteen patients showed no evidence of intra-abdominal disease. True negative results were confirmed in 14 patients. Two patients with a negative DPL died within two weeks without confirmatory interventions. Diagnostic accuracy of DPL in this series was 95%.

Peritoneal tap and paracentesis were initially described in the 50's as diagnostic aids for acute abdominal disease [16]. Later, it was suggested that lactic acid determination in ascitic fluid from cirrhotic patients would indicate the presence of spontaneous bacterial peritonitis. A subsequent study reported on the value of lactic acid determination in the peritoneal fluid as a means of identifying patients with acute intra-abdominal catastrophes, specifically in the setting of bowel ischemia [17]. This study compared the values of lactic acid measured simultaneously in serum and in the abdominal fluid. Forty four patients were entered in the study, 3 were ultimately excluded because no confirmatory information could be obtained before death. Intra-abdominal sepsis was confirmed in 19 patients, they had intra-abdominal abscesses, gangrenous bowel, perforation and/or peritonitis. The average lactic acid in peritoneal fluid was 9.9±5.3 versus 4.0±3.3 mmol/L in plasma. The difference between plasma and peritoneal fluid in 24 patients who had non-inflammatory intra-abdominal pathology was not statistically significant (2.6±3.2 in peritoneal fluid versus 2.5±3.1 in serum). The difference and the ratio between peritoneal fluid and plasma were both significantly different among those patients with intra-abdominal catastrophes and those without. Sensitivity and specificity was calculated for the PF-plasma difference. In this series, a peritoneal minus plasma lactic acid difference greater than 1.5 mmol/L predicted the presence of acute intra-abdominal pathology. Smaller differences suggested the absence of those conditions [17].

Walsh published *(Abstract Form)* a series of critically ill patients in which DPL was performed before laparoscopy and laboratory and laparoscopic findings were later corre-

lated. A positive DPL was defined as having greater than 200 WBC cell/mm³. No negative laparoscopy was positive by lavage. Eight patients underwent laparoscopy for diagnosis of intra-abdominal catastrophes. Four were found to have positive findings including 2 patients with ischemic bowel, one with perforated diverticulitis and one with thickened terminal ileum suggestive of inflammatory bowel disease. Ventilatory parameters changed during laparoscopy with an average increase of 9 mm Hg in Peak Airway (1 to 23). No hemodynamic changes were seen in mean arterial pressure, central venous pressure or pulmonary capillary wedge pressure. A similar publication reporting on the use of DPL included 7 patients, 4 with severe burns, 2 with respiratory failure and one patient with a drug overdose. Positive DPL was defined as WBC count greater than 500 cells/mm³. Three patients had positive lavage and were found to have necrotic bowel at the time of laparotomy. The other four patients with negative DPL showed no evidence of intra-abdominal infection at laparotomy. Thus peritoneal lavage proved accurate in every case.

The role of intra-abdominal infection as a possible initiator or perpetuator of organ failure requires a sensitive and accurate diagnostic algorithm for intra-abdominal sepsis. DPL offers a safe, practical, and inexpensive technique [18,19].

3.2. Diagnostic Laparoscopy in the ICU

Undoubtedly, general surgeons have become familiar with laparoscopic procedures. All residency programs are graduating residents whose laparoscopic experience initiated during their elective surgical rotation as medical students [14]. The advances in techniques and the progression and evolution of the surgical literature has faster than ever placed what was considered a "new" procedure in general surgery as a landmark of today's surgical practice. However, a cursory look at history indicates that the role of laparoscopy and more specifically diagnostic laparoscopy was recognized many years ago by physicians like John C. Ruddock, an internist who introduced the "Ruddock peritoneoscope" and completed more than 5000 laparoscopies by 1957 [20]. Despite Ruddock's contributions, the value of minimally invasive procedure as part of routine diagnostic algorithms in septic ICU patients has not been clearly defined. This chapter will summarize the experience published in the recent years. Special attention will be given to information relating to the sensitivity and safety of these procedures.

Bender et al in 1992 published a study of the use of laparoscopy in the ICU [21]. He presented 7 patients in which laparoscopy was performed for diagnostic purposes. Two of these procedures where performed in the ICU. Patients were admitted to the ICU for management of myocardial infarction, severe pneumonia, Gram negative sepsis, severe burn and post-operative care for coronary bypass. Mechanical ventilation was used in 6.7 patients, 2 had abdominal pain and 5 had unexplained sepsis. Most patients required general anesthesia, however, four cases were carnied out under IV sedation (midazolam) and Pavulon. Pneumoperitoneum was created with CO2 to a pressure of 10 mm H20. Two patients required 15 mm H20 to complete. Five patients had positive findings, acalculous cholecystitis occurred in two, gangrenous colon was seen in two patients and one had severe cirrhosis with ischemic liver. Two patients had normal laparoscopy. Although this is a small group of

patients and the mortality was high (5/7), the authors conclude that laparoscopy was safe, no hemodynamics or respiratory complications occurred during the procedure and no diagnoses were missed.

Brandt in 1993, reported on 25 ICU patients who underwent diagnostic laparoscopy to evaluate a suspected acute intraabdominal process [22]. The overall accuracy of laparoscopy was 96% as confirmed by subsequent laparotomy autopsy or clinical course. Non-therapeutic laparotomy was avoided in five patients and early diagnosis and laparotomy was done in 4 patients. There were no hemodynamic effects and the procedure related morbidity as 8%. The authors concluded that laparoscopy is safe, may help in avoiding non-therapeutic laparotom, and confirm the need for early operative intervention.

3.3. Role of ICU Laparoscopy in Acalculous cholecystitis (ACC)

Acute inflammation of the GB in the absence of gallstones has long been recognized as a source of intra-abdominal sepsis in the critically ill patient [10,11,12,23,24]. The incidence has been calculated between 5% to 18%, depending on the type of ICU studied [25,26]. The incidence of ACC is higher in patient, on TPN as well as in patients receiving high doses of narcotics [12,27]. Ultrasound is the most common diagnostic modality. Classical sonographic findings described include biliary sludge, hydrops, GB wall thickening, and pericholecystic fluid collections. These findings are usually described after 7 to 12 days of ICU admission and may or may not be associated with systemic signs of infection such as fever leukocytosis and right upper quadrant pain. Sonographic findings are often non-specific [28,29]. The examination is operator dependent and findings such as the sonographic Murphy sign may not always be elicited in comatose patients [30,22]. Diagnosis can be difficult with an estimated rate of failure of ultrasound close to 42%. Mortality may be as high as 50% [31]. CT of the abdomen has also been suggested as a diagnostic tool for ACC [12]. ACC has also been described following cardiac surgery with a mortality rate of 32% [23]. In this series, gangrene and perforation was seen in 87% of patients in whom surgery was delayed. Laparoscopic cholecystectomy appears to be well tolerated in patients with severe cardiac dysfunction [24]. The difficulties in accurately diagnosing AC, as well as, the lack of consensus on the indications for cholecystostomy versus cholecystectomy suggest that laparoscopy might play a definitive role in the management algorithm of ICU patients with possible AC.

Shapiro emphasizes that early diagnosis with rapid intervention is crucial in managing this disease if the outcome is to be improved [32]. Establishing the presence of gangrene and/or necrosis of the gallbladder, which occurred in close to 59% of patients, suggests that cholecystectomy may be the best approach to management. The diagnostic pitfalls of AC, as well as, the role of ultrasound and scintigraphy will be discussed in this chapter. A review of the available series on laparoscopic approach to AC in the ICU patient will also be presented.

3.4. Ultrasound as a screening tool in the ICU

The diagnostic findings for ACC using ultrasound include the presence of hydrops, biliary sludge, and wall thickening. However, several factors common to a number of ICU patients such as fasting, sedation, parenteral nutrition, high doses of narcotics and mechanical ventilation may induce gallbladder stasis and lead to changes in the gallbladder that do not necessarily require cholecystostomy or cholecystectomy [29]. A study using routine right upper quadrant ultrasound reported on the *prevalent* findings of gallbladder abnormalities in 28 medical ICU patients [28]. Three of the main diagnostic criteria used for ACC were evaluated in these patients. Seventeen (61%) patients were found to have abnormal GB. None of these patients required surgical intervention during the study because of GB disease. Gallstones were seen in 5 patients. None of them were symptomatic before admission to the ICU. In an attempt to better differentiate between patients with an abnormal GB and patients with AC a scoring system has been proposed [29]. In this study, a scoring system based on longitudinal and transversal diameter, wall thickening, contents, and pericholecystic fluid was developed. The score ranges from 0 to 8. The US findings were correlated with clinical findings as well as histology at cholecystectomy or autopsy. Of 77 US follow up examinations carriet out on 21 patients, GB distention was identified in 19 patients, wall thickening in 18, sludge in 15, striated thickening of the GB in 13 and pericholecystic fluid in 12. Of these, 41 (53%) examinations were scored > or = 6 and 36 (47%) examinations < or = 5. None of the patients (8) with a maximum score of 5 developed AC or died from GB complications. Of the 11 patients with a score > 6, 4 went on to develop histopathologic proven AC. Four patients survived with normalization of GB morphology. One patient had a normal GB at autopsy and 2 could not be confirmed surgically or pathologically.

Although this is an interesting study, it does not obviate the variability of the scoring system when performed by different radiologists or other examiners with non-comparable experience.

3.5. Cholescintigraphy in the critically ill

Radionuclide cholescintigraphy (RC) has been proposed as an adjunctive diagnostic tool for the identification of AC [44]. The studies available showed controversial results. Some series indicate that the use of morphine-augmented RC (MRC) may help to reduce the rates of false positive results characteristically found in critically ill patients [34,35]. However, Fig et al, indicated that MRC must be used with caution in the critically ill. A 40% rate of false positive diagnosis of AC was reported in this study [36]. These findings contrast with those reported by Flancbaum, in which a positive predictive value of 0.89 was described for MRC in this series. The rate of no visualization of the GB decreased from 40% to 5% with the use of morphine [33].

In summary, analysis of the literature suggests that non-visualization of the gallbladder on the delayed images of cholescintigraphy is a non-specific finding. Morphine augmentation has a reasonably good, though imperfect, specificity and positive predictive value that are significantly better than for delayed imaging in addition to its logistical advantage (shortening the imaging time). Sincalide cholecystokinin (CCK) pretreatment, when administered at the physiologic rate, is helpful in conditions in which functional resistance to tracer flow into the gallbladder are present [34]. The critical care physician should be aware that certain conditions and medications may affect gallbladder contraction. Failure to recognize such effects can lead to incorrect interpretations.

3.6. Laparoscopy experience

Brandt again reported on ten trauma patients with suspected ACC [37]. Four procedures were considered positive and 5 negative and there was no procedure related morbidity. Accuracy was 100% and laparoscopy was proposed as the definitive diagnostic intervention for ACC in critically ill patients.

A subsequent series presented in 1995 also reported on the use of laparoscopy for the diagnosis of acalculous cholecystitis [38]. Ten critically ill patients were entered in the study. Nine of the patients were trauma victims. All patients were on ventilatory support, the laparoscopy was carried out after a mean of 15 days after ICU admission. Six laparoscopies were done in the ICU and 4 in the operating room. No complications were reported. Two patients were found to have gangrenous cholecystitis and underwent laparoscopic cholecystectomies in the OR. These authors had similar conclusions regarding the safety and accuracy of the procedure, specifically for the evaluation of patients with risk factors for acalculous cholecystitis.

3.7. Role of cholecystostomy

Despite the widespread use of percutaneous cholecystostomy as an acceptable method for the treatment of AC in critically ill patients, specific criteria regarding indications for cholecystostomy have not been agreed upon. The use of PCC as a "trial" for ICU patients with persistent unexplained sepsis was proposed by Lee 1991 [39]. Persistent high fevers were present in all patients, elevated WBC count was present in 18 patients, vague abdominal tenderness in 11 and septic shock requiring vasopressors in 15. Sonographically, all patients had distended, spherical gallbladders, six had gallstones, eight had wall thickening, three had pericholecystic fluid and four had Murphy's sign. All patients were seen by a general surgeon, who agreed to a trial of percutaneous cholecystostomy. Fourteen patients (58%) responded to percutaneous cholecystostomy, as evidenced by a decrease in WBC count, defervescence and the ability to be weaned off vasopressors. Bile cultures were positive in four patients. Ten patients (42%) did not respond to percutaneous cholecystostomy; five eventually died of unrelated causes. A respiratory source of infection was eventually found in three of these 10 patients, with no proved source of infection in the remainder. No complications related to catheter insertion occurred in this group of patients. Bile leaks occurred in two patients when the percutaneous cholecystostomy catheter was removed, but without serious consequence. The author concluded that a lower threshold for performing percutaneous cholecystostomy in this difficult clinical subset of patients is worthwhile.

Browning reported in 49 patients with sepsis [40]. The PCC was performed under us guidance and carried out on 40 patients at bedside. The mortality in this group of patients was high (51%). However, 31 of 49 (63%) improved after PCC based on absence of fever, normalization of white count and resolution of abdominal pain within 72 hours after the procedure. Complication rate was 12% including catheter dislodgment, hematoma and severe pain. The efficacy of PCC was further evaluated in 82 ICU patients. All patients were febrile. Sonographic findings were not helpful in predicting response to percutaneous cholecystostomy. Improvement in clinical condition was observed in 48 patients (59%) within 48 hrs. No clinical response was observed in 34

patients (41%). No complications related to catheter insertion occurred.

The suspected source of sepsis. A response rate to percutaneous cholecystostomy of 59% was seen in this study.

The efficacy of PCC was retrospectively evaluated in 33 critically ill patients (mean age 52, range 5-87) univariant analysis was performed to identify which patients might benefit from PCC. No major complications were reported in this series. Failure to improve within 24 hours was associated with increased mortality (P = 0.02). A total of 22/33 patients improved, 17/33 survived, and 8/33 required surgery. PC delayed definitive operation in two patients. Cholelithiasis was associated with surgical intervention (P = 0.01) but not increased mortality. Predictors of improvement included gallbladder non-visualization on hepatobiliary scan (P = 0.047), positive bile cultures (P = 0.017) and initial drainage of greater than 100 cc (P = 0.009). Age, laboratory data, the use of total parenteral nutrition and intubation did not predict outcome. Nine positive bile cultures prompted antibiotic changes in five cases. Finally, PC was less expensive than open cholecystostomy ($1620 versus $3155). The authors proposed that PCC is a safe, cost-effective, minimally invasive procedure that has diagnostic and therapeutic value in critically ill patients with acute cholecystitis. The involvement of a general surgeon is important to ensure that those patients who do not improve within 24 hours receive early surgical intervention and provide long-term definitive care for those patients with cholelithiasis [41] . In an attempt to identify clinical or radiologic features predictive of response to PCC, a retrospective review of 66 PCC was recently published [42]. A response to percutaneous cholecystostomy was defined as an improvement in clinical symptoms and signs of or a reduction in fever and WBC to normal within 72 hours of percutaneous cholecystostomy. The presence of gallstones, gallbladder wall thickening, distention and pericholecystic fluid was recorded. The clinical and radiologic findings were analyzed for their relationship in response to percutaneous cholecystostomy. Thirty-one patients had gallstones. Thirty-one patients were in the intensive care unit and 15 were ventilated. Complications occurred in six (10%) including misplacement of the percutaneous cholecystostomy catheter in the colon (one), exacerbation of sepsis (three) and bile leakage (two). The mortality rate was 2%. Forty-three patients (73%) responded to PCC. Patients with gallstones and symptoms and signs localized to the right upper quadrant of the abdomen were more likely to respond (P = .006). The only individual radiologic feature predictive of a positive response was the presence of pericholecystic fluid in patients with gallstones (P = .03). The presence of all four radiologic findings was also associated with a positive response (P = .039). The results of bile cultures were not predictive of response. Of the 16 non-responder, six had documented biliary sepsis and cholecystitis. It is likely that a comparative study in which correlation between sonographic findings and laparoscopic findings will definitely aid in identifying those patients with a higher likelihood of positive response to PCC. Unfortunately, such a trial is not available.

med gallbladder. The gallbladder was decompressed with a trocar inserted in the fundus. Subsequently, a 16 French Foley catheter was inserted and secured with an Endoloop by tightening the loop around a cuff of GB. Sepsis resolved in all six patients and only one required cholecystectomy [31]. Several of these patients underwent laparoscopic placement of gastric or enteral feeding tubes at the same time of the cholecystostomy. The authors emphasize the diagnostic significance of demonstrating the omentum wrap around a distended gallbladder. This finding was exclusively seen in the inflamed gallbladders. Their recommendation is not to attempt a laparoscopic resection of the GB but proceed with drainage except in the case of necrotic GB in which immediate cholecystectomy must be carried out. Haicken published a similar report earlier on the use of tube cholecystostomy in 3 patients with gallstones cholecystitis [43]. In this study, patients scheduled for laparoscopic cholecystectomy who were suspected of having significant cholecystitis were given the option of performing a cholecystostomy. Although these were not critically ill patients, it is interesting to review the technique as well as the proposed long term management of these patients. They were admitted for 48 hours and received intravenous antibiotics. Tube drainage was done for 4-6 weeks as outpatients. Interval laparoscopic cholecystectomy was performed successfully in all three patients.

3.8. Laparoscopic Cholecystostomy

The use of laparoscopic cholecystostomy has been reported in six trauma ICU patients. The diagnosis was confirmed during laparoscopy based on the presence of an omentum drawn up over a distended/infla-

3.9. Proposed Role For Laparoscopy: "Present And Future"

The role of diagnostic and therapeutic laparoscopy for critically ill patients is summarized in the algorithm (Figure 1). The majority of acute ill patients may give equivocal

Figure 1

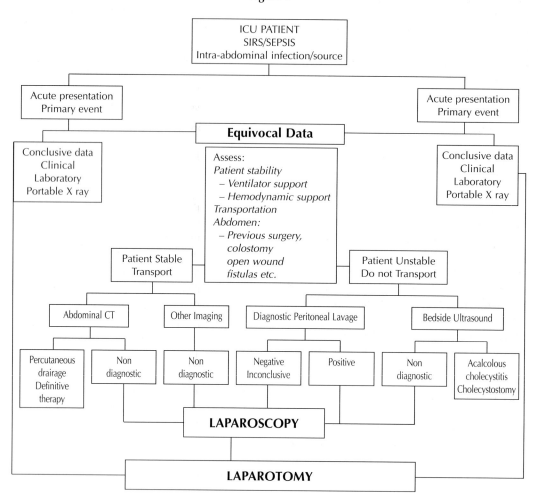

or inconclusive data placing themselves in the central area of the flow chart. The physician will assess the patient guided by questions related to hemodynamic and ventilatory support. What kind of ventilator mode does the patient require? Is there a requirement for high peep and/or Pressure control ventilation? Is the pulmonary compliance changing? How does the patient tolerate changes in position? Is the patient dependent on inotropic support?, etc. This type of assessment will aid in deciding the risk and benefits of sending the patient to the radiology suite. It is also important to establish whether the patient is a good candidate for laparoscopy. The presence of open wounds, fistulas, ostomies, etc., may preclude the use of standard laparoscopy. It is possible however, that new technology in the area of optics and scopes may permit limited visualization of certain anatomical compartments using micro laparoscopic devices, however, the value of such interventions remain to be investigated. The role of diagnostic peritoneal lavage remains unclear. There is no sufficient data in the literature to accurately determine the sensitivity and specificity of the test. However, the combined use of DPL and laparoscopy may minimize the number of false positive and false negative results.

To establish a definitive role for laparoscopy in the algorithm of diagnosis of occult intra-abdominal infections will require further clinical trials with systematic protocols comparing other diagnostic techniques with laparoscopy and stratifying patients according to type of intra-abdominal infection and severity of illness. Nonetheless, laparoscopy continues to be a valuable and safe technique that used appropriately can facilitate early diagnosis of intra-abdominal catastrophes and minimize the incidence of non-therapeutic laparotomy in the ICU.

REFERENCES

1. Aranha, G.V., Boone-Goldberg, N. Surgical problems on ventilators. Crit Car Med, 1981. 9(6) (June): p. 478-480.

2. Merrell, R.C. The abdomen as source of sepsis in critically ill patients. Crit Care Clin, 1995. 11(2) (Apr): p. 255-272.

3. Sinanan, M., Maier, R.V., Carrico, C.J. Laparotomy for intra-abdominal sepsis in patients in an intensive care unit. Arch Surg, 1984. 119(6)(Jun): p. 652-658.

4. Hamilton, S.M. Mead Johnson Critical Care Symposium for the Practicing Surgeon. 3. Monitoring and investigation of intra-abdominal sepsis. Can J Surg, 1988.31(5)(Sep): p. 327-330.

5. Buunt, T.J. Non-directed laparotomy of intra-abdominal sepsis. A futile procedure. Am Surg, 1986. 52(6)(June): p. 294-298.

6. Anderson, I.D., Fearon, K.C., Grant, I.S. Laparotomy for abdominal sepsis in the critically ill. Br J Surg, 1996. 83(4)(Apr): p. 535.539.

7. Ferraris, V.A. Exploratory laparotomy for potential abdominal sepsis in patients with multiple-organ failure. Arch Surg, 1983. 118(10)(Oct): p. 1130-1133.

8. McCrory, C., Crowley, K. Is repeat laparotomy of value in patients with suspected intra-abdominal sepsis in the intensive care unit? Ir J Med Sci, 1997. 166(2)(Apr): p. 88-91.

9. Renz, B., Feliciano, D.V. The length of hospital stay after an unnecessary laparotomy for trauma: a prospective study. J Trauma, 1996. 40(2)(Feb): p. 187-190.

10. Long, T.N., Helmbach, D.M., Carrico, C.J. Acalculous Cholecystitis in Critically Ill Patients. Amer J Surg, 1978. 136(July): p. 31-35.

11. Savino, J.M., Scalea, T.M., Del Guercio, L.R. Factors encouraging laparotomy in acalculous cholecystitis. Crit Care Med, 1985. 13(5)(May): p. 377-380.

12. Cornwell, E., ed, Rodriguez, A., Mirvis, S.E., Shorr, R.M. Acute acalculous cholecystitis in critically injured patients. Preoperative diagnostic imaging. Ann Surg, 1989. 210(1)(Jul): p. 52-55.

13. Geis, W., Kim, H.C. Use of laparoscopy in the diagnosis and treatment of patients with surgical abdominal sepsis. Surg Endosc, 1995. 9(2)(Feb): p. 178-182.

14. Lekawa, M., Shapiro, S.J., Gordon, L.A., Rothbart, J., Hiatt, J.R. The laparoscopic learning curve. Surg Laparosc Endosc, 1995. 5(6)(Dec): p. 455-458.

15. Bailey, R.L., Laws, H.L. Diagnostic peritoneal lavage in evaluation of acute abdominal disease. South Med J, 1990. 83(4)(Apr): p. 4220-424.

16. Moretz, W., Erickson, W.G. The diagnostic peritoneal tap. Am Surg, 1956. 22: p. 1095-107.

17. DeLaurier, G.A., Ivey, R.K., Johnson, R.H. Peritoneal fluid lactic acid and diagnostic dilemmas in acute abdominal disease. Amer J Surg, 1994. 167(March): p. 302-305.

18. Richardson, J.D., Flint, L.M., Polk, H.C. Peritoneal lavage: A useful diagnostic adjunct for peritonitis. Surg, 1983. 94(November): p. 826-829.

19. Larson, F.A., Haller, C.C., Romano, D., James, H.T. Diagnostic peritoneal lavage in acute peritonitis. 1992. 164(Nov): p. 449-452.

20. Morgenstern, L. No surgeon he: John C. Ruddock, M.D., FACP, pioneer in laparoscopy. Surg Endosc, 1996. 10: p. 617-618.

21. Bender, J.S., Talamini, M.A. Diagnostic laparoscopy in critically ill intensive-care-unit patients. Surg Endosc, 1992. 6(6)(Nov): p. 302-304.

22. Brandt, C.P., Priebe, P.P., Eckhauser, M.L. Diagnostic laparoscopy in the intensive care patients. Avoiding the nontherapeutic laparotomy. Surg Endosc, 1993. 7(3)(May): p. 168-172.

23. Sessions, S., Scoma, R.S., Sheikh, F.A., McGeehin, W.H., Smink, R.D., Jr. Acute acalculous cholecystitis following open heart surgery. Am Surg, 1993. 59(2)(Feb): p. 74-77.

24. Carroll, B., Chandra, M., Phillips, E.H., Margulies, D.R. Laparoscopic cholecystectomy in critically ill cardiac patients. Am Surg, 1993. 59(12)(Dec): p. 783-785.

25. Romero Ganuza, F., LaBanda, G., Montalvo, R., Mazaira, J. Acute acalculous cholecystitis in patients with acute traumatic spinal cord injury. Spinal Cord, 1997. 35(2)(Feb): p. 124-128.

26. Hiatt, J., Kobayashi, M.R., Doty, J.E., Ramming, K.P. Acalculous candida cholecystitis: a complication of critical surgical illness. Am Surg, 1991. 57(12)(Dec): p. 825-829.

27. Raunest, J., Imhof, M., Rauen, U., Ohmann, C., Thou, K.P., Burrig, K.F. Acute cholecystitis: a complication in severely injured intensive care patients. J Trauma, 1992. 32(4)(Apr): p. 433-440.

28. Molenat, F., Boussuges, A., Valantin, V., Sainty, J.M. Gallbladder abnormalities in medical ICU patients: an ultrasonographic study. Intensive Care Med, 1996. 22(4)(Apr): p. 356-358.

29. Helbich, T., Mallek, R., Madl, C., Wunderbaldinger, P., Breitenseher, M., Rscholakoff, D., Mostbeck, G.H. Sonomorphology of the gallbladder in critically ill patients. Value of a scoring system and follow-up examinations. Acta Radiol, 1997. 38(1)(Jan): p. 129-134.

30. MacGahan, J., Lindfors, K.K. Acute cholecystitis: diagnostic accuracy of percutaneous aspiration of the gallbladder. Radiology, 1988. 167(3)(Jun): p. 669-671.

31. Yang, H.K., Hodgson, W.J.B. Laparoscopic cholecystostomy for acute acalculous cholecystitis. Surg Endo, 1996. 10: p. 673-675.

32. Shapiro, M., Luchtefeld, W.B., Kurzweil, S., Kaminski, D.L., Durham, R.M., Mazuski, J.E. Acute acalculous cholecystitis in the critically ill. Am Surg, 1994. 60(5)(May): p. 335-339.

33. Flancbaum, L., Wilson, G.A., Choban, P.S. The significance of a positive test of morphine cholesinitigraphy in hospitalized patients. Surg Gynecol Obstet, 1993. 177(3)(Sep): p. 227-230.

34. Kim, C. Pharmacologic intervention for the diagnosis of acute cholecystitis: cholecystokinin pretreatment of morphine, or both? J Nucl Med, 1997. 38(4)(Apr): p. 647-649.

35. Flancbaum, L., Alden, S.M., Trooskin, S.Z. Use of cholesintigraphy with morphine in critically ill patients with suspected cholecystitis. Surgery, 1989. 106(4)(Oct): p. 668-673.

36. Fig, L., Wahl, R.L., Stewart, R.E., Shapiro, B. Morphine-augmented hepatobiliary scintigraphy in the severely ill: caution is in order. Radiology, 1990. 175(2)(May): p. 467-473.

37. Brandt, C.P., Priebe, P.P., Jacobs, D.G. Value of laparoscopy in trauma ICU patients with suspected acute acalculous cholecystitis. Surg Endosc, 1994. 8(5)(May): p. 361-364.

38. Almeida, J., Sleeman, D., Sosa, J.L., Puente, I., McKenney, M., Martin, L. Acalculous cholecystectomy: the use of diagnostic laparoscopy. J Laparoendosc Surg, 1995. 5(4)(Aug): p. 227-231.

39. Lee, M., Saini, S., Brink, J.A., Hahn, P.F., Simeone, J.F., Morrison, M.C., Rattner, D., Mueller, P.R. Treatment of critically ill patients wih sepsis of unknown cause: value of percutaneous cholecystostomy. AJR Am J Roentgenol, 1991. 156(6)(Jun): p. 1163-1166.

40. Browning, P., McGahan, J.P., Gerscovich, E.O. Percutaneous cholecystostomy for suspected acute cholecystitis in the hospitalized patient. J Vasc Interv Radiol, 1993. 4(4)(Jul): p. 531-537.

41. Hultman, C., Herbert, C.A., McCall, J.M., Mauro, M.A. The efficacy of percutaneous cholecystostomy in critically ill patients. Am Surg, 1996. 62(4)(Apr): p. 263-269.

42. England, R., McDermott, V.G., Smith, T.P., Suhocki, P.V., Payne, C.S., Newman, G.E. Percutaneous cholecystostomy: who responds? AJR Am J Roentgenol, 1997. 168(5)(May): p. 1247-1251.

43. Haicken, B.N. Laparoscopic tube cholecystostomy. Surg Endo, 1992. 6: p. 285-288.

44. Garner, W., Marx, MV, Fabri, PJ. Cholescintigraphy in the critically ill. Am J Surg, 1988. 155(6)(Jun): p. 727-729.

Monitoring Intra-abdominal Infection

Harry van Goor and R. Jan A. Goris

INTRODUCTION

Despite recent advances in diagnosis and treatment, mortality from several forms of intra-abdominal infection remains high. For example, patients with large bowel perforation, anastomotic leakage and pancreatic necrosis have mortality rates, varying from 20% to 60% (Mc Lauchlan et al 1995). Despite aggressive eradication of the primary source of infection by surgery and appropriate powerful antibiotics, followed by planned relaparotomies, eventually some of these patients suffer from persistent or recurrent intra-abdominal infection and eventually die with multiple organ dysfunction syndrome (MODS)(Mc Lauchlan et al 1995, Bohnen et al 1983). Others may die from the same syndrome in the absence of recurrent intra-abdominal infection. It is not well understood why these patients die from an untoward local (intraperitoneal) and/or systemic reaction to the primary insult, rather than from the primary infection.

Awareness of the current shortcomings in the studying, monitoring and treating of severe intra-abdominal infection, has stimulated the search for new approaches. Recent studies have focused on the specific behaviour of micro-organisms in the abdominal cavity, on the peritoneal inflammatory response that bacteria and abdominal surgery themselves elicit, on the systemic response to severe intra-abdominal infection and on possible genetic factors predisposing to an accelerated systemic response.

1. THE LOCAL RESPONSE OF THE ABDOMINAL CAVITY TO INFECTION

After bacterial contamination of normal sterile peritoneal tissue, a complex series of events is initiated by the host in order to eradicate invading bacteria. These local defense mechanisms are: mechanical clearance of fluid and bacteria via the diaphragmatic lymphatics (Autio 1964, Zinsser et al 1952), phagocytosis and destruction by phagocytic cells (Marchesi 1961, Hau 1979) and sequestration of bacteria by fibrin (Zinsser et al 1952, Hau et al 1979a, Ahrenholz et al 1980, Dunn et al 1982).

These defense mechanisms, in conjunction with surgery and antibiotics, are capable of sterilizing the peritoneal cavity and halting peritoneal inflammatory response in the majority of intra-abdominal infections. In some cases of severe intra-abdominal infection peritoneal defense mechanisms fail and infection will spread throughout the abdominal cavity. In other cases, intra-abdominal infection is cured but intra-abdominal inflammation persists. Such a condition may be accompanied by systemic inflammation representing 'tertiary peritonitis', a term coined to describe the condition of a subgroup of patients who develop MODS and die despite 'successful initial local host defense' and 'successful' operation and antibiotic and supportive therapy (Marshall et al 1988, Rotstein et al 1986a).

Failure of peritoneal defense mechanisms to control infection is caused by at least six interacting mechanisms.

(1) Large amounts of protein-rich exudate into the abdominal cavity impairs bacterial opsonization by diluting opsonins and reducing the ability of phagocytic cells to reach and phagocytose bacteria (Dunn et al 1984).

(2) Impairment of peritoneal immunological defense by dilution of chemotactic factors and opsonins, by adjuvant substances and by fibrin. Adjuvant substances, such as bile salts, gastrin mucin, faeces, necrotic tissue, blood components and foreign bodies inhibit migration and killing capacity of neutrophils and result in premature release of oxygen radicals by these cells (Hau et al 1978, Schneierson et al 1961, Zimmerli 1982, Rotstein et al 1986b). Fibrin inhibits phagocytic killing of *E. coli* by neutrophils and impedes macrophage migration (Rotstein et al 1986b, Ciano et al 1986).

(3) Adjuvant substances not only impair immunological defense mechanisms but promote bacterial growth. Haemoglobin, for example, enhances bacterial growth and increases bacterial virulence. In vitro addition of iron to a culture medium enhances growth of *E. coli* (Bullen 1981).

(4) In most intra-abdominal infections both anaerobic and aerobic infections bacterial synergism are present. Synergism between these bacteria attribute to the failure to control infection. The possible mechanisms of synergy are the ability of one species to provide growth nutrients for its bacterial partner, the ability of one species to impair host defenses, permitting its co-pathogen to survive and exerts it's intrinsic virulence and the ability of the species to optimize local environment, thereby enhancing bacterial proliferation (Rotstein et al 1987, Rotstein et al 1988a).

(5) Fibrin entraps bacteria and provides a protected environment, in which bacteria may proliferate almost unaffected by neutrophils and as has been mentioned above, also impairs neutrophil function (Rotstein et al 1986b).

(6) Bacterial translocation from the bowel lumen to the peritoneal cavity may provide for an extra source of intra-peritoneal bacteria. Though this phenomenon has been extensively documented experimentally and clinically under various circumstances, its clinical relevance remains unclear (Nieuwenhuijzen et al 1996, Lemaire et al 1997). For example, in an experimental model of zymosan-induced peritonitis, elimination of peritoneal macrophages significantly increased bacterial translocation but decreased mortality (Nieuwenhuijzen et al 1993).

Table 1
Parameters of coagulation and fibrinolysis in the peritoneal fluid of patients
with peritonitis (n=25) and control patients (n=7). Median values.

	peritonitis peritoneal fluid		control peritoneal fluid	peritonitis plasma		control plasma
tPA antigen	66	*	1	8		6
PAI-1 antigen	395	*	0,5	15		14
uPA antigen	740	*	78	204	*	120
TAT	5500	*	89	5		3
PAP	10952	*	57	709		381
FbDP	40360	*	126	1201	*	350
PAP	10952	*	57	709		381

* $p < 0,05$ peritonitis versus controls

The impairment of neutrophil function due to bacteria, fibrin and adjuvant substances, includes premature extracellular release of neutrophil enzymes. These enzymes are capable of damaging viable tissue resulting in necrosis (Rudek et al 1976). In necrotic tissue, characterized by hypoxia and a low pH, neutrophil function is further impaired and bacterial growth is stimulated (Klempner et al 1983, Raju et al 1976, Rotstein et al 1988b, Hohn et al 1976, Knighton et al 1984). Tissue necrosis, fibrin and bacteria augment the severity of the peritoneal inflammatory process with a continuous influx of neutrophils, macrophages, local release of (pro)-inflammatory cytokines and exudation of fibrin-rich fluid. This process may readily become self-perpetuating, even in the absence of bacteria. Then, intra-abdominal infection is 'cured' but an uncontrolled peritoneal inflammation persists.

We seem to be unable to predict in which patients intra-abdominal infection will be cured by appropriate surgery and local inflammation is well controlled, or in which infection is controlled but inflammation persists, or in which both intra-abdominal infection and inflammation will persist. Proper monitoring of local peritoneal infection and/or inflammation is a prerequisite to distinguish between such patients. These peritoneal processes have thus far seldom been investigated. The peritoneal adherence of micro-organisms, the peritoneal immunological host responses and the coagulation and fibrinolytic responses in the peritoneal cavity will be discussed in more detail in the following paragraphs.

1.1. Adherence and invasion of micro-organisms in the peritoneum

Little is known on the adherence to and the invasion of bacteria in the peritoneum during intra-abdominal infection. Bacterial adherence is predominantly investigated in relation to prostheses. Many bacteria are capable of generating a fibrous exopolysaccharide glycocalyx (slime capsule) that allows them to adhere to prosthetic surfaces and grow on them (Gristina et al 1984). Presumably this slime production may be turned on and off randomly: organisms with active slime production colonize the surface whereas non-producer cells (so-called swarmer cells) may migrate away from the colony to generate invasive infection (Mills et al 1984). Production of the glycocalyx appears to protect bacteria from the local host defense in several ways, including inhibition of neutrophil phagocytosis and chemotaxis, suppression of mononuclear cell lymphoproliferative response and reduction of antibiotic efficacy (Meddens et al 1984).

In vitro adherence of Staphylococci to mesothelial cells and the mesothelial extracellular matrix has been studied by Betjes et al (1992). Mesothelial cells were isolated from peritoneal dialysis effluents and cultured. The presence of an extracellular matrix was demonstrated 10 days post-confluency of mesothelial cells. The matrix contained fibronectin, laminin and vitronectin. Staphylococcus aureus adhered well to both mesothelial cells and the extracellular matrix, whereas and mesothelial extracellular matrix was a poor substrate for Staph. epidermidis. There was no increased risk for adherence of Staphylococci when the mesothelial extracellular matrix was exposed. This latter finding is important since in intra-abdominal infection the mesothelial cell layer has been damaged and has disintegrated, exposing the submesothelial connective tissue. In other studies, however, it has been shown that fibronectin and collagen layers promote adherence (Dougherty 1994).

The adherence of aerobic and anaerobic enteric bacteria, being the predominant bacteria causing intra-abdominal infection, has not extensively been studied. In a

rat study of bacterial peritonitis, Edminston et al. demonstrated adherence to and invasion of various aerobic and anaerobic species in the serosal mesothelium (Edminston et al 1990). The majority of bacteria in the mesothelium appeared to be resistant to abdominal lavage with saline, whereas bacterial concentration in the peritoneal fluid was significantly reduced. Antimicrobial lavage (cephazolin, kanamycin, metronidazole) initially lowered the bacterial concentration in mesothelial tissue but after 48 hours mesothelial microbial recovery was equal to or preceded prelavage values. Currently a similar study in humans is being performed in our department and preliminary data reveal the same results as those of Edminston et al. Thus, the finding of negative peritoneal fluid cultures does not imply that local infection has subsided.

Visser et al. examined whether mesothelial cells can ingest and digest bacteria (Visser et al 1996). They showed that Staphylococcus aureus and epidermidis, and E. coli strains were ingested. In contrast to staphylococci, E. coli was digested early after incubation, whereafter the mesothelial cells disintegrated and bacteria proliferated. These findings indicate that ingestion of bacteria by the cells lining the abdominal cavity may maintain intra-abdominal infection.

So far, no antiadhesive agents directed against bacterial adherence are developed. One might think of covering the mesothelial layer with various surface proteins to prevent bacterial adherence. For example, albumin coating of a prothesis reduces bacterial adherence (Dougherty et al 1982). Another point of impact might be modulation or blocking the slime production of bacteria.

1.2. The local immunological host responses

As aforementioned, local host defense mechanisms to bacterial invasion in the abdominal cavity are complex, involving both stimulating and blocking local immunological response.

Restoration of immunological host defense, which is impaired in intra-abdominal infection, for example 1. by supplementation of intact opsonins and immunoglobulins, 2. by administration of granulocyte colony stimulating factor (G-CSF), 3. by neutralizing free oxygen radicals, 4. by increasing intra-abdominal pH or 5. by modulating cytokines, which would improve bacterial elimination.

1. In a prospective randomized trial of 30 patients with intra-abdominal infection, of whom 15 received one unit of fresh frozen blood compatible donorserum intra-abdominally, it was demonstrated that opsonin function was enhanced leading to increased bacterial elimination. The treatment group showed more improvement during follow-up as measured by the APACHE II score and mortality was lower (33%) compared to the controls (53%) (Billing et al 1994).

2. Improved availability and function of granulocytes is another approach to restore immunological defense. G-CSF is a nonglycosylated protein that stimulates bone marrow stem cell differentiation and acts on differentiated granulocytes and macrophages to enhance phagocytosis and the killing of bacteria. In several animal models the effect of G-CSF has been demonstrated, although emphasis has been put on white blood cells and not on peritoneal leucocytes (Bauhofer et al 1995, Weitzel et al 1994a, Weitzel et al 1994b). It has recently been demonstrated that the effect of G-CSF is en-

hanced when administered directly at the site of a subsequent intraperitoneal infective challenge (Molloy et al 1995).

In a dog model of severe acute pancreatitis, Rao and associates showed that G-CSF significantly increased the white blood cell count, mature polymorphonuclear leucocytes in particular, thereby decreasing the rate of distant infection (Rao et al 1996). However, peritoneal leucocytes were not assessed and an effect on translocation of bacteria to the local inflammatory process was not found.

Treatment with G-CSF of patients with intra-abdominal infection has rarely been carried out (Lorenz et al 1994). Currently there is more interest in prophylaxis of intra-abdominal infection after surgery with G-CSF. Administration of restorative proctomucosectomy G-CSF was seen to cause a great reduction of inflammation in the abdominal cavity at planned relaparotomy in a case report of leukopenic sepsis (Reimund et al 1995). Unfortunately, in this patient blood leucocyte counts and several serum cytokines were monitored and not the peritoneal cells and cytokines.

3. Installation of free oxygen radical scavengers to counteract the deleterious effects of premature release of granulocytes may be useful. Continuous sampling of peritoneal fluid in patients with peritonitis for determination of peroxidation of haemoglobin, revealed an increased production of reactive oxygen intermediates early after laparotomy. This increase correlated with the clinical picture, as a secondary increase correlated with a poor outcome (Heinzelmann et al 1997).

4. During intra-abdominal infection peritoneal pH is decreased (Klempner et al 1993,

Raju et al 1976). In such an environment of low pH, phagocyte function is impaired, bacterial growth is stimulated and various toxic cascades are activated. Restoration of normal pH, which might be achieved by intra-abdominal instillation of bicarbonate, is likely to improve immunological defense and to stop these toxic cascades. Imhof et al. achieved restoration of normal pH after intra-abdominal lavage with sodium bicarbonate (pH 8) in experimental peritonitis (Imhof et al 1987). Furthermore, they demonstrated reduction of leucocyte migration, a diminished premature release of lysosomal enzymes in the abdominal cavity and reduced peritoneal permeability after lavage with bicarbonate in comparison with control rats and rats treated with normal saline. In vitro studies using human neutrophil and mesothelial cells, showed better preserved intracellular ATP content, enhancement of phagocytosis and IL-6 production after exposure of the cells with bicarbonate buffered dialysis solution (pH 7.2) in comparison with lactate buffered solution (pH 5.5) (Topley et al 1996).

5. In 'ongoing' intra-abdominal infection immunological response is established and most likely exaggerated with a continuing inflammatory process. Increased intra-abdominal levels of TNF-alpha, IL-1, IL-6, IL-8, neopterin and elastase associated with bacterial peritonitis and inflammation have been reported in several experimental and clinical studies (Holzheimer et al 1995). These levels were much higher than systemic levels, indicating a compartmentalized inflammatory process and suggesting that cytokines do not equilibrate between the abdominal cavity and the systemic circulation (Shein et al 1996). In vitro results of peritoneal and splenic macrophage cytokine production in experimental peritonitis support the concept of compartmentalized cy-

tokine production (Battafarano et al 1994, Jansen et al 1996) (Fig 1).

Increased plasma levels of cytokines in intra-abdominal infections are considered to be 'spillover' from the peritoneal cavity or produced systematically. This hypothesis of compartmentalization might explain the lack of success of systemic modulation of inflammation resulting from intra-abdominal infection (Stack et al 1995, Freeman et al 1995). Novel anticytokine strategies directed at the site of cytokine production e.g. the abdominal cavity, are probably more effective. Thus far, such a manner of modulating the peritoneal immunological host response has barely been investigated. Hence, it has been shown that a decrease of peritoneal TNF-alpha and elastase levels during planned relaparotomies is associated with increased patient survival after severe intra-abdominal infection (Holzheimer et al 1995).

1.3. Coagulation and fibrinolysis in the abdominal cavity

Fibrin in the abdominal cavity plays a pivotal role in residual intra-abdominal infection and inflammation. Fibrin walls off infection by incorporating bacteria in its matrix and by the creating a physical barrier against dissemination through formation of adhesions. Fibrin stimulates the inflammatory response by increasing vascular permeability and chemotaxis of neutrophils and monocytes. By these actions fibrin protects the host against early systemic spread of bacteria and subsequent death. An adverse effect of fibrin is the impairment of phagocyte function. Fibrin inhibits phagocyte migration and induces premature release of oxygen radicals by phagocytes. This may result in tissue ischemia and necrosis,

Figure 1a
Plasma levels of immunoreactive TNF-α at various time points after intraperitoneal administration of zymosan in mice.
C = values in controls

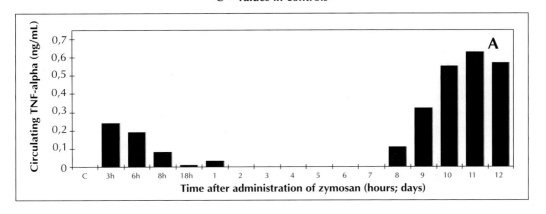

Figure 1b
TNF-α production by peritoneal macrophages. Comparison of LPS-stimulatd (open bars) and non-stimulated (closed bars) in vitro release of immunoreactive TNF-α by mouse peritoneal cells.
C = values in controls

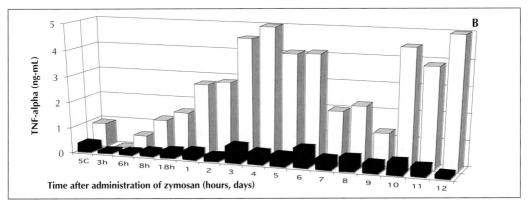

which in turn stimulates bacterial growth and the inflammatory process with continuing influx of phagocytes. This process may readily become self-perpetuating and may result in ongoing infection and/or inflammation.

Prevention of fibrin deposits may limit the inflammatory process and thereby contribute to more rapid recovery from intra-abdo-

minal infection. Both inhibition of intra-abdominal coagulation and stimulation of fibrinolysis has been investigated.

In experimental peritonitis, the fibrinolytic activity of the peritoneum is decreased (Hau 1979b). In the abdominal cavity of patients with bacterial peritonitis, both the coagulation system and the fibrinolytic system, including inhibitors of fibrinolysis, are stimulated, as shown by significantly elevated peritoneal fluid concentrations of thrombin-antithrombine III (TAT) complex, tissue-type plasminogen activator (tPA), urokinase-type plasminogen activator (uPA), plasminogen activator inhibitor (PAI), plasmin-∂_2-antiplasmin (PAP) complex, and fibrin degradation products (FbDP) (van Goor et al 1996)(Table 1). The resultant fibrin deposition probably reflects a relative deficit of fibrinolytic activity, due to strongly enhanced inhibition of plasminogen activators.

In this study it was also demonstrated that plasma levels of coagulation and fibrinolysis parameters were not elevated in peritonitis patients, except for a relatively small increase of uPA and FbDP (Table 1). The finding of predominantly normal plasma levels, as well as the absence of correlations between plasma and peritoneal levels, again suggests that the abdominal cavity with its surrounding peritoneum is a separate compartment.

Recently, an attempt has been made to inhibit intra-abdominal coagulation during infection in patients by intravenous administration of antithrombin-III (AT-III) combined with intraperitoneal installation of fresh frozen serum (Siebeck et al 1996). It appeared that the AT-III concentration in the peritoneal fluid was enhanced for several days after administration. However, preliminary results on morbidity and mortality were not different between control patients and patients treated with AT-III.

In several experimental studies, tissue plasminogen activator (tPA) has been used to enhanced intra-abdominal fibrinolytic activity in order to prevent intra-abdominal abscess formation and residual infection (van Goor et al 1994, Rotstein et al 1988c, McRitchie et al 1989).

Abscess formation could be successfully reduced by intraperitoneal administration of tPA. Bacteraemia as a side effect of the use of tPA during infection, could be treated by antibiotics (van Goor et al 1995). Thus far, no controlled human studies using tPA in the treatment of peritonitis have been carried out.

2. THE SYSTEMIC RESPONSE

In the last decade, much attention has been paid to the systemic inflammatory response to trauma, major surgery and peritonitis. This response results in life threatening complications such as ARDS, SIRS, MODS and sepsis. Although inflammation is intended to be a localized process, a systemic activation of inflammatory cells and a systemic spillover of inflammatory products and mediators may be expected in patients with peritonitis. In bacteraemia and endotoxemia such intravascular activation is logical.

2.1. Clinical monitoring

The "classical" method of clinical (pulse, blood pressure, physical examination of the abdomen etc.) and biochemical (blood gases, leucocyte count, etc.) monitoring of the peritonitis patient will not be discussed here. Specific scores for monitoring peritonitis patients are the Mannheim Peritonitis Index and Peritonitis Index Altona, based on pre- and intraoperative data (for review see Ohmann and Hau 1997). Other systems have been developed to monitor the severity of the systemic response in peritonitis-patients (for review see Nikken and Goris 1997). The first system described was the Acute Physiology and Chronic Health Evaluation (APACHE I)(Knaus et al 1981). It consisted of 34 physiological variables, each awarded a value between 0 and 4, depending on the severity of the disturbance. The sum of the worst value of each variable during the initial 24 hours after ICU admission yielded the Acute Physiology Score (APS). The complexity of the system led to the development of APACHE II, consisting of three components: 12 variables containing APS obtained within 24 hours of ICU admission, an age score and a chronic health score, assigning points to severe health problems already present before the actual illness. (Knaus et al 1985). APACHE II has been shown to predict hospital mortality (ROC = 0,85), to reliably quantify severity of disease. In 1991, APACHE III was introduced as a refinement of the prognostic abilities of APACHE II, with the aim of predicting the risk of death in individual patients (Knaus et al 1991). The "risk of death predictive equation" together with a computerized program, to be used in the APACHE III model, is the property of APACHE Medical Systems Inc. and is not released for general use. The reported ROC as to outcome was 0.90 versus 0.85 for APACHE II.

The Sepsis Severity Score was developed as a method to classify patients with sepsis, using easily obtainable data and tested in a population of 15 ICU patients (Elebute and Stoner 1983). The score uses a combination of physiological, anatomical and laboratory findings. Four groups of clinical features are defined : local effects of infection, pyrexia, secondary effects of sepsis and laboratory data. It appeared, however, that only the organ dysfunction and laboratory data correlated with outcome (Ponting et al 1987). The sepsis score has only been used in small studies and showed no predictive value in septic shock patients (Arregui et al 1991).

"Pure" organ dysfunction scores, not including age and/or previous diseases, are the

Sepsis Severity Score (SSS), the MOF score, the SOFA-score, the Legall-score and the MODS score (Marshall et al 1995). Only the first two scores will be discussed here. The SSS grades dysfunction in 7 organ systems with a value between 0 and 5 (Stevens et al 1983). The organ functions scored are the pulmonary, cardiovascular, renal, hepatic, haematological, gastro-intestinal and central nervous system. The SSS is calculated by summing the squares of the 3 highest values obtained, in analogy of the Injury Severity Score, yielding a maximum score of 75. The intensity of treatment, necessary to support the function of each organ system is incorporated in the weighting of severity. The authors tested the score in a population of 30 "septic" surgical patients. Several studies showed a good correlation of SSS with outcome and with length of ICU stay (Nerlich et al 1991, Roumen et al 1992a).

The MOF-score was introduced in 1985, based on the daily observation of 92 MODS patients, 37 with MODS from peritonitis, 55 with MODS after severe trauma, for a total data base of some 2500 ICU days (Goris et al 1985). The 'MOF score' grades severity of dysfunction (0 = not present, 1 = present, 2 = severe) in the same seven organ systems as the SSS (maximum score = 14). A MOF score of 5 or more indicates severe MOF (Roumen et al 1992a). In septic shock patients, the MOF score has been shown to be a better predictor of outcome than several other scores (Arregui et al 1991). Furthermore, the MOF score has been validated for patient populations with severe pancreatitis (Roumen et al 1992a), severe peritonitis (Ohmann et al 1997) and mixed surgical ICU-populations (The Nijmegen-Cologne Study Group). All studies available have shown a good correlation between the severity of organ failure and mortality.

From our work within the Nijmegen-Cologne Study Group, it became evident that actually two types of scores are necessary for peritonitis, depending on their purpose. The first one is a "pure" organ dysfunction score, reflecting only the severity of illness, especially MODS. By necessity, such an organ dysfunction score should have a reasonable correlation to outcome, though such correlation is not the primary purpose of such a score. The second type is a predictive score, which should additionally include a variety of prognostic factors such as age and pre-existing diseases.

2.2. The biochemical response

Excessive complement activation may lead to a generalized inflammatory reaction and organ injury (Mollnes and Fosse 1994). Elevated plasma levels of $C3_a$desArg have been found before the development of ARDS by several authors (Tennenberg et al 1987, Heideman et al 1988, Roumen et al 1993, 1995) but in most studies these elevated levels were only found during the first 24 to 48 hours. Elevated levels of the stable split product of C3, C3d, were predictive for MODS in one study (Nuytinck et al 1986). In patients with sepsis, elevated plasma levels of the cytolytic terminal complement complex were found, normalizing in successfully treated patients, or further increasing in patients developing ARDS.

In patients with SIRS, the relative contribution of endothelial cells in the process of PMN-endothelial adherence appears to be far more important than from activated PMN's (Chen and Christou 1996). In patients with peritonitis, skin biopsies from remote areas revealed substantial ELAM-1 expression (Engelberts et al 1992).

In ARDS patients, circulating pulmonary artery PMNs are activated as shown by increased CD11b/CD18 expression and increased hydrogen peroxide and superoxide production (Simms and D'Amico 1991). After major surgery, PMN adhesion is significantly increased (Morris et al 1985).

At the site of inflammation, PMNs release numerous active substances, such as proteolytic enzymes (e.g. elastase), toxic oxygen radicals, vasoactive substances (PAF, leukotrienes, PGE_2) and wound hormones (M-CSF, GM-CSF). The local concentrations of these substances are much higher than the plasma levels, while plasma levels may not reflect the local situation at all (van Goor et al 1996, Keel et al 1996, Jansen et al 1996). However, plasma levels may even not reflect the cytokine-output of circulating monocytes (Munoz et al 1991). Assessing the local production of these substances in clinical patients is limited to the sampling of BAL-fluid (Keel et al 1996) or peritoneal fluid in peritonitis patients (van Goor et al 1996). For all these reasons, interpreting the results of plasma-levels of pro-and anti-inflammatory substances should be performed with caution. Finally, measuring these substances as an index of PMN activity in clinical patients only recently has become clinically practicable, such as with elastase. A positive correlation between persistently elevated plasma elastase levels and the occurrence and severity of the systemic inflammatory response has consistently been found in various conditions (Duswald et al 1985, Nuytinck et al 1986, Waydhas et al 1992, Roumen et al 1995).

The involvement of free radicals in patients prone to ARDS and MOF is still poorly documented because of the difficulty of demonstrating the presence or effects of free radicals in vivo. Free radicals have an extremely short half-life and are rapidly inactivated by ubiquitous radical scavengers. On the other hand, human PMNs generate much higher concentrations of free radicals in response to inflammatory stimuli than bovine, ovine, and porcine PMNs (Young and Beswick 1986), possibly explaining why the human race is so sensitive to inflammatory stimuli. Malondialdehyde, a stable end-product of lipid-peroxidation, is elevated in pulmonary tissue of trauma patients dying of ARDS and sepsis/SIRS (Nerlich et al 1986). In patients with severe trauma or ruptured aortic aneurysm, plasma levels of lipofuscin –another product of lipid peroxidation– positively correlated with the incidence of ARDS and MODS (Roumen et al 1994). In another study, no elevated levels of malondiadehyde or conjugated dienes could be detected the first 6 hours after severe trauma (Girotti et al 1991).

Macrophages, as well as PMNs, exert their inflammatory activities locally. Monitoring macrophage activity thus requires measuring their cytokines (TNF-·, IL-1, IL-6) or metabolic products (e.g. neopterin). Again, caution is necessary as local production of these substances may not be reflected in the systemic circulation (Jansen et al 1996). In some studies, sustained high plasma TNF-· levels correlated well with severity of illness and mortality but not with positive blood cultures, endotoxin levels or subsequent septic shock (Offner et al 1990, Marks et al 1990, Meduri et al 1995). In other studies, plasma TNF-· levels were significantly higher in patients with ARDS than in patients at risk but without ARDS (Roten et al 1991, Roumen et al 1993). In two studies no relation to outcome was found (Calandra et al 1990, Hyers et al 1991). Therefore, at present the TNF data in this setting are confusing. A reason may be that soluble TNF-receptors have a variable effect on the ability

of the different TNF assay to detect TNF (Engelberts et al 1991a). A recent study, however, showed that the only independent predictor of death in critically ill patients was the presence of biologically active TNF (Friedland et al 1996). Furthermore, a positive correlation between outcome and elevated concentrations of soluble TNF-receptors or a decrease in cell surface TNF-receptor values has been demonstrated (Calvano et al 1996).

IL-1 probably acts merely as a local paracrine pro-inflammatory cytokine and no consistent correlations could be demonstrated between plasma IL-1 levels and severity or mortality of ARDS, SIRS or MODS (Roumen et al 1993, Blackwell and Christman 1996). In addition, recent data have shown that the presence of nonspecific immunoactivity in sera may confound IL-1 and other cytokine assays resulting in false positive serum activity (Herzyk et al 1993). One study reported that persistent elevation of IL-1 concentrations in BAL and plasma appears related to outcome in patients developing ARDS (Meduri et al 1995). As for IL-1ß, elevated plasma levels have been reported in septic patients however levels in survivors were higher than in nonsurvivors (Cannon et al 1991). In ARDS patients, lower levels of plasma IL-1ß correlated with survival (Meduri et al 1995).

High circulating levels of IL-6 were found early in sepsis and ARDS patients, correlating with the outcome (Calandra et al 1991, Roumen et al 1993,1995, Goldie et al 1995, Meduri et al 1995). Also, a markedly increased synthesis of IL-6 was found in T cells isolated from patients with major trauma (Ertel et al 1991). After conventional cholecystectomy, plasma IL-6 and C-reactive protein levels were elevated but this was not the case after laparoscopic cholecystec-

Table 2
Incidence of MODS and mortality in patients with and without HLA-DR6 serotype.

43 peritonitis patients	HLA-DR6	MODS	mortality
11	–	–	o
4	+	–	1
18	–	+	6
10	+	+	7 *

* p < 0,001

tomy (Roumen et al 1992b), indicating that the systemic response correlates with the extent of injury.

Interleukin-10 is a potent inhibitor of monocyte and macrophage proinflammatory cytokine production. In critically ill patients, high plasma IL-10 levels were higher in the presence of septic shock and correlated well with APACHE II scores (Gomez-Jimenez et al 1995, Sherry et al 1996). In the lung fluids of patients with the ARDS, decreased concentrations of Interleukin-10 and of Interleukin-1 receptor antagonist were associated with increased mortality rates (Donnelly et al 1996).

Neopterin is a stable, inactive end product of macrophage metabolism. After administration of endotoxin to normal human subjects, a delayed but sustained elevation of serum neopterin levels was found (Bloom et al 1990). In all clinical studies available, plasma levels of neopterin were an excellent marker of the severity of ARDS, MOF and sepsis/SIRS and accurately predicted nonsurvivors several days before the event (Pacher et al 1989, Waydhas et al 1992, Roumen et al 1995, Delogu et al 1995). In one study, plasma neopterin levels correlated well with the clinical signs of sepsis/SIRS but not with plasma endotoxin

levels (Aasen et al 1989). Plasma neopterin levels above 30 mg/dL on day 3 after injury predicted subsequent severe MODS with 70% sensitivity and 93% specificity. The negative predictive value was 93% (Waydhas et al 1992). Differentiation among survivors without MODS, survivors with MODS and nonsurvivors (all with MODS) was possible as early as the first hours after injury, using the plasma levels of elastase, lactate and antithrombin III, or after a few days with the help of neopterin, C-reactive protein and phospholipase A values (Waydhas et al 1992).

Plasma phospholipase A2 was assessed daily in a large series of patients with peritonitis (Uhl et al 1995). High values were found from the onset, with a high predictive value for the development of subsequent MODS, thus providing for an estimate of the individual risk.

3. GENETIC FACTORS

The impossibility to predict the postoperative course in patients with severe bacterial insults to the peritoneum remains a major puzzle. Why do some patients recover uneventfully, while others, with the same cause, severity and duration of peritonitis go on developing MODS and subsequently die. This enigma has prompted the studying of interindividual differences in the inflammatory response to severe stimuli. Only a few studies so far have addressed this topic.

After uncomplicated surgery, neutrophil activation is downregulated, as is hypochlorous acid production (Carey et al 1992). However, in patients who subsequently developed sepsis seven to ten days later, neutrophil HOCl production was augmented to supra-normal values on post-operative day one, independently from any nutritional, metabolic or technical factor. Wakefield et al (1992) found that in patients destined to develop post-operative sepsis, neutrophil activation is an early event in the post-operative course. Patients developing sepsis were constitutively high expressors of CD16 on their neutrophils.

Evidence from in vitro studies suggests that the production of cytokines is related to the HLA-DR type of the individual. Various investigators found stable interindividual differences of in vitro human monocyte LPS-stimulated production of TNF-a, IL-1 and PGE2, correlating with the HLA-DR phenotype. HLA-DR2 homozygotes and HLA-DR2/DR1 genotypes were low secretors (Molvig et al 1988, Santamaria et al 1989, Bendtzen 1988).

Recently we performed HLA-DR typing in 89 ICU patients at risk of developing MODS, including 43 peritonitis patients. The actual incidence of MODS in the study population was 48% and mortality was 46% in the MODS group versus 9% in the non-MODS group. Mortality was significantly higher in the peritonitis patients with the HLA-DR6 serotype (table 3) (Kouwenberg et al 1997).

In another study, homozygous TNFB2 patients seemed to have a higher risk of developing a severe sepsis after a severe insult, as well as a higher mortality rate than heterozygous patients. Homozygous TNFB2 patients displayed higher circulating TNF-a concentrations as well as higher MOF scores compared with heterozygous (TNFB1/TNFB2) patients (Stüber et al 1996, Flohé et al 1997). Thus, further studies are warranted to determine individual risk factors related to the development of severe complications after peritonitis.

CONCLUSIONS

Despite various efforts, better antibiotics, improvements in Intensive Care, and more or less aggressive surgical approaches, survival after severe peritonitis has not substantially improved during the last 20 years. New paths of research should, therefore, be opened to study the underlying problem. New approaches address the peritoneal defence mechanisms against bacteria, the local inflammatory process, the systemic inflammatory response and interindividual genetically determined differences in this systemic response.

REFERENCES

1. Aasen AO, Rishovd AL, Stadaas JO (1988) Role of endotoxin and proteases in multiple organ failure (MOF). In: Schlag G, Redl H (eds) Second Vienna Shock Forum. Liss, New York, pp 315-322.

2. Ahrenholz DH, Simmons RL (1980) Fibrin in peritonitis. I:beneficial and adverse effects of fibrin in experimental E. Coli peritonitis. Surgery 88:41-47.

3. Arregui M, Moyes DG, Lipman J, Fatti LP (1991) Comparison of disease severity sco-

ring systems in septic shock. Crit Care Med 19: 1165-1171.

4. Autio V (1964) The spread of intraperitoneal infection: studies with roentgen contrast medium. Acta Chir Scand 123:1-31.

5. Battafarano RJ, Burd RS, Kurrelmeyer KM, Ratz CA, Dunn DL (1994) Inhibition of splenic macrophage tumor necrosis factor alpha secretion in vivo by antilipopolysaccharide monoclonal antibodies. Arch Surg 29:179-180.

6. Bauhofer A, Celik I, Reimund KP, Rothmund M, Lorenz W (1995). G-CSF and antibiotic sepsis profylaxis in a rat infectious model for the development of a consensus assisted study protocol. Shock 3:60(S).

7. Bendtzen K, Morling N, Fomsgaard, Svenson M, Jakobsen B, Ødum N, Svejgaard A (1988) Association between HLA-DR2 and production of Tumour Necrosis Factor-a and Interleukin 1 by mononuclear cells activated by lipopolysaccharide. Scand J Immunol 28:599-606.

8. Betjes MG, Tuk CW, Struijk DG, Krediet RT, Arisz L, Beelen RH (1992). Adherence of *Staphylococci* to plastic, mesothelial cells and mesothelial extracellular matrix. Adv Perit Dial 8:215-218.

9. Billing AG, Fröhlich D, Konecny G, et al (1994). Local serum application: restoration of sufficient host defence in human peritonitis. Eur J Clin Invest 24:28-35.

10. Blackwell TS, Christman JW. Sepsis and cytokines: current status. Br J Anaesth 1996;77:110-117.

11. Bloom JN, Suffredini AF, Parillo JE, Palestine AC (1990) Serum neopterin levels following intravenous endotoxin administration to normal humans. Immunobiol 181:317-323.

12. Bohnen J, Boulanger M, Meakins JL et al (1983). Prognosis in generalized peritonitis; relation to cause and risk factors. Arch Surg 118:285-290.

13. Bullen JJ (1981). The significance of iron in infection. Rev Infect Dis 3:1127-1138.

14. Calandra T, Baumgartner J-D, Grau GE et al. (1990) Prognostic values of tumor necrosis factor/cachectin, Interleukin-1, Interferon-a and Interferon-y in the serum of patients with septic shock. JID 161:982-987.

15. Calvano SE, van der Poll T, Coyle SM et al (1996) Monocyte tumor necrosis factor receptor levels as a predictor of risk in human sepsis. Arch Surg 131:434-437.

16. Cannon JG, Tompkins RG, Gelfand JA et al. (1990) Circulating interleukin-1 and tumor necrosis factor-a in septic shock and experimental endotoxin fever. JID 161:79-84.

17. Carey PD, Wakefield CH, Thayeb A, Monson JRT, Guillou PJ (1992) Preservation of neutrophil antimicrobial function after laparascopic surgery. Br J Surg 79:1223.

18. Caruana JA, Montes M, Camara DS, Ummer A, Potmesil SH, Gage AA (1982) Functional and histopathologic changes in the liver during sepsis. Surg Gynecol Obstet 154:653-656.

19. Chen X, Christou NV (1996) Relative contribution of endothelial cell and polymorphonuclear neutrophil activation in their interactions in systemic inflammatory response syndrome. Arch Surg 131:1148-11154.

20. Ciano PS, Colvin RB, Dvorak AM et al (1986). Macrophage migration in fibrin gel matrices. Lab Invest 54:62-70.

21. Delogu G, Casula MA, Mancini P et al (1995) Serum neopterin and soluble IL-2 receptor for prediction of a shock-state in gram-negative sepsis. J Crit Care 10:64-71.

22. Donnelly SC, Strieter RM, Reid PT et al (1996) The association between mortality rates and decreased concentrations of Interleukin-10 and Interleukin-1 receptor antagonist in the lung fluids of patients with the Adult Respiratory Distress Syndrome. Ann Intern Med 125:191-196.

23. Dougherty SH, Simmons RL (1982). Infections in bionic man: the pathobiology of infections in prosthetic devices. Curr Probl Surg 19:217.

24. Dougherty SH (1994). Diagnoses and management of prosthesis infection. In: Surgical infections: Diagnoses and treatment. Ed. Meakins JL. Scientific American, Inc., New York 262.

25. Dunn DL, Simmons RL (1982). Fibrin in peritonitis. III: the mechanism of bacterial trapping by polymerizing fibrin. Surgery 92:513-519.

26. Dunn DL, Barke RA, Ahrenholz DL et al (1984). The adjuvant effect of peritoneal fluid in experimental peritonitis: mechanism and clinical implications. Ann Surg 199:37-43.

27. Duswald KH, Jochum M, Schramm W, Fritz H (1985) Released granulocytic elastase: an indicator of pathobiochemical alterations in septicemia after abdominal surgery. Surgery 98:892-899.

28. Edminston CE Jr, Goheen MP, Kornhall S et al (1990). Fecal peritonitis: microbial adherence to serosal mesothelium and resistance to peritoneal lavage. World J Surg 14:176-183.

29. Elebute EA, Stoner HB (1983) The grading of sepsis. Br J Surg 70:29-31.

30. Engelberts I, Stephens S, Francot GJM, van der Linden CJ, Buurman WA (1991) Evidence for different effects of soluble TNF-receptors on various TNF measurements in human biological fluids. Lancet ii:515-516.

31. Engelberts I, Hoof van SCJ, Samyo SK, Buurman WA, van der Linden CJ (1992) Generalized inflammation during peritonitis evidenced by intracutaneous ELAM-1 expression. Clin Immunol Immunoth 65:330-334.

32. Ertel W, Morrison MH, Wang P, Zheng F, Ayala A, Chaudry IH (1991) The complex pattern of cytokines in sepsis. Ann Surg 214:141-148.

33. Flohé S, Majetschak M. Obertacke U, Stueber F, Flach R, Schade FU (1997) Polymorphism within TNF gen locus : correlation with severe sepsis after polytrauma. Shock S8:38.

34. Freeman BD, Yatsiv I, Natanson C et al (1995). Continuous arterial venous hemofiltration does not improve survival in a canine model of septic shock. J Am Coll Surg 180:286-292.

35. Friedland JS, Porter JC, Daruanani S et al (1996) Plasma proinflammatory cytokine concentrations, Acute Physiology and Chronic Health Evaluation (APACHE) III scores and survival in patients in an intensive care unit. Crit Care Med 24:1775-1781.

36. Girotti MJ, Khan N, McLellan BA (1991) Early measurements of systemic lipid peroxidation products in the plasma of major blunt trauma patients. J Trauma 31:32-35.

37. Goldie AS, Fearon KC, Ross JA et al (1995) Natural cytokine antagonists and endogenous anti-cytokine core antibodies in sepsis syndrome. JAMA 274:172-177.

38. Gomez-Jimenez J, Martin MC, Sauri R et al (1995) Interleukin-10 and the monocyte-macrophage-induced inflammatory response in septic shock. J Infect Dis 171:472-475.

39. Goor H van, Graaf JS, Kooi K et al (1994). Effect of recombinant tissue plasminogen activator on intra-abdominal abscess formation in rats with generalized peritonitis. J Am Coll Surg 179:407-411.

40. Goor H van, Graaf JS de, Kooi K, Bleichrodt RP (1995). Gentamicin reduces bacteraemia and mortality associated with the treatment of experimental peritonitis with recombinant tissue plasminogen activator. J Am Coll Surg 181:38-42.

41. Goor van H, Borm VJJ, Meer van der J, Sluiter WJ, Bleichrodt RP (1996) Coagulation and fibrinolytic responses in human peritoneal fluid and plasma to bacterial peritonitis. Brit J Surg 83:113-1135.

42. Goris RJA, te Boekhorst TPA, Nuytinck JKS, Gimbrere JSP (1985) Multiple organ failure. Generalised autodestructive inflammation? Arch Surg 120: 1109-1115.

43. Gristina AG, Costerton JW (1984). Bacterial adherence and the glycocalyx and their role in musculoskeletal infection. Orthop Clin North Am 15:517.

44. Hau T, Hoffman R, Simmons RL (1978). Mechanisms of the adjuvant effect of haemoglobin in experimental peritonitis. I: *in vivo* inhibition of peritoneal leucocytes. Surgery 83:223-229.

45. Hau T, Payne WD, Simmons RL (1979) Fibrinolytic activity of the peritoneum during experimental peritonitis. Surg Gynecol Obstet 148:471-477.

46. Hau T, Ahrenholz DH, Simmons RL (1979a). Secondary bacterial peritonitis: the biologic basis of treatment. Curr Probl Surg 16:1-65.

47. Hau T, Payne WD, Simmons RL (1979b). Fibrinolytic activity of the peritoneum during experimental peritonitis. Surg Gynecol Obstet 148:415-418.

48. Heideman M, Norder-Hanssen B, Bengtson A, Mollnes TE (1988) Terminal complement complexes and anaphylatoxins in septic and ischemic patients. Arch Surg 123:188-192.

49. Heinzelmann M, Simmen HP, Battaglia H, Friedl HP, Trentz O (1997) Inflammatory response after abdominal trauma, infection, or intestinal obstruction measured by oxygen radical production in peritoneal fluid. Am J Surg 174:445-447.

50. Herzyk DJ, Wewers MD (1993) ELISA detection of IL-beta in human sera needs independent confirmation. False positives in hospitalized patients. Am Rev Respir Dis 147:139-142.

51. Hohn DC, MacKay RD, Halliday B et al (1976). Effect of O2 tension on microbicidal function of leukocytes in wounds and in vitro. Surg Forum 27:18-21.

52. Holzheimer RG, Shein M, Wittmann DH (1995). Inflammatory response in peritoneal exudate and plasma of patients undergoing planned relaparotomy for severe secondary peritonitis. Arch Surg 130:1314-1320.

53. Hyers TM, Tricomi SM, Dettenmeier PA, Fowler AA (1991) Tumor necrosis factor levels in serum and bronchoalveolar lavage fluid of patients with the adult respiratory distress syndrome. Am Rev Resp Dis 144:268-271.

54. Imhof M, Schmidt E, Bruch HP et al (1987). Neue therapeutische Aspekten in der Behandlung der diffusen Peritonitis. Chirurg 58:590-593.

55. Jansen MJ, Hendriks Th, Vogels MT et al (1996) Inflammatory cytokines in an experimental model for the multiple organ dysfunction syndrome. Crit Care Med 24:1196-1202.

56. Keel M, Ecknauer E, Stocker R et al (1996) Different patterns of local and systemic release of proinflammatory and anti-inflammatory mediators in severely injured patients with chest trauma. J Trauma 40:907-914.

57. Khighton Dr, Halliday B, Hunt TK (1984). Oxygen as an antibiotic. The effect of inspired oxygen on infection. Arch Surg 119:199-204.

58. Klempner MS, Styrt B (1983). Alkalinizing the intraliposomal PH inhibits degranulation of human neutrophils. J Clin Invest 72:1793-1800.

59. Knaus WA, Zimmerman JE, Wagner DP et al (1981) APACHE - acute physiology and health evaluation: A physiologically based classification system Crit Care Med 9:591-597.

60. Knaus WA, Draper EA, Wagner DP, Zimmerman JE (1985) APACHE II: a severity of disease classification system. Crit Care Med 13,818-829.

61. Knaus WA, Wagner DP, Draper EA et al (1991) The APACHE III Prognostic System; risk prediction of hospital mortality for critically ill hospitalized adults. Chest 100:1619-1636.

62. Kouwenberg PP, Reemst PH, Allebes WA, Tijssen H, Mulier S, Goris RJA (1997) Is there a genetic predisposition to cause multiple organ dysfunction syndrome. Shock S8:72.

63. Lemaire LCJM, van Lanschot JJB, Stoutenbeek CP, van Deventer SJH, Wells CL, Gouma DJ (1997) Bacterial translocation in multiple organ failure : cause or epiphenomenon still unproven. Brit J Surg 84:1340-1350.

64. Lorenz W, Reimund KP, Wietzel F, Celik I, Kurnatowski M, Schneider C, Mannheim W, Heiske A, Neumann K, Sitter H, Rothmund M (1994). Granulocyte colony-stimulating factor prophylaxis before operation protects against lethal consequences of postoperative peritonitis. Surgery 116:925-934.

65. Marchesi VT (1961). The site of leucocyte emigration during inflammation. Q J Exp Physiol 46:115-118.

66. Marks JD, Marks CB, Luce JM et al. (1990) Plasma tumor necrosis factor in patients with septic shock. Am Rev Resp Dis 141:94-97.

67. Marshall JC, Christou NV, Horn R (1988). The microbiology of multiple organ failure. The proximal gastrointestinal tract as a reservoir of pathogens. Arch Surg 123:309-315.

68. Marshall JC, Cook DJ, Christou NV et al (1995) Multiple Organ Dysfunction Score: a reliable descriptor of a complex clinical outcome (1995) Crit Care Med 23:1638-1652.

69. McLauchlan GJ, Anderson ID, Grant IS, Fearon KCH (1995). Outcome of patients with abdominal sepsis treated in an intensive care unit. Br J Surg 82:524-529.

70. McRitchie DI, Cummings D, Rotstein OD (1989). Delayed administration of tissue plasminogen activator reduces intra-abdominal abscess formation. Arch Surg 124:1406-1410.

71. Meddens MJ, Thompson J, Leij PC et al (1984). Role of granulocytes in the induction of an experimental endocarditis with a dextran-producing Streptococcus sanguis and its dextran-negative mutant. Br J Exp Pathol 65:257.

72. Meduri GU, Headley S, Kohler G et al (1995) Persistent elevation of inflammatory cytokines predicts a poor outcome in ARDS. Chest 107:1062-1072.

73. Mills J, Pulliam L, Dall L, et al (1984). Exopolysaccharide production by viridans stretococci in experimental endocarditits. Infect Immun 43:359.

74. Mollnes TE, Fosse E. The complement system in trauma-related and ischemic tissue damage: a brief review. Shock 1994;2:301-310.

75. Molloy RG, Holzheimer R, Nester M et al (19954). Granulocyte-macrophage colony-stimulating factor modulates function and improves survival after experimental termal injury. Br J Surg 82:770-776.

76. MØlvig J, Baek L, Chrisyensen P, Manogue KR, Vlassara H, Platz P, Nielsen LS, Svejgaard A, Nerup J (1988) Endotoxin-stimulated human monocyte secretion of Interleukin-1, Tumour Necrosis Factor, and prostaglandin E2 shows stable interindividual differences. Scand J Immunol 27:705-716.

77. Morris JS, Meakins JL, Christou NV (1985) In vivo neutrophil delivery to inflammatory sites in surgical patients. Arch Surg 120:205-209.

78. Munoz C, Carlet J, Fitting C et al (1991) Dysregulation of in vitro cytokine production by monocytes during sepsis. J Clin Invest 88:1747-1754.

79. Nerlich ML, Seidel J, Regel G, Nerlich AG, Sturm AJ (1986) Klinische experimentelle Untersuchungen zum oxidativen Membranschaden nach schwerem Trauma. Langenbecks Arch Chir (Suppl) 217-222.

80. Nerlich ML, Holch M, Maghsudi M (1991) Comparison of APACHE II, Sepsis Severity Score and MOF-score (Goris) in posttraumatic organ failure. Circ Shock 34:41.

81. Nikken JJ, Goris RJA Scoring systems in critically ill patients. In : Trauma Care, an update. B Risberg (Ed). Pharmacia and Upjohn Stockholm 1997, pp 56-67.

82. Nieuwenhuijzen GAP, Haskel Y, Lu Q, Deitch EA, Goris RJA (1993) Macrophage elimination increases bacterial translocation and gut-origin septicemia but attenuates symptoms and mortality rate in a model of systemic inflammation. Ann Surg 218:791-799.

83. Nieuwenhuijzen GAP, Deitch EA, Goris RJA (1996) Infection, the gut and the development of the multiple organ dysfunction syndrome. Eur J Surg 162:259-273.

84. Nijmegen-Cologne Study Group. Revision of the MOF-score. Personnal communication.

85. Nuytinck JKS, Goris RJA, Redl H, Schlag G. van Munster PJJ (1986) Posttraumatic complications and inflammatory mediators. Arch Surg 121: 886-890.

86. Ohmann C, Hau T (1997) Prognostic indices in peritonitis. Hepatogastroenterology 44:937-946.

87. Ohmann Chr, Yang Q, Hau T, Wacha H, and the Peritonitis Study Group of the Surgical Infection Society Europe. (1997) Prognostic Modelling in Peritonitis. Eur J Surg 163:53-60.

88. Offner F, Phillipe J, Vogelaers D et al. (1990) Serum tumor necrosis factor levels in patients with infectious disease and septic shock. J Lab Clin Med 116:100-105.

89. Pacher R, Redl H, Frass M, Petzl DH, Schuster E, Woloszczuk W. Relationship between neopterin and granulocyte elastase plasma levels and the severity of multiple organ failure. Crit Care Med 1989;17:221-226.

90. Ponting GA, Sim AJW, Dudley HAF (1987) Comparison of the local and systemic effects of sepsis in predicting survival. Br J Surg 74:750-752.

91. Raju R, Weiner M, Enauist IF (1976). Quantitation of local acidosis and hypoxia produced by infection. Am J Surg 132:64-66.

92. Rao R, Prinz RA, Kazantsev GB et al (1996). Effects of granulocyte colony-stimulating factor in severe pancreatitis. Surgery 119:657-663.

93. Reimund KP, Lorenz W, Celik I, Bauhofer A, Greger B, Seitz R, Rothmund M (1995). Management of leucopenic sepsis. Lancet 346:382-383.

94. Roten R, Markert M, Feihl F, Schaller M-D, Tagan M-C, Perret C (1991) Plasma levels of tumor necrosis factor in the adult respiratory distress syndrome. Am Rev Resp Dis 143:590-592.

95. Rotstein OD, Pruett TL, Simmons RL (1986). Microbiologic features and treatment of persistent peritonitis in patients in the intensive care unit. Can J Surg 29:247-250.

96. Rotstein OD, Pruett TL, Simmons RL (1986b). Fibrin in peritonitis. V: fibrin inhibits phagocytic killing of *Escherichia coli* by human polymorphonuclear leukocytes. Ann Surg 203:413-419.

97. Rotstein OD, Pruett TL, Wells CL, Simmons RL (1987). The role of *Bacteroides* encapsulation in the lethal synergy between *Escherichia coli* and *Bacteroides* species studied in a rat fibrin clot peritonitis model. J Infect 15:135-146.

98. Rotstein OD, Kao J (1988a). The spectrum of *Escherichia coli-Bacteroides fragilis* pathogenic synergy in an intra-abdominal infection model. Can J Microbiol 34:352-357.

99. Rotstein OD, Fiegel VD, Simmons RL et al (1988b). The deleterious effect of reduced pH and hypoxia on neutrophil migration in vitro. J Surg Res 45:298-303.

100. Rotstein OD, Kao J (1988c). Prevention of intra-abdominal abscesses by fibrinolysis using recombinant tissue plasminogen activator. J Infect Dis 158:766-772.

101. Roumen RM, Schers TJ, de Boer HH, Goris RJA (1992a) Scoring systems for predic-

ting outcome in acute hemorrhagic pancreatitis. Eur J Surg 158:167-171.

102. Roumen RMH, van Meurs PA, Kuypers HJC et al (1992b) Serum Interleukin-6 and C reactive protein responses in patients after laparoscopic or conventional cholecystectomy. Eur J Surg 158:541-544.

103. Roumen RMH, Hendriks Th, van der Ven-Jongekrijg J et al (1993) Cytokine patterns in patients after major vascular surgery, hemorrhagic shock and severe blunt trauma : relation with subsequent ARDS and MOF. Ann Surg 218:769-776.

104. Roumen RMH, Hendriks Th, De Man BM et al (1994) Serum lipofuscine as a marker of ARDS and MOF. Br J Surg 81:1300-1305.

105. Roumen RMH, Redl H, Schlag G et al (1995) Inflammatory mediators in relation to the development of multiple organ failure in patients after severe blunt trauma. Crit Care Med 23:474-480.

106. Rudek W, Hague R (1976). Extracellular enzymes of the genus *Bacteroides*. J Clin Microbiol 4:458-460.

107. Santamaria P, Gehrz RC, Bryan MK, Barbosa JJ (1989) Involvement of class II MHC molecules in the LPS-induction of IL-1/TBNF secretions by human monocytes. Quantitative differences at the polymorphic level. J Immunol 143:913-922.

108. Schneierson SS, Amsterdam D, Perlman E (1961). Enhancement of intraperitoneal staphylococcal virulence for mice with different bile salts. Nature 190:829-830.

109. Shein M, Wittmann DH, Holzheimer RG et al (1996). Hypothesis: compartimentalisation of cytokines in intra-abdominal infection. Surgery 119:694-700.

110. Sherry RM, Cué JI, Goddard JK et al (1996) Interleukin-10 is associated with the development of sepsis in trauma patients. J Trauma 40:613-617.

111. Siebeck M, Schorr M, Welcker K et al (1996). Antithrombin III und locale Serum-gabe als adjuvante Therapie bei Patienten mit diffuser, sekundärer Peritonitis. Langenbecks Arch Chir Suppl 1287-1288.

112. Simms HH, D'Amico R (1991) Increased PMN CD11b/CD18 expression following post-traumatic ARDS. J Surg Res 50:362-367.

113. Stack AM, Saladino RA, Thompson C et al (1995). Failure of prophylactic and therapeutic use of murine anti-tumour necrosis factor monoclonal antibody in Escheria coli sepsis in the rabbit. Crit Care Med 23:512-518.

114. Stevens LE (1983) Gauging the severity of surgical sepsis. Arch Surg 118:1190-1192.

115. Stüber F, Petersen M, Bokelman F, Schade U. (1997) A genomic polymorphism within the tumor necrosis factor locus influences plasma tumor necrosis factor-a concentrations and outcome of patients with severe sepsis. Crit Care Med 24:381-384.

116. Tennenberg SD, Jacobs MP, Solomkin JS (1987) Complement-mediated neutrophil activation in sepsis- and trauma-related adult respiratory distress syndrome. Arch Surg 122:26-32.

117. Topley N, Kaur D, Petersen MM et al (1996). Biocompatibility of bicarbonate buffered peritoneal dialysis fluids: influence on mesothelial cell and neutrophil function. Kidney Int 49(5):1447-1456.

118. Uhl W, Beger HG, Hoffman G, Hanisch E, Schild A, Waydhas C, Entholzer E, Muller K, Kellermann W, Vogeser M et al (1995) A multicenter study of phospholipase A2 in patients in intensive care units. J Am Coll Surg 180:323-331.

119. Visser CE, Brouwer-Steenbergen JJ, Schadee-Eestermans IL, Meijer S, Krediet RT, Beelen RH (1996). Ingestion of *Staphylococcus aureus*, *Staphylococcus epidermidis*, and *Escherichia coli* by human peritoneal mesothelial cells. Infect Immun 64(8):3425-3428.

120. Wakefield CH, Carey PD, Foulds S, Monson JRT, Guillou PJ (1992) Surgical significance of neutrophil phosphatidylinositol-glycan-tailed receptors. Br J Surg 79:1225.

121. Waydhas C, Nast-Kolb D, Jochum M, Trupka A, Lenk S, Fritz H, Duswald K-H, Schweiberer L (1992) Inflammatory mediators, infection, sepsis, and multiple organ failure after severe trauma. Arch Surg 127:460-467.

122. Weitzel F, Schneider C, Heymanns J, Celik I, Reimund KP Lorenz W (1994a). G-CSF treatment results in an increase of TNF receptors both in serum and on the surface of neutrophils in man. Eur Surg Res 36:4(S).

123. Weitzel F, Reimund KP, Lorenz W, Schneider M, Kurnatowski M, Rothmund M (1994b). G-CSF prophylaxis protects against lethal consequences of post-operative peritonitis. Abstracts of the Fifty-Fifth Annual Meeting and Ninth Tripartite Meeting of the Society of University of Surgeons, Jackson, Mississippi: 17.

124. Young S, Beswick P (1986) A comparison of the oxidative reactions of neutrophils from a variety of species when stimulated by opsonized zymosan and FMLP. J Comp Pathol 96:189-196.

125. Zimmerli W, Waldvogel FA, Vaudaux P et al (1982). Pathogenesis of foreign body infection: description and characteristics of an animal model. J Infect Dis 146:487-497.

126. Zinsser HH, Pryde AW (1952). Experimental study of physical factors, including fibrin formation, influencing the spread of fluids and small particles within and from the peritoneal cavity of the dog. Ann Surg 136:818-827.

Issues in the Design of Clinical Trials of Anti-Infectives for Intra-abdominal Infections

Joseph S. Solomkin, MD and Randeep S. Jawa, MD

1. INTRODUCTION

The development of new anti-infectives is integral to the practice of modern medicine. Aside from the search for safer and more convenient drugs and drug formulations, antimicrobial resistance to older agents continues to occur and new pathogens continue to emerge. Furthermore, changes in treatment approaches to other, non-infectious diseases result in a continuing evolution of the patient groups developing infection. The review of investigational anti- infectives by the FDA for marketing approval is similarly a continuously evolving process, driven by these factors as well as by new insights in the design of clinical trials.

A regulatory decision to approve a new drug is based upon the results of wellcontrolled studies providing substantial evidence of effectiveness. Clinical trial results must show the product is safe under the conditions of use in the proposed labeling; that is, the benefits of the drug appear to outweigh its risks. For anti-infectives, the meaning of the term, "substantial evidence of effectiveness" most often means that the agent was tested in prospective, controlled trials. There are, however, a variety of issues regarding how such trials are designed, ranging from the disease processes entered into the study or excluded from the trial to whether the study is blinded.

These issues of adequate trial design and regulatory approval have developed a global dimension. Considerable benefits would accrue to patients around the world if agreement was reached on the nature of an adequate trial; large studies would not have to be repeated in each country. Management of intra-abdominal infections is similar, if not identical, in most developed countries. To achieve consistency on a larger scale, the International Conference on Harmonization is bringing together pharmaceutical industry representatives and the drug regulating agencies of the European Union, Japan and the United States to establish common procedures to speed up the availability of new medicines worldwide.

It is, therefore, worth reviewing material on FDA procedures to provide a background

Figure 1a
A schematic flow chart for the various stages of the FDA group approval process.
See tables 1 and 2 for additional information.

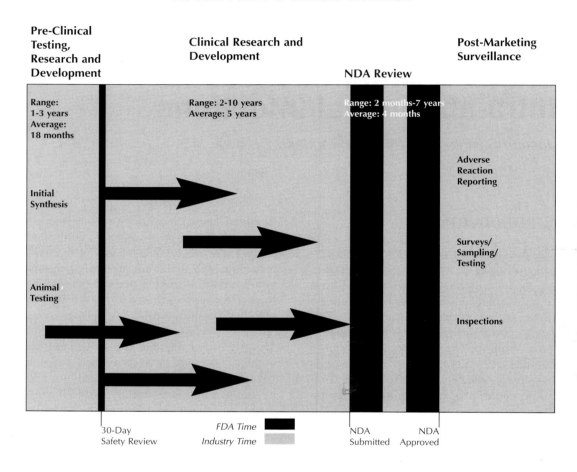

for a discussion of clinical trial design. These procedures are quite similar to those in use elsewhere.

The overall process for development and testing of new compounds is displayd in Figure 1. Further information about these various phases is provided in Table 1. A glossary is provided in Tables 2 and 3. Most

physicians will become involved in clinical trials in Phase II and III.

2. THE IDSA/FDA GUIDELINES

In 1991, a contract was developed between the Infections Disease Society of America (IDSA) and the U.S. Food and Drug Admi-

Table 1
The standard phases of drug testing for FDA marketing approval.

	Number of Patients	Purpose	Length	Per cent of Drugs Successfully Tested*
Phase 1	20-100	Mainly safety	Several months	70 per cent
Phase 2	Up to several hundred	Some short-term safety but mainly effectiveness	Several months to 2 years	33 per cent
Phase 3	Several hundred to several thousand	Safety, dosage, effectiveness	1-4 years	25-30 per cent

*For example, of 100 drugs for which investigational new drug applications are submitted to the FDA, about 70 will successfully complete phase 1 trials and go on to phase 2; about 33 of the original 100 will complete phase 2 and go to phase 3; and 25 to 30 of the original 100 will clear phase 3; and 25 to 30 of the original 100 will clear phase 3 (and, on average, about 20 of the original 100 will ultimately be approved for marketing).

nistration which described a process for creation of position papers on clinical anti-infective trial design in several specific disease areas. Thomas Beam, Calvin Kunin and David Gilbert from the IDSA and Bruce Burlington and Matthew Lumpkin from the FDA directed this activity [11]. The product of this work was published in a supplement to Clinical Infectious Deseases in 1992, and consisted of a set of general guidelines which were applicable to most if not all trial areas and a series of area-specific guidelines [8].

The regulatory status of these documents has remained somewhat vague. It is important to note that federal law specifies the criteria for drug approval. A complex administrative process exists for development. There has, however, been considerable reluctance to translate this first effort into a regulatory requirement because the ideas have in many cases not been tested.

An additional issue countervailing the rigid application of process guidelines is the importance of regulatory flexibility. Specific compounds may require modified trial design because of unique activities or unique

problems in applying the guidelines. Also, there may be additional data available in support of an agent that modifies the data requirements for approval.

The IDSA/FDA guidelines, published six years ago, have provided structure to the evaluation of anti-infective therapy and have rationalized various aspects of study design. These guidelines also began an ongoing dialogue between interested physicians and the FDA. However, since publication of the guidelines, specific problems have been identified with them and new study elements have appeared. This article is an effort to provide an individual perspective on these issues.

2.1. Rationale for specific design elements

An important concept in understanding regulatory issues is the definition of a "valid" or "evaluable" patient. Anti-infectives are developed to cure infections. Efficacy can, therefore, only be established for patients with documented infections and without

Table 2
Terminology used in the drug approval process

Investigational New Drug Application, or IND: An application that a drug sponsor must submit to FDA before beginning tests of a new drug on humans. The IND contains the plan for the study and is supposed to give a complete picture of the drug, including its structural formula, animal test results and manufacturing information.

New Drug Application, or NDA: An application requesting FDA approval to market a new drug for human use in interstate commerce. The application must contain, among other things, from data specific technical viewpoints for FDA review-including chemistry, pharmacology, medical, biopharmaceutics, statistics and, for anti-infectives, microbiology.

Abbreviated New Drug Application, or ANDA: A simplified submission permitted for a duplicate of an already approved drug. ANDAs are for products with the same or very closely related active ingredients, dosage form, strength, administration route, use and labeling as a product that has already been shown to be safe and effective. An ANDA includes all the information on chemistry and manufacturing controls found in a new drug application (NDA) but does not have to include data from studies in animals and humans.

Accelerated Approval: A highly specialized mechanism intended to speed approval of drugs promising significant benefit over existing therapy for serious or life-threatening illnesses. It incorporates elements aimed at making sure that rapid review and approval is balanced by safeguards to protect both the public health and the integrity of the regulatory process. This mechanism may be used when approval can be reliably based on evidence of a drug's effect on a surrogate endpoint or when the FDA determines an effective drug can be used safely only under restricted distribution or use. Usually, such a surrogate can be assessed much sooner than such an endpoint as survival. In accelerated approval, FDA approves the drug on condition that the sponsor study the actual clinical benefit of the drug.

Action Letter: An official communication from the FDA to an NDA sponsor that informs of a decision by the agency. An approval letter allows commercial marketing of the product. An approvable letter can list minor issues to be resolved before approval can be given. A not approvable letter describes important deficiencies that preclude approval unless corrected.

Advisory Committe: A panel of outside experts convened periodically to advise the FDA on safety and efficacy issues about drugs and other FDA-regulated products. The FDA is not bound to take committee recommendations but usually does.

Effectiveness: The desired measure of a drug's influence on a disease condition. Effectiveness must be proven by substantial evidence consisting of adequate and well-controlled investigations, including human studies by qualified personnel which proves the drug will have the effect claimed in its labeling.

Parallel Track Mechanism: A U.S. Public Healt Service Policy that makes promising investigational drugs for AIDS and other HIV-related diseases more widely available under "parallel track" protocols while the controlled clinical trials essential to establish the safety and effectiveness of new drugs are carried out. The system established by this policy is designed to make the drugs more widely available to patients with these illnesses who have no therapeutic alternatives and who cannot participate in the controlled clinical trials.

Preclinical Studies: Studies that test a drug on animals and other non-human test systems. They must comply with the FDA's good laboratory practices. Data about a drug's activities and effects in animals help establish boundaries for safe use of the drug in subsequent human testing (clinical studies). Also, because animals have a much shorter lifespan than humans, valuable information can be gained about a drug's possible toxic effects over an animals life cycle and on offspring.

Table 2 (cont.)
Terminology used in the drug approval process

Supplement: A marketing application submitted for changes in a product that already has an approved NDA. The FDA must approve all important NDA changes (in packaging or ingredients, for instance) to ensure that the conditions originally set for the product are not adversely affected.
Treatment IND: A mechanism that allows promising investigational drugs to be used in "expanded access" protocols-relatively unrestricted studies in which the intent is both to learn more about the drugs, especially their safety and to provide treatment for people with immediately life-threatening or otherwise serious diseases for which there is no real alternative.
But these expanded access protocols also require researchers to formally investigate the drugs in well-controlled studies and to supply some evidence that the drugs are likely to be helpful. The drugs cannot expose patients to unreasonable risk.

confounding factors that would prevent evaluation of the efficacy of the anti-infective being studied. Documentation of infection for intra-abdominal infection requires an intervention, either operative, percutaneous or laparoscopic, which documents an infection by radiographic appearance.

The section of these guidelines dealing with intra-abdominal infections was based on work done through the Surgical Infection Societies of North America and of Europe [1,5,6,13]. An important goal was to develop a study design that would allow identification of predictors of failure independent of the anti-infective agent being studied. Without a clear understanding of the factors which independently affect outcome, it would not be possible to attribute success or failure to the agent under study. It was apparent that this would result in evolution of both the data items required and the entry and exclusion criteria, as information was gained from completed trials.

To accomplish these initial goals, certain modifications were required from the previous approach to anti-infective evaluation. Perhaps most important was the separation of established infection from prophylactic

settings. For gastrointestinal perforations, this was accomplished by defining times from perforation to operation. The specific cases were gastroduodenal ulcer perforation operated upon within 24 hours and traumatic bowel perforation greater than 12 hours. These are arbitrary time frames that reflected a consensus opinion. They might be validated by prospective observational research.

2.2. Effect Of Prior Anti-Infective Therapy On Eligibility

An issue of considerable regulatory concern is whether an anti-infective can be evaluated in patients who have received antimicrobial therapy prior to obtaining the index culture (the culture to be used for defining the organisms being treated). The previous prohibition of prior (non-protocol determined) anti-infective treatment had two unwanted consequences. Firstly, if patients were to be enrolled prior to confirmation of the diagnosis of intra-abdominal infection requiring intervention, they would have to be entered on the study as soon as they received clinical attention. Since many of these patients (approximately half) are ultimately found not to have complicated

Table 3
FDA classifies investigational new drug applications (INDs) and new drug applications (NDAs) to assign review priority on the basis of the drug's chemical type and potential benefit.

Chemical Type

1. **New molecular entity, or NME:** An active ingredient that has never been marketed in this country.

2. **New derivative:** A chemical derived from an active ingredient already marketed (a "parent" drug).

3. **New formulation:** A new dosage form or new formulation of an active ingredient already on the market.

4. **New combination:** A drug that contains two or more compounds, the combination of which has not been marketed together in a product.

5. **Already marketed drug product but a new manufacturer:** A product that duplicates another firm's already marketed drug product: same active ingredient, formulation or combination.

6. **Already marketed drug product but a new use:** A new use for a drug product already marketed by a different firm.

Treatment Potential

P: Priority review drug: A drug that appears to represent an adavance over available therapy.

S: Standard review drug: A drug that appears to have therapeutic qualities similar to those of an already marketed drug.

Other Designations (may apply simultaneously)

AA: AIDS drug: A drug indicated for treating AIDS or other HIV-related disease. E. Subpart E drug: A drug developed or evaluated under special procedures for drugs to treat life-thrreatening or severely debilitating illnesses. (The name refers to Title 21 of the Code of Federal Regulations, Part 312, Subpart E, which governs this classification).

V: Designated orphan drug: A drug for which the sponsor received orphan designation under the Orphan Drug Act. Such a sponsor is eligible for tax credits and exclusive marketing rights for the drug.

---

intra-abdominal infections, a number of patients would be exposed to the investigational agent with no possibility of benefit. This raises obvious ethical concerns. Secondly, the enrollment of patients with certain clinically important infections would be prohibited. Evaluation of the investigational anti-infective in settings where new agents are needed would be hampered from both efficacy and safety perspectives.

The IDSA/FDA guidelines, therefore, specified that patients who had received anti-infectives could be entered onto the study. The evidence to support this were data showing that anti-infective therapy did not change the bacterial flora of abscesses in an animal model [4,9,10]. We have since performed an analysis of patients from two clinical trials in which patients could be treated with non-protocol agents prior to intervention [2,3]. We found that there was no substantial change in the organisms recovered.

The general guidelines allowed for non-protocol therapy *after* the index culture was obtained. The duration of such therapy a patient could receive was keyed to the expected duration of overall treatment. For intra-abdominal infections, which generally require 5-7 days of treatment, up to 24 hours of treatment could be given. However, recent clinical trials have either not allowed such treatment or have limited it to one or two doses.

The primary reason to allow such treatment is to increase the percentage of patients in a clinical trial whose outcome sheds light on the drug's efficacy. Anti-infectives, intended to kill infecting micro-organisms, have no effect on the outcome of conditions other than infections. Inclusion of patients with signs and symptoms of infection but who are ultimately shown to have inflammatory but not infectious diseases actually hampers evaluation of efficacy. Such cases lessen the per cent incidence of failure, thereby lessening the likelihood of finding statistical difference. Clinical trials are first analyzed by examining outcome results for all patients entered into the trial, whether or not they receive any therapy and whether or not they have the disease under study. This is termed an "intention to treat" analysis. An accepted corollary is that a subgroup analysis has no validity if the intention to treat analysis does not show a significant effect. The rationale for this type of analysis is to prevent patient exclusions for reasons related to the agent(s)

they receive from affecting interpretation of the study. An example would be the consequences of excluding from analysis patients infected with organisms resistant to a study regimen. This would make an agent with a narrow spectrum of activity appear similar in efficacy to a similar agent with a broader spectrum of activity.

The particular issue for intra-abdominal infections is that enrollment of patients prior to operative or percutaneous intervention results in inclusion of patients with inflammatory but not infectious diseases. Such conditions as acute, non-perforated appendicitis, small bowel obstruction without infarction, pancreatitis or inflammatory bowel disease without abscess or peritonitis, certainly present with signs and symptoms of infection and are commonly initially treated with anti-infectives until the diagnosis is established. The simple solution to this problem would be to enroll patients after gross confirmation of infection by operative or percutaneous findings.

Whether one or two doses of non-protocol anti-infective therapy would alter the outcome of the trial is unlikely. For example, in a large study we performed in which such therapy was allowed, substantial differences were identified in the regimens employed (3).

Aside from the statistical issues, the ethical problems of exposing patients to investigational agents when they cannot benefit must also be recognized. The general presumption that agents which have reached Phase III testing have already been shown to be safe is not true. Phase II testing does not involve the range of patients, severity of illness, and associated diseases which may have substantial impact on the agent's toxicity. The clearest example is moxalactam, which appeared safe when given to patients without severe infections but caused significant bleeding problems in patients in acute renal failure.

Provision of anti-infective treatment for multi-resistant organisms such as methicillin resistant Staphylococci, Enterococci and fungi while the patient is receiving study therapy remains an area of discussion. The problem with allowing such therapy is that there may be effects on outcome that cannot be identified since there is no true control group. For example, marginally active agents against Gram negatives might appear more effective if vancomycin or some other "specific" agent interrupts synergistic interactions between Gram negatives and Gram positives. Conversely, there is no evidence that provision of such therapy alters the outcome of polymicrobial infection. The simplest approach might be to allow such therapy only when cultures identify such organisms in settings where the organism is known to be pathogenic.

2.3. Appendicitis

Perforated appendicitis is a common condition and patients with this disease frequently constitute a numerically important component of the study population. Use of appendicitis as a disease model is attractive because the pathology and surgical treatment are uniform, the population is generally young and not suffering other diseases which would complicate outcome assessment and treatment failure is not accompanied with mortality.

However, appendicitis is not representative of other, more complex intra-abdominal infectious processes. While the range of organisms is similar, their density is substantially lower and a need for more than brief

prophylactic treatment has not been demonstrated for perforated appendicitis not accompanied by a defined abscess. Furthermore, "peritonitis" in this condition does not have the same clinically ominous meaning as it does in colon-derived infections.

It is certainly reasonable to include patients with appendicitis with abscess formation in general intra-abdominal infection studies since they represent a common intra-abdominal infection. However, if the study population includes a large percentage of such cases, there may be insufficient power to determine efficacy in the non-appendiceal cases. One approach to this problem would be to require sample size calculations based on a lower incidence of failure, proportionate to the number of appendicitis cases enrolled. If the number of non-appendicitis cases was insufficient to meet the sample size requirements for the desired level or significance, efficacy could not be claimed if there was no difference between control and investigational therapy.

2.4. Inclusion of Nosocomial Infections

Since publication of the IDSA/FDA guidelines, logistic regression analyses of relatively large patient populations have been performed (7, 12). These have demonstrated that post-operative infections or infections occurring in patients recently treated with anti-infective agents are important risk factors for treatment failure. One explanation is that the microbial flora is more difficult to eradicate; non-exclusive alternatives include more difficult anatomic, physiologic or immunologic circumstances.

The decision to include such patients in clinical trials must be based on an awareness of the organism likely to be encountered and the activity of the agents against them. If a proposed regimen does not have activity against *Pseudomonas aeruginosa, Enterobacter species* and other common nosocmial organisms, such patients should be prohibited from study entry.

2.5. Use of sequential intravenous/oral therapy

The increasing need for cost control in health care has led to interest in conversion of intravenous anti-infective regimens to oral. Cost savings for patients remaining in hospital are substantial and include reduction or elimination of the need for intravenous access and use or oral *vs* parenteral product formulations. Hospitalization for the sole purpose of receiving anti-infective therapy has also been reduced by the use of home infusion therapy and conversion to oral regimens.

Whether clinical trials intended to support registration of parenteral anti-infectives should routinely include provisions for sequential parenteral/oral therapy is unclear. There is a presumption that anti-infective therapy given following treatment with an investigational agent may mask defects in the anti-microbial activity of the study agent. This becomes even more of a concern if there is no period of time when no treatment is given which might allow emergence of dormant organisms.

Sequential treatment is less of an issue if the same agents are used for both the parenteral and oral therapies. In this case, absorption of the oral agent(s) in the population being studied should be documented since overgrowth, provision of other agents such as antacids and anatomic factors might alter drug absorption.

If no oral form of the agent is available, studies involving oral regimens with other, approved agents should be carried out only after a standard comparative parenteral study is completed which documents efficacy.

2.6. Testing of anti-infectives in previously restricted groups

In recent years there has been growing interest at the FDA and by the public in drug testing in patient populations that have been relatively neglected in clinical trials, especially women and children. Children are generally not included in trials at all until the drug has been fully evaluated in adults, unless the drug is intended for a pediatric disease. Without pediatric studies or other sources of scientific information, labeling cannot include guidance about dosage, side effects and when a drug should or should not be used in children. In October 1992, the FDA proposed changes in its regulations governing drug labeling for "pediatric use". The proposal is aimed at encouraging drug sponsors to develop pediatric information –through clinical trials in children or by extrapolation of findings in adults– that can be included in drug labeling.

Although both sexes now are generally represented in clinical trials in proportions that reflect gender patterns of disease, the FDA and women's health advocates agree that less care has been taken to develop information about significant differences in the way men and women respond to drugs. A new FDA guideline on the study and evaluation of gender differences in clinical drug trials, issued in July 1993, encourages drug companies to include appropriate numbers of women in drug development programs and to pay particular attention to factors that can affect drug behavior, such as phases of the menstrual cycle, menopause and the use of oral contraceptives or estrogens. Another focus is discovering gender-related differences in how a drug is absorbed, metabolized or excreted and its mechanisms of action.

The guideline also does away with an FDA policy dating from 1977 that excluded women of childbearing potential from participation in early clinical studies. The agency believes that institutional review boards, as well as clinical investigators and women themselves, can gauge whether women's participation in clinical trials is appropriate and make sure that fetuses are not unduly exposed to potentially toxic agents.

3. Summary and Conclusions

The regulatory approval for marketing of new anti-infectives is an important area both because of the commercial aspects of drug development and because this process substantially affects how physicians care for patients. This may become even more meaningful as health maintenance organizations and insurers move towards standardized formularies based on approved indications. It is important for physicians interested in infections to participate in the testing of investigational anti-infectives because the outcome of any clinical study is utlimately determined by the quality of investigator participation.

REFERENCES

1. Solomkin JS, Meakins JL, Alo MD, Dellinger EP, Simmons RL. Antibiotic trials in intra-abdominal infections. A critical evaluation of study design and outcome reporting. Ann Surg 1984; 200: 29-39.

2. Solomkin JS, Dellinger EP, Christou NV, Busuttil RW. Results of a multicenter trial comparing imipenem/cilastatin to tobramycin/clindamycin for intra-abdominal infections. Ann Surg 1990; 212: 581-591.

3. Solomkin JS, Reinhart HH, Dellinger EP, Bohnen JM, Rotstein OD, Vogel SB, Simms HH, Hill CS, Bjornson HS, Haverstock DC, Coulter HO, Echols RM. Results of a randomized trial comparing sequential intravenous/oral treatment with ciprofloxacin plus metronidazole to imipenem/cilastatin for intra-abdominal infections. The Intra-Abdominal Infection Study Group. Ann Surg 1996; 223: 303-315.

4. Bartlett JG, Onderdonk AB, Louie T, Kasper DL, Gorbach SL. A review. Lessons from an animal model of intra-abdominal sepsis. Arch Surg 1978; 113: 853-857.

5. Meakins JL, Solomkin JS, Allo MD, Dellinger EP, Howard RJ, Simmons RL. A proposed classification of intra-abdominal infections. Stratification of etiology and risk for future therapeutic trials. Arch Surg 1984; 119: 1372-1378.

6. Dellinger EP, Wertz MJ, Meakins JL, Solomkin JS, Allo MD, Howard RJ, Simmons RL. Surgical infection stratification system for intra-abdominal infection. Multicenter trial. Arch Surg 1985; 120: 21-29.

7. Montravers P, Gauzit R, Muller C, Marmuse JP, Fichelle A, Desmonts AM. Emergence of Antibiotic-Resistant Bacteria in Cases of Peritonitis After Intra-abdominal Surgery Affects the Efficacy of Empirical Antimicrobial Therapy. Clin Infect Dis 1996; 23: 486-494.

8. Beam TR Jr., Gilbert DN, Kunin CM. General guidelines for the clinical evaluation of anti-infective drug products. Infectious Diseases Society of American and the Food and Drug Administration. Clinical Infectious Diseases 1992; 15 Suppl. 1: S5-32.

9. Onderdonk AB, Weinsteins WM, Sullivan NM, Bartlett JG, Gorbach SL. Experimental intra-abdominal abscess in rats: quantitative bacteriology of infected animals. Infect Immun 1974; 10: 1256-1259.

10. Bartlett JG, Louie TJ, Gorbach SL, Onderdonk AB. Therapeutic efficacy of 29 antimicrobial regimens in experimental intra-abdominal sepsis. Rev Infect Dis 1981; 3: 535-542.

11. Gilbert DN, Beam TR Jr., Kunin CM. The path to new FDA guidelines for clinical evaluation of anti-infective drugs. Reviews of Infectious Diseases 1991; 13 Suppl. 10: S890-4.

12. Burnett RJ, Hverstock DC, Delinger EP, Reinhart HH, Bohnen JM, Rotstein OD, Vogel SB, Solomkin JS. Definition of the role of enterococcus in intra-abdominal infection: analysis of a prospective randomized trial. Surgery 1995; 118: 716-21; discussion 721-3.

13. Nystrom PO, Bax R, Dellinger EP, Dominioni L, Knaus WA, Meakins JL, Ohmann C, Solomkin JS, Wacha H, Wittmann DH. Proposed definitions for diagnosis, severity scoring, stratification and outcome for trials on intra-abdominal infection. Joint Working Party of SIS North American and Europe. [Review]. World J Surg 1990; 14: 148-158.

14. Joseph S, Solomkin MD. Department of Surgery, University of Cincinnati College of Medicine, 231 Bethesda Avenue Cincinnati, OH 45267-0558 (USA). Tel. +1 513 558 4427. Fax +1 513 558 2585. E-mail: joseph.solomkin@uc.edu.

Primary Peritonitis

Miguel Navasa, MD

Primary peritonitis is considered when, in contrast to secondary peritonitis, the infection of the peritoneum is not associated with the loss of the integrity of the gastrointestinal tract and, therefore, there is no leakage of the intestinal content in the peritoneal cavity. The most characteristic primary peritonitis is the so-called spontaneous bacterial peritonitis in cirrhosis, in which the peritoneum is infected via the bloodstream. Infections of the abdominal cavity in patients on peritoneal dialysis or with ventriculoperitoneal shunts, although the route by which micro-organims reach the peritoneal cavity is not well understood, are also considered to be primary peritonitis, indicating that peritonitis is not associated with a perforation of an intra-abdominal organ. The present chapter, although mainly focused on cirrhosis, discusses the pathogenesis, treatment and prevention of these clinical entities.

1. SPONTANEOUS BACTERIAL PERITONITIS

Spontaneous bacterial peritonitis (SBP) is the infection of a previously sterile ascitic fluid, with no apparent intra-abdominal source of infection. This type of infection is the most characteristic infective complication in cirrhotic patients. The incidence of SBP in cirrhotic patients admitted to hospital with ascites has been estimated to range between 7% and 23% [1,2]. The diagnosis is established on the basis of clinical signs and symptoms and/or a polymorphonuclear cell count in ascitic fluid higher than 250 cells/ mm^3. This diagnosis is confirmed by a positive culture in approximately 70 % of the cases. The remaining 30% are considered culture negative SBP but are empirically treated with antibiotics because no treatment is associated with the development of severe peritonitis and death [3]. The outcome of cirrhotic patients with SBP has dramatically improved during the last 15 years. In studies published before 1980, the rate of SBP resolution ranged between 25% and 50% and the survival of patients ranged between 0% and 20% [1]. The corresponding values in the latest studies are 70%-90% and 50%-70%, respectively [1]. An early diagnosis of SBP due to a better knowledge of the signs and symptoms associated with the infection, the routine use of diagnostic paracentesis in patients admitted to hospital with ascites and, specially, the use of a more adequate antibiotic therapy are the most likely reasons for this improvement in prognosis.

1.1. Pathogenesis

According to the most accepted hypothesis on the pathogenesis of SBP, the mechanism by which cirrhotic patients with ascites develop spontaneous bacterial peritonitis is the colonization of the ascitic fluid from an episode of bacteraemia [1,4]. Although the passage of micro-organisms from the bloodstream to the ascites has never been documented, it can be assumed that bacteria present in the circulation may easily reach the ascites because of the constant fluid exchange between these two compartments. Once micro-organisms have colonized the ascites, the development of spontaneous bacterial peritonitis would depend on the defensive capacity of ascitic fluid. Patients with a decreased antimicrobial activity of ascitic fluid would develop spontaneous bacterial peritonitis (Fig 1). The passage of enteric organisms from the bowel lumen to the peritoneal cavity through the intestinal wall, another possible mechanism for deve-

lopment of SBP, has never been clinically or experimentally demonstrated.

Spontaneous bacterial peritonitis is caused predominantly by enteric organisms [1,2,4,5], and there are three most accepted pathogenic mechanisms which explain the passing of enteric organisms from the lumen of the bowel to the systemic circulation: 1) The depression of the hepatic reticuloendothelial system, which represents a failure of the liver "filtering" these bacteria, thereby allowing the passage of micro-organisms from the bowel lumen to the systemic circulation via the portal vein; 2) The relative increase of aerobic Gram-negative bacilli in the jejunal flora in cirrhosis and the possible alteration in the intestinal barrier caused by circumstances decreasing mucosal blood flow (e.g. acute hypovolemia or

Figure 1
Pathogenesis of Spontaneous Bacterial Peritonitis (SBP).

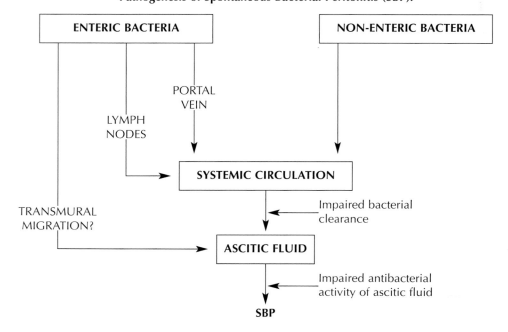

splanchnic vasoconstrictor drugs) ; 3) Bacterial translocation, or the process by which enteric bacteria normally present in the gastrointestinal tract, can cross the mucosa and infect the mesenteric lymph nodes and reach the bloodstream through the intestinal lymphatic circulation. To explain the mechanism of SBP caused by non-enteric bacteria, it can reasonably be assumed that these micro-organisms enter the circulation from the skin or the upper respiratory tract, the pathogenesis being aided in many cases by therapeutic or diagnostic procedures which rupture the natural mucocutaneous barriers. Whatever the source of the bacteria reaching the bloodstream, a bacteraemic event could be more prolonged and, therefore, could more readily become clinically significant in cirrhotic patients than in non-cirrhotic subjects, because of the marked depression of the reticulendothelial system in the former. As indicated above, once micro-organisms have colonized the ascites, the development of spontaneous bacterial peritonitis would depend on the defensive capacity of ascitic fluid (Fig 1).

1.2. Predisposing factors of SBP in Cirrhosis

1.2.1. Latrogenic factors

In addition to procedures well known to predispose to infection such as intravenous or urethral catheters, cirrhotic patients are frequently subjected to other diagnostic or therapeutic maneuvers which may alter the natural defense barrier and, therefore, increase the risk of bacterial infection. Endoscopic sclerotherapy for bleeding esophageal varices, particularly emergency sclerotherapy, seems to be associated with bacteremia with an incidence ranging from 5 to 30 per cent [6,7]. Despite in some ca-

ses sclerotherapy being implicated in the development of serious infective complications such as purulent meningitis [8] and bacterial peritonitis [9], bacteremia is usually a transient phenomenon and the use of prophylactic antibiotics is not recommended. The placement of a transjugular intrahepatic portosystemic stent for the treatment of bleeding esophageal varices is not associated with the development of significant bacterial infections. Cirrhotic patients with a peritoneovenous shunt (LeVeen shunt) frequently develop infective complications, particularly spontaneous bacteremia and peritonitis. In several series the incidence of bacterial infections after the insertion of a LeVeen shunt for the treatment of ascites was approximately 20 per cent [10,11]. Finally, there is a very low risk of clinically relevant infection with other invasive techniques often performed in these patients, such as diagnostic or therapeutic paracentesis and endoscopy.

1.2.2. Changes in the intestinal flora and in the intestinal barrier

Whereas aerobic (facultative) Gram-negative bacilli are present in low numbers in the small bowel of normal subjects, these micro-organisms have been found to be significantly increased in the jejunal flora of many cirrhotic patients [12]. The change in the intestinal flora caused by the abnormal small bowel colonization in cirrhosis may increase the chance that aerobic Gram-negative bacteria will invade the bloodstream and cause infections of enteric origin in these patients. In addition, it has been shown in CCl4 induced cirrhotic rats with ascites, that there is an increased passage of bacteria from the intestinal lumen to extraintestinal sites, including regional lymph nodes and the systemic circulation [13-15]. Causes for bacterial translocation are a disruption of the intestinal permeability barrier, bacterial overgrowth and/or a decrease in host immune defenses. The submucosa of the cecum of cirrhotics rats with ascites becomes markedly edematous and inflamed suggesting that in these animals, portal hypertension could produce a rupture in the intestinal permeability barrier and thus favor bacterial translocation [15]. Changed permeability of the intestinal mucosa has been seen in hemorrhagic shock, sepsis, injury or administration of endotoxin [16]. In portal hypertensive rats [13,17] it has been shown that hemorrhagic shock is followed by an increased bacterial translocation to mesenteric lymph nodes suggesting that the hemorragic shock, a non infrequent event in cirrhotic patients, could alter the intestinal barrier in these animals.

1.2.3. Depression of activity of the reticuloendothelial system

Although the reticuloendothelial system is widely distributed throughout the body, approximately 90 per cent of this defensive system is in the liver, where Kupffer cells and endothelial sinusoidal cells are the major components. The special location of the reticuloendothelial system is thus considered to be the main defensive mechanism against bacteria and other infections acquired through a hematogenous route, such as SBP [18]. Several groups have demonstrated that many cirrhotic patients show marked depression of reticuloendothelial system function, particularly of the hepatic reticuloendothelial system fraction. In addition, it has been shown that the risk of acquiring bacteraemia and SBP in cirrhosis is directly related to the degree of dysfunction of the reticuloendothelial system in these patients [19,20].

The pathogenesis of the depression of phagocytic activity of the reticuloendothelial system in cirrhosis is not clear. However, several mechanisms have been proposed to explain the impairment of the reticuloendothelial system. The majority of studies suggest that this impairment could be due to the intrahepatic shunting of blood, which escapes the phagocytic action of the reticuloendothelial system cells located in the sinusoids. According to this theory, a significant amount of hepatic blood flow would circulate through anatomical or functional intrahepatic shunts which, therefore, would not be available for blood-tissue exchange [1]. Other mechanisms may also be involved including a reduction in the phagocytic capacity of monocytes, which are considered as the Kupffer cell precursors and an impaired function of macrophage Fc gamma receptors in alcoholic cirrhosis [18,21,22]. Serum opsonic activity has been found to be markedly reduced in most cirrhotic patients, probably as a consequence of a decreased serum concentration of complement and fibronectin, substances that normally stimulate the phagocytosis of micro-organisms by enhancing their adhesiveness to the reticuloendothelial cell surface.

1.2.4. Decreased Opsonic activity of the ascitic fluid

In the last few years it has been demonstrated that the non-specific antimicrobial capacity of ascitic fluid in cirrhosis varies greatly from patient to patient and this variability may be involved in the pathogenesis of SBP. Runyon reported the existence of an inverse and highly significant correlation between the opsonic activity of ascitic fluid and the risk of developing peritonitis in patients admitted to hospital with ascites

[23]. In this study, 15 per cent of patients with opsonic activity lower than normal developed SBP during their hospital stay, whereas this complication did not occur in any patient with increased opsonic activity in ascitic fluid.

Opsonic activity of ascitic fluid in cirrhosis is directly correlated with the concentration of defensive substances, such as immunoglobulins, complement and fibronectin and with the concentration of total protein in ascites [23-27]. Interestingly, several investigators have found that concentration of total protein in ascitic fluid, a very easy measurement in clinical practice, correlated very well with the risk of SBP in cirrhosis with ascites. It has been demonstrated that patients with protein concentration in ascitic fluid below 1 g/dl developed peritonitis during their hospital stay with a significantly higher frequency than those with a greater protein content in ascites [15 per cent versus 2 per cent, respectively) [24] and that the cumulative probability of developing peritonitis during long-term follow-up is significantly greater in cirrhotics with ascites whose ascitic fluid concentration of total protein was below 1 g/dl than in those with an ascitic protein concentration over 1g/dl [20 versus 2 per cent, respectively after 1 year) [26]. Finally, the probability of the first episode of SBP in cirrhotic patients with ascites is significantly influenced by the antimicrobial capacity of ascitic fluid and hepatic function with ascitic fluid protein levels and serum bilirubin levels being the most single and useful indicators of a high risk of peritonitis [27].

The reason for the variation in the antimicrobial properties, the concentration of defensive substances and the total protein content in ascitic fluid in cirrhotic patients is unknown, although several authors have suggested that all these indices could be related (a) to the serum levels of the defensive proteins involved in antibacterial mechanisms of ascitic fluid; (b) to the degree of portal hypertension and hepatic insufficiency and (c) to the volume of water diluting ascitic fluid solutes. This last possibility is supported by the finding that diuretic-induced reduction of water in ascitic fluid increases the total protein concentration and the antibacterial power of ascites [28] and by the common observation in clinical practice that SBP occurs predominantly in cirrhotics with large volume ascites.

1.2.5. Neutrophil leucocyte dysfunction

A high proportion of cirrhotic patients show altered neutrophil leucocyte function at different levels. The most frequent disturbance is a marked reduction of chemotaxis, probably caused by the presence of substances in the serum that are capable of inhibiting granulocyte migration. The nature of these chemotactic inhibitory substances has not yet been determined. Furthermore, the phagocytic and bacterial killing capacity of neutrophils has been found to be reduced in many cirrhotic patients [29]. Leucocyte dysfunction has not been investigated adequately in relation to the risk in cirrhotic patients of acquiring bacterial infections. However, since the types of infection frequently developed by patients with congenital or acquired neutrophyl-function abnormalities (mainly chronic granulomatous diseases and recurrent staphylococcal and fungal infections) are very different from the infections developed by cirrhotic patients, it seems very unlikely that leucocyte dysfunction plays a major role in the susceptibility of cirrhosis to bacterial infections.

Table 1
Micro-organisms isolated in 123 episodes of spontaneous
bacterial peritonitis (SBP) in cirrhosis (39).

Culture positive SBP	82 (67%)
Gram-negative bacilli	61
E. Coli	45
Klebsiella spp.	7
Other	9
Gram-positive cocci	21
S. pneumoniae	12
Other sptreptococci	8
S. aureus	1
Culture negative SBP	41 (33%)

1.3. Treatment

Antibiotic therapy in spontaneus bacterial peritonitis has to be started once the diagnosis is established on the basis of a polymorphonuclear cell count higher than 250 cells/mm3 [30]. Table 1 shows the most common organisms isolated in patients with SBP. The empirical treatment should cover all this organism without causing adverse effects. Third generation cephalosporins are considered the gold standard in the treatment of SBP complicating cirrhosis. However, other antibiotics are also effective in the treatment of this infective complication.

1.3.1. Treatment of SBP with cefotaxime (Table 2)

In 1985 Felisart et al [31] published the first investigation assessing the efficacy of cefotaxime in patients with SBP. It consisted in a randomized controlled trial comparing cefotaxime (2g every 4 hrs in patients without renal failure) with a combination of ampicillin plus tobramycin in a large series of cirrhotic patients with SBP or other severe bacterial infections. Cefotaxime was more effective in achieving SBP resolution than ampicillin plus tobramycin and whereas no patient treated with cefotaxime developed nephrotoxicity and superinfections, these two complications occurred in more that 10% of the patients treated with ampicillin plus tobramycin. Following this study, cefotaxime is considered as one of the first-choice antibiotic therapies in the empirical treatment of SBP in patients with cirrhosis.

Two randomized controlled trials assessing the optimal duration of therapy and dosage of cefotaxime in cirrhotic patients with SBP have recently been reported. Runyon et al [32] randomized 90 patients with SBP to receive cefotaxime (2g i.v. every 8 h.) during 10 days (43 patients) or during 5 days (47 patients). Resolution of the infection (93.1% vs 91.2%), recurrence of SBP during hospitalization (11.6% v.s. 12.8%) and hospital

Table 2
Cefotaxime in the treatment of spontaneous bacterial peritonitis (SBP)

	SBP Resolution	Superinfection	Hospital Survival
FELISART et al (31) (2 g/ 4h)	86%	—	73%
ARIZA et al (34) (1 g/ 6h)	81%	—	42%

RUNYON et al (32)
  * 5 DAYS TREATMENT
  * 10 DAYS TREATMENT
	93%
	91%
		—
		—
			67%
			42%

RIMOLA et al (33)
  * 2 g/ 6h
  * 2 g/ 12h
	75%
	79%
		—
		—
			69%
			79%

mortality (32.6% vs 42.5%) was comparable in the two groups. Short-course treatment with cefotaxime is, therefore, as efficacious as long-course therapy in cirrhotic patients with SBP. Rimola et al [33] have reported the results of a randomized multicenter controlled trial in 143 patients with SBP treated with cefotaxime comparing two different dosages: 2g every 6h (71 cases) vs 2g every 12 h (72 cases). The rate of SBP resolution (77% vs 79%) and patient survival (69% vs 79%) were similar in both groups. Therefore, doses of cefotaxime lower than those usually recommended are very effective in SBP.

1.3.2. Treatment of SBP with other parenteral antibiotics (Table 3)

Several investigations have been carried out to assess the efficacy of other antibiotic regimes in these patients. In 1986, Ariza et al [34] evaluated the use of aztreonam in 16 episodes of SBP caused by enterobacteria. Overall mortality during hospitalization was 62%. Superinfections due to resistant organisms were detected in 3 cases (19%).

These results, together with the fact that aztreonam is only capable of covering approximately 75% of the potential organism causing SBP, suggest that this antibiotic is probably not adequate for the empirical treatment of cirrhotic patients with SBP. In 1989, Mercader et al [35] reported that ceftriaxone 2g/day, was effective in 83% of 18 episodes of SBP in cirrhotic patients. Three patients developed superinfections *(Candida* in 2 and *Enterococcus* in one). More recently ceftriaxone (2g/24h) and cefonicid 2g/12h.) have been compared in an open randomized trial [36]. Both antibiotics showed similar efficacy in the treatment of SBP, with a resolution rate of 100% for ceftriaxone and 94% for cefonicid. Despite this high efficacy, hospital mortality rate was 30% and 37% respectively. Three patients treated with ceftriaxone and two patients treated with cefonicid developed colonizations with *Enterococcus faecalis* or *Candida albicans*. Finally, in an investigation published in 1990 by Grange et al [37], the administration of 1g/6h of amoxicillin associated to clavulanic acid was found to be effective in 85% of 27 episodes of SBP. One patient developed superinfection.

Table 3
Other parenteral antibiotics in the treatment of spontaneous bacterial peritonitis (SBP)

	SBP Resolution	Superinfection	Hospital Survival
CEFTRIAXONE (35,36)	91%	—	70%
CEFONICID (36)	94%	—	63%
AZTREONAM (34)	66%	16%	50%
AMOXICILLIN + CLAVULANIC ACID (37)	85%	4%	63%

1.3.3. *Treatment of SBP with oral antibiotics*

In most instances, patients with SBP are in relatively good clinical condition and could be treated orally. Two studies have been reported assessing the effectiveness of oral antibiotics in SBP. Both studies used wide spectrum quinolone which are almost completely absorbed after oral administration and rapidly diffuse to the ascitic fluid. Silvain et al [38] reported the effectiveness of oral pefloxacin alone (1 case) or in combination with other oral antibiotics (cotrimoxazole, 9 cases; amoxicillin, 3 cases; cefadroxil, 1 case; and cotrimoxazole plus metronidazole, 1 case) in 15 SBP episodes. The rate of infection resolution was 87%. Two patients developed superinfections and the survival at the end of hospitalization was 60%. Navasa et al [39] have recently reported the results of a randomized controlled trial in patients with non-severely complicated SBP (no septic shock, ileus or serum creatinine >3 mg/dl) comparing oral ofloxacin (400 mg/12 h) vs intravenous cefotaxime (2g every 6 h). The rate of infection resolution and patient survival were similar in the two groups. In addition, the incidence of superinfections and the length of antibiotic treatment were also similar in both groups, suggesting that oral ofloxacin is as effective as intravenous cefotaxime in

the treatment of non-severely complicated SBP in cirrhosis.

1.4. Predictors of SBP resolution and survival

Two hundred and thirteen consecutive episodes of SBP empirically treated with cefotaxime in 185 cirrhotic patients were retrospectively analyzed by Toledo et al [40] to identify predictors of infection resolution and patients survival at the time of diagnosis. In a multivariate analysis 4 out of 51 clinical and laboratory variables considered at the time of diagnosis of infection (band neutrophils in white blood cell count, community-acquired vs hospital acquired SBP, blood urea nitrogen and serum aspartate aminotransferase levels) were identified as independent predictors of infection resolution and six (blood urea nitrogen serum aspartate aminotransferase level, community acquired vs hospital acquired SBP, age, Child-Pugh score and ileus) as independent predictors of survival. A study by Follo et al [41] in 252 consecutive episodes of SBP has shown that the development renal of impairment following diagnosis of SBP is the strongest independent predictor of patient mortality in those episodes responding to cefotaxime. Renal impairment occurred in 83 episodes (33%) and in every instance it fulfilled the criteria of functional renal failure. Renal impairment was progressive in 35 episodes, steady in 27 and transient in 21. Mortality rate was 100% in episodes associated with progressive renal impairment, 31% in episodes associated with steady renal impairment, 5% in episodes with transient renal impairment and 7% in episodes without renal impairment. Other independent predictors of mortality in this series were age, blood urea nitrogen at diagnosis, isolation of the responsible organism in the ascitic blood culture and peak serum bilirubin during the antibiotic treatment.

Severe infection of SBP, promotes the inflammatory response, characterized by the activation of macrophages and PMN and release of cytokines. Recent studies [42,43] have shown that the plasma and ascitic fluid concentration of cytokines (tumor necrosis factor and interleukin-6) are markedly increased in cirrhotic patients with SBP and that they have prognostic value in cirrhotic patients with severe bacterial infections.

1.5. Prophylaxis of SBP

Cirrhotic patients with gastrointestinal hemorrhage are predisposed to develop severe bacterial infections during or immediately after the bleeding episode. Rimola et al [44] and Soriano et al [45] have shown that short-term intestinal decontamination is effective in preventing SBP in cirrhotic patients with gastrointestinal hemorrhage. In a recent study, systemic antibiotic therapy was evaluated in the prevention of infections in cirrhotic patients with gastrointestinal hemorrhage [46]. Ofloxacin 400 mg/day for ten days and amoxicillin plus clavulanic acid before each endoscopy performed during hemorrhage, significantly re-

duced bacterial infections in cirrhotic patients with gastrointestinal hemorrhage caused by ruptured esophageal varices (20% treated group vs 66% control group).

Cases with low ascitic fluid total protein concentration may be a second group of cirrhotic patients who may benefit from short-term intestinal decontamination. This contention has been proved by Soriano et al [47] in a randomized controlled study in 63 patients admitted to hospital for the treatment of an episode of ascites with an ascitic fluid total protein concentration lower than 1.5 g/dl. Thirty-two patients received oral norfloxacin (400 mg/day) throughout all the hospitalization period. The remaining 31 patients did not receive norfloxacin. The incidence of SBP was 0% in patients treated with norfloxacin and 22% in the control group.

Patients recovering from an episode of SBP represent a unique population assessing the effect of long-term intestinal decontamination in the prophylaxis of SBP. Ginés et al [48] have investigated in a double-blind placebo-controlled trial the effect of long-term administration of norfloxacin in 80 cirrhotic patients who had recovered from an episode of SBP. The overall probability of SBP recurrence at 1 year of follow-up was 20% in the norfloxacin group and 68% in the placebo group and the probability of SBP caused by aerobic Gram-negative bacilli at 1 year of follow-up was 3% and 60%, respectively. Only one patient treated with norfloxacin experienced side effects related to treatment (oral and esophageal candidiasis). Long-term selective intestinal decontamination, therefore, dramatically decreases the rate of SBP recurrence in patients with SBP. A recent study has shown that cirrhotic patients with ascites on long-term selective intestinal decontamination with norfloxacin often develop fecal organisms resistant to fluoroquinolones within the first 45 days of treatment [49]. The clinical relevance of this finding regarding the development of SBP, however, is uncertain since, as indicated previously, Ginés et al have demonstrated that long-term norfloxacin administration drastically reduces the incidence of SBP recurrence. In addition, a very recent study has shown that micro-organisms isolated from feces of patients receiving ciprofloxacin for the prevention of the SBP did not develop resistance to this antibiotic after 6 months of treatment [50]. In this study that included cirrhotic patients with protein concentration in ascitic fluid <1.5 g/dl, ciprofloxacin 750 mg once a week reduced the incidence of SBP during follow-up from 22% (placebo group) to 3.6%. Trimethoprim-sulfamethoxazol, 1 double-strength tablet 5 times/wk, was also effective in the prevention of SBP in cirrhotic patients with ascites [51]. In this randomized controlled trial with a medium follow-up of only 90 days, the incidence of SBP was 26.7% in the control group and 3.3% in the group of patients receiving trimethoprim-sulfamethoxazole prophylaxis. These two studies suggest that the cost of the antibiotic prophylaxis in the prevention of SBP may be significantly reduced by administering ciprofloxacin once a week, instead of the proposed administration of norfloxacin once a day, or by using cheaper antibiotics. However, it should be kept in mind that the best way of doing prophylaxis is to select patients very carefully. Among cirrhotic patients with ascites, those who have recovered from a SBP episode and those with low protein content in the ascitic fluid may benefit from antibiotic prophylaxis. In those cirrhotic patients with ascites and protein concentration higher than 1 g/dl, the risk of SBP is very low and therefore they are not good candidates for antibiotic prophylaxis.

Two studies have been performed assessing the incidence and predictive factors of a first episode of SBP in cirrhotic patients with ascites. Llach et al [26] showed in a series of 127 patients admitted to hospital for the treatment of an episode of ascites that the appearance probability of first-SBP is 11% at one year and 15% at three years of follow-up. Five variables obtained at admission were significantly associated with a higher risk of SBP appearance during follow-up (poor nutritional status, increased serum bilirubin levels, decreased prothrombine activity, increased serum AST levels and low ascitic fluid protein concentration) but only one (low ascitic fluid protein concentration) showed independent predictive value. The 1-year and 3-year probabilities of first episode of SBP in patients with ascitic fluid protein content lower than 1 g/dl and equal to or greater than 1 g/dl were 0% and 4% and 20% and 24%, respectively. In a similar study performed in 110 consecutive cirrhotic patients hospitalized for the treatment of an episode of ascites, Andreu et al [27] identified 6 variables associated with a higher risk of first SBP appearance during follow-up (serum bilirubin > 2.5 mg/dl, prothrombin activity < 60%, ascitic fluid total protein concentration <1 g/dl, serum sodium concentration < 130 mEq/l, platelet count < 116,000/mm³ and serum albumin concentration < 26 g/l) but only two (ascitic fluid protein concentration and serum bilirubin) showed independent predictive value. Using these two variables a relative risk index of a first SBP episode was constructed. The one year cumulative probability for a first episode of SBP in all patients was 29% The corresponding values in the 55 patients with risk index higher and lower than the median value were 8% and 50%, respectively. Both studies, therefore, indicate that cirrhotic patients with ascites who are at risk of developing a first episode of

SBP can be identified using routine biochemical parameters and suggest that these patients might benefit from selective intestinal decontamination. Finally, since the prognosis of patients recovering from a SBP episode is very poor, liver transplantation should be considered in these patients [30].

2. PERITONITIS IN PATIENTS ON PERITONEAL DIALYSIS

Peritonitis in patients on peritoneal dialysis is characterized by the appearance of cloudy fluid and abdominal pain [52]. The presence of peritonitis is strongly suggested by an effluent dialysate leukocyte count exceeding 100 cells/mL with more than 50% polymorphonuclear leuckocytes. The culture of the cloudy dialysate is generally positive for bacteria or fungi. However, 20% of the episodes that meet the criteria for peritonitis based on cell count are culture negative. Main reasons for culture negative dialysates are inadequate culture technique or antibiotic therapy at the time of the culture. Other causes include chemical peritonitis, intra-abdominal malignancy, chyloperitoneum, eosinophilic peritonitis, pancreatitis and sclerosing peritonitis. Peritonitis rates have decreased over time. The actual rate of peritonitis in patients on continuous ambulatory peritoneal dialysis (CAPD) using disconnect systems range from 0.4 to 1.1 episodes/patient/year [52].

2.1. Pathogenesis

The pathogenesis of peritonitis in patients on CAPD is not well known. It is possible that for the development of peritonitis in these patients the complementary action of two factors is required. One is the arrival of the micro-organism in the peritoneal cavity due to contamination at the time of an exchange, equipment malfunction, catheter related infection, enteric or gynecological source or after a bacteremic episode. The second factor required is a decrease in the immunological defenses of the peritoneum [53]. The main defenses of the peritoneum depend upon macrophages, B lymphocytes and the concentration of opsonic proteins such as IgG, complement and fibronectin. Both the number of macrophages per unit volume and the concentration of opsonic proteins are reduced when dialysis fluid is continuously present in the peritoneal sac [53,54]. In addition, the fluids used for CAPD are toxic to both macrophages and to mesothelial cells [54]. Whether clinical peritonitis appears depends on the perturbation in the balance between host defenses and the micro-organism.

2.2. Risk factors

Different factors have been identified as potential risk factors for the development of peritonitis in patients on CAPD including race (black), low education levels, diabetes mellitus, age > 60 years, connection device, previous episodes of peritonitis, lower effluent opsonic activity, HIV-infected patients and serum albumin levels [52]. Most of them are controversial but probably reflect that the arrival of a virulent micro-organism and an impaired peritoneal immune status are required for the development of peritonitis.

2.3. Treatment

Most of the micro-organisms causing peritonitis in patients on CAPD are Gram-positive (65%), followed by Gram-negative (25%), fungi (6%) and anaerobes (4%) [55-59]. For this reason, the empirical treatment usually includes vancomycin and ceftazidime, with the intention of covering the two most prominent groups of micro-organisms responsible for peritonitis. This empirical treatment can be appropriately modified according to the results of the culture of the dialysate and the in vitro susceptibility of the isolated organisms, always considering the diffusion of the proposed antibiotic from blood into the peritoneum and the possibility of chemical peritonitis after intraperitoneal administration. The most adequate antibiotic therapy according to the isolated organism and the convenience of antibiotic prophylaxis are discussed below.

Gram-positive:

Peritonitis due to *Staphylococcus epidermidis* is mainly caused by contamination at the time of a peritoneal dialysis exchange and rarely due to catheter infection [56,58]. However, *S. epidermidis* can colonize peritoneal catheter, producing a slime layer, which can extend from the exit site through the cuff into the peritoneal cavity. This biofilm is the result of the exopolysaccharide production by the micro-organisms which promotes adhesion of the organism to the plastic and protects them against phagocytic attack and the penetration of antibiotics [60]. This biofilm may play a role in recurrent *S. epidermidis* peritonitis episodes.

Vancomycin is probably the most convenient antibiotic treatment of S epidermidis peritonitis. However, in the biofilm phase, vancomycin resistance is common and then rifamycin is a reasonable alternative [61]. It should be taken into account that the activity of rifamycin is antagonized by heparin, insulin, urokinase and calcitriol within the peritoneal fluid and these drugs should, therefore, not be administered concomitantly with rifamycin [61,62].

Staphylococcus aureus peritonitis is frequently associated with a catheter infection due to *S. aureus* and catheter removal is often required to resolve the peritonitis [63]. In addition, *S. aureus* catheter infections and peritonitis are associated with colonization of skin, catheter exit site and nose. Patients with a positive nose culture of *S. aureus* at the initiation of CAPD have higher rates of *S. aureus* exit site infection, tunnel infection and peritonitis than those without *S aureus* nasal carriage [64]. Intranasal mupirocin in patients who had positive nose cultures for *S. aureus* was effective in reducing the rate of *S. aureus* catheter infections and peritonitis episodes compared with retrospective controls [65,66]. Prophylactic trimethoprim-sulfamethoxazole has been also shown to be effective in reducing rates of *S. epidermidis* and *S. aureus* peritonitis [67].

The treatment of *S. aureus* peritonitis includes 3 weeks of therapy with vancomycin, adding rifamycin if the dialysate is not clearing by day 4 [68]. If a concomitant catheter infection is present, the peritoneal catheter must be removed for resolution of the peritonitis episode or prevention of recurrence. Teicoplanin has recently been introduced as a potentially less toxic alternative glycopeptide antibiotic with similar antimicrobial efficacy.

Gram-negative:

Approximately 20 to 25 % of the peritonitis in patients on CAPD are caused by Gram-negative organism. *Pseudomonas aeruginosa* is a common Gram-negative bacilli causing peritonitis in these patients and it is frequently due to a catheter infection with the same organism. Therapy with two antibiotics active against *P. aeruginosa* should be used in order to avoid antibiotic resistance [68]. Peritonitis due to *Acinetobacter* usually oc-

curs within a few months of a previous episode of peritonitis and is infrequently associated with catheter infection [69]. *Neisseria
meningitidis* and *Campylobacter* are infrequent examples of Gram negative cocci and
Gram negative bacilli respectively causing
peritonitis in patients on CAPD.

Fungal infection is an uncommon cause of
peritonitis in patients on CAPD with a rate
that ranges from 0.01 to 0.11 per year [52].
Many different fungi have been reported as
a cause of fungal peritonitis in patients on
CAPD, particularly *Candida species, Crip-
tococcus neoformans* and *Aspergillus species* [70-72]. Antibiotic therapy without
catheter removal is not generally successful and many investigators favor rapid removal of the catheter once the diagnosis of
fungal peritonitis is confirmed to maintain
peritoneal membrane function and allow a
return to effective peritoneal dialysis. The
Ad Hoc Committee on Peritonitis Management recommends the use of flucitosine 1
g orally each day and fluconazole 150 mg
per one exchange intraperitoneally every
other day with catheter removal if there is
no clinical improvement in 4 to 7 days
[68]. It has been suggested that prophylaxis with oral nystantin during antibiotic
therapy may be effective in preventing
fungal peritonitis [73], although prior antibiotic therapy has been suggested but not
confirmed as a predisposing cause of fungal peritonitis.

Polymicrobial. When the culture of the
dialysate indicates the presence of two
gram-negative bacilli, anaerobes or combination of a fungus plus a Gram-negative bacilli, the bowel as the source of the peritonitis must be suspected and, although
polymicrobial peritonitis is not exclusively
due to bowel pathology, a secondary peritonitis has to be ruled out [74].

Other organisms. Mycobacterium Tuberculosis and other Mycobacterium Species are
very infrequent causes of peritonitis in patients on CAPD. Documented viral peritonitis is also rare in these patients.

3. PERITONITIS IN PATIENTS WITH VENTRICULOPERITONEAL SHUNTS

Infection remains a serious complication of
cerebrospinal fluid (CSF) shunt implantation
with an actual incidence that ranges between
5 and 10% [75]. Abdominal pain and tenderness characterize the initial clinical presentation of the ventriculoperitoneal (VP) shunt infection. It is important to note that patients
with VP shunt infections usually present without central nervous symptomatology, often
leading physicians to disregard the possibility
of shunt infection and to consider other diagnostic possibilities including acute appendicitis [76]. Furthermore, some shunt infections
are insidious, causing few or no symptoms in
which patients may have only intermittent
low-grade fever or general malaise. The culture of the CSF obtained from the shunt reservoir is positive in a high proportion of the
cases and it is the most accurate diagnostic
test for infection. Blood cultures are positive
in less than 50% of the cases with VP shunt
infections. Unlike other piogenic infections
involving the meninges, there is a modest inflammatory reaction and leucocyte counts
may be less than 100 cells/mm^3 in many cases [76]. The development of CSF ascites
complicating VP shunts is rare and only few
cases have been reported [77].

3.1. Pathogenesis

Different studies have shown that more
than 90% of the CSF shunt infections are

diagnosed within 6 months of shunt implantation, supporting the hypothesis that infection of a shunt is a complication of shunt surgery and colonization at the time of surgery is probably the most frequent cause of CSF shunt infections [75]. Hematogenous seeding and infection of shunts is possible but probably is not a frequent occurrence. The hematogenous route might be the cause of VP infection occurring after 6 months of shunt implantation and this would be the case of traditional meningitides caused by *H. influenzae, S. pneumoniae* and *N. meningitidis* [78]. Retrograde infection from the distal end is the most likely mechanism involving infection of externalized devices. In the case of PV shunts perforation of the bowel wall by the distal end of the VP shunt may lead to a polymicrobial infection of the shunt. *Ascaris lumbricoides* infestation has also been reported [79]. Another mechanism postulated is the breakdown of the surgical wounds or the skin overlying the shunt hardware. This may be the case of infants that scratch open the wound or debilitated or immobile patients in whom a decubitus ulcer may develop over the shunt [75].

3.2. Risk factors

Many factors have been associated with shunt infection, including the age of the patient, the etiology of hydrocephalus, skin bacterial density, the type of shunt implanted, surgeon's experience and poor operative technique [80]. Although the reason why every one of these factors may promote a higher incidence of PV shunt infections is not well known, it is possible that there is a synergistic effect between them. In fact, the use of a protocol involving all personnel concerned with pre, intra, and post-operative care of patients undergoing a shunt pro-

cedure and that includes measures with special attention to patient and skin preparation, theater schedules and timing, theater staff, shunt material, surgical technique and postoperative period, has demonstrated an important reduction in the incidence of infection per procedure, from 7.75% to 0.17% [80]. A no touch technique protocol has been shown to be also useful in reducing the incidence of shunt infection from 9.1% to 2.9% [81].

3.3. Treatment

Numerous methods of treating CSF shunt infections have been reported. However, parenteral antibiotic treatment with external drainage and infected shunt removal appears to be the most effective treatment [75,82]. The ventriculitis of shunt infections appears to clear more quickly with external drainage and the status of the infection can be regularly monitored. External drainage also allows intraventricular antibiotic administration if needed.

Since the most frequent causative organisms of CSF shunt infections are Stafilocci (*S. epidermidis* and *S. aureus* -65-80%-) and Gram negative organisms (*E. Coli, Klebsiella sp. Proteus, Pseudomonas sp*, 5-20%) [75-76], empirical antibiotic therapy might include vancomycin and ceftaxidime. This empirical antibiotic regime should be modified according to the susceptibility of the isolated organism. CSF shunt infections caused by coagulase-negative staphylococci, the most commonly encountered organism, should be treated with vancomycin. Rifampin should be added if the patient fails to improve. An increasing number of fungal infections of the CFS shunts is currently being reported. The approach to fungal shunt infections is similar to that described above. In

addition to the appropriate intravenous antifungal therapy, the infected shunt should be
removed and an external ventriculostomy
placed. The later allows drainage of purulent material, intraventicular administration
of antifungal agents and treatment of underlying hydrocephalic condition.

3.4. Prophylaxis

The efficacy of different antibiotics administered prophylacticaly during shunt implantation in the prevention of CSF shunt infections has been evaluated by many
investigators [83-91]. However, none of
these studies show clear and definitive results. On the contrary, they have produced
confusing and inconclusive results and although the use of prophylactic antibiotics in
this kind of surgery is a common practice
there is a week evidence for its use, based
on the results of the published studies. Finally, two meta-analysis including randomized clinical trials [92,93] have shown that
perioperative antimicrobial prophylaxis decreases the risk of subsequent shunt infection in patients who require placement of
internal CSF shunts in approximately 50%.
Different antibiotics have been used including oxacillin, cloxacillin, vancomycin,
meticillin, cefotiam, ceftriaxone, cefamandole and rifampin/trimethoprim [83-93].
On the basis of the published reports it is
not possible to establish the best prophylactic antibiotic regime.

REFERENCES

1. Rimola A. Infections in liver disease. En: "Oxford Textbook of Clinical Hepatology".
McIntyre N, Benhamou JP, Bircher J, Rizzetto
M, Rodés J (eds). Oxford Medical Press. Oxford 1991; 1272-1284.

2. Caly W.R, Strauss E. A prospective study of
bacterial infections in patients with cirrhosis. J Hepatol 1993; 18:353-358.

3. Runyon BA, Hoefs JC. Culture-negative
neutrocytic ascites: a variant of spontaneous
bacterial peritonitis. Hepatology 1984;
4:1209-1211.

4. Runyon B.A, Squier S, Borzio M. Translocation of gut bacteria in rats with cirrhosis to
mesenteric lymph nodes partially explains
the pathogenesis of spontaneous bacterial
peritontis. J Hepatol 1994; 21: 792-796.

5. Rimola A, Arroyo V, Rodes J. Infective complications in acute and chronic liver failu-
re:Basis and control. In:Williams R (ed). Crit
Care Medicine, Liver Failure. London:
Churchill-Livingstone 1986;93-11.

6. Rolando N, Gimson A, Philpott-Howard J,
Sahathevan M, Casewell M, Fagan E, Wes-
taby D, Williams R. Infectious sequelae after endoscopic sclerotherapy of oesophage-
al varices: role of antibiotic prophylaxis. J
Hepatol 1993; 18:290-4.

7. Selby WS, Norton ID, Pokorny CS, Bernn
RA. Bacteremia and bacteriascitis after
esophageal varices and prevention by intravenous cefotaxime: a randomized trial.
Gastrointest Endosc 1994; 40:680-4.

8. Toyoda K, Saku YU, Sadoshima S, Fujishima
M. Purulent meningitis after endoscopic injection sclerotherapy for esophageal varices. Intern Med 1994; 33:706-9.

9. Bac DJ, de Marie S, Siersema PD, Snobl J,
van Buuren HR. Post-sclerotherapy bacterial peritonitis: a complication of sclerotherapy or of variceal bleeding?. Am J Gastroenterol 1994; 89:859-62.

10. Arroyo V, Gines P, Planas R. Treatment of ascites in cirrhosis. Diuretics, peritoneovenous
shunt and large-volume paracentesis. Gastroenterol Clin North Am 1992; 21:237-256.

11. Gines A, Planas R, Angeli P, et al. Treatment
of patients with cirrhosis and refractory ascites using LeVeen shunt with titanium tip:

comparison with therapeutic paracentesis. Hepatology 1995; 22:124-131.

12. Morencos FC, de las Heras Castano G, Martin Ramos L, Lopez Arias ML, Ledesma F, Pons Romero F. Small bowel bacterial overgroth in patients with alcoholic cirrhosis. Dig Dis Sci 1995; 40:1252-6.

13. Sorell WT, Quigley EMM, Jin G, Johnson TJ, Rikkers LF. Bacterial translocation in the portal-hypertensive rat: studies in basal conditions and on exposure to hemorrhagic shock. Gastroenterology 1993; 104:1722-1726.

14. Llovet JM, Bartoli R, Planas R, Cabre E, Jimenez M, Urban A, Ojanguren I, Arnal J, Gassull MA. Bacterial translocation in cirrhotic rats. Tis role in the development of spontaneous bacterial peritonitis. Gut 1994; 35:1648-1652.

15. Garcia-Tsao G, Lee F-Y, Barden GE, Cartun R, West B. Bacterial translocation to mesenteric lymph nodes is increased in cirrhotic rats with ascites. Gastroenterology 1995; 108:1835-1841.

16. Van Leeuwen P.A.M, Boermeester M.A, Houdijk A.P.J, et al. Clinical significance of translocation. Gut 1994; Supplement 1:S28-S34.

17. Llovet JM, Bartoli R, Planas R, et al. Selective intestinal decontamination with norfloxacin reduces bacterial translocation in ascitic cirrhotic rats exposed to hemorrhagic shock. Hepatology 1996; 23:781-787.

18. Jones EA, Summerfield JA. Kupffer cells. In: Arias IM, Jakoby WB, Popper H, Schacter D, Shafritz DA, eds. The liver: biology and pathobiology. 2nd ed. New York: Raven Press 1988: 683-704.

19. Rimola A, Soto R, Bory F, Arroyo V, Piera C, Rodes J. Reticuloendothelial system phagocytic activity in cirrhosis and its relation to bacterial infections and prognosis. Hepatology 1984; 4:53-58.

20. Bolognesi M, Merkel C, Bianco S, et al. Clinical significance of the evaluation of hepatic reticuloendothelial removal capacity in patients with cirrhosis. Hepatology 1994; 19:628-634.

21. Guarner C, Runyon BA. Macrophage function in cirrhosis and the risk of bacterial infection. Hepatology 1995; 22:367-369.

22. Gomez F, Ruiz P, Schreiber AD. Impaired function of macrophage Fc gamma receptors and bacterial infection in alcoholic cirrhosis. N Engl J Med 1994: 331:1122-1128.

23. Runyon BA. Patients with deficient ascitic fluid opsonic activity are predisposed to spontaneous bacterial peritonitis. Hepatology 1988; 8:632-635.

24. Runyon BA. Low-protein-concentration ascitic fluid is predispossed to spontaneous bacterial peritonitis. Gastroenterology 1986, 91:1343-1346.

25. Tito Ll, Rimola A, Gines P, Llach J, Arroyo V, Rodes J. Recurrence of spontaneous bacterial peritonitis in cirrhosis: frequency and predictive factors. Hepatology 1988; 8:27-31.

26. Llach J, Rimola A, Navasa M,et al. Incidence and predictive factors of first episode of spontaneous bacterial peritonitis in cirrhosis with ascites: relevance of ascitic fluid protein concentration. Hepatology 1992; 16:724-727.

27. Andreu M, Solá R, Sitges-Serra A, et al. Risk factors for spontaneous bacterial peritonitis. Gastroenterology 1993; 104:1133-1138.

28. Runyon BA, Antillon MR, McHutchinson JG. Diuresis increases ascitic fluid opsonic activity in patients who survive spontaneous bacterial peritonitis. J Hepatol 1992; 14:249-252.

29. Garcia-Gonzalez M, Boixeda D, Herrero D, Burgaleta C. Effect of granulocyte-macrophage colony-stimultating factor on leukocyte function in cirrhosis. Gastroenterology 1993; 105:527-531.

30. Navasa M. Treatment of spontaneous bacterial peritonitis and other severe bacterial infections in the setting of cirrhosis. In: Treat-

ments in Hepatology. V. Arroyo, J. Bosch and J. Rodes, Eds. MASSON S.A. Barcelona (Spain) 1995, pp 109-115.

31. Felisart J, Rimola A, Arroyo V, et al. Cefotaxime is more effective than is ampicillin-tobramycin in cirrhotics with severe infections. Hepatology 1985; 5:457-462.

32. Runyon BA, McHutchison JG, Antillon MR, Akriviadis EA, Montano AA. Short- course versus long-course antibiotic treatment of spontaneous bacterial peritonitis. A randomized controlled study of 100 patients. Gastroenterology 1991; 100:1737-1742.

33. Rimola A, Salmeron JM, Clemente G, et al. Two different dosages of cefotaxime in the treatment of spontaneous bacterial peritonitis in cirrhosis: results of a prospective, randomized, multicenter study. Hepatology 1995; 21:674-679.

34. Ariza J, Xiol X, Esteve M, et al. Aztreonam vs Cefotaxime in the treatment of Gram-negative spontaneous peritonitis in cirrhotic patients. Hepatology 1991; 14:91-98.

35. Mercader J, Gómez J, Ruiz J, Garre MC, Valdés M. Use of ceftriaxone in the treatment of bacterial infections in cirrhotic patients. Chemotherapy 1989; 35(suppl 2):23-26.

36. Gómez-Jimenez J, Ribera E, Gasser I, Artaza MA, Del Valle O, Pamissa A, Martínez-Vázquez JM. Randomized trial comparing ceftriaxone with cefonicid for treatment of spontaneous bacterial peritonitis in cirrhotic patients. Antimicrob Agents Chemother 1993; 37:1587-1592

37. Grange JD, Amiot X, Grange V, et al. Amoxicillin-Clavulanic acid therapy of spontaneous bacterial peritonitis: a prospective study of twenty-seven cases in cirrhotic patients. Hepatology 1990; 11:360-364.

38. Silvain C, Breux JP, Grollier G, Rouffineau J, Breq-Giraudon B, Breauchant M. Les septicémies et les infections du liquide d°ascite du cirrhotique peuvent-elles être traitées exclusivement par voie orale?. Gastroenterol Clin Biol 1989; 13:335-339.

39. Navasa M, Planas R, Clemente G, et al. Oral ofloxacin vs intravenous cefotaxime in the treatment of non-complicated spontaneous bacterial peritonitis (SBP) in cirrhosis. Results of a multicenter, prospective, randomized trial. J Hepatol 1994; Suppl 1:S-11.

40. Toledo C, Salmerón JM, Rimola A, et al. Spontaneous Bacterial peritonitis in cirrhosis: predictive factors of infection resolution and survival in patients treated with cefotaxime. Hepatology 1993; 17: 251-257.

41. Follo A, Llovet JM, Navasa M, et al. Renal impairment after spontaneous bacterial peritonitis in cirrhosis: incidence, clinical course, predictive factors and prognosis. Hepatology 1994; 20:1495-1501.

42. Byl B, Roucloux I, Crusiaux A, Dupont E, Devière J. Tumor necrosis factor alpha and interleukin-6 plasma levels in infected cirrhotic patients. Gastroenterology 1993; 104:1492-1497.

43. Zeni F, Tardy B, Vindimian M, et al. High levels of tumor necrosis factor alpha and interleukin-6 in the ascitic fluid of cirrhotic patients with spontaneous bacterial peritonitis. Clin Infect Dis 1993; 17:218-223.

44. Rimola A, Bory F, Terés J, Pérez-Ayuso R.M, Arroyo V, Rodés J. Oral non-absorbable antibiotics prevent infection in cirrhosis with gastrointestinal hemorrhage. Hepatology 2985; 5:463-467.

45. Soriano G, Guarner C, Tomás A, et al. Norfloxacin prevents bacterial infection in cirrhotics with gastrointestinal hemorrhage. Gastroenterology 1992; 103:1267-1272.

46. Blaise M, Pateron D, Trinchet J-C, Levacher S, Beaugrand M, Pourriat J-L. Systemic antibiotic therapy prevents bacterial infection in cirrhotic patients with gastrointestinal hemorrhage. Hepatology 1994; 20:34-38.

47. Soriano G, Guarner C, Teixidó M, et al. Selective intestinal decontamination prevents spontaneous bacterial peritonitis. Gastroenterology 1991; 100:477-481.

48. Ginès P, Rimola A, Planas R, et al. Norflo-
    xacin prevents spontaneous bacterial perito-
    nitis recurrence in cirrhosis: results of a dou-
    ble-blind,   placebo-controlled   trial.
    Hepatology 1990; 12:716-724.

49. Dupeyron C, Mangeney N, Sedrati L, Cam-
    pillo B, Fouet P, Leluan G. Rapid emergen-
    ce of quinolone resistance in cirrhotic pa-
    tients treated with norfloxacin to prevent
    spontaneous bacterial peritonitis. Antimi-
    crob Agents Chemother 1994; 38:340-344.

50. Rolanchon A, Cordier L, Bacq Y, et al. Ci-
    profloxacin and long-term prevention of
    spontaneous bacterial peritonitis: results of
    a prospective controlled trial. Hepatology
    1995; 22:1171-1174.

51. Singh N, Gayowski T, Yu VL, Wagener MM.
    Trimethoprim-sulfamethoxazole for the pre-
    vention of spontaneous bacterial peritonitis
    in cirrhosis:a randomized trial. Ann Intern
    Med 1995 Apr 15; 122:595-598.

52. Piraino B,M. Infections in peritoneal dyali-
    sis. In: Nissenson AR, Fine RN and Gentle
    DE, eds. Clinical Dialysis.Appleton & Lan-
    ge, East Norwalk, Connecticut 1995: 426-
    449.

53. Cameron JS. Host defences in continuous
    ambulatory peritoneal dialysis and the ge-
    nesis of peritonitis. Pediatr Nephrol 1995,
    9:647-662.

54. Holmes C, Lewis S. Host defense mecha-
    nisms in the peritoneal cavity of continuous
    ambulatory peritoneal dialysis patients. Se-
    cond of two parts 2. Humoral defenses. Pe-
    rit Dial Int 1991; 11:112-117.

55. Golper TA, Hartstein AI. Analysis of the cau-
    sative pathogens in uncomplicated CAPD-
    associated peritonitis: duration of therapy,
    relapses and prognosis. Am J Kidney Dis
    1986; 7:141-145.

56. Eisele G, Bailie GR, Lomaestro B. Relations-
    hip between peritonitis and exit site infec-
    tions in CAPD. Adv Perit Dial 1992; 8:227-
    229.

57. Piraino B, Bernardini J, Sorkin M. A five ye-
    ar study of the microbiologic results of exit
    site infection and peritonitis in continuous
    ambulatory peritoneal dialysis. Am J Kidney
    Dis 1987; 4:281-286.

58. Holley JL, Beranrdini J, PIraino B. Infecting
    organisms in continuous peritoneal dialysis
    patients on the Y-set. Am J Kidney Dis 1994;
    23:560-573.

59. Echeverria MJ, Ayarza R, Lopez de Goicoe-
    chea MJ, et al. Comparative study of 2 cul-
    ture methods by seeding, in hemoculture
    bottles, the dialysis fluid from patients on
    continuous ambulatory peritoneal dialysis.
    Enf Inf Mic Clin 1995; 13:506-510.

60. Richards GK, Prentis J, Gagnon RF. Antibio-
    tic activity against *Staphylococcus epider-
    midis* biofilms in dialysis fluids. Adv Perit
    Dial 1989; 5:133-137.

61. Gagnon RF, Harris AD, Prentis J, Richards
    GK. The effects of heparin on rifampin acti-
    vity against *Staphylococcus epidermidis*
    biofilms. Adv Perit Dial 1989; 5:138-142.

62. Gagnon RF, Richard GK, Obst G. Modula-
    tion of rifampin action against *Staphylococ-
    cus epidermidis* biofilms by drug additives
    to peritoneal dialysis solutions. Perit Dial Int
    1993; 13:S345-S347.

63. Davies SJ, Ogg CS, Cameron JS, Ponton S,
    NOble WC. *Staphylococcus aureus* nasal
    carriage, exit-site infection and catheter loss
    in patients treated with continuous ambula-
    tory peritoneal dialysis (CAPD). Perit Dial
    Int 1989; 9:61-64.

64. Piraino B, Perlmutter JA, Holley KL, Bernar-
    dini J. Staphylococcus aureus peritonitis is
    associated with *Staphylococcus aureus* na-
    sal carriage in peritoneal dialysis patients.
    Perit Dial Int 1993; 13(suppl2):S332-S334.

65. Perez-Fontan M, Rosales M, Rodriguez-Car-
    mona A, et al. Treatment of *Staphylococcus
    aureus* nasal carriers in CAPD with mupiro-
    cin. Adv Perit Dial 1992; 8:242-245.

66. Perez-Fontan M, Garcia-Falcon T, Rosales
    M, et al. Treatment of *Staphylococcus au-*

reus nasal carriers in continuous ambulatory peritoneal dialysis with mupirocin: long-term results. Am J Kidney Dis 1993; 22:708-712.

67. Swartz R, Messana J, Starmann B, Weber M, Reynolds J. Preventing *Staphylococcus aureus* infection during chronic peritoneal dialysis. J Am Soc Nephrol 1991; 2:1085-1091.

68. The Ad Hoc Advisory Committee on Peritonitis Management. Peritoneal dialysis related peritonitis treatment recommendations 1993 update. Perit Dial Int 1993; 13:14-28.

69. Ruiz A, Ramos B, Burgos D, Frutos MA, Lopez de Novales E. *Acinetobacter calcoaceticus* peritonitis in continuous ambulatory peritoneal dialysis (CAPD) patients. Perit Dial Int 1988; 8:285-286.

70. Miles AM, Barth RH. *Aspergillus* peritonitis: therapy, survival, and return to peritoneal dialysis. Am J Kidney Dis 1995; 26:80-3.

71. Hoch BS, Namboodiri NK, Banayat G, et al. The use of fluconazole in the management of *Candida* peritonitis in patients on peritoneal dialysis. Perit Dial Int 1993; 13(suppl 2):S357-S366.

72. Yinnon AM, Solages A, Treanor JJ. *Cryptococcal* peritonitis: report of a case developing during continuous ambulatory peritoneal dialysis and review of the literature. Clin Infect Dis 1993; 17:736-741.

73. Zaruba K, Peters J, Jungbluth H. Succesful prophylaxis for fungal peritonitis in patients on continuous ambulatory peritoneal dialysis: six years experience. Am J Kidney Dis 1991; 17:43-46.

74. Holley JL, Bernardini J, Piraino B. Polymicrobial peritonitis in patients on continuous peritoneal dialysis. Am J Kidney Dis 1992; 19:162-166.

75. Kaufman B.A, Tunkel A.R, Pryor J.C, Dacey Jr R.G, Meningitis in the neurosurgical patient. Infect Dis Clin North Am 1990; 4:677-701.

76. Forward K.R, F.R.C.P. (C), Derek Fewer H, Grant Stiver H. Cerebrospinal fluid infections. J Neurosurg 1983; 59:389-394.

77. Yount R.A, Glazier M.C, Mealey J, Kalsbeck J.E. Cerebrospinal fluid ascites complicating ventriculoperitoenal shunting. J Neurosurg 1984; 61:180-183.

78. Ronan A, Hogg GG, Klug GL. Cerebrospinal fluid infection in children. Pediatr Inf Dis J 1995; 4:782-786.

79. Peter JC, Lamprecht J, Rode H. Ascaris lumbricoides: an unusual cause of shunt infection. Childs Nervous System 1992; 8:294-296.

80. Choux M, Genitori L, Lang D, F.R.C.S., Lena G. Shunt implantation: reducing the incidence of shunt infection. J Neurosurg 1992; 77:875-880.

81. Faillace WJ. A no-touch technique protocol to diminish cerebrospinal fluid shunt infection. Surg Neurol 1995; 43:344-350.

82. Yogev R. Cerebrospinal fluid shunt infections: A personal view. Pediatr Infect Dis J 1985; 4:113-117.

83. Zentner J; Gilsbach J, Felder T. Antibiotic prophylaxis in cerebrospinal fluid shunting: a prospective randomized trial in 129 patients. Neurosurg Rev 1995; 18:169-172.

84. Wlaters BC, Goumnerova L, Hoffman HJ, Hendrick EB, Humphreys RP, Levinton C. A randomized controlled trial of perioperative rifampin/trimethoprim in cerebrospinal fluid shunt surgery. Childs Nervous System 1992; 8:253-257.

85. Ajir F, Levin AB, Duff TA. Effect of prophylactic methicillin on cerebrospinal fluid infections in children. Neurosurgery 1981; 9:6-8.

86. Alvares-Garijo JA, Mengual MV. Infection rate with and without prophylactic antibiotic therapy after shunt infection. Monogr Neurol Sci 1982; 8:66-68.

87. Blomstedt GC. Results of trimethoprim-sulfamethoxazole prophylaxis in ventriculostomy and shunting procedures. A double-blind randomized trial. J Neurosurg 1985; 62:694-697.

88. Haines SJ. Antibiotic prophylaxis in neurosurgery. The controlled trials. Neurosurg Clin North Am 1992; 3:355-358.

89. Haines SJ, Taylor F. Prophylactic methicillin for shunt operations: effects on incidence of shunt malfunction and infection. Childs Brain 1982; 9:10-22.

90. Schmidt K, Gjerris G, Osgaard O, et al. Antibiotic prophylaxis in cerebrospinal fluid shunting: a prospective randomized trail in 152 hydrocephalic patients. Neurosurgery 1985; 17:1-5.

91. Young RF, Lawner PM. Perioperative antibiotic prophylaxis for prevention of postoperative neurosurgical infections. A randomized clinical trial. J Neurosurg 1987; 66:701-705.

92. Langley JM, LeBlanc JC, Drake J, Milner R. Efficacy of antimicrobial prophylaxis in placement of cerebrospinal fluid shunts: meta-analysis. Clin Infect Dis 1993; 17:98-103.

93. Haines SJ, Walters BC. Antibiotic prophylaxis for cerebrospinal fluid shunts: a meta-analysis. Neurosurgery 1994; 34:87-92.

Secondary Peritonitis

Daniel E. Swartz and Nicolas V. Christou

The gut can be seen as an extension of the external surface of the body in which the resident bacterial flora exist symbiotically and in balance with the tissues of the host. It is when the normal host defense mechanisms are compromised or overwhelmed that the epithelial barrier is predisposed to breakdown resulting in peritonitis and its complications.

1. DEFINITION

Secondary peritonitis is defined as inflammation of the peritoneum, secondary to perforation of a hollow viscus or transmural necrosis of, gastrointestinal tract. Secondary peritonitis is usually but not always, caused by a mono- or polymicrobial inoculum, at which point it fulfills the definition of intra-abdominal infection. Examples include perforated appendicitis, perforated duodenal ulcer, perforated sigmoid colon secondary to diverticulitis, volvulus or cancer, strangulation obstruction of the small bowel and post-operative anastomotic disruption.

The terms sepsis, infection and systemic inflammatory response syndrome (SIRS) are distinct, non-interchangeable terms as defined by the 1992 Consensus Conference of the American College of Chest Physicians and the Society of Critical Care Medicine. Infection is the documented evidence of microbial growth in culture or presence in staining. SIRS is defined as two or more of the following: a temperature higher than 38°C or lower than 36°C; a pulse greater than 90 beats per minute; a respiratory rate greater than 20 breaths per minute or an arterial carbon dioxide pressure of less than 32 mm Hg and a white blood cell count greater than 12,000 or less than 4,000 per mm^3 or greater than 10% bands on differential. This definition is valid only in the absence of any other cause such as the immediate post-operative state. Sepsis is defined as the presence of SIRS with documented infection.

An intra-abdominal abscess is a well-defined collection of pus walled-off from the rest of the peritoneal cavity by inflammatory adhesions, loops of intestine, mesentery, greater omentum and other viscera. The abscess may be located intra- or extra-viscerally within the peritoneal cavity or within the retroperitoneum. Extravisceral abscesses occur after resolution of diffuse peritonitis when a loculation of infection persists or after visceral perforations, such as anastomotic breakdowns and become walled off by peritoneal defense mechanisms. Visceral abscesses usually occur secondary to hematogenous or lymphatic spread of bacteria. Retroperitoneal abscesses are the result of hematogenous or lymphatic spread to retroperitoneal tissues or perforations of retropertioneal viscera of the gastrointestinal tract.

2. EPIDEMIOLOGY OF SECONDARY PERITONITIS

Mortality rates have changed little since the advent of antibiotics in the 1930's. Reported mortality rates vary from 0 to 70% reflecting a variety of etiologies and severities of peritonitis in patients with varying degrees of chronic diseases and immunocompetency. The improvements in surgical therapy and in identifying patients at risk of

mortality as well as the enhanced bactericidal capacity in antibiotic regimens are offset by a greater number of older, more severely ill patients with weakened immune defenses. Table 1 reviews the most recently reported mortality rates and mean APACHE II scores in clinical studies of intra-abdominal infections.

The risk of mortality appears to correlate more with the capacity of the host to respond, rather than the cause or severity of the infection or of the regimen of antibiotics used. A recent prospective, consecutive, observational study of 239 adult patients with intra-abdominal infections requiring surgery and APACHE II scores greater than 10 demonstrated a 32% mortality. Significant independent risk factors

Table 1
Reported mortality rates of intra-abdominal infections

Author	Year	N	Design	Entry Criteria	Mean APACHE II	Mortality (%)
Koperna	1996	92	P,O	Pro IAI	12.7	18.5
Pacelli	1996	604	R,O	Pro IAI	11	21.3
Ercan	1993	14	R,O	Pro IAI		29
Ohmann	1993	271	P,O	Pro IAI	30.3	21
Christou	1993	239	P,O	Pro IAI, APII > 10	18.4	32
Hakkiluoto	1992	21	P,O	Pro IAI	22	52
Sawyer	1992	29	R,O	Pro IAI, APII ≥ 15	21	52
Poenaru	1991	118	P,O	Sus IAI	14.5	18.6
Schein	1990	87	P,RCT	Pro IAI	9	17
Wittmann	1990	117	P,O	Pro IAI, > 48 hrs	16.5	24
Kumar	1989	50	R,O	Sus IAI		30
Garcia-Sabrido	1988	15	R,O	Pro IAI, APII > 15	24.3	27
Total	—	**1657**	—	—	**18**	**16**

Abbreviations: number of study participants (N), prospective (P), retrospective (R), observational (O), randomized controlled trial (RCT), proven (Pro) or suspected (Sus) intra-abdominal infections (IAI).

included the APACHE II score, serum albumin level and the New York Heart Association level [1]. The relative importance of host defense mechanisms in intra-abdominal infections has been reproduced in animal studies. In one controlled porcine study in which 63 animals were inoculated intraperitoneally with varying concentrations of stool, E coli and B fragilis cultures, the most sensitive independent predictor of mortality at 24 hours was the serial acute physiology score (positive predicted value of 75%) [2]. When this value was combined with the area under the curve of bacterial concentration in the presence of feces which takes into account bacterial dose, elimination and proliferation, the positive predicted value for 24-hour mortality increased to 84%.

3. SCORING SYSTEMS

The utility of scoring systems in evaluating patients with intra-abdominal infection is to stratify groups of patients according to risk of mortality, define inclusion and exclusion criteria in clinical trials and to make comparisons of treatment regimens. Similar to statistical values, scores are assessments of populations, not individuals and thus are not intended to guide therapeutic decisions relating to individual patients.

Many scoring systems have been used in predicting outcomes in patients with intra-abdominal infections. They include the Acute Physiology and Chronic Health and Evaluation (APACHE) II score [3,4,5,6,7], the Multiple Organ System Failure (MOSF) or Goris score [4,8], Multiple Organ Dysfunction Syndrome (MODS) Score [9], Mannheim Peritonitis Index (MPI) [6,10] and Peritonitis Index Altona (PIA) II [11]. These scores are usually calculated prior to

treatment but the predictive value may be improved if serial scores are calculated after treatment has been administered. In one study, twenty-nine patients with severe intra-abdominal infections (mean APACHE II ≥ 15, predicted mortality = 50%) were prospectively observed. While preoperative APACHE II scores among survivors and patients who died were not significantly different, an increase in mean of APACHE II on post-operative days 3 and 7 was associated with 91% risk of mortality, while a decrease on those days was associated with 22% mortality [7]. Other authors concur with use in sequential scoring [5].

The ideal scoring system combines simplicity with optimal predictive value and it has long been an object of controversy. One of the principal purposes of these systems is to allow interstudy comparisons of treatment which is predicated on investigators using the same system. Despite the fact that each system has its own group of proponents, most studies to date use the APACHE II system. Investigations which compare scoring systems in their ability to predict outcome have determined that the APACHE II is at least equivalent to and usually more accurate, than any other system [4,6]. The strongest supporting data from this comes from Ohmann and co-workers who compared the predictive accuracy for mortality of APACHE II, MPI and PIA II in a prospective observational study of 271 patients with confirmed intra-abdominal infection. They demonstrated that APACHE II was superior with respect to discriminating ability (as determined by area under receiver-operator curve) and reliability in which there were no significant differences between predicted and observed mortality rates. Although the best of the three, the APACHE II discriminating ability is still associated with unacceptably high false positive and false negative rates when applied to individuals. The Surgical Infection Society as well as most investigators of intra-abdominal infections and the authors of this chapter advocate the use of APACHE II in defining risk groups but not for making therapeutic decisions for individual patients [12].

The APACHE II score, introduced in 1985 by Knaus, was designed to be less cumbersome than the original APACHE score [3]. The scoring is comprised of three parts: an acute physiology score grading eleven physiological and laboratory variables from zero to four with a twelfth variable reflecting neurologic status using the Glasgcow Coma Scale, a point system for age of the patient and an assessment of chronic disease in five organ systems. The estimated risk of death can be calculated from the APACHE II score as follows [5]:

$$ln(R/1-R) = -3.517 + (APACHE\ II \times 0.146)$$
$$+ 0.603(if\ emergency\ surgery)$$
$$+ diagnostic\ weight$$

Methods to improve the accuracy of APACHE II include combining the score with the delayed-type hypersensitivity (DTH) score and by intradermal skin testing with recall antigens. DTH is a measure of both cell-mediated immunity as well as nonspecific host defense and correlates to the immunocompetency of the patient. Previous studies have demonstrated that an impaired DTH skin-test response is associated with increased mortality in critically ill patients [13]. When DTH is combined with the APACHE II score, a more accurate prediction of mortality can be derived than by using only APACHE II [14]. Although this combined score has been tested on a wide variety of disease

states over a broad range of severities, the DTH score which is required to calculate the risk of death, takes two days to obtain. Currently the APACHE II score alone is the most rapid, simple and accurate method to stratify outcome, define inclusion criteria in clinical trials and compare treatment regimens in patient populations with intra-abdominal infections.

4. CLINICAL PRESENTATION

Abdominal pain, either acute or insidious, has been reported in 100% of patients with peritonitis in a large prospective study [1]. Patients will often prefer to lie still in fetal position or supine with knees bent and head elevated to minimize painful irritation of the peritoneum. Anorexia and nausea are commonly present as well.

On physical examination, the patient is frequently *in extremis*; appearing toxic and in distress. Low grade fever is often present but the temperature may be higher than 40°C or the patient may be hypothermic. The clinical manifestations of shock with tachycardia and a narrowed pulse pressure may be straightjorward. In septic shock, a hyperdynamic state prevails accompanied by high cardiac output, diminished peripheral vascular resistance, bounding pulses and warm extremities. Abdominal tenderness is variable; it is diffuse in the presence of generalized peritonitis or if localized, the point of maximal tenderness overlies the diseased organ. Varying amounts of distension, absent bowel sounds and increased abdominal muscle tone secondary to voluntary guarding may be elicited. In a recent large prospective study of patients with intra-abdominal infections, abdominal tenderness was elicited in approximately 80% of patients, distension and guarding in 50% and rebound tenderness in about 40% [1]. Localized peritonitis is associated with less extreme symptoms and signs and normal abdominal findings are often appreciated distant to the diseased site.

A prospective observational study has established the sensitivity, specificity and positive predicted value for the cough test for diagnosing peritonitis as 78%, 79% and 76%, respectively [15]. The cough test, in which a patient is asked to cough and is positive if they show any signs of pain, is not confounded by the apprehension or voluntary guarding associated with manual palpation by the diagnostician [16].

The clinical presentation of an intra-abdominal abscess differs from secondary peritonitis in that the former is a clinical diagnosis while the latter requires imaging techniques such as ultrasound or computed tomography for diagnosis. Usually the signs and symptoms of peritonitis are present in varying degrees and the diagnosis is based on clinical suspicion with radiological confirmation. Classically, there is mild abdominal pain and localized tenderness. Previous peritonitis, recent operation or antecedent gastrointestinal disease are important historical findings. On examination, one may appreciate a more diffuse mass, rather than a discrete mass, indicative of an abscess with adherent viscera or omentum. Low-grade fever and leucocytosis with greater than 3% bands, particularly in the patient receiving antibiotics or in the wake of recent bowel anastomosis or peritonitis, should prompt a thorough investigation.

5. MANAGEMENT OF INTRA-ABDOMINAL INFECTIONS

In general, the diagnosis of secondary peritonitis warrants urgent surgical treatment but many non-surgical causes of peritonitis should first be ruled out (Table 2). Rapidly fatal ruptured ectopic pregnancy and ruptured abdominal aortic aneurysm are good examples.

5.1. Preoperative Therapy

The first step in the management of secondary peritonitis is crystalloid fluid resuscitation since all patients have some degree of hypovolemia. Lactated Ringer's is an appropriate balanced salt solution which most approximates the electrolyte content of plasma. In generalized peritonitis, two peripheral large-bore intravenous catheters should be placed with an initial bolus of two liters if there is no sign of renal or cardiovascular deficiency. Monitoring of adequate end-organ perfusion should include frequent examinations of mental status and vital signs and an indwelling urinary catheter to monitor hourly urine output. In the elderly and critically ill, one should consider more invasive monitoring devices such as an arterial and central venous catheter. Pulmonary artery catheterization has been indicated in patients with severe cardiorespiratory disease states, in hypotensive individuals unresponsive to fluid administration as occurs in sepsis and in multiorgan failure when the status of the cardiac, respiratory and renal systems is unclear [17]. The benefit of pulmonary artery catheterization has not been established in randomized controlled trials and recent data suggests that its use, at least in the initial care of critically ill patients, may be associated with increased mortality, cost and hospital stay [18].

Antibiotics should be initiated as soon as the diagnosis is made. Antibiotic therapy in secondary peritonitis is covered elsewhere.

Table 2.
Non-surgical causes of peritonitis by anatomic location

Right Upper Quadrant	Epigastrium	Left Upper Quadrant	Right Lower Quadrant	Left Lower Quadrant	Diffuse
Acute cholecystitis	Pancreatitis	Splenic infarction	Crohn's disease	Acute diverticulitis	Gastroenteritis
Choledocho-lithiasis	Gastritis	Pancreatits	Ovarian cyst	Colorectal cancer	Pancreatitis
Pancreatitis	Acute cholecystitis	Herpes zoster	Ovarian torsion	Splenomegaly	Acute cholecystitis
Hepatitis	Myocardial ischemia	Pneumonia	Pelvic inflam-matory disease	Ovarian cyst	Colitis
Congestive hepatomegaly	Pericarditis	Myocardial ischemia	Endometriosis	Ovarian torsion	Crohn's disease
Hepatic metastases		Pericarditis	Mittelschmerz	Seminal vesiculitis	Ulcerative colitis
Herpes zoster		Empyema	Renal calculi		Leukemia
Pneumonia		Pulmonary infarction	Seminal vesiculitis		Sickle cell disease
Myocardial ischemia		Splenomegaly	Cystitis		Addisonian crisis
Pericariditis			Acute diverticulitis		Mesenteric adenitis
Empyema			Mesenteric adenitis		

5.2. Surgical Therapy

Secondary peritonitis mandates timely surgical intervention. The cardinal principles of treatment of intra-abdominal infections are:

1. Eliminate the source of contamination

2. Reduce microbial inoculum

3. Prevent the development of persistent sepsis

The incision used for generalized peritonitis is classically the midline vertical laparo-tomy. With this incision, the peritoneal cavity is rapidly opened with good exposure and access to the entire abdomen. For localized peritonitis, incisions are commonly directly over the site of inflammation such as the Rocke-Davis in acute appendicitis and the right sub-costal in acute cholecystitis.

The first step after the abdomen is opened is to take a culture of the peritoneal fluid or pus. Many surgeons are reluctant to perform this inexpensive, simple task because of the relative success of broad-spectrum antibiotics and that the usual polymicrobial flora grown from cultures does not alter the management. Despite this popular sentiment, intra-abdominal pus cultures have been shown to be more sensitive and lead to appropriate limited spectrum antibiotic treatment than blood cultures [19]. A recent double-blinded, prospective, randomized multicenter trial comparing limited and broad-spectrum antimicrobial therapy in 213 patients with suspected intra-abdominal infections found microbial resistance to the assigned regimen in 57% of the patients who failed treatment [20]. The authors recommended that intra-operative cultures be routinely taken and antibiotic therapy adjusted to eliminate the recovered organisms in order to reduce the number of treatment failures.

Goal 1: Eliminate the source of contamination

The options for eliminating the infectious source, usually a perforated viscus, include primary closure with suture or stapler, resection, exclusion or exteriorization. If the patient's condition contraindicates a prolonged operation, one may postpone anastomosis, colostomy or repair until a subsequent laparotomy. Such "damage control laparotomies" have proven particularly effective in the traumatically injured abdomen [21]. Bleeding may be controlled by packing.

The choice of repair or resection as well as how to manage the ends of retained bowel (anastomosis, exteriorization or simple closure) depend on the anatomic source of infection, the viability of the bowel, the degree of peritonitis and the patient's capacity to mount an effective local and systemic response. Resection is preferred if the disease process is likely to continue.

Self-limited inflammatory processes such as acute exacerbation of Crohn's disease, ischemic but viable bowel and acute phelgmonous diverticulitis may be left in-situ.

For gastric ulcer with perforation, it is preferable to include the ulcer in the resected portion of the stomach wall. The gastrotomy may then be closed primarily with or without omentopexy or, for larger resections, antrectomy, hemigastrectomy or total gastrectomy with Billroth I or II repair may be required. Types II, III and IV gastric ulcers mandate vagotomy and pyloroplasty.

The treatment of small bowel perforation involves few options. Perforated duodenal ulcer is treated on an emergency basis by omentopexy and definitive treatment is reserved for patients with a history of chronic peptic ulcer disease especially when the operation is performed early when there has been minimal peritoneal soiling.

Smithwick popularized the three-staged repair for perforated sigmoid diverticulitis in the 1940's which comprised transverse colostomy and mucus fistula initially followed at a later date by resection and primary anastomosis and finally closure of the colostomy [22]. This procedure was replaced several decades later by the Hartman 2-staged repair, whereby primary resection, end-colostomy and closure of the rectal stump was followed by closure of the colostomy. Most authors advocate resection and Hartmann's procedure for perforated diverticulitis [23] rather than the three-staged repair since the first principle of treatment, removal of the source of infection, is omitted in the initial operation of the latter. In the last two decades, increasing numbers of surgeons have been promoting single-staged primary repair alone or with intracolonic bypass tubes.

Some authors advocate resection and primary anastomosis in selected patients, usually with localized inflammation, by experienced surgeons [23,24].

Primary anastomosis of the colon in the face of diffuse peritonitis has traditionally been shunned due to the high risk of anastamotic dehiscence. However many factors contribute to anastamotic breakdown other than infection such as hypoperfusion, technical failure, fluid resuscitation and nutritional status. Gutman investigated the role of infection on anastamotic breakdown in a rat fecal peritonitis model by semicircular incision of the sigmoid colon [25] Mortality and anastomosis burst strength was measured in 70 animals assigned to four groups: one group had creation of fecal peritonitis only, a second had the same with the addition of resection and primary anastomosis, a third group had, in addition to the second, resuscitation with saline and systemic broad-spectrum antibiotics and the fourth (sham) group had resection and primary anastomosis only. Anastomosis burst strength after seven days was not significantly different between the groups, while mortality was reduced by 43% (from 84% to 48%) by the addition of fluid resuscitation and broad spectrum antibiotics, suggesting that infection plays a minor role in anastomosis failure when the systemic manifestations of sepsis are adequately managed. Thus the choice of surgical procedure may correlate more with the condition of the host and less with the severity of injury to the bowel or peritoneal cavity.

One retrospective study of 39 consecutive patients undergoing emergency left colon resection compared primary anastomosis with (n=17) or without (n=5) intraoperative colonic lavage versus Hartman procedure (n=17) with the outcome defined as morbidity, mortality and duration of hospital stay. There were no significant difference between mortality and morbidity with patients receiving Hartmann procedure resulting in a 50% increase in hospital stay. When compared with a group of 69 patients undergoing the same resections but under elective situation, the results were no different [26]. Resection and primary anastomosis are utilized more frequently in colonic perforation with secondary peritonitis.

One retrospective study of 136 patients with perforation of the colon from diverticulitis or tumor compared primary resection with anastomosis (n=81), primary resection and Hartmann procedure (n=33) or simple colostomy (n=22). Mean APACHE II scores and mortality rates were 9.4 and 6.2% for primary anastomosis, 14.0 and 33% for Hartmann's and 31.3 and 59% for simple colostomy (three-staged repair) [27]. There are insufficient data from randomized control trials to support one repair over another. Current standards of practice permit one-staged and two-staged depending on the experience and judgment of the operator. The first principle, eliminating the infectious source, mandates primary resection and, depending primarily on the patient's condition, one may elect to perform primary anastomosis or a procedure involving a colostomy. Other factors traditionally used to select the type of repair are duration of peritonitis, amount of fecal spillage and severity of peritonitis, however, there are no data from multivariate logistic regression analyses supporting these factors as independent determinants of morbidity, mortality or anastomosis dehiscence. Severely ill, unstable patients appearing moribund will not benefit from a lengthy operation which places undue stress on the already compromised cardiovascular and immune systems. These patients may tolerate little more than proximal fecal diversion and drainage in the initial operation with definitive repair conducted over several laparotomies after correction of hypothermia, coagulopathy and dehydration.

Intracolonic bypass devices, such as Coloshield®, for use in one-stage repairs have not achieved broad popularity but results from the only two clinical studies suggest a possible role. In a prospective observational study, 28 patients with sigmoid diverticulitis requiring operation underwent resection, primary anastomosis and placement of a latex bypass tube 3 cm proximal to the anastomosis affixed with absorbable sutures. The distal end was fashioned to lie in the rectal ampulla. Ten of the 28 patients had generalized peritonitis. The authors reported no anastomosis leaks or deaths following this procedure [28]. In another prospective observational study, 29 consecutive patients required left colon surgery on unprepared bowel. Patients with septic shock or a colonic lumen too narrow to use the tube were excluded. Two of the 29 patients had anastomotic leaks (8.7%) which were associated with the one mortality in the study (4.3%) [29]. The relatively few numbers of subjects of which only two had preoperative diagnoses of generalized fecal peritonitis and the lack of controlled trials of intracolonic bypass devices precludes definitive support for these devices, for use in the treatment of secondary peritonitis at this time.

Laparoscopy continues to play progressively greater roles in the diagnosis and treatment of secondary peritonitis. Cholecystitis may be safely treated laprascopically even in its acute stage with minimal complications in skilled hands. Appendicitis has been successfully treated by laparoscopy and compared well to traditional appendec-tomy in a prospectively randomized trial. There were no significant complications in the laparoscopy group and authors noted a conversion rate of only 7-12.5% [30].

One study has investigated a potential role for laparoscopy in the diagnosis and treatment of acute perforated diverticulitis [31]. This retrospective series of 8 patients presenting with acute abdomen and diagnosed on laparoscopy as stage III diverticulitis defined as in the presence of generalized purulent peritonitis [32]. Each underwent laparoscopic irrigation and aspiration without complication. Although the theory behind minimally invasive treatment of acute abdominal conditions is appealing, randomized controlled trials are needed to determine the role of laparoscopy with respect to morbidity and mortality.

Closure of the laparotomy wound is dictated by the degree to which the three goals of treatment have been achieved. If the infectious source has been completely eliminated, the microbial inoculum reduced and there is a low risk for persistent or recurrent infection, then the fascia may be closed with a single layer of non-absorbable monofilament suture such as polypropylene. In general the surgeon must consider the condition of the patient at three levels: the viscus, the abdomen and the patient as an immunocompetent host. In cases where the viability of the bowel is questioned, there is significant risk of persistent or recurrent peritonitis, or it the overall condition of the patient is poor, temporary closure may be undertaken (see below). Furthermore, if the abdominal wall can not be apposed without tension, then temporary closing devices are also indicated. In malnourished, immunocompromised or elderly patients, the use of retention sutures is encouraged. Skin and subcutaneous tissue should be managed by delayed primary closure or, if infection is questioned, allowed to close secondarily as the risk of associated wound infection exceeds 20%.

A variety of temporary closure mechanisms have been used successfully in uncontrolled trials. Retention sutures or Marlex® mesh sheets which may be closed by suturing, embedding a zipper, a plastic slide fastener or a Velcro® adhesive sheet. One prospective observational study compared four temporary abdominal closure devices in 117 patients with diffuse, long-standing purulent intra-abdominal infections. They reported the highest rate of complications in retention sutures (n=51) related to abdominal wall necrosis secondary to its inability to allow for adequate decompression of the abdomen. The mesh-zipper (n=32) was associated with similar complications. The slide fastener (n=18) was found to open with minimal patient movement and thus portend a high risk of evisceration. The authors favored the Velcro® fastener in multiple repeat operations since it may be trimmed to account for resolution of peritoneal and abdominal wall edema [33].

Goal 2: *Reduction of microbial inoculum*

Once the source of infection is eliminated, efforts are directed to limiting the bacterial contamination. Gross purulent exudates and particulate matter should be removed by swabbing or manual extraction and all fluids should be aspirated. Loculations in the pelvis, paracolic gutters and subphrenic areas should be opened and debrided. Fibrin, the building block of adhesions, is believed to act as a nidus for infection. This was the historical rationale for radical peritoneal debridement which has long since fallen from fa-

vor. It is tedious, time-consuming, leads to significant blood loss and the only randomized controlled trial demonstrated no benefit over the conservative approach [34].

Intraoperative peritoneal lavage is the standard procedure, although its efficacy is not documented. The aim of lavage is to reduce the quantity of bacteria and remove adjuvant substances. The theoretical risks are that lavage may dilute opsonins and disseminate bacteria, the latter of which is unlikely since bacteria is rapidly spread throughout the peritoneum by physiologic mechanisms. The risk of leaving a collection of infectious fluid with persistence of peritonitis and its consequences, outweigh any risk of not performing lavage. Fluid acts as an adjuvant to infection by impairing phagocytosis and inflammatory cell migration. More important than lavage itself is probably aspiration of all fluid including that used to lavage. The benefit of antibiotics or antiseptics added to the lavage fluid, a common clinical practice due to positive results in uncontrolled series [35], has not been effectively borne out in clinical or animal trials. Not for lack of trials do we state this but for lack of trials in which an acceptable model is used.

The only clinically or experimentally relevant model to the treatment of intra-abdominal infections is one in which the subjects and controls are at the very least treated with fluid resuscitation and systemic antibiotics, followed by laparotomy and elimination of gross infection. Human or animal studies which omit one or more of these factors have little relevance to the treatment of intra-abdominal infections [36,37,38,39]. Unfortunately, the vast majority of animal studies fail to meet this minimal criteria and their respective results must be considered with extreme caution, if not overt skepticism. The difficulty of performing clinical trials lies in the heterogenous etiologies and severities that fall under the diagnosis of secondary peritonitis. Scoring systems have been created to stratify study participants, not to direct therapy of individuals since they are themselves models prone to inaccuracy. The reader is referred to an excellent treatise on the principles of designing and performing clinical investigations in intra-abdominal infections including the appropriate use of scoring systems [5].

One animal study demonstrated that lavage with or without antibiotics failed to reduce the inoculum of bacteria. Using a cecal ligation and puncture model in rats, Edmiston and co-workers demonstrated through serial peritoneal biopsies that intraoperative saline lavage resulted in no difference in the amount of colony-forming units per milliliter of aerobic and anaerobic pathogens cultured immediately following lavage. When cephazolin (250 µg/ml), cephazolin plus metronidazole (100 µg/ml) or metronidazole plus kanamyucin (100 µg/ml) were added to 250 ml of saline lavage, a transient decrease in pathogens was obtained on post-lavage biopsies which returned to prelavage values 24 hours later. When kanamycin or metronidazole were used alone in the lavage fluid, there was no reduction of pathogens post-lavage. Although the results point to a transient benefit at best with antibiotic lavage, the contact time of the lavage fluid in the study, 4-7 minutes, may have been inadequate for the antimicrobials to act effectively [36]. Unfortunately the authors failed to treat the animals with systemic antibiotics or hydration and thus although interesting from an anatomist's standpoint, the results add little to the treatment of intra-abdominal infections.

The only randomized controlled trial comparing no lavage to saline lavage with or without antibiotics in patients with proven intra-abdominal infections was performed by Schein and co-workers [40]. Eighty-seven patients operated on for diffuse or localized peritonitis were randomly assigned to one of the three aforementioned groups (n=29 in each group). Age, gender and mean APACHE II scores were equivalent in each group. There were no differences in mortality, morbidity or length of hospital stay between the three groups. Although the authors appropriately excluded appendectomies and non-ruptured abscesses, they also excluded diffuse fecal peritonitis and infected pancreatic necrosis which are the severe types of injury most likely to benefit from intraoperative peritoneal lavage.

These results contrast with a similarly designed animal study to examine the efficacy of intraoperative lavage alone or with cephalopthin in rats with fecal peritonitis which showed a survival benefit with saline lavage not significantly enhanced with the addition of antibiotics [37]. The investigators also examined the effect of ozonated saline, known to possess rapid antimicrobial oxidizing properties, which showed no benefit over lavage alone. Although the greatest survival benefit was associated with the more severe peritonitis in animals, the study failed to include the first principle in the treatment of secondary peritonitis: elimination of the source of infection by aspiration or manually debridement. With respect to treating intra-abdominal infections, these results add little.

Several antiseptics added to the lavage fluid have been studied in the treatment of secondary peritonitis. These include providone-iodine, noxythiolin, hydrogen peroxide, taurolin and chlorhexidine. No benefit has been demonstrated with any and many were found to be injurious. One animal study examined the outcome of mice inoculated intraperitonieally with E. coli six hours prior to no lavage, saline lavage, providone-iodine (1:20 Ringer's lactate) and determined that there was no difference in mortality rate at one week between controls and antiseptic whereas saline lavage resulted in a 50% reduction in mortality rates. They also noted that systemic absorption occurred resulting in significantly elevated levels of iodine in the blood and liver for 24 hours [41]. Previous authors have determined that this antiseptic caused chemical burns in the peritoneum and was toxic to mesothelial cells [42] and fibroblasts [43]. Use of proviodine was associated with increased mortality secondary to damaged host defense mechanisms [44,45]. There is no role for antiseptic lavage of the peritoneal cavity.

Use of lavage volumes in excess of five liters has been erroneously thought to be associated with deleterious fluid and electrolyte shifts from peritoneal absorption. Large-volume lavage has been investigated with the use of mechanical assist devices which permit a rapid influx of volume up to thirty liters. One retrospective case-control study examined the effect of mechanically-assisted large volume versus manual lavage in perforated gastric and duodenal ulcers on the development of infectious complications. The operation, volume of warmed saline lavage, decision to leave a drain and decision to use manual or mechanical lavage was left up to the surgeon. Although the authors noted a negative trend relating volume of lavage fluid and the incidence of infectious complications, the small numbers of subjects and the presence of confounding variables (such as time to operation, non-randomized use of drains, lavage fluid and type of operation) prevented con-

clusive evidence supporting its benefit in peritonitis from perforated peptic ulcers [46]. The same group of investigators did find a benefit with large-volume lavage in preventing infectious complications following blunt traumatic small bowel rupture. Other significant risk factors for post-operative infectious complications included time to operation, distal site of perforation and positive peritoneal cultures. The mechanical device allowed rapid (11.3 litres/min) infusion of warm saline lavage which was associated with a positive outcome [47].

The reader is referred to thorough review of intraoperative peritoneal lavage either alone or modified by large volumes or the addition of antibiotics or antiseptics [48].

Goal 3: Prevent the development of persistent sepsis

The decision whether or not to place a drain in the post-operative abdomen following secondary peritonitis has long been a matter of controversy. The indications for drainage are: evacuation of an abscess, establishment of a controlled fistula and, if indicated, to provide post-operative lavage. Previous authors have pointed out that it is virtually impossible to drain the peritoneal cavity in diffuse peritonitis. Furthermore, by providing a site for bacterial adherence and fibrin formation, drains or other foreign bodies appear to act as adjuvants for infection [49]. The disadvantages of using drains is that they may erode into the bowel or vessels or provide external bacteria access into peritoneum. The guidelines for the usage of drains have been previously reported [50].

1. No drain is better than any drain.

2. Drain selection should consider anticipated risk of complication.

3. Active closed-system suction drains are better than simple passive drains.

4. Drain placement should be in a dependent area (Douglas Pouch, Morrison pouch, subdiaphragmatic spaces) and exit near watertight anastomosis through a separate stab wound.

5. Drains require careful observation for malfunction, frequent irrigation and early removal when no longer required.

The type of material used to drain also impacts on the complication rate. Experimental evidence clearly demonstrates rubber drains in E. coli peritonitis to be associated with significantly greater amounts of bacterial translocation to mesenteric lymph nodes, serum IL-6 levels and morphologic degree of peritonitis than no drain [51]. Rubber drains should not be used in the treatment of intra-abdominal infections.

The options for the treatment of severe, fecal or purulent peritonitis with multiple loculations, extensive fibrinous adhesions or ischemic bowel not amenable to a complete removal of infection at the initial operation include: continuous or intermittent post-operative peritoneal lavage, open drainage (laparostomy) and planned or on-demand relaparatomy.

Continuous or intermittent post-operative peritoneal lavage (POPL) is thought to reduce the inoculum and adjuvants to infection. The procedure is employed most commonly for acute hemorrhagic pancreatitis with infected necrotic tissue but some surgeons advocate its use in fecal or purulent peritonitis [52]. The lavage is performed as a continuous flow or intermittently with exchange volumes of at least two liters, commonly including antibiotics and heparin, intermittently for 48 to 72 hours or until effluent clear. The disadvantages are that the procedure is labor intensive and requires monitoring in a critical care setting.

One group of investigators using a fecal inoculation-induced peritonitis model in rabbits compared the efficacy of continuous POPL for 72 hours with and without clindamycin/gentamycin in rabbits exposed to high (HFI) or low (LFI) fecal inocula. The animals were assigned to six groups of HFI and LFI: no lavage and no antibiotics; lavage and no antibiotics; lavage and intramuscular antibiotics; lavage containing antibiotics; and both lavage containing antibiotics and intramuscular antibiotics. The results demonstrated the greatest survival advantage when antibiotics are provided both systemically and included in the lavage, less so if they are only in the lavage fluid and a possible worsening of the outcome with lavage in the absence of any antibiotics [38]. In this study, continuous POPL with antibiotics and systemic antibiotics as the only means of treatment correlated with improved survival. Although this study was appropriately controlled for all variables, the relevance of this model to the patient undergoing the current standard of treatment is limited by the authors' neglect to eliminate the source of infection in this animal model. Despite the apparent benefit demonstrated for continuous POPL, data are lacking to support its use in clinical practice. The one prospective, randomized controlled trial of patients with purulent peritonitis treated with systemic cefuroxime and metronidazole and operative debridement and intra-operative lavage compared 72-hour continuous saline POPL with no lavage. The authors noted no outcome benefit was associated with continuous POPL and the cost in time, labor and material resources were substantial [53]. A similar retrospective study also failed to demonstrate improvement in morbidity, mortality and duration of hospital stay [54]. The data do not support the use of continuous or intermittent POPL in the treatment of secondary peritonitis, however, its use in acute hemorrhagic pancreatitis is accepted.

Open drainage, also known as laparostomy, was first advocated by Steinberg in 1979 [55] and has enjoyed widespread popularity in the treatment of severe intra-abdominal infections [33, 52, 55, 56, 57, 58, 59, 60, 61, 62]. Steinberg and co-workers reported on a series of 14 patients in which the abdominal wound was left open and covered only with gauze and an abdominal binder for 48-72 hours [55]. No complications or recurrent infections developed in twelve of the 14 patients. The rationale for open treatment was to permit open drainage of pus and decompression of high intra-abdominal pressures resulting from edema, inflammation and fluid resuscitation.

The goals of open drainage include promoting improved ventilation and abdominal organ perfusion while preventing an abdominal compartment syndrome. The disadvantages are increased rate of enteric fistulization, evisceration, prolonged ventilation and hernia formation. An additional hypothetical disadvantage is that subsequent laparotomies may act as additional traumatic insults to an already depleted host defense system. A minimum of a 24 hour interval between laparotomies is recommended not only since bacteria regrow to initial inoculum by this time but to minimize the effect on the systemic inflammatory response [36]. Initial complications such as massive fluid loss, evisceration, spontaneous enteric fistulas and abdominal wall defects were significantly reduced with temporary closure devices, such as mesh-zipper or Velcro® adhesive sheets, which do not inhibit decompression or drainage. The mesh may provide an exit site for stomas or drains.

One non-randomized prospective observational study of intra-abdominal infections demonstrated no difference in survival or morbidity between 18 patients who were left open or could not be closed and 221 patients were closed after initial laparotomy [1]. This association was confounded by the selection of techniques by the treating surgeon in each case. A retrospective series of 14 patients presenting with delayed suppurative peritonitis and mean APACHE II score of 30.3 (70-90% expected mortality) and treated by laparotomy, lavage and placement of mesh-zipper apparatus. Daily lavages were carried out in the ICU by opening the zipper. When peritoneal healing was adequate as determined by the formation of adhesions as to prevent evisceration, negative peritoneal cultures and resolution of SIRS criteria, the mesh-zipper was removed and the fascia closed. Mortality was 57% and significantly better than the expected mortality of 70-90% [63]. Other authors have also reported diminished mortality rates in patient series treated in a similar manner [33,58,60,62, 64]. A metanalysis of 22 reported series involving 642 patients with secondary peritonitis concluded that insufficient evidence exists to determine whether open drainage or closing the abdomen between laparotomies improves outcome [65]. Open drainage should include placement of a temporary closure device and the indications for open drainage are: generalized peritonitis with incomplete elimination of the infectious source or its adjuvants, massive abdominal wall loss or inability to close the abdominal fascia without undue tension, critical condition preventing definitive repair, high intra-abdominal pressures impairing visceral perfusion or ventilation, uncertainty of viable bowel, the presence of MODS and when subsequent laparotomies are planned [66].

Planned or staged relaparotomy mandates re-exploration every 24 to 72 hours regardless of patient condition until there is clinical and microbiolgical resolution of sepsis and the peritoneal cavity is clean of infection. The rationale for planned relaparotomy is the lack of clinical signs indicating on-going sepsis or MODS in sedated, intubated patients with large dressings. On-demand relaparotomy uses the patient's clinical or radiological evolution to mandate returning to the operating room. The trade-off is the risk of missing persistent infection of the development of MODS versus the risk of a negative laparotomy effectuating repeated "hits" on an already traumatized system of host defense [67].

Data supporting planned relaparotomy over on-demand relaparotomy, derived from retrospective or observational studies, demonstrate a 30 to 40% reduction from mortality predicted by APACHE II scores [33,68].

Ettappenlavage, a variant of planned relaparotomy advocated by Wittmann for patients with diffuse purulent peritonitis at high risk of mortality, consists of open drainage and planned daily irrigation and debridements. The focus of infection is first eliminated by suture, staple, closure, excision or exteriorization and packs are often left *in-situ*. The first reoperation is performed in an operating room when packs are removed and subsequent debridements of necrotic and infected tissue take place in the intensive care unit at bedside. Prosthetic mesh is used unless the fascia can be approximated without tension and the skin may be closed with low risk of wound infection primarily or with a split-thickness skin graft or may be left open to heal by secondary intention. One hundred and seventeen patients prospectively observed and treated with ettappenlavage for diffuse,

long-standing purulent peritonitis had a lower observed mortality (24%) than predicted by APACHE II (45%) [33].

6. MANAGEMENT OF INTRA-ABDOMINAL ABSCESS

The ability to wall off an infection and form an abscess demonstrates a success of the host defenses and correlates with survival. In a prospective non-randomized trial of 239 patients who underwent an operation for intra-abdominal infection with APACHE II score greater than 10, 24% of patients who formed abscesses died as opposed to 38% of patients who did not (p=0.033) [1]. Other prospective studies have confirmed the association with abscess and survival [4].

Three principles guide the treatment of intra-abdominal abscesses:

1. General patient care

2. Antibiotics

3. Drainage

General patient care comprises adequate rehydration and monitoring to the extent mandated by each individual condition. Hypoxemia is commonly present as a consequence of atelectasis, impaired ventilation from abdominal distension or pulmonary effusions from subdiaphragmatic or subphrenic abscesses. Malnutrition is commonly associated with prolonged infection and may require enteral or parenteral supplementation.

Combination or monotherapy antimicrobials should be directed against the specific pathogen but both aerobes and anaerobes should be covered. Antibiotics without drainage are usually ineffective because of poor penetration into the abscess cavity and inactivation by the hypoxic and acidotic. Cultures should always be taken since pus provides a higher recovery of bacteria and more accurately directs antibiotic treatment than blood cultures alone [19]. Antibiotic therapy is discussed elsewhere.

Drainage is the sine qua non of treatment of intra-abdominal abscesses and improves the effectiveness of antibiotics. Sumps are preferred and rubber or Penrose drains should be avoided. Computed tomography (CT) or ultrasound is required for diagnosis localization and is usually effective for guiding drainage. Percutaneous drainage by CT or ultrasound guidance is the treatment of choice for single, well-defined abscesses. If there is no clinical improvement within 48 hours after drainage, CT scan should be repeated with percutaneous drainage of any new or residual fluid collection. In the absence of radiographic findings or if drainage is not possible, exploratory laparotomy should follow. For a single, well-defined abscess cavity or to establish a controlled fistula for an intestinal leak, percutaneous drainage is 80-90% successful. Acceptable criteria for percutaneous drainage also include multiple or loculated abscesses and infected tumor mass.

Drainage can be curative if complete resolution is achieved without the need of an operation or palliative, if it improves patient's condition prior to performance of a definitive repair. Percutaneous drainage is preferred but surgical drainage is particularly useful for abscesses which are multiple, multiloculated or associated with enteric communication, neoplasia or tissue necrosis and those located in the lesser sac or between loops of bowel. Data from randomized controlled trials supporting percutaneous over surgical drainage with respect to patient outcome are lacking.

The use of drains is not without risk as erosion into the vessels or bowel with massive hemorrhage or peritonitis are recognized complications. Also included are enteric fistulae to the skin or other organs and empyema. Drains should be removed as early as possible when the clinical condition, temperature and white count improve; output is minimal and there is radiological evidence of resolution.

7. NUTRITION MANAGEMENT

In severe intra-abdominal infections, as in other forms of systemic inflammation, the metabolic response of the patient is divided into an initial catabolic 'ebb' phase characterized by normal or decreased energy expenditure, hypoglycemia and diminished tissue perfusion and a subsequent anabolic 'flow' phase with hypermetabolism, negative nitrogen balance, and hyperglycemia [69]. The former usually lasts several hours while the latter can last up to several weeks. Fever caused by increased IL-1 release will further increase the metabolic rate.

The stress hormone response involving ACTH, cortisol, catecholamines, glucagon, growth hormone, arginine-vasopressin and elevations of TNF, IL-1, and IL-6 lead to altered metabolism of lipids, carbohydrates and proteins. Furthermore, glutamine, a major source of energy for the gut, lympmhocytes, fibroblasts and plays an important role in restoring the mucosal barrier and immune system of the gastrointestinal tract, is preferentially used by the gut as an energy source. A reduced supply of glutamine is associated with increased bacterial translocation and MODS. The enteral route of glutamine administration is superior to the intravenous.

The guidelines for nutritional support in intra-abdominal infections are as follows:

1. The enteral route of administration should be used whenever possible and include glutamine. When the gut cannot be used, parenteral nutrition can be an adequate energy source.

2. The goal of nutritional support is to restore nitrogen balance. Carbohydrates up to 5 g/kg/day; proteins as 45% branched-chain amino acids enriched with high leucine solutions up to 2g/kg/day; and lipids as medium-chain triglycerides up to 1g/kg/day. Total calorie supply up to 168 kJ/kg/day [50].

8. SUMMARY

Secondary peritonitis remains a therapeutic challenge for the surgeon and intensivist as the mortality has changed little over half a century, hovering around 30%. The diagnosis is a clinical one and once made, mandates adequate crystalloid resuscitation, monitoring and antimicrobial therapy. The three cardinal principles of management are to eliminate the source of infection, reduce the inoculum and prevent the development of persistent sepsis.

The first principle ideally comprises complete resection and primary repair of the viscus, however, variations may be tailored to the condition of the patient. The literature documents a trend towards primary repair regardless of the location of injury, even in left colon perforations with fecal spillage. Laparoscopy may be useful in diagnosis as well as irrigational therapy for stage III acute diverticulitis (with peritonitis).

The second principle mandates intra-operative irrigation with warm saline of an adequate volume to remove all infectious debris. Complete aspiration of all fluid is vital and no benefit has been demonstrated by the addition of antibiotics or antiseptics to the lavage fluid.

The third principle deals with the type of closure and whether or not to leave a drain. Aside from acute hemorrhagic pancreatitis, post-operative peritoneal lavage is rarely indicated in secondary peritonitis. Drains are used either to evacuate an abscess or residual source of infection not removed during the initial laparotomy or to establish a controlled fistula. They must be of the closed, suction type, placed in a dependent area of the abdomen, vigilently monitored and removed as early as possible. If the source of contamination is completely eliminated and the abdomenal fascia may be closed without undue tension, primary closure is appropriate. Temporary closure is indicated when there is incomplete removal of infectious debris, inability to close without tension, high intra-abdominal pressures impairing visceral perfusion, malnourished or immunocompromised state, critical condition preventing definitive repair, uncertainty of viable bowel or if there are subsequent laparotonies planned. The device should be a type of mesh with a Velcro® fastener which may be trimmed to accomodate variations in the approximation of the fascia. Drains and temporary stomas may be fashioned to the mesh and relaparotomies should be "planned" to take place every 24 to 48 hours since physical or investigative signs of complications in these patients are often masked, unnoticed or delayed. Patients managed by the latter "on demand" approach to re-laparotomy have been shown to have a significantly greater survival than that predicted by their APACHE II scores. Although technically considered a complication of secondary peritonitis, the ability of the patient to form an abscess is associated with survival. The diagnosis is a radiological one, although an abscess may be suspected clinically. Treatment falls into three areas: general patient care, antibiotics and drainage. General patient care requires fluid hydration, supplemental oxygenation, monitoring of ongoing sepsis and providing adequate nutrition. Antimicrobial therapy, either combination or monotherapy, should cover anaerobes and Gram negative aerobes. Drainage should be attempted percutaneously with computed tomographic or ultrasonic guidance, even in multiple or multiloculated abscesses. Indications for surgical drainage include failed percutaneous drainage, interloop or lesser sac abscesses, or when associated with neoplasia, tissue necrosis or extensive enteric communication.

REFERENCES

1. Christou NV, Barie PS, Dellinger EP, Waymack JP, Stone HH. Surgical Infection Society intra-abdominal infection study. Prospective evaluation of management techniques and outcome. Arch Surg1993; 128:193-8; discussion 198-9.

2. Jonsson B, Berglund J, Skau T, Nystrom PO. Outcome of intra-abdominal infection in pigs depends more on host responses than on microbiology. Eur J Surg 1993; 159:571-8.

3. Knaus WA, Draper EA, Wagner DP, Zimmerman JE. APACHE II: A severity of disease classification system. Knaus: Crit Care Med 1985:13;818-29.

4. Koperna T, Schulz F. Prognosis and treatment of peritonitis. Do we need new scoring systems? Arch Surg 1996; 131:180-6.

5. Nystrom P-O, Bax R, Dellinger EP, et al. Proposed definitions for diagnosis, severity scoring, stratification and outcome for trials on intra-abdominal infection. World J Surg 1990; 14:148-58.

6. Pacelli F, Doglietto GB, Alfieri S, et al. Prognosis in intra-abdominal infections. Multivariate analysis on 604 patients. Arch Surg 1996; 131:641-5.

7. Sawyer RG, Rosenlof LK, Adams RB, May AK, Spengler MD, Pruett TL. Peritonitis into the 1990s: changing pathogens and changing strategies in the critically ill. Am Surg 1992; 58:82-7.

8. Goris RJA, Boekhorst TPA, Nuytinck KS, Gimbere JSF. Multiple-organ failure: generalized autodestructive inflammation? Arch Surg 1985; 120:1109-15.

9. Marshall JC, Cook DJ, Christou NV, Bernard GR, Sprung CL, Sibbald WJ. Multiple Organ Dysfunction Score: A reliable descriptor of a complex clinical outcome. Crit Care Med 1995; 23:1638-52.

10. Wacha H, Linder MM, Feldmann U. Mannheim peritonitis index — prediction of risk of death from peritonitis. Theor Surg 1987; 1:169-77.

11. Wittmann DH, Teichmann W, Muller M. Development and validation of the Altona peritonitis index - PIA II. Langenbecks Arch Chir 1987; 327:834-5.

12. Ohmann C, Wittmann DH, Wacha H. Prospective evaluation of prognostic scoring systems in peritonitis. Peritonitis Study Group. Eur J Surg 1993; 159:267-74.

13. MacLean LD, Meakins JL, Taguchi K, Duignan JP, Dhillon KS, Gordon J. Host resistance in sepsis and trauma. Ann Surg 1975; 182:207-16. Discussion pp 216-7.

14. Poenaru D, Christou NV. Clinical outcome of seriously ill surgical patients with intra-abdominal infection depends on both physiological (APACHE II score) and immunological (DTH score) alterations. Ann Surg 1991; 213:130-6.

15. Bennett DH, Tambeur LJMT, Campbell WB. Use of coughing test to diagnose peritonitis. BMJ 1994; 308:1336.

16. Kovachev LS. 'Cough sign': a reliable test in the diagnosis of intra-abdominal inflammation. Br J Surg 1994; 81:1542.

17. Abrams JH, Cerra F, Holcroft JW. Cardiopulmonary monitoring. In Wilmore DW et al. (eds.) Scientific American Surgery 1994, Scientific American, Inc., New York, USA.

18. Connors AF Jr, Speroff T, Dawson NV, et al. The effectiveness of right heart catheterization in the initial care of critically ill patient. JAMA 1996; 276:889-97.

19. Filice C, Brunetti E, Dughetti S. Diagnostic yield of abscess drainage. Dig Dis Sci 1995; 40:1582.

20. Christou NV, Turgeon P, Wassef R, Rotstein O, Bohnen J, Potvin M. Management of intra-abdominal infections. The case for intraoperative cultures and comprehensive broad-spectrum antibiotic coverage. The Canadian Intra-abdominal Infection Study Group. Arch Surg 1996; 131:1193-201.

21. Morris JA Jr, Eddy VA, Rutherford EJ. The trauma celiotomy: the evolving concepts of damage control. Current Problems in Surgery 1996; 33:611-700.

22. Smithwick RH. Experiences with surgical management of sigmoid diverticulitis. Ann Surg 1942; 115:969-85.

23. Khan AL, Ah-See AK, Crofts TJ, Heys SD, Eremin O. Surgical management of the septic complications of diverticular disease. Ann R Coll Surg Eng 1995; 77:16-20.

24. Medina VA, Papanicalou GK, Tadros RR, Fielding LP. Acute perforated diverticulitis: primary resection and anastomosis. Conn Med 1991; 55:258-61.

25. Gutman M, Klausner JM, Lelcuk S. Fecal peritonitis—the effect on anastomotic healing. Eur Surg Res 1993; 25:366-9.

26. Kressner U, Antonsson J, Ejerblad S, Gerdin B, Pahlman L. Intra-operative colonic lavage and primary anastomosis—an alternative to Hartmann procedure in emergency surgery of the left colon. Eur J Surg 1994; 160:287-92.

27. Nespoli A, Ravizzini C, Trivella M, Segala M. The choice of surgical procedure for peritonitis due to colonic perforation. Arch Surg 1993; 128:814-8.

28. Ravo B, Mishrick A, Addei K, et al. The treatment of perforated diverticulitis by one-stage intracolonic bypass procedure. Surg 1987; 102:771-6.

29. Rosati C, Smith L, Deitel M, Burul CJ, Baida M, Borowy ZJ, Bryden P. Primary colorectal anastomosis with the intracolonic bypass tube. Surg 1992; 112:618-23.

30. Attwood SEA, Hill ADK, Murphy PG, Thornton J, Stephens RB. A prospective randomized trial of laparoscopic versus open appendectomy. Surg 1992; 112:497.

31. O'Sullivan GC, Murphy D, O'Brien MG, Ireland A. Laparoscopic management of generalized peritonitis due to perforated colonic diverticula. Am J Surg 1996; 171:432-4.

32. Hinchey EJ, Schaal PGH, Richards MB. Treatment of perforated diverticulitis of the colon. Adv Surg 1978; 12:85-105.

33. Wittmann DH, Aprahamian C, Bergstein JM. Etappenlavage. Advanced diffuse peritonitis managed by planned multiple laparotomies utilizing zippers, slide fastener, and Velcro analogue for temporary abdominal closure. World Journal of Surgery 1990; 14:218-26.

34. Polk HC Jr, Fry DE. Radical peritoneal debridement for established peritonitis: the result of a prospective randomized clinical trial. Ann Surg 1980; 192:350-5.

35. Saha SK. Efficacy of metronidazole lavage in treatment of intraperitoneal sepsis. A prospective study. Dig Dis Sci 1996; 41:1313-8.

36. Edmiston CE, Jr., Goheen MP, Kornhall S, Jones FE, Condon RE. Fecal peritonitis: microbial adherence to serosal mesothelium and resistance to peritoneal lavage. World J Surg 1990; 14:176-83.

37. Ozmen V, Thomas WO, Healy JT, et al. Irrigation of the abdominal cavity in the treat-

ment of experimentally induced microbial peritonitis: efficacy of ozonated saline. Am Surg 1993; 59:297-303.

38. Dobrin PB, O'Keefe P, Tatarowicz W, Stachowski M, Freeark RJ. The value of continuous 72-hour peritoneal lavage for peritonitis. Am J Surg 1989; 157:368-71; discussion 371.

39. Browne MK, Leslie GB. Animal models of peritonitis. Surg Gynecol Obstet 1976; 143:738-40.

40. Schein M, Gecelter G, Freinkel W, Gerding H, Becker PJ. Peritoneal lavage in abdominal sepsis. A controlled clinical study. Arch Surg 1990; 125:1132-5.

41. Oguz M, Bektemir M, Dulger M, Yalin R. Treatment of experimental peritonitis with intraperitoneal povidone-iodine solution. Can J Surg 1988; 31:169-71.

42. Ahrenholz DH. The treatment of intra-abdominal sepsis. In Najarian JS, Delaney JP (eds.) Advances in Gastrointestinal Surgery, : Year Bk Med., Chicago 1984; 393-7.

43. Lineaweaver W, Howard R, Soucy D, et al. Topical antimicrobial toxicity. Arch Surg 1985; 120:267-70.

44. Lally KP, Nichols RL. Various intraperitoneal irrigation solutions in treating experimental fecal peritonitis. South Med Journal 1981; 74:789-91.

45. Ahrenholz DH, Simmons RL. Providone-iodine in peritonitis. 1. Adverse effects of local instillation in experimental E. coli peritonitis. J Surg Res 1979; 26:458-63.

46. Sugimoto K, Hirata M, Takishima T, Ohwada T, Shimazu S, Kakita A. Mechanically assisted intra-operative peritoneal lavage for generalized peritonitis as a result of perforation of the upper part of the gastrointestinal tract. J Am Coll Surg 1994; 179:443-8.

47. Sugimoto K, Hirata M, Kikuno T, Takishima T, Maekawa K, Ohwada T. Large-volume intraoperative peritoneal lavage with an assistant device for treatment of peritonitis cau-

sed by blunt traumatic rupture of the small bowel. J Trauma 1995; 39:689-92.

48. Schein M, Saadia R, Decker G. Intraoperative peritoneal lavage. Surg Gynecol Obstet 1988; 166:187-95.

49. Nathans AB, Rotstein OD. Therapeutic options in peritonitis. Surg Clin N Am 1994; 74:677-92.

50. Pissiotis CA, Klimopoulos S. Recent advances in the management of intra-abdominal infections. Surg Annual 1993; 25:59-83.

51. Guo W, Soltesz V, Ding JW, et al. Abdominal rubber drain piece aggravates intra-abdominal sepsis in the rat. Eur J Clin Invest 1994; 24:540-7.

52. Pick AW, Mackay J. Laparostomy: a technique for the management of severe abdominal sepsis. Aust NZ J Surg 1993; 63:888-93.

53. Hallerback B, Andersson C, Englund N, et al. A prospective randomized study of continuous peritoneal lavage post-operatively in the treatment of purulent peritonitis. Surg Gynecol Obstet 1986; 163:433-6.

54. Kumar GV, Smile SR, Sibal RN. Post-operative peritoneal lavage in generalized peritonitis. A prospective analysis. International Surgery 1989; 74:20-2.

55. Steinberg D. On leaving the peritoneal cavity open in acute generalized suppurative peritonitis. Am J Surg 1979; 137:216-20.

56. Ivatury R, Nallathambi M, Prakaschanda R, et al. Open management of the septic abdomen: therapeutic and prognostic consideration based on APACHE II. Crit Care Med 1989; 17:511-5.

57. Teichmann W, Wittmann DH, Andreone A. Scheduled reoperations (Etappenlavage) for diffuse peritonitis. Arch Surg 1986; 121:147-52.

58. Wouters DB, Krom RAF, Slooff MJH, Kootstra G, Kuijjer PJ. The use of Marlex mesh in patients with generalized peritonitis and multiple organ failure. Surg Gynecol Obstet 1983; 156:609-14.

59. Bose SM, Kalra M, Sandhu NP. Open management of septic abdomen by Marlex mesh zipper. Aust NZ J Surg 1991; 61:385-8.

60. Hedderrich GS, Wexler MJ, McLean APH, et al. The septic abdomen: Open management with Marlex mesh with a zipper. Surgery 1986; 99:399-407.

61. Sleeman D, Sosa JL, Gonzalez A, et al. Reclosure of the open abdomen. J Am C Surg 1995; 180:200-4.

62. Hakkiluoto A, Hannukainen J. Open management with mesh and zipper of patients with intra-abdominal abscesses or diffuse peritonitis. Eur J Surg 1992; 158:403-5.

63. Ercan F, Korkmaz A, Aras N. The zipper-mesh method for treating delayed generalized peritonitis. Surg Today 1993; 23:205-14.

64. Garcia-Sabrido JL, Tallado JM, Christou NV, Polo JR, Valdecantos E. Treatment of severe intra-abdominal sepsis and/or necrotic foci by an 'open abdomen' approach. Zipper and zipper-mesh techniques. Arch Surg 1988; 123:152-6.

65. Schein M, Hirshberg A, Hashmonai M. Current surgical management of severe intra-abdominal infection. Surgery 1992; 112:489-96.

66. Wittmann DH, Schein M, Condon RE. Management of secondary peritonitis. Ann Surg 1996; 224:10-8.

67. Wilson SE. A critical analysis of recent innovations in the treatment of intra-abdominal infection. Surg Gynecol Obstet 1993; 177:11-7; discussion 35-40.

68. Penninckx FM, Kerremans RP, Lauwers PM. Planned relaparotomies in the surgical treatment of severe generalized peritonitis from intestinal origin. World J Surg 1983; 7:762-6.

69. Gann DS, Foster AH. Endocrine and metabolic responses to injury. In Schwartz SI, Shires GT, Spencer FC, Husser WC (eds.) Principles of Surgery, 6th ed., 1994, pp. 3-59, McGraw-Hill, Inc., New York, USA.

Intra-abdominal Infections: Antibiotics in Secondary Peritonitis

Jesús Esquivel, John Mihran Davis and Robert Wood

1. INTRODUCTION

Intra-abdominal infections are relatively common clinical problems in hospital-based practice and are especially common in general surgery and in surgical intensive care units. Secondary peritonitis is defined as the presence of purulent exudate in the abdominal cavity derived from an enteric source and usually there is polymicrobial flora as a result of hollow viscus perforation.

Others suggest that the mortality of intra-abdominal infection was about 90 per cent when treated non-operatively [1]. The occurrence of wartime injuries, particularly penetrating abdominal wounds, gave impetus to developments in surgical techniques for managing these infections. Adjuvant therapy with antibiotics was first introduced in the 1930's and was widely applied in the treatment of peritonitis after the middle of this century. However, mortality did not improve substantially and continued to be reported in the 30 to 70 per cent range [1].

Major advances occurred after World War II when usage of antibiotics was accompanied by aggressive surgical management of penetrating abdominal wounds. Standardization of surgical methods led to major improvements in survival of soldiers with these injuries; mortality dropped to the range of 40 to 50 per cent.

These principles were extended to the civilian population in the late 1960's with the introduction of trauma centers where expeditious surgical intervention for penetrating abdominal wounds were widely applied [2]. Misconceptions of the complex microbial populations in an abdominal wound and lack of understanding of the underlying pathophysiologic processes in peritonitis and the pharmacodynamics of antibiotics, limited the effective use of antibiotics. As a result, the acute phase of peritonitis was successfully managed, leaving in its wake a huge amount of intra-abdominal abscesses [2].

Improved understanding of the pathophysiology of these infections, scanning techniques that have revolutionized diagnosis, percutaneous drainage techniques that have radically altered management of abscesses as well as the ability to give better respiratory and cardiac support, the correction of hypoxia and hypovolemia and giving the appropriate antimicrobial drugs by the appropriate route and for the appropriate time, have all translated in an improvement in into mortality from secondary peritonitis that in the 1990's has decreased to the range of 10 to 20 per cent.

2. DEFINITION AND SOURCE OF CONTAMINATION

Secondary peritonitis occurs as a result of perforation of an intra-abdominal viscus such as the large intestine. Because the initial inoculum consists of those microorganisms present within the lumen, these infections are almost invariably polymicrobial and involve both aerobic and anaerobic micro-organisms.

Successful treatment of intra-abdominal sepsis entails the removal of the source of infection, eradication of residual bacteria and metabolic and hemodynamic support to counteract the physiologic alterations that occur during sepsis. Source control is perhaps the most important of these treatment modalities. By definition, the underlying problem is caused by a disease process that leads to gastrointestinal tract necrosis and perforation and that, therefore, requires surgical intervention. The Surgical Infection Society has agreed to exclude from this definition peptic ulcer perforation of less than 12 hours duration, enteric perforations due to trauma of less than 24 hours duration, non-perforated appendicitis, simple acute cholecystitis and simple bowel necrosis [3]. Surgical treatment generally consists of removal or resection of necrotic or diseased tissue, drainage of obvious areas of infection and diversion or reconstitution of gastrointestinal tract continuity. Although small

perforations are occasionally sealed by the inflammatory response in association with omental containment, natural closure is inhibited by ongoing leakage of succus entericus coupled with the growth of micro-organisms derived from the perforated viscus. As the peritoneal defense response compartmentalizes infected fluid, neutrophils and monocytes that are able to enter the area invariably release cytokine and lysosomal enzymes that contribute to both the formation of abscesses and the systemic response. Thus, it is common to find an open viscus perforation with ongoing spillage during the course of an operation for intra-abdominal sepsis, as well as loculation of infected fluid or discrete abscesses scattered throughout the abdomen.

Abscesses and necrotic tissue are largely inaccessible to the normal host defense processes and antimicrobial agents and, therefore, must be physically removed because the ability of the host to combat infection that is concentrated and localized within an internal body cavity is relatively poor [4].

Although the primary mode of therapy consists of surgical intervention to remove the source of peritoneal contamination, antimicrobial agents play a critical role in eradication of intraperitoneal pathogens. Therefore, antibiotic therapy should be initiated as soon as the diagnosis of intra-abdominal infection is made. The choice of antibiotics is empirically based on the most likely micro-organisms causing infection. The spectrum of micro-organisms inoculating the peritoneal cavity after perforation of the gastrointestinal tract depends on the level of perforation (Figure 1) [5].

The terminal ileum and the colon contain more than 500 different species of bacteria

Figure 1
Type of bacteria present as it relates to the site of gastrointestinal perforation

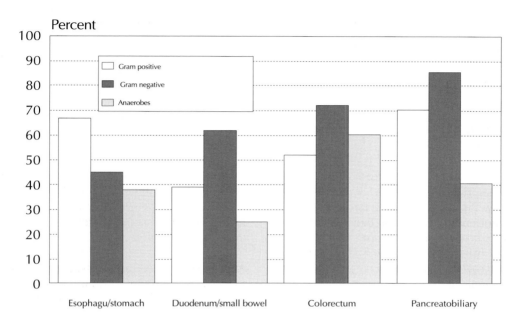

at a concentration of 10^{12} bacteria per gram, with an anaerobe: aerobe ratio of 100:1. Thus, distal perforation leads to a massive bacterial inoculum. By contrast, the stomach and duodenum are relatively sterile, and consequently initially cause a sterile, chemical peritonitis. However, the relative achlorhydria associated with gastric ulcers or the use of antacids and H_2 receptor antagonists which permit gastric colonization with Gram-positive oral anaerobes, Candida species and facultative Gram-negative bacilli lead to greater contamination at the time of perforation [6].

The gastrointestinal flora becomes relatively well established at 1 year of age, there are minimal differences based on dietary habits and the flora in an individual gene-

rally remains stable according to sequential sampling unless perturbed by administration of antibiotics or H_2 blockers as mentioned above. Hospitalization may also result in at least transient colonization by extraneous bacteria, presumably from environmental sources, that may become the source of pathogens or the source of genetic material that confers resistance to antibiotics by the original colonizing strains [7].

Despite the diverse bacterial inoculum released into the peritoneal cavity at the time of gastrointestinal perforation, the spectrum of isolates recovered at the time of laparotomy is markedly simplified. Most commonly, the resultant infection is polymicrobial, containing a mixture of aerobic and anaerobic bacteria (Table 1) [5]. Polymicrobial infec-

Table 1
Peritoneal isolates at laparotomy

Organism	Solomkin et al[*]	Mosdell et al[+]
Gran-negative aerobic and facultative anaerobes		
Escherichia coli	56.8	68.4
Enterobacter species	13.5	6.1
Klebsiella species	15.4	17
Pseudumonas aeruginosa	14.8	19.1
Proteus species	6.2	2.7
Serratia marcescens	1.2	4.1
Morganella morganii	1.2	–
Citrobacter species	3.1	3.4
Others	3.7	7.5
Yeast		
Candida species	18.6	4.1
Gran-positive aerobic and facultative anaerobes		
Nonenterococcal streptococci	35.8	25.9
Enterococci	23.5	10.5
Staphylococcus aureus or S. epidermidis	10.5	10.5
Anaerobic organisms		
Bacteroides fragilis	22.8	44.5
Other Bacteroids	21	–
Clostridium species	17.9	5.8
Peptococci/streptococci	7.4	16
Fusobacterium species	6.2	5.1
Lactobaclilius	5.6	–
Eubacterium species	4.3	–
Others	12.4	3.7

Adapted from Solomkin JS, Dellinger EP, Christou NV, eta al: Results of a multi cesnter trial comparing imipenem/cilastin to ro-
bramycin/clindamycin for intraabdominal infections. Ann Surg. 212:581. 1990 (56); *and* Mosdell DM, Voltura A, et al: Antibiotic
for surgical peritonitis. Ann Surg 214:543 (9); with permission.
[*]Data represent percent of all patients.
[+]Data represent percent of all cultures.

tions are present in about 2/3 of patients, with an average of 2.9 to 3.9 isolates per patient at the time of initial laparotomy. In a recent study of 339 peritoneal culture specimens in patients with peritonitis, 76% contained mixed aerobic and anaerobic bacteria, with the most frequent combination being Escherichia coli and Bacteroides fragilis. Anaerobic organisms were present alone in only 13% and aerobic in only 11% of specimens. The predominant Gram-posi-

tive organisms were the non-enterococcal streptococci and enterococci [9].

3. SUPPORT FOR BROAD SPECTRUM BACTERIAL COVERAGE

Antimicrobial therapy is a critical adjunctive treatment that combats bacteremia during the operation, limits spread of peritonitis, and speeds resolution of the intra-abdominal infectious process. Accordingly, selection of efficacious antimicrobial therapy can result in reduced superficial and deep operative-site infection, early recovery of intestinal function and timely discharge from the hospital. On the other hand, selection of antimicrobial which do not have an effective spectrum or to which the organisms are resistant, can result in post-operative infectious complications and longer periods of hospitalization [10].

Optimal empiric antibiotic therapy for the treatment of secondary bacterial peritonitis should include an agent or agents active against both Gram-negative enteric bacilli such as E. coli and anaerobic bacteria such as B. fragilis. Several facts constitute the basis for this selection. First, it is difficult to predict the level of intestinal perforation based on clinical grounds. Thus, therapy is directed against the more complex bacterial inoculum derived from colonic perforation [5]. A second fact is documented by the excellent work of Bartlett [7], Gorbach et al. [11] in the study of the pathogenesis of intra-abdominal sepsis using a rodent model designed to simulate the sequence of events following colonic perforation using an inoculum of stool. Their initial studies were designed to determine the natural history of the infection in terms of anatomic changes and quantitative microbiology and showed a two-stage disease process: The first stage was peritonitis characterized by a free-flowing peritoneal exudate, E. coli bacteremia and a 39% mortality. The second stage of infection was characterized by multiple intra-abdominal abscesses with grossly purulent exudate within a collagen wall capsule that became well formed at five days after challenge. Bacteriologic studies of the abscesses showed the numerically dominant bacteria to be B. fragilis. The conclusion of this work was the concept of

the biphasic disease with two major microbial pathogens. E. coli (and presumably other coliform bacteria) represented the major pathogen in the early-stage disease, characterized by generalized peritonitis. Supporting data were the high rates of E. coli bacteremia, protection afforded with gentamicin treatment and early lethality with monomicrobial challenge; B. fragilis (and possibly other encapsulated anaerobes) represented the major pathogen in the second stage of disease. Supporting evidence was the numeric dominance of this organism in abscesses, protection afforded with clindamycin or metronidazole treatment and reproduction of abscesses with monomicrobial challenge. The obvious therapeutic implications of these observations is that treatment should be directed against both E. coli and B. fragilis [11]. No pathogenic role could be assigned to the enterococcus because treatment against this organism had no impact on outcome and monomicrobial challenge produced no detectable pathological effects [7]. The modern era of treating intra-abdominal infections was inaugurated in the late 1960's, driven by three lines of scientific inquiry confirmed by a new generation of surgeons and physicians committed to the study of infection [2]. Each of these developments relied on the others for support. The first was the improvement in techniques in anaerobic bacteriology that allowed the isolation of fastidious anaerobic bacteria that failed to grow in the conventional microbiology laboratory. Subsequent studies of the principal anaerobic culprits, Bacteroides species, showed that a virulence factor - the polysaccharide capsule - could explain, in part, the selection advantage that facilitated the emergence of these organisms as pathogens.

The second, as mentioned above, was the animal model, simulating the clinical course of abdominal infection and, therefore, providing insights into a better understanding of the pathophysiologic events and the host defense mechanisms in secondary peritonitis.

The third element in defining the current approach was the discovery of anti-anaerobe antimicrobial agents. Clindamycin, a drug originally developed for treating staphylococcal and streptococcal infections, was found to suppress anaerobic bacteria in the normal intestinal flora when given by mouth. The drug was then tried in selected anaerobic infections with outstanding results. The first randomized, comparative trial that examined the need for an anti-anaerobe antibiotic was carried out in 1970-1972 in patients with penetrating abdominal trauma [12]. The regimens were clindamycin/kanamycin versus cephalothin/kanamycin, the standard treatment of that era. The cephalothin/kanamycin group had a 22% incidence of anaerobic infections (11 of 52 patients) compared with an incidence of only 2% in the clindamycin/kanamycin group (1 of 48 patients). In Europe, metronidazole was recognized for its unique anti-anaerobe activity and several clinical trials established its superiority over other antibiotic regimens that lacked such activity. Once more, it was demonstrated that adjuvant therapy with the appropriate antibiotics played a crucial role in maximizing the likelihood of a successful outcome in treating patients with secondary peritonitis. The increasingly broad number and classes of drugs, left clinicians looking for a drug or drug combination that would provide patients with the best opportunity in the immediate term to avoid invasive sepsis and to preclude the locally destructive effects of infection. A variety of new antibiotics that might be useful in the management of intra-abdominal infections have been introduced in the past several years, leaving surgeons with a extensive range of choices of antimicrobial agents for the treatment of secondary peritonitis. Many of these antibiotics are approved by the Food and Drug Administration, however, few have sufficient published clinical experience to recommend their use. Also, the decision to use a particular regimen should be based on the underlying pathologic condition, concurrent patient risk factors (e.g. major organ dysfunction, immunosuppression, etc.), risk of adverse drug effects and published clinical experience with a particular regimen [13].

4. PROBLEMS WITH CLINICAL STUDIES

It is important to mention that when attempting to extrapolate published data on antimicrobial agents to the general patient population, the disease status and risk factors of the study population must be assessed carefully. Published clinical trials frequently do not include patients at the highest risk for mortality, therefore, application of these studies to critically ill patients must be limited. Some important risk factors to assess with clinical trials include age, malnutrition, concurrent organ failure, location of abscess, presence of positive blood culture and the presence of multiple abscesses [14-16]. Nosocomial pneumonia also has been demonstrated to be an important risk factor for mortality with intra-abdominal infection [17].

Comparison of trials of antimicrobial agents and application of the findings to patients would be aided by the universal use of scoring systems such as APACHE II, penetrating abdominal trauma index (PAT I) and sepsis severity score (SSS) [3].

5. COMPARATIVE STUDIES

Combination treatment regimens in which either clindamycin or metronidazole with an aminoglycoside are used, enjoy an unbroken record of efficacy in the treatment of serious intra-abdominal infections. Each of the anti-anaerobe drugs has its supporters; clindamycin is favored by some authorities because of its added spectrum of activity against staphylococci and streptococci, although it is recognized that resistant strains of anaerobes have developed and there is concern about gastrointestinal side effects. Metronidazole has excellent activity against a broad range of anaerobic bacteria but not against microaerophilic or facultative streptococci. In several comparative trials (Table II) both clindamycin and metronidazole performed equally well as therapy for intra-abdominal infections and they still rank among the favorite treatment choices for mixed infections [2].

Monotherapy became feasible since the advent of broad-spectrum antimicrobial drugs that cover both the aerobic/facultative and anaerobic components of mixed infection. Cefoxitin has been most widely studied as a monotherapy for intra-abdominal infections. In thirteen studies of appendicitis, trauma or peritoneal infection, cefoxitin has compared favorably with either aminoglycoside-containing regimen or another broad spectrum antibiotic. Imipenem has been used as the single agent in eight studies in which the comparison group contained an anti-anaerobe drug and an aminoglycoside. The results with imipenem were as good as and in some cases superior to, the alternative regimen. Three studies employed cefotetan as a single agent and one study used piperacillin, with results equivalent to those in the comparison group [2].

In general, the studies conducted in established intra-abdominal infection do not demonstrate significant differences in efficacy between combination regimens and single agents. Solomkin et al [18] published an evaluation of antimicrobial clinical trials in intra-abdominal infection and examined study design and outcome reporting. Sixteen articles were included in the review that met their screening criteria. In the studies reviewed, 1,275 patients had a mortality rate of 3.5%, which was clearly related to enrollment of low-mortality infections of the infections, 25% were classified as acute appendicitis, which has reported mortality rates of 0 - 2%. Conditions known to be associated with high mortality rates were rarely enrolled in these trials. Because of this problem and the small sample sizes used in most studies, the authors concluded that the various regimens may not be of equal efficacy but rather that the studies were designed in such a way that they failed to distinguish between regimens.

Some other studies compared the anaerobic component of the antimicrobial regimen. In a trial conducted by the Canadian Metronidazole-Clindamycin Study Group [19], the outcomes of 141 patients treated with either metronidazole plus gentamicin or clindamycin plus gentamicin for intra-abdominal peritonitis or abscess were evaluated. This study, in addition to a smaller trial by Smith et al [20], demonstrated that metronidazole and clindamycin are equally effective as anti-anaerobic agents for the treatment of intra-abdominal infections. At present, most clinicians accept that clindamycin and metronidazole are equivalent in efficacy for treatment of intra-abdominal infections when added to aminoglycosides.

A well-designed clinical trial published in 1985 by Lennard et al [21] compared clin-

Table 2
Combination antibiotic therapy in intra-abdominal infection

Reference	Patient Population	Agents	No.	Failures (%)
Harding et al, 1980 (23)	Adults (mean age, 52.2 years) and children (mean age, 10.3 years) with peritonitis abscess, or wound infection due to various inciting events and surgeries including appendicitis, small bowel or colonic perforation	Clindamycin/gentamicin Chloramphenico/gentamicin Ticarcillin/gentamicin	42 53 39	9 (21.4) 10 (18.9) 4 (10.3)
Smith et al, 1980 (20)	Intra-abdominal infections due to appendicitis, bowel perforation, diverticular disease, gangrenous bowel, inflammatory bowel disease	Clindamycin/tobramycin Metronidazole/tovramycin	23 34	3 (13.0) 6 (17.6)
Stone and Fabian, 1980 (22)	Peritoneal and soft tissue infections, including appendicitis, cholecystitis, peritoneal abscesses. Average agr, 42.6 years	Clindamycin/gentamicin Metronidazole/gentamicin Erythomycin/cefamandole	68 60 60	2 (2.9) 1 (1.7) 2 (3.3)
Tallery et al, 1981 (24)	Mixed infections at various sites, including intraabdominal, cutaneous, bone, and lung. Median ages, 51 and 56 years	Cefoxilin with or without amikacin Clindamycin/anikacin	37 37	3 (8.1) 8 (21.6)
Canadian Metronidazole-Clindamycin Study Group, 1983 (19)	Peritonitis (30% secondary to appendicitis) or abscess. Mean age, 50 years	Metronidazole/gentamicin Clindamycin/gentamicin	72 69	4 (5.5) 3 (4.3)
Harding et al, 1984 (25)	Compilation of four studies. Peritonitis and/or abscess or wound infection from apprendiz, colon, or small bowel. Mean ages: Clindamycin/toramycin, 44 years; cefoxitin/tobramycin, 42 years; clindamycin/tobramycin, 41 years; Ceftzoxime, 54 years	Cefoxitin/tobramycin Clindamycin/tobramycin Ceftizoxime Clindamycin&tobramycin	30 29 24 15	2 (6.7) 3 (12.5) 2 (13.3)
Lennars et al, 1985 (21)	Intra-abdominal sepsis at laporotomy; patients with appendicitis or cholecystitis Without gangrene or perforation were excluded: Patient groups stratified by age, snock, alcoholism, gastrointestinal bleeding, steroid use, diabetes, obesity, organ dysfunction. Mean age, approximately 52 years	Clindamycin/gemtamycin Chloramphenicol/gentamicin	124 124	23 (18.5) 20 (16.1)

damycin/gentamicin with chloramphenicol/gentamicin for treatment of established intra-abdominal infections. The investigators carefully stratified the treatment groups for risk factors such as malnutrition, age, shock, alcoholism, diabetes and organ dysfunction. Although the two regimens were demonstrated to be equally effective, chloramphenicol is generally not considered for treatment of intra-abdominal infection due to potential hematologic side effects. However, with changing pathogens and changing strategies in the critically ill patient with peritonitis, chloramphenicol may again play a crucial role in the antibiotic armamentarium for the treatment of patients with established intra-abdominal infections, especially those with multi-drug resistant organisms.

Over the past several years, interest in new antibiotic combinations and the desire to avoid the nephrotoxicity and ototoxicity caused by aminoglycosides has led to the use of alternate agents that have comparable efficacy and less toxic side effects. It should be noted that the added cost attributable to the use of aminoglycosides, incurred through monitoring of drug levels and treatment of adverse reactions, also argues against their use.

Aztreonam is a monobactam antibiotic that is effective against aerobic Gram-negative organisms, is stable to beta-lactamase and is a weak inducer of beta-lactamase production. It is an appropriate substitute for aminoglycosides in patients in whom it is necessary to avoid nephrotoxicity and ototoxicity. When given in combination with clindamycin, aztreonam can be used to treat intra-abdominal infections [26]. It should not be given with metronidazole alone as metronidazole lacks coverage of Gram positive facultative organisms.

At least six clinical trials using aztreonam have appeared in the literature and are summarized in Table III [7,12]. One trial of aztreonam/clindamycin versus tobramycin/clindamycin for treatment of intra-abdominal infections demonstrated similar clinical responses in the two groups but the patient populations studied had a high percentage of relatively low-risk patients, including those with appendicitis and cholecystitis [27]. Birolini et al, [28-29] reported in two different trials the effectiveness of aztreonam/clindamycin versus tobramycin/clindamycin. The patients were stratified according to diagnosis and surgical procedure; however, a large proportion of patients were at relatively low risk. Berne et al [30], reported in a randomized study of patients with surgically treated gangrenous or perforated appendicitis that aztreonam plus clindamycin was equal in efficacy to gentamicin plus clindamycin. Although the authors stated that patients with more advanced peritonitis should be studied, the results are encouraging, since the trial was conducted in a relatively homogenous group of patients with serious infections and aztreonam was shown to be as effective as gentamicin. More recently, Barboza et al [31], published in 1994 a prospective, randomized, single blind study to evaluate the efficacy and safety of clindamycin plus amikacin versus clindamycin plus aztreonam in treating intra-abdominal infections in adults with perforated appendicitis or intra-abdominal abscess. Both combinations were highly effective in managing intra-abdominal sepsis. The clindamycin-aztreonam group showed a slight advantage because of absence of renal toxicity and shorter time to apyrexia.

The combination of ceftazidime plus clindamycin was studied by Bubrick et al [32], in comparison with tobramycin plus clin-

Table 3
Clinical Trials with Alternative Combination Therapy

Reference	Patient Population	Agents	No.	Failures (%)	
Henry, 1985 (54)	Pooled data from open and randomized trials. Peritonitis and intra-abdominal abscess confirmed by positive culture. Mean age not stated	Aztreonam/antianaerobic agent (usually clindamycin) Tobramycin/antianaerobic agent (usually clindamycin)	59 56	4 11	(6.8) (19.6)
Birolini et al, 195 (28)	Varoius intra-abominal infections including acute appendicitis and cholecystitis Surgery specified. Mean ages, 36.4 years and 31.4 years	Aztreonam/clindamycin Tobramycin/clindamycin	36 30	3 4	(8.3) (13.3)
Berne et al, 1987 (30)	Gangrenous or perforated appendix. Mean age 27 years	Aztreonam/clindamycin Gentamicin/clindamycin	56 28	2 0	(3.6) (0)
Birolini et al, 1989 (29)	Various intra-abdominal infections, including appendicitis (50%), perforated small and large bowel, and abscess. Mean age about 37 years	Aztreonam/clindamycin Tobramycin/clindamycin	76 80	10 11	(13.2) (13.8)
Williams and Hatchkin, 1991 (27)	Various intra-abdominal infections. Appendicitis and cholecystitis more common in aztreonam group; peptic ulcer disease with duodenal perforation more common in tobramycin group. Mean age, 43 years	Aztreonam/clindamycin Tobramycin/clindamycin	104 105	16 16	(15.4) (15.2)
Bubrick et al, 1990 (32)	Intra-abdominal sepsis, 50% traumatic wound. Mean age, 29 years	Ceftazidime/clindamycin Tobramycin/clindamycin	34 34	3 4	(8.8) (11.8)
Barboza et al, 1994 (31)	62 patients with perforated apprendicitis or intra-abdominal abscess	Clindamycin + amikacin Clindamycin + aztreonam	31 31	2 0	(6.3) (0)

Table 4

Antimicrobial Sensitivities of Commonly Encountered Pathogens to Parenteral Antibiotics Used in Abdominal Infection

	Gram-negative	Enterococci	Other Streptococcus Species	Gram-negative Bacilli	Gram-positive Bacilli	Gram-positive Cocci
Penicillin	0	++	+++	+	+++	+++
Ampicillin	+	+++	+++	+	+++	+++
Piperacillin	+++	+++	+++	+	+++	+++
Ticarcillin*	++	++	+++	++	++	++
Cefazolin	++	0	+++	+++	++	+++
Cefamandole	++	0	+++	+	++	+++
Cefoxilin	++	0	++	++	+++	+++
Cefotaxime	+++	0	++	+	++	+++
Imipenem	+++	++	+++	+++	+++	+++
Aztreonam	+++	0	0	0	0	0
Aminoglycosides	+++	0	0	0	0	0
Clindamycin	0	0	++	+++	+++	+++
Metronidazole	0	0	0	+++	+++	+++
B-lactamase inhibitor-B-lactam combinations						
Ampicillin-sulbactam	++	+++	+++	+++	+++	+++
Ticarcillin-clavulanic acid	++	++	+++	+++	+++	+++

*0 Indicates little or no activity; +, some activity; ++, moderate to good activity; and +++, excellent activity.
+ Azlocillin, mezlocillin, and carbenicillin have similar spectra.
Includes cephalothin, cephapirin, and cephradine.
Includes cefuroxime, cefonicid, cefotiam, and ceforanide.
Includes cefotetan and cefmetazole.
Includes ceftriaxone, ceftazidime, cefoperazone, and ceftizoxime.
#Includes gentamicin, tobramycin, netilmicin, and amikacin.

Ref. (3) - Bohnen JM, Solomkin JS, Dellinger EP, et al; Guidelines for clinical care: Anti-infective Agents for intra-abdominal infection. Arch Surg- Vol 127. Januar 1992.

damycin in 94 patients, approximately 50% of whom were trauma patients who received treatment for acute contamination. A variety of infections were treated and surgical procedures were not specified. Ceftazidime appeared to be an effective substitute for aminoglycosides in the treatment of intra-abdominal infections.

All the above mentioned trials document once more that antimicrobial agents are important elements of therapy, service to reduce the incidence of persistent or recurrent abscess or peritonitis and to decrease the incidence of infective wound complications. The true value of one anti-infective regimen versus another has, however, become difficult to substantiate in current practice because of the potency of currently available antibiotics.

Rationale for the selection of antibacterial agents is supported also by the in vitro data, especially antimicrobial susceptibility tests which are predictive of the in vivo response of infecting bacteria to particular antibacterial agents. Although a variety of susceptibility testing techniques are available,

disk or automated testing is appropriate for bacteria isolated from intra-abdominal infections except in extraordinary circumstances [3]. Table IV summarizes the in vitro susceptibilities of important pathogens to commonly used anti-infective agents in abdominal infection. Other issues in the selection of antimicrobial regimens for treatment of established intra-abdominal infections include adverse drug effects and cost.

6. ADVERSE DRUG EFFECTS

An important factor in selecting agents for the treatment of intra-abdominal infection is adverse drug effects. It is well known that adverse drug effects are common, particularly in critically ill patients. Common or important adverse effects of antimicrobial agents used to treat intra-abdominal infections are listed in Table V.

Nephrotoxicity is an important risk with aminoglycosides even when serum concentrations are within "acceptable" ranges. Factors such as older age, pre-existing renal

Table 5
Adverse Drug Effects of Antimicrobial Agents Used for Treatment of Instra-Abdominal infections

Nephrotoxity	Aminoglycosides
Coaggulopathy	Penicilina Cephalosporins
Diarrhea or psudomembranous colitis	Clindamycin Cephalosporins
Seizures	Imipenem/cilastatin Penicilina
Hypersensitivity	Penicilins Imipenem/cilastatin

Ref. (13) - DiPiro, JT, Fortson JS: Combination Antibiotic Therapy in the Management of Intra-abdominal infection. Am J of Surg, Vol 165, No. 2A, Feb. 1993.

disease, hypovolemia, diuretic use or concurrent use of other nephrotoxic drugs increase the risk of nephrotoxic reactions. Two large epidemiologic studies have placed in perspective the costs associated with aminoglycoside nephrotoxicity [33-34]. Aminoglycoside use was identified as one of four significant risk factors for development of acute renal failure in hospitalized patients, along with intravascular volume depletion, congestive heart failure and septic shock. Development of acute renal failure in these patients, increased mortality by a factor of 10 and was associated with prolongation of hospital stay. It is important to remember that the usage of relatively low doses to avoid this complication can increase the likelihood of therapeutic failure.

Many antimicrobial agents have been reported to cause coagulation defects. Coagulopathy may occur with cephalosporins, particularly those that have the N-methylthiotetrazole ring on the side chain (e.g. cefamandole, moxalactam, cefoperazone, cefotetan) or with penicillins that in high doses can inhibit platelet function (e.g. ticarcillin). Clearly, the risk is greater in patients who already have underlying liver dysfunction.

Hypersensitivity reactions traditionally have been problems with beta-lactam antibiotics, particularly the penicillins and may also occur infrequently with aminoglycosides. Saxon and associates [33] have reported that aztreonam, a monobactam, does not cross-react with penicillins and cephalosporin and can be given to patients with allergies to these compounds. Imipenem is, however, likely to result in hypersensitivity reactions in penicillin-allergic patients.

Anti-anaerobic agents, particularly clindamycin, ampicillin and some cephalospo-

rins, can dramatically alter gastrointestinal flora, thereby permitting overgrowth of pathogenic Gram-negative bacilli and fungi or organisms such as Clostridium difficile that are responsible for pseudomembranous colitis.

With combination regimens, there may be a greater risk of adverse events, since the effects of the agents are additive. Some "single-agent" regimens such as imipenem/cilastatin, ampicillin/sulbactam, ticarcillin/clavulanic acid or piperacilliri/Tazobactam are combinations of drugs, even though there is only one antimicrobial agent. These added agents may be valuable in some respects but the exposure to two drugs will increase the risk of adverse effects compared with either drug given alone. Also, when adverse drug effects do occur, it may be impossible to distinguish the causative agent.

7. COST

A major consideration in the treatment of intra-abdominal infection is cost. There is a wide range of costs associated with antimicrobial regimens. Single agents are perceived to be less expensive than combinations but this is not always true. In fact, the least expensive antimicrobial regimen is the combination of gentamicin and clindamycin [13].

When considering costs, more than just the simple drug expense should be considered; costs associated with treatment also should be included. For example, aminoglycosides require monitoring of serum drug concentrations and this can add considerably to the cost of antimicrobial therapy. Delays in achieving adequate aminoglycoside peak levels can contribute significantly to costs by causing treatment failures [18]. Costs associated with drug administration should also be added. Drugs that require more frequent administration have higher costs associated with infusion fluids and devices as well as nursing time. Finally, the cost of adverse effects should be factored in.

Looking for the ideal antimicrobial regimen, a wide variety of anti-infective agents have been marketed for treatment of patients with intra-abdominal infections, often with marked differences in their anti-bacterial spectra, toxic effects and cost. Guidelines for use of specific agents were not available because of problems in clinical research. Most notably, a variety of patient-specific factors that are independent of anti-infective therapy affect outcome. Such factors include pre-existing medical conditions that may impair adaptive physiologic responses to the effects of infection, the patient's resistance to the infection, the source and density of micro-organisms and the severity of infection.

In order to provide considered guidance to physicians caring for patients with intra-abdominal infection in regard to selection of appropriate anti-infective therapy and based on analysis of in vitro activity against enteric bacteria, results of experiments in animal models, review of prospective randomized, clinical trials and certain theoretical concerns regarding pharmacokinetics, mechanisms of action and safety profile, the Antimicrobial Agents Committee of the Surgical Infection Society (SIS) published in 1992 guidelines for the use of anti-infective agents in intra-abdominal sepsis [3]. These guidelines are summarized in Table VI.

The SIS recommendations stratified intra-abdominal infection into two categories, the first being community acquired, mild-to-moderate intra-abdominal infections,

such as the complications of appendicitis, perforated duodenal ulcer older than 24 hours and complicated diverticulitis. The second category of more severely ill patients included advanced peritonitis, nosocomial infections and immunocompromised hosts. For first-level severity peritonitis, the recommendations are for single-Agent ß-lactam therapy, either a broad-spectrum second generation cephalosporin or a ß-lactam/ß-lactamase inhibitor combination. For severe or nosocomial infections, STS guidelines recommend a carbapenem or combination of agents. For each level of peritonitis, however, antimicrobial agents must be effective against the spectrum of aerobic and anaerobic bacteria encountered in enterogenous peritonitis (Table VII).

Also addressed in these guidelines are antimicrobial regimens that are not recommended in the treatment of intra-abdominal infections. Because of inadequate coverage of both aerobic and anaerobic organisms, cefazolin and other first generation cephalosporin, penicillin, cloxacillin and other antistaphylococcal penicillins, ampicillin, erythromycin and vancomycin should not be used as empiric therapy unless combined with acceptable agents listed above.

Metronidazole and clindamycin should not be used alone because they lack activity against facultative enteric organisms. The following agents should not be used alone because of inadequate coverage of anaerobic Gram-negative bacilli: aminoglycosides, aztreonam, polymyxins, cefuroxime, cefonicid, cefamandole, ceforanide, cefotiam, cefotaxime, ceftizoxime, cefoperazone, ceftriaxone, ceftazidime [3] and the new 4th generation cephalosporin cetepime [36].

Because of inadequate clinical data documenting efficacy and concerns about resis-

Table 6
Acceptable Antimicrobial Regimens

Single Agents

Community-acquired infections of mild to moderata severity
        Cefoxitin
        Cefotetan
        Cefmetazole
        Ticardilin-clavulanic acid
 	
Severe infections
        Imipenem-cilastatin

Combinations
Antianaerobe˙ plus aminoglycoside+ (young patients, no   hypotension or renal compromise) Antianaerobe˙ plus third-generation cephalosporin Clindamycin plus monobactam

˙Antianaerobes include clindamycin or metronidazole.
+Aminoglycosides include gentamycin, tobramycin, netilmicin and amikacin.
Cefotaxime and ceftizoxime. Ceftazidime and ceftriaxone are logical alternatives because of similar antimicrobial properties and lack of adverse effects; clinical data are insuficient.
Aztreonam.

Ref. (3) - Bohnen JM, Solomkin JS, Dellinger EP, eta al: Guidelines for clinical Care: anti-infective Agents for intra-abdominal infection.
Arch Surg - Vol. 127, January 1992.

Table 7
Microorganisms Included in This Guideline

Facultative Gram-negative Bacilli	Obligate Anaerobes	Facultative Gram-positive Cocci	Aerobic Gram-negative Bacilli
Escherichia coli	Bacteroides fragilis	Enterococci	Pseudomonas aeruginosa
Klebsiella species	Bacteroides species	Staphylococcus species	
Proteus species	Fusobacterium species	Streptococcus species	
Enterobacter species	Clostridium species		
Morganella moranii	Peptococcus species		
Other enteric gram-negative species	Peptostreptococcus species Lactobacillus species		

Ref. (3) - Bohnen JM, Solomkin JS, Dellinger EP, et al: Guidelines for Clinical Care: Anti-infective Agents for Intra-abdominal ionfection. Arch Surg - Vol 127 January 1992.

tance, the following drugs should not be used as single agents for empiric therapy despite their relative safety and broad in vitro antibacterial spectra: piperacillin, mezlocillin, azlocillin, ticarcillin and carbenicillin.

For patients whose abdominal infection develops in the hospital after previous antibiotic therapy, cefoxitin, cefotetan, cefmetazole, cefotaxime, ceftriaxone and ceftizoxime should not be used because of the risk of resistant facultative Gram-negative organisms [3].

The time has come when we should desist from using what many institutions consider the "gold standard" empiric triple-drug regimen of clindamycin, gentamicin and ampicillin or metronidazole, gentamicin and ampicillin for patients with community acquired intra-abdominal infection. Ampicillin is the gratuitous insurance policy for enterococcal infection. In the only clinical trial in which this combination has been put to the test, 119 patients with abdominal trauma were randomized to receive the triple-drug regimen or cefoxitin [2]. Infectious complications were noted in 18% of the triple drug group compared with 14.5% in the cefoxitin group. There are, of course, special situations in which an aminoglycoside should be used in the treatment of intra-abdominal infections: Previous use (within 30 days) of antibiotics, isolation of resistant Gram-negative bacilli; reoperation or recurrence of infections and prolonged pre-operative hospitalization. Yet, these situations account for only a minority of patients treated for intra-abdominal infections and therefore, the potent activity of aminoglycosides should be

Figure 2
Type of bacteria present as it relates to the site of gastrointestinal perforation

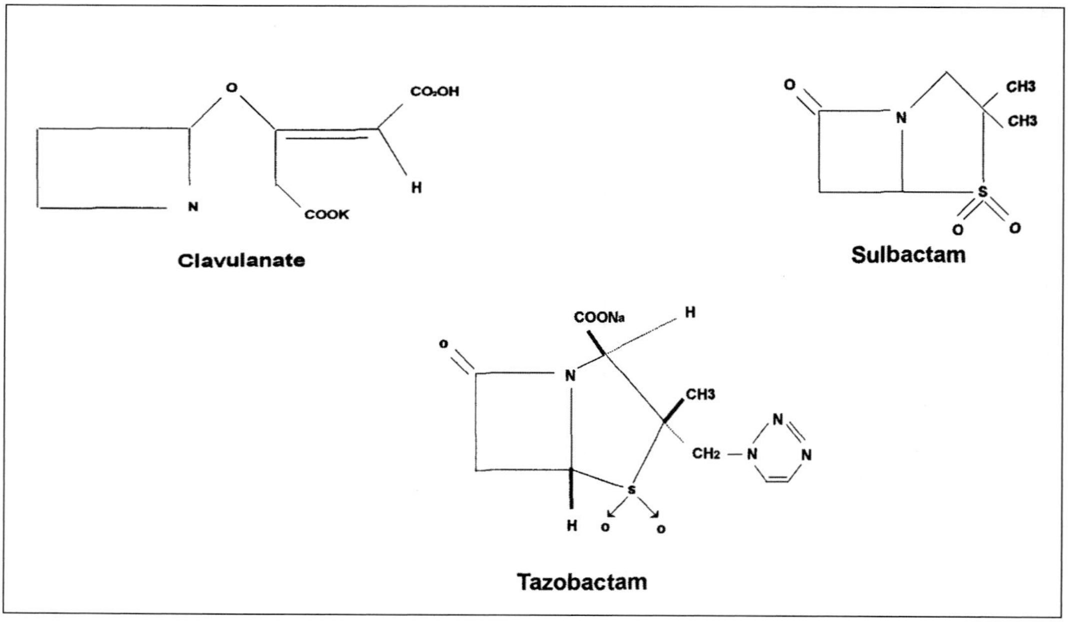
O
CO₂OH
N
COOK
H
Clavulanate
O
N
CH3
CH3
S
O
O
Sulbactam
COONa
H
O
N
CH3
CH2 — N
N
N
S
H
O
O
Tazobactam

"saved" for special circumstances that involve resistant Gram-negative bacilli.

Since the SIS guidelines were published, numerous reports have focused on the role of ß-lactam/ß-lactamase inhibitors in the treatment of intra-abdominal infection. This important new class of antimicrobial agents has resulted from the addition of ß-lactamase inhibitors to extended spectrum penicillins (Figure 2).

The imperative for development of these agents was the emergence of high rates of resistance in gram-positive and gram-negative organisms caused by their production of ß-lactamase enzymes, which activated previously effective penicillins, such as ampicillin, carbenicillin, and the cephalosporin [10]. Three ß-lactamase inhibitors have undergone clinical trial: sulbactam, clavulanate and tazobactam. When combined with their respective penicillins (ampicillin/sulbactam, ticarcillin/clavulanate, and piperlacillin/tazobactam), the resulting agents are effective against a broad variety of gram-positive and gram-negative organisms, including the bacteria of enterogenous peritonitis [37].

Table VIII reviews the clinical trial experience from both North America and Europe with the extended-spectrum penicillin/ß-lactamase inhibitor combinations in the treatment of intra-abdominal infections.
These studies demonstrate that the principal advantages of the three agents clinically available are a broad spectrum of antimicrobial activity against the gram-positive aerobes, gram-negative Enterobacteriaceae, and anaerobic flora. These compounds have low toxicity (except for those patients with penicillin allergy) and do not adversely affect renal function. Treatment of community-acquired intra-abdominal infections with the extended-spectrum penicillin/(-

lactamase inhibitors yields results comparable to those of the aminoglycoside plus antianaerobic agents, the carbapenems, and broad-spectrum cephalosporin therapies.

8. UNRESOLVED ISSUES AND SPECIAL CONSIDERATIONS RESISTANCE

The use of anti-infective agents may result in the development of bacterial resistance. This can take the form of initially susceptible isolates becoming resistant during treatment or the appearance of other organisms resistant to the antimicrobial agents used. Individual patients may develop extra-abdominal nosocomial infections with resistant organisms. Clearly, the emergence or antibiotic-resistant pathogens is on the rise, and therefore continual evaluation of new antimicrobial agents and resistance patterns to current antimicrobial in use should be carefully studied in each individual institution [37]. Sanders and colleagues [38] have pointed out that the importance of the ß-lactamase mechanism in the resistance of gram-negative pathogens to ß-lactam antimicrobial, illustrated by the resistance to ampicillin in approximately 50 percent or more of E. coli in certain high-risk populations. They also pointed out that TEM-1 and SHV-1 continue to be the two most commonly encountered plasmid-mediated (-lactamases among the Enterobacteriaceae and are responsible for much of the resistance to penicillin and the older cephalosporin.

An important factor promoting resistance of bacteria to antimicrobial is the inappropriate use of such agents both inside and outside of hospitals. Indiscriminate use must be avoided and therapy should be continued only as long as necessary.

Table 8
Summary of Clinical Data Obtained from Randomized Prospective Trials of Beta-lactam/Beta-lactamase Inhibitors in the Treatment of Community-Acquired intra-Abdominal Infections

Clinical Trial	Authorm yr	No. of Pts.	No. Evaluable	% Clinical Cures	% Bacteriological Cures
Ampicillin/sulbactam vs cefoxitin[*]	Walker et al, 1993	194	96	86	85
		191	101	78	83
Ampicillin/sulbactam vs gentamicin/clindamycin[+]	Yellin eta al, 1985	67	(ns)	88	(ns)
		90	(ns)	98	(ns)
Ticardillin/clavulanate vs gentamicin/clindamycin[*]	Sirinek and Levine, 1991	56	(ns)	86	98
		43	(ns)	84	92
Piperacillin/tazobactam vs clindamycin/gentamicin[*]	Polk et al, 1993	217	104	88	86
		114	43	77	75
Piperacillin/tozobactam vs imipenem/cilastin	Brismar et al, 1992	69	55	91	93
		65	58	69	76
Piperacillin/tazobactam vs imipenem/cilastin	Minikoski et al, 1993	47	30	87	100
		39	26	77	89
Piperacillin/tazobactam vs gentamicin/metronidazole	Karran et al, 1994	88	81	79	93
		86	75	81	94

[*]p = not significant; [*]p < 0.05; p = 0.05
ns = not stated
Ref. (10) - Wilson SE, Nord CE: Clinical Trials of Extended Spectrum Penicillin/Beta-lactamase inhibitors in the Treatment of intra-abdominal infections. Am of Surg. Vol 169, No. 5A, May 1995.

9. DURATION OF ANTIBIOTIC TREATMENT

In patients with established infections, the recommendations of the Advisory Group representing the Food and Drug Administration and the Infectious Diseases Society of America is 5 to 14 days for complicated infections, 3 to 7 days for uncomplicated infections, and 2 to 5 days for postoperative wound infections [7]. However, duration of therapy for secondary bacterial peritonitis should be based on objective criteria [4]. Unfortunately, only rather crude indicators are available to direct clinical judgement. Lennard, et al, observed patients in whom fever was still present at the conclusion of a standard course of antimicrobial therapy and found that 8 of 11 patients (57%) developed recurrent intra-abdominal infections [39]. Recurrent intra-abdominal infections developed in 7 of 21 (33%.) of patients who were afebrile with persistent leukocytosis, at the termination of antimicrobial therapy, and there were no recurrences in patients in whom both of these factors were normal. In a large review by Stone, et al, no patients exhibiting a normal rectal temperature, white blood cell count, with a normal differential blood smear, had recurrent sepsis [40]. If the differential smear was not included as a criterion, 3% of patients had recurrent sepsis, and if only rectal temperature was taken into account, 19% of patients had recurrent sepsis. On the basis of these studies, it is clear that antimicrobial therapy for the treatment of established, severe intra-abdominal infection should be continued until the patient's temperature, white blood cell count, and differential smear are within normal limits, rather than discontinuing therapy after a predetermined length of treatment has been administered. If clinical improvement is not evident within 4 days, or if fever or leukocytosis persists after more than 5 days of therapy, undrained abdominal infection or an inadequately treated extra-abdominal infection should be sought.

PSEUDOMONAS

Pseudomonas aeruginosa is isolated in initial cultures of appendiceal specimens and specimens collected after penetrating trauma at rates that vary from 5% to 20% in various hospitals. Several studies have shown that it is not necessary to administer an aminoglycoside or another drug with specific activity against P. aeruginosa in the management of patients with intra-abdominal sepsis. In. two separate studies relatively resistant strains of Pseudomonas and Enterobacter were isolated in initial cultures [41, 42] These studies reported no advantage for a clindamycin-aminoglycoside regimen over a single agent such as cefoxitin or moxalactam, on the other hand, Heseltine and colleagues examined the results of treatment when P. aeruginosa was recovered from initial culture. This study showed P. aeruginosa in 30% of peritoneal cultures from patients with peritonitis and supported the need for treatment when it was present. While specific anti-Pseudomonal therapy controversial prudent care would advise adding coverage in the setting of a positive culture especially if a patient's were complicated.

ANTIFUNGAL TREATMENT

Candida is considered normal flora of the gastrointestinal tract and consequently is relatively common in intra-abdominal sepsis. This organism often poses the controversy regarding indications for treatment [7]. Solomkin, et al reviewed 56 patients with peritonitis involving Candida [44]. Approximately half had previous abdominal surgery, and 82% had Candida recovered as a component of a polymicrobial infection. Of the 10 patients with pure culture of Candida, 9 expired, and the overall mortality for the entire series was 73%. The authors concluded that this organism should be aggressively pursued. Subsequent data, however, has given great diversity of opinion. Rutledge and coworkers retrospectively reviewed 24 patients with intra-abdominal sepsis involving Candida species; 20 were treated with drainage and antibiotics directed exclusively against bacteria, and there was only one death [45]. Marsh and coworkers reported a similar experience, suggesting that polymicrobial intra-abdominal abscesses could be treated simply with drainage plus antibiotics directed against bacteria [46]. More recently, Calandra and associates attempted to identify prospectively the patients with intra-abdominal sepsis involving Candida that might be of clinical significance [47]. An analysis of 49 patients showed that the major indicator suggesting clinical significance was the recovery of the fungus in high concentrations or increasing concentrations with sequential cultures. Other factors of probable importance include the recovery of Candida species from blood cultures or distant sites, suggesting disseminated disease or the recovery of this organism in pure culture. While a localized collection involving Candida species that is adequately drained does not require antifungal treatment, a patient with clinical deterioration and a single positive culture should receive anti-fungal therapy.

ENTEROCOCCUS

The gastrointestinal tract is the major reservoir for enterococcus. Enterococcus faecalis accounts for about 90% of all clinical isolates in this genus, and Enterococcus faecium accounts for most of the remaining 10%. Studies of intra-abdominal sepsis usually show that the enterococcus is recovered in 10% to 20% of cases, and a continuing debate is whether these organisms require treatment when involved in polymicrobial infections [7]. Animal studies have failed to define any role of enterococci in intra-abdominal sepsis, and therapeutic trials have failed to show any difference in outcome between regimens that did and did not include activity versus this organism. Enterococci, however, have become major pathogens during the past 15 to 20 years and are now second only to E. coli as nosocomial pathogens in the National Nosocomial Infections Surveillance System (NNIS) [48]. E. faecium has attracted special attention because many strains are resistant to vancomycin and also resistant to virtually all other antimicrobial agents. Some authorities believe the extraordinary escalation in rates of E. faecalis and E. faecium is the reflection of the extensive use of antibiotics, primarily third-generation cephalosporin. A review of six reports of enterococcal bacteremia published from 1980 through 1991 showed and abdominal or pelvic portal of entry in 11% to 38% [49].

When considering the pathogenic role of Enterococcus, it is important to distinguish between monomicrobic and polymicrobic infections. In monomicrobic infections,, such as bacterial endocarditis, in which enterococcus is the only organism recovered, it clearly is acting as a pathogen and requires primary treatments [50]. However, in the context of abdominal infections that are polymicrobial in nature, and in which enterococcus is only one of many species of bacteria present, it rarely acts as a primary pathogen. However, it will persist if initial treatment of the infection fails. When such a clinical course is predictable, as immuno-compromised patients, then coverage of enterococcus as a part of initial therapy is reasonable. But, for most patients, antibiotic therapy covering enterococci in intra-abdominal infections is not necessary, nor is the addition of antienteroccocal coverage needed if initial peritoneal cultures yield enterococci but the patient clinically is doing well.

As noted earlier, enterococcus, has emerged as a major pathogen of nosocomial infections in the 1990's and future strategies in intra-abdominal sepsis will need to deal with the issue of enterococcus as an important superinfecting pathogens.

QUINOLONES

The fluoroquinolones include ciprofloxacin, enoxacin, norfloxacin, ofoxacin, and pefloxacin. The most widely studies of these and the one with most activity in vitro, is ciprofloxacin. These compounds have a unique antibacterial action: they inhibit deoxyribonucleic acid gyrase of bacteria (but not of mammalian cells), thus preventing the super-coiling of bacterial deoxyribonucleic acid [51]. Ciprofloxacin is potentially a very useful agent because its spectrum of activity includes aerobic gram-negative bacterial isolates such as Pseudomonas species that have been implicated as a cause of antimicrobial treatment failures during intra-abdominal sepsis [52]. Using an experimental model of intra-abdominal sepsis in rats, Lahnborg and Nord demonstrated that ciprofloxacin plus clindamycin was as effective as gentamicin plus clindamycin in preventing mortality [53]. Only 5% of the animals in these two groups died, while untreated animals suffered an 80% mortality, and animals treated with ciprofloxacin alone exhibited a 30%

mortality. While ciprofloxacin cannot be recommended for clinical use in secondary bacterial peritonitis in the absence of clinical trial data, this agent may be of some utility as a nontoxic alternative to the aminoglycosides. Clinical trials are currently underway to assess the efficacy of this drug in combination with anti-anaerobic agents for the treatment of secondary bacterial peritonitis.

REFERENCES

1. Wittman DH, Walker AP and Condon RE: Peritonitis and Intraabdominal Infection; in Principles of Surgery, by S. Schartz, G.T.Shires and F. Spencer, Sixth Edition 1994.

2. Gorbach SL: Intraabdominal Infections; Clinical Infectious Diseases 1993; 17:961-7.

3. Bohnen.JM, Solomkin JS, Dellinger EP, et al: Guidelines for Clinical Care: Anti-infective Agents for Intra-abdominal Infection; Arch Surg - Vol. 127: 83-39, January 1992.

4. Sawyer MD and Dunn DL: Antimicrobial Therapy of Intra-abdominal Sepsis; Infectious Disease Clinics of North America; Vol. 6, No. 3: 545-570, Sept. 1992.

5. Nathens and Rotstein: Therapeutic Options in Peritonitis; Surgical Clinics of North America; Vol. 74, No. 3: 677-692, June 1994.

6. Ruddel WSJ, Axon ATR, Findlay JM, et al: Effect of Cimetidine on the Gastric Bacterial Flora. Lancet 1:672, 1980.

7. Bartlett JG: Intra-abdominal Sepsis; Medical Clinics of North America; Vol. 79, No. 3: 599-617, May 1995.

8. Brook I: A 12 Year Study of Aerobic and Anaerobic Bacteria in Intra-abdominal and Postsurgical Abdominal Wound Infections. Surg Gynecol Obstet 169:387, 1989.

9. Mosdell DM, Morris DM, Voltura A, et al: Antibiotic Treatment for Surgical Peritonitis. Ann Surg 241:543, 1991.

10. Wilson SE, Nord CE: Clinical Trials of Extended Spectrum Penicillin/Betalactamase Inhibitors in the Treatment of Intra-abdominal Infections. Am J of Surg, Vol. 169, No. 5A: 215-265, May 1995.

11. Bartlett JG, Louie TJ, Gorbach SL, et al: Therapeutic Efficacy of 29 Antimicrobial Regimens in Experimental Intra-abdominal Sepsis. Rev Infect Dis 3:535-542, 1981.

12. Thadepalli H, Gorbach SL, Broido PW, et al: Abdominal Trauma, Anaerobes and Antibiotics. Surgery 137:270, 1973.

13. DiPiro JT, Fortson NS: Combination Antibiotic Therapy in the Management of Intra-Abdominal Infection. Am J of Surg, Vol. 165, No. 2A: 82S-88S, February 1993.

14. Bohnen J, Boulanger M, Meakins JL, McLean AP: Prognosis in Generalized Peritonitis: Relation to Cause and Risk Factors.Arch Surg 1983, 118:285-90.

15. Dellinger EP, Wertz MJ, Meakins JL, et al: Surgical Infection Stratification Sustem for Intra-Abdominal Infection. Arch Surg 1985; 120:21-9

16. Fry DE, Garrison RN, Heitsch RC, Calhoun K, Polk HC Jr.: Determinants of Death in Patients with Intra-abdominal Abscess. Surgery 1980; 88: 517-23.

17. Mustard RA, Bohnen JMA, Rosati C, Souten BD: Pneumonia Complicating Abdominal Sepsis: An Independent Risk for Mortality. Arch Surg 1991; 126: 170-5

18. Solomkin JS, Meakins JL, Allo MD, Dellinger EP, Simmons RL: Antibiotic Trials in Intra-Abdominal Infections: A Critical Evaluation of Study Design and Outcome Reporting. Ann Surg 200:29-39, 1984.

19. Canadian Metronidazole Clindamycin Study Group. Prospective, Randomized Comparison of Metronidazole and Clindamycin, Each with Gentamicin, for the Treatment of Serious Intra-Abdominal Infection. Surgery 1983; 93:221-9.

20. Smith JA, Skidmore AG, Forward AD, Clarke AM, Sutherland E: Prospective, Randomized, Double-Blind Comparison of Metronidazole and Tobramycin with Clindamycin and Tobramycin in the Treatment of Intra-Abdominal Sepsis. Ann Surg: 190:213-20, 1980.

21. Gennard ES, Minshew BH, Dellinger EP, Wertz MN, et al: Stratified Outcome Comparison of Clindamycin-Gentamicin Versus Chloramphenicol-Gentamicin for Treatment of Intra-abdominal Sepsis. Arch Surg; 120:889-98, 1985.

22. Stone HH, Fabian TC: clinical comparison of Antibiotic Combinations in the Treatment of Peritonitis and Related Mixed Aerobic-Anaerobic Surgical Sepsis. World J Surg; 4:415-21, 1980.

23. Harding GKM, Buckwold FJ, Ronald AR, et al: Prospective, Randomized Comparative Study of Clindamycin, Chloramphenicol and Ticarcillin, Each in Combination with Gentamicin, in Therapy for Intra-Abdominal and Femal Genital Tract Sepsis. Rev Infect Dis; 142:384-393, 1980.

24. Tally FP, McGowan K, Kellum JM, Gorbach SL, O'Donnel TF: A Randomized Comparison of Cefoxitin with or without Amikacin and Clincamycin plus Amikacin in Surgical Sepsis. Ann Surg; 193:318-323, 1981.

25. Harding GKM, Nicolle LE, Haose DA: Prospective Randomized, Comparative Trials in the Therapy for Intra-Abdominal and Female Genital Tract Infections. Rev Infect Dis; 6:S283-92, 1984.

26. Malangoni MA: Pathogenesis and Treatment of Intra-Abdominal Infection. Surg Gynecol Obstet; Supp. Vol. 171: 31-34, Dec. 1990.

27. Williams RR, Hotchkin D: Aztreonam plus Clindamycin Versus Tobramycin plus Clindamycin in the Treatment of Intra-Abdominal Infections. Rev Infect Dis 1991; 13 (suppl. 7):S629-33.

28. Birolini D, Moraes MF, DeSousa OS. Aztreonam plus Clindamycin versus Tobramycin plus Clindamycin for the Treatment of Intra-Abdominal Infections. Rev Infec Dis 7 (suppl. 4):S724-8, 1989.

29. Birolini D, Moraes MF, DeSousa OS: Comparison of Aztreonam plus Clindamycin with Tobramycin plus Clindamycin in the Treatment of Intra-Abdominal Infections. Chemotherapy; 35 (suppl. 1):49-57, 1989.

30. Berne TV, Appleman MD, Chenella FC, Yellin AE, Gill MA, Heseltine PNR: Surgically Treated Gangrenous or Perforated Appendicitis: A Comparison of Aztreonam and Clindamycin Versus Gentamicin and Clindamycin. Ann Surg; 205:133-7, 1987.

31. Barboza E, Castillo M, Yi A and Gotuzzo E: Clindamycin plus Amikacin Versus Clindamycin plus Aztreonam in Established Intra-Abdominal Infections. Surgery; Vol. 116: 28-35. Mp/ 1, July 1994.

32. Bubrick MP, Heim-Duthoy KL, Yellin AE, et al. Ceftazidine/Clindamycin Versus Tobramycin/Clindamycin in the Treatment of Intra-Abdominal Infections. Ann Surg;56:613-7, 1990.

33. Eisenberg JM, Koffer H, Glick HA, et al: What is the Cost of Nephrotoxicity Associated with Animoglycosides? Ann Intern Med; 107:900-9, 1987.

34. Shusterman N, Strom BL, Murray TG, Morrison G, West SL, Maislin G: Risk Factors and Outcome of Hospital-Acquired Acute Renal Failure: Clinical Epidemiologic Study. Am J Med; 83:65-71, 1987.

35. Saxon A, Beall GN, Rohr AS, Adelman DC: Immediate Hypersensitivity Reactions to Beta-Lactam Antibiotics. Ann Intern Med; 107:204-15, 1987.

36. Wilson SE: A Critical Analysis of Recent Innovations in the Treatment of Intra-Abdominal Infection. Surg Gynecol Obstet, Suppl. Vol 177: 11-17, Dec 1993.

37. Applebaum PC, Spangler SK, Jacos MR. Susceptibilities of 394 Bacteroides Fragilis, Non-B. Fragilis Group, Bacteroides Species, and Fusobacterium Species to Newer Antimicrobial Agents. Antimicrobial Agents and Chemother 1991; 35:1214-8.

38. Sanders CC and Sanders WE, Jr.: Beta-Lactam Resistance in Gram-Negative Bacteria: Global Trends and Clinical Impact. Clin Infect Dis, 1992, 15:824-839.

39. Lennard ES, Dellinger EP, Wertz MJ, et al: Implications of Leukocytosis and Fever at Conclusion of Antibiotic Therapy for Intra-Abdominal Sepsis. Ann Surg 195:19-24, 1982.

40. Stone HH, Bourneuff AA, Stimson LD: Reliability of Criteria for Predicting Persistent or Recurrent Sepsis. Arch Surg 120:17-20, 1985.

41. Nichols RL, Smith JW, Klein DB, et al: Risk of Infection After Penetrating Abdominal Trauma. N Engl J Med 311:1066-1070, 1984.

42. Schentagg JJ, Wells PB, Reitberg DP, et al: A Randomized Clinical Trial of Moxalactam Alone Versus Tobramycin Plus Clindamycin in Abdominal Sepsis. Ann Surg 198:35-41, 1983.

43. Heseltine PNR, Yellin AE, Appleman MD, et al: Perforated and Gangrenous Appendicitis: An Analysis of Antibiotic Failures. J Infect Dis 148:322-329, 1983.

44. Solomkin JS, Flohr AB, Quie PG, et al: The Role of Candida in Intraperitoneal Infections. Surgery 88:524-530, 1980.

45. Rutledge R, Mandel SR, Wild RE: Candida Species: Insignificant Contaminant or Pathogenic Species. Ann Surg 52:299-302, 1986.

46. Marsh PK, Tally FP, Kelum J, et al: Candida Infections in Surgical Patients. Am Surg 198:42-47, 1983.

47. Calandra T, Bille J, Schneider R, et al: Clinical Significance of Candida Isolated from Peritoneum in Surgical Patients. Lancet 2:1437-1440, 1989.

48. Schaberg DR, Culver DL, Gaynes RP: Major Trends in the Microbial Etiology of Nosocomial Infection. Am J Med 91:(suppl. 3B):725-755, 1991.

49. Shales DM, Levy J, Wolinsky E: Enterococcal Bacteremia Without Endocarditis. Arch Intern Med 141:578-581, 1981.

50. Barie PS, Christou NV, Dellinger EP, et al: Pathogenecity of the Enterococcus in Surgical Infections. Ann Surg, Vol 212, No. 2, 155-159, Aug. 1990.

51. Pollock AV: Non-operative Anti-infective Treatment of Intra-Abdominal Infections. World J Surg, 14, 227-230, 1990.

52. Yellin AE, Heseltine PNR, Berne TV, et al: The Role of Pseudomonas Species in Patients Treated with Ampicillin and Subactam for Gangrenous and Perforated Appendicitis. Surg Gynecol Obstet. 161:303-307, 1985.

53. Lahnborg G, Nord CE: Effect of Ciprofloxacin Compared to Gentamicin in the Treatment of Experimental Intra-Abdominal Infections in Rats. Scand J Infect Dis 60:S35-8, 1989.

54. Poenaru D, DeSantis M, Christou NV: Imipenem versus tobramycin-antianaerobe therapy in intra-abdominal infections. Can J Surg. 33:415-422, 1990.

Tertiary Peritonitis

Dietmar H. Wittmann, MD, PhD

1. INTRODUCTION

Primary and secondary intra-abdominal infections (IAI) are well defined [1]. Both forms of IAI usually respond to treatment and resolve, or form distinctive abscesses. The term tertiary peritonitis, on the other hand, is much less familiar. It describes an infective intra-abdominal syndrome that, because of impaired host defenses following overwhelming infection, cannot be contained [2].

2. HISTORICAL PERSPECTIVES

With the increased awareness during the 1960s and 1970s that remote organ failure is a valid sign of occult infection, an ever increasing aggressiveness was practiced in the search for adequate management of IAI [3-7].

During the 1980s, improved intensive care, organ support, total parenteral nutrition, and broad-spectrum antibiotics, in combination with energetic operative efforts to search for "undrained pus", have produced a "new" subgroup of critically ill patients that survived the abdominal catastrophes and its initial treatment but whose subsequent course is characterized by multiple surgical procedures and sequential organ failure [8-14].

A common scenario is a patient in a surgical intensive care unit after one or multiple operations for severe intra-abdominal infection, trauma, or acute pancreatitis. The patient continues to show clinical and laboratory signs of sepsis despite administration of effective antibiotics. An intensive search for occult infectious focus is conducted and a directed or exploratory laparotomy is performed. The operation does not reveal definite collections of pus or necrotic material; instead, some thin cloudy fluid is present. Postoperatively, clinical sepsis persists and the patient dies in multiple organ failure. Endotoxin generally is not found in circulating blood. At autopsy, no foci of infection are demonstrated [15-19]. To account for the emerging and increasingly common syndrome, a new term was deemed necessary. Tertiary peritonitis was offered by Rotstein and Meakins [2] and accepted by the North American and European Surgical Infection Societies [20,21].

3. DEFINITION

Tertiary peritonitis is a sepsis-like syndrome not induced by endotoxin and seen in patients where severe bacterial peritonitis follows. The definition for the syndrome is not uniformly accepted. Marshall, et al consider it the "persistence or recurrence" of culture-positive IAI at least 72 hours after apparently adequate therapy for an episode of primary or secondary peritonitis [22]. Their definition, however, is rather simplified and too-broad. It includes the relatively easily treatable post-operative abdominal abscesses and does not address the disturbed interplay of immunological factors involved, nor does it exclude endotoxin production as its cause. A better definition of the complex syndrome of tertiary IAI would encompass the following:

1. Occurs after optimal operative treatment of peritonitis

2. Exhibits clinical signs of sepsis

3. No infectious focus of endotoxin production is found

4. Micro-organism of questionable pathogenicity or none are isolated and it may be defined as follows:

Tertiary peritonitis is a post-operative syndrome of an ongoing but altered systemic inflammatory response with clinical signs similar to (systemic) sepsis but without a focus for bacterial toxin or endotoxin release.

3.1. Post-operative State

At least one operation and frequently multiple procedures, have been performed and have eradicated IAI. Typically, as Fry noted [23], patients who develop early post-operative organ failure tend to have undrained abscesses. Patients who show signs of infection late, i.e. two weeks or more following their initial operation, exhibit immunological collapse and thus, tertiary peritonitis.

3.2. Clinical Sepsis

The clinical picture is that of "septic" response: tachycardia, low grade fever, increased respiratory rate, decreased urine output, platelet aggregation and altered mentation. The circulation is hyperdynamic with peripheral vasodilatation due to the cellular inability to utilize oxygen. The hypermetabolic, autocannibalistic response eventually leads to death [5,24-34].

Clinically "non-specific" intraperitoneal findings are predominant. At abdominal exploration in patients suffering from tertiary peritonitis, characteristics of diffuse purulent or fecal peritonitis are not found, nor are there localized abscesses. Instead, tertiary peritonitis may consist of diffuse, poorly localized collections of cloudy or serosanguinous fluid. The pathogenic importance of the fluid is questionable. Data are not available.

3.3. Peculiar microbiology

The monomicrobial of primary - and polymicrobial microbiology of secondary peritonitis, respectively, are predictable. In secondary forms of IAI, the peritoneal cultures are dominated by a few organisms such as E.coli and B.fragilis [4,35-40]. The microbiology of tertiary peritonitis is different and not so well-defined and consistent. Cultures taken from patients who died of persistent peritonitis in the intensive care units, after multiple surgical procedures, grew no or few peculiar organisms of mostly low pathogenicity such as Staphylococcus epidermidis, Enterococcus faecalis and faecium, and Candida albicans. The classical endotoxin producing bacteria of secondary peritonitis are rarely encountered [2, 16, 19, 25, 30].

3.4. Etiology

The low virulence of the organisms typical to tertiary peritonitis reflects the global immunodepression in the face of ongoing extended spectrum antibiotic therapy. In fact, the primary insult, be it secondary peritonitis or abdominal injury, as well as its medical-supportive treatments, produce immunocompromised hosts [17].

How do these organisms enter the peritoneal cavity? One possibility is direct exogenic contamination through drains that may take place during the repeated abdominal entries or represent bacterial contamination of the peritoneal cavity through an open-abdomen (laparostomy) wound.

Another source of the organisms is probably the patient's own gastrointestinal tract. Marshall and associates performed quantitative cultures of proximal gastrointestinal fluid in surgical intensive care patients and found a significant number of specimens contaminated with the above mentioned micro-organisms. Positive cultures correlated with invasive infections with the same organisms [19].

Translocation from the distal intestinal tract [41-43] is not a likely explanation because occasional organisms typical for tertiary peritonitis do not generally live in the distal bowel. Hematogeneous spread is open to speculation. Because tertiary peritonitis does not include endotoxinemia, the notion that the gastrointestinal tract functions like the so-called "undrained abscess" [22] or the "hidden wound" [42] of multiple organ failure may not be true.

Cause-effect relationship of these bacteria and the infectious morbidity experienced by the patients is not clear. Currently, the consensus tends to view the organisms of tertiary peritonitis as "markers" or "associates" of the immunodepression and not its cause [16,19,22,42]. Indeed, tertiary peritonitis can be considered as a subclass of the so-called systemic inflammatory response syndrome (SIRS) [44]. The latter, a syndrome of numerous names [45], probably represents a "mediator effect" and a common pathway toward multiple organ failure and death in the critically ill surgical patient [46]. It does not distinguish between systemic inflammatory responses from infectious and non-infectious causes such as trauma and burns nor does it specifically address features of tertiary peritonitis with ongoing systemic inflammation without a definable cause. Intraperitoneal injection of an inflammation stimulant (zymosan), which activates macrophages and the complement system, produces clinical sepsis in absence of endotoxin and multi-organ damage in rats [25,47].

A name such as defense failure syndrome (DFS) would more precisely describe the untamed systemic inflammation seen in tertiary peritonitis patients. Tertiary peritonitis, indeed, would then belong to the category of defense failure syndrome rather than SIRS [4,48]. (Figure 1)

SIRS represents a host-determined response which may follow a multitude of infective and non-infective causes such as bacterial, fungal and viral infections, endotoxins, trauma, burns, necrotic tissue, injury and others [30,32,49-51]. It is mediated by multiple endocrine and inflammatory mediators [52]. Mediators of SIRS are released by the host's own immune system such as macrophages and endothelium and other cells [53]. Thus, it is believed that SIRS signifies a physiological event that may turn in an exaggerated immune response of the host and that may

Figure 1
Relation between systemic inflammatory response syndrome,
sepsis, sepsis syndrome and defense failure syndrome

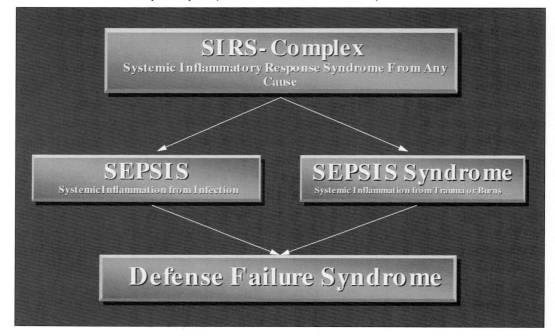

lead to generalized autodestructive inflammation [54]. Tertiary peritonitis, on the other hand, seems to always signify an exaggerated inflammatory response that invariable leads to autodescruction.

Clearly, the mediators of sepsis released by the immune system possess dose-dependent, beneficial and adverse effects and act, therefore, as a double-edged sword. Bacteria and its products, which escape from the patient's own intestinal tract (the "motor of multiple organ failure") [32,53], have been thought to contribute to SIRS but are not typical for tertiary peritonitis because of missing endotoxin levels. Maybe bacteria are dead, causing jelly like colorless stools often seen in patients with tertiary peritonitis.

The main mechanisms causing intestinal barrier failure and translocation of bacteria and endotoxin release are ischemic disruption of intestinal mucosal barrier of an intact ecological bowel flora. Antibiotics and impaired host immune defenses disturb the ecological balance of the intestine, resulting in bacterial overgrowth [32,41,46,53]. The primary insults found to enhance translocation are shock, thermal injury and early intra-abdominal infection and contributory iatrogenic factors, such as systemic antibiotics and prolonged non-enteral nutrition [41,55]. In tertiary peritonitis, none of these factors apply because the syndrome is seen late: all pathogens have been eliminated by multiple regimen of broad spectrum antibiotics, leaving only those micro-organims that are poorly covered by our potent antibiotic armamentarium. Such germs are of low pathogenectity and represent just a marker of a disease unrelated to its cause.

4. TERTIARY PERITONITIS, DEFENSE FAILURE SYNDROME AND NITRIC OXIDE

The common terminal pathway of septic shock is sequential organ failure from cellular death of various organs due to oxygen depletion [56-63]. While the circulation is hyperdynamic there is no or very little difference between arterio-venous oxygen saturation. The macro-organism increases cardiac output to its natural limits to transport sufficiant oxygen to cells.

Nitric oxide, in this situation, is generated on the helpful direction of mediators to relax vascular smooth muscles and dilate vessels to enhance flow of oxygen carriers. [57,59,62-65]. At a cellular level, however, mitochondria do not seem to consume oxygen that is excessively provided by circulation and, resulting in high oxygen content of post cellular venous blood. The reason for this inability to utilize oxygen may well be in a defective mitochondrial Krebs cycle. There is evidence that nitric oxide inhibits iron containing enzymes such as aconitase and complex I and II. Those enzymes are essential for aerobic energy production and if inhibited, energy must be gained from the very inefficient anaerobic glycolysis. [41,55-57,59,66].

The process seem to be gradual and depends on numerous other factors that are not well understood. Defense failure syndrome and more specifically, tertiary peritonitis, seem to share exactly that process of cellular asphyxia with sepsis and other systemic inflammatory response syndromes; the phenomenom of Krebs cycle failure.

The mediator pattern, in tertiary peritonitis, however, may be different, because it always follows a physiological inflammatory response. Follwing SIRS various factors including up and down, regulating cytokines may be in dysbalance due to shorter half lives, disproportional degradation, substrate deficits and synthesis deficiencies by the failing liver. This may explain differences of cytokine levels. For example, increased platelet activating factor (PAF) levels is often seen in tertiary peritonitis. This may lead to peripheral and pulmonary platelet aggregations and thrombotic occlusion of pulmonary and peripheral microvasculature [67,68] (see Figure 2). Cellular death happens gradually and therefore correlates with the hyperdynamic circulation and sequential organ failure eventually leading to death.

The imbalances between agoniststic and antagonistic physiological or biochemical actions that fail to terminate the immunological response to infection adequately, result in the clinical disaster of tertiary peritonitis when bacteria no longer challenge the host. Since during evolution, humans always died before reaching this situation, nature has not developed a response for a syndrome that we see as we further advance therapy.

5. MANAGEMENT

Therapeutic answers to these syndromes are under intensive investigation. The research, which concentrates on arresting the "roller coaster" of the sytemic inflammatory response using drug manipulations and im-

Figure 2
Peripheral microthrombosis seen in tertiary peritonitis

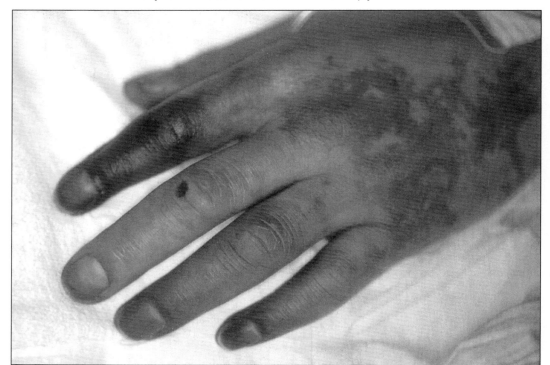

munomodulation, has not as yet achieved a breakthrough [69]. In the absence of effective treatment, what should we offer to these patients? Clearly, minimizing iatrogenic contributory factors is a possiblility. In this regard, anecdotal experience suggests that ceasing all antibiotics and intensive enteral feeding may reverse sepsis-induced multiple organ failure in patients who are thought to be dying of this disorder [70]. It seems, however, that the selection of resistant strains fueling ongoing infection may not simply be controlled by discontinuing antibiotics. More logical appears to be the concept of eliminating bacterial initiators of secondary peritonitis early and radically by aggressive early operative therapy combi-

ned with high doses of the most potent antibiotics to eliminate the bacterial challenge early and consequently moderate ongoing sytemic inflammation. Tertiary peritonitis affects patients in whom there may have been halfhearted use of a combination of supportive medical treatment and mechanical-surgical options. Once it is present, no options are available. At present, the best treatment remains prevention: only the early and effective treatment of abdominal catastrophes can avoid the cascade of events leading to whole body inflammation, which requires additional therapy, which in turn promote the syndromes, a cycle that ends in organ failure and death by tertiary peritonitis.

REFERENCES

1. Wittmann DH, Walker A, Condon R. Peritonitis and intra-abdominal infection. In: Schwartz SI, Shires GT, Spencer FC, eds.Principles of Surgery. 6th ed. McGraw-Hill, Inc. 1994:1449-83.

2. Rotstein OD, Meakins JL. Diagnostic and therapeutic challenges of severe peritonitis. World J Surg. 1990;14:159-66.

3. Wachsmuth W. Peritonitis. Langenb Arch Chir. 1965;313:146-69.

4. Wittmann DH, Schein M, Condon RE. Current management of secondary peritonitis. Ann Surg. 1996;224:10-8.

5. Baue AE. Multiple, Progressive, or Sequential Systems Failure. A Syndrome of the 1970's. Arch Surg. 1975;110:779-81.

6. Fry DE, Pearlstein L, Fulton RL, Polk HC. Multiple system organ failure: the role of uncontrolled infection. Arch Surg. 1981; 115:136.

7. Polk HC, Shields CL. Remote organ failure: A valid sign of occult intra-abdominal infection. Surgery. 1977;81:310-3.

8. Harbrecht PJ, Garrison RN, Fry DE. Early Urgent Relaparotomy. Arch Surg. 1984; 119:369-74.

9. Butler JA, Huang J, Wilson SE. Repeated laparotomy for post-operative intra-abdominal sepsis. Arch Surg. 1987;122:702-6.

10. Ferraris VA. Exploratory laparotomy for potential abdominal sepsis in patients with multiple-organ failure. Arch Surg. 1983; 118:1130-3.

11. Sinanan M, Maier RV, Carrico CJ. Laparotomy for intra-abdominal sepsis in patients in an intensive care unit. Arch Surg. 1984; 119:652-8.

12. Bunt TJ. Non-direct relaparotomy for intra-abdominal sepsis: A futile procedure. Am Surg. 1986;52:294-8.

13. Makela J, Kairaluoma MI. Relaparotomy for post-operative intra-abdominal sepsis in janudiced patients. Br J Surg. 1988;75:1157-9.

14. Hindsdale JC, Jaffe EM. Reoperations for intra-abdominal sepsis. Ann Surg. 1984; 199:31-6.

15. Schein M. Planned reoperations and open management in critical intra-abdominal infections: prospective experience in 52 cases. World J Surg. 1991;15:537-45.

16. Rotstein OD, Pruett TL, Simmons RL. Microbiologic features and treatment of persistent peritonitis in patients in the intensive care unit. Can J Surg. 1986;29:247.

17. Meakins JL, Wicklund B, Forse RA, McLean APH. The surgical intensive care unit: Current concepts in infection. Surg Clin North Am. 1980;60:117-32.

18. Norton LW. Does drainage of intra-abdominal pus reverse multiple organ failure? Am J Surg. 1985;149:347-50.

19. Marshall JC, Christou NV, Horn R, Meakins JL. The microbiology of multiple organ failure. Arch Surg. 1988;123:309-15.

20. Nyström PO, Knaus WA, Meakins JL, et al. A proposed standard for trials on intra-abdominal infection. World J Surg. 1990;14: 148-56.

21. Wittmann DH. Symposium of intra-abdominal infections: Introduction. World J Surg. 1990;14:145-230.

22. Marshall JC, Christou NV, Meakins JL. The gastrointestinal tract: The "undrained abscess" of multiple organ failure. Ann Surg. 1993;218:111-9.

23. Fry DE. The microbiology of multiple organ failure. Arch Surg. 1988;1123:309-15.

24. Manship L, McMillin RD, Brown JJ. The influence of sepsis and multisystem and organ failure on mortality in the surgical intensive care unit. Am Surg. 1984;50:94-101.

25. Goris RJA, Boekholz WKF, Van Bebber IPT, Nuytinck HKS, Schillings PHM. Multiple-or-

gan failure and sepsis without bacteria. An experimental model. Arch Surg. 1986; 121:897-900.

26. Goris RJA. Mediators of multiple organ failure. Intensive Care Med. 1990;16:S192-6.

27. Hack CE, Nuijens JH, Strack van Schijndel RJM, Abbink JJ, Erenberg AJM, Thijs LG. A model for the interplay of inflammatory mediators in sepsis -a study in 48 patients. Intensive Care Med. 1990;16:S187-91.

28. Stadler J, Billiar R, Curran RD, Stuehr DJ, Ochoa JB, Simmons RL. Effect of exogenous and endogenous nitric oxide on mitochondrial respiration of rat hepatocytes. Am J Physiol. 1991;260:C910-6.

29. Hebert PC, Drummond AJ, Singer J, Bernard GR, Russell JA. A simple multiple system organ failure scoring system predicts mortality of patients who have sepsis syndrome. Chest. 1993;104:230-5.

30. Marshall JC, Sweeney D. Microbial Infection and the septic response in critical illness: sepsis, not infection, determines outcome. Arch Surg. 1990;125:17-23.

31. Schottmüller H. Wesen und Behandlung der Sepsis (Nature and therapy of sepsis). Verhandl d dtsch Kongr f inn Med. 1914;31:17-280.

32. Wiles JB, Cerra FB, Siegel JH, Border JR. The systemic septic response: Does the organism matter? Crit Care Med. 1980;8:55-60.

33. Bone RC. Sepsis, the sepsis Syndrome, Multi-Organ Failure: A Plea for Comparable Defintions. Ann Intern Med. 1991;114, No. 4:332-3.

34. Ayres SM. SCCM's new horizons conference on sepsis and septic shock. Crit Care Med. 1985;13:864-6.

35. Shinagawa N, Mizuno A, Mashita K, et al. [Bacteria isolated from intra-abdominal infection and their susceptibilities to antimicrobial agents]. [Japanese]. Japanese Journal of Antibiotics. 1994;47:1329-43.

36. Schoeffel U, Jacobs E, Ruf G, Mierswa F, von Specht BU, Farthmann EH. Intraperitoneal micro-organisms and the severity of peritonitis. European Journal of Surgery. 1995;161:501-8.

37. Wilson SE, Hopkins JA. Clinical correlates of anaerobic bacteriology in peritonitis. [Review]. Clinical Infectious Diseases. 1995;20 Suppl 2:S251-6.

38. Bartlett JG, Onderdonk AB, Louie TJ, Kasper DL. A review. Lesson from an animal model of intra-abdominal sepsis. Arch Surg. 1978; 113:853-7.

39. Aprahamian C, Schein M, Wittmann D. Cefotaxime and metronidazole in severe intra-abdominal infection. Diagnostic Microbiology & Infectious Disease. 1995;22:183-8.

40. Gorbach SL. Normal bowel flora in intra-abdominal sepsis in bacteriology of the gut and its clinical implication. West J Med. 1974;121:390.

41. Saadia R, Schein M, McFarlan C, Bofard K. The gut barrier function and the surgeon. Br J Surg. 1990;77:487-92.

42. Border JR. Multiple systems organ failure. Ann Surg. 1992;216:111-6.

43. Kraft R, Ruchti C, Burkhardt A, Cottier H. Pathogenetic Principles in the development of gut-derived infectious-toxic shock (GITS) and multiple organ failure. In: Cottier H, Kraft R, eds.Gut-derived infectious-toxic shock (GITS). Basel: Curr Stud Blood Transf. Karger, 1992:204-40.

44. Wittmann DH, Syrrakos B, Wittmann MM. Advances in the diagnosis and treatment of intra-abdominal infection. In: Nyhus L, Nichols RL, eds.Problems in General Surgery: Surgical Sepsis, 1992 and beyond. 10th ed. Philadelphia: J.B. Lippincott Company, 1993:604-27.

45. Baue AE. What's in a name? Acronym or a response? Am J Surg. 1993;165:299-301.

46. Jenkins CD, Stanton BA, Jono RT. Quantifying and predicting recovery after heart sur-

gery [see comments]. Psychosomatic Medicine. 1994;56:203-12.

47. Steinberg S, Flynn W, Kelly K. Development of a bacteria-independent model of multiple organ failure syndrome. Arch Surg. 1989; 124:1390-5.

48. Gerhart KA, Koziol-McLain J, Lowenstein SR, Whiteneck GG. Quality of life following spinal cord injury: knowledge and attitudes of emergency care providers. Annals of Emergency Medicine. 1994;23:807-12.

49. Trunkey DD. Inflammation and Trauma. Arch Surg. 1988;123:1517.

50. Nuytinck HKS, Offermans JM, Kubat K, Goris RJA. Whole-Body Inflammation in Trauma Patients. An Autopsy Study. Arch Surg. 1988;123:1519-24.

51. Marano MA, Fong Y, Moldawer LL. Serum cachectin/tumor necrosis factor in critically ill patients with burns correlates with infection and mortality. Surg Gyencol Obstet. 1990;170:33-8.

52. Watters JM, Bessey PQ, Dinarello CA, Wolff SM, Wilmore DW. Both inflammatory and endocrine mediators stimulate host responses to sepsis. Arch Surg. 1986;121:179-90.

53. Border JR. Hypothesis: Sepsis, multiple organ failure, and the macrophage. Arch Surg. 1988;123:285-6.

54. Schaefer A, Neugebauer E, Bouillon B, Tiling T, Troidl H. [Instruments for measuring the quality of life of severely injured patients]. [Review] [German]. Unfallchirurg. 1994;97:223-9.

55. Dionigi R, Cremaschi RE, Jemos V, Dominioni L, Monico R. Nutritional Assessment and Severity of Illness Classification Systems: A Critical Review on Their Clinical Relevance. World J Surg. 1986;10:2-11.

56. Drapier JC, Hibbs JFJ. Differentiation of murine macrophages to express non specific cytotoxicity for tumor cells results in L-arginine dependent inhibition of mitrochondrial iron-sulfur enzymes in the macrophage effector cell. J Immunol. 1988;140:2829-38.

57. Palmer RMJ, Ashton DS, Moncada S. Vascular endothelial cells synthesize nitric oxide from L-arginine. Nature. 1988;333:664-6.

58. Bredt DS, Snyder SH. Isolation of nitric oxide synthetase, a calmodulin-requiring enzyme. Proc Natl Acad Sci. 1990;87:682-5.

59. Moncada S, Palmer RMJ, Higgs EA. Nitric Oxide: Physiology, Pathophysiology, and Parmacology. Pharmacological Reviews. 1991;43:109-42.

60. Lancaster JR. Nitric Oxice in Cells - This simple molecule plays Janus-faced roles in the body, acting as both messenger and destroyer. American Scientist. 1992;80:248-59.

61. Lancaster JR, Langrehr JM, Bergonia HA, Murase N, Simmons RL, Hoffman RA. EPR Detection of Heme and Nonheme Iron-containing Protein Nitrosylation by Nitric Oxide during Rejection of Rat Heart Allograft. J Biol Chem. 1992;267:266-10998.

62. Palmer RMJ. The discovery of nitric oxyde in the vessel wall. Arch Surg. 1993; 128: 396-401.

63. Vallance P, Moncada S. Role of Endogenous Nitric Oxide in Septic Shock. New Horizons. 1993;1:77-86.

64. Nava E, Palmer RMJ, Moncada S. Inhibition of nitric oxide synthesis in septic shock: how much is beneficial? Lancet. 1991; 338:1555-8.

65. Pellat C, Henry Y, Drapier JC. Detection by electron paramagnetic resonance of a nitrosyl-iron-type signal in interferon-Y-activated macrophages. In: Moncada S, Higgs EA, eds.Nitric oxide from L-arginine: a bioregulatory system. Elsevier Science Publishers (Biomedical Division), 1990:281-9.

66. Drapier JC, Pellat C, Henry Y. Generation of EPR-detectable Nitrosyl-Iron Complexes in Tumor Target Cells Cocultured with Activated Macrophages. J Biol Chem. 1991; 266:10162-7.

67. Kotai M, Hosford D, Braquet PG. Platelet-Activating Factor in Septic Shock. New Horizons. 1993;1:87-95.

68. Pinckard RN, Ludwig JC, McManus LM. Platelet-activating factors. In: Gallin JI, Goldstein IM, Snyderman R, eds.Inflammation: Basic Principles and Clinical Correlates. New York: Raven Press, 1988:139-68.

69. Lynn WA, Cohne J. Adjunctive therapy for septic shock: A review of experimental approaches. Clin Inf Dis. 1995;20:143-58.

70. Offenbartl K, Bengmark S. Intraabdominal Infections and Gut Origin Sepsis. World J Surg. 1990;14:191-5.

Newer Methods of Operative Therapy for Peritonitis: Open Abdomen, Planned Relaparotomy or Staged Abdominal Repair (STAR)

Dietmar H. Wittmann, MD, PhD.

1. PRINCIPLES OF OPERATIVE THERAPY FOR PERITONITIS

Treatment of intra-abdominal infections (Acute Suppurative Peritonitis) includes operative and non-operative management of pathophysiological changes as well as antimicrobial therapy. The operation, however, remains the most important therapeutic modality. If it fails, all supporting non-operative measures will fail and the patient may die. Operative management of suppurative peritonitis follows four Principles:

1. Conclude/occlude leak of infectious material (**REPAIR, SOURCE, CONTROL**)

2. Evacuate bacteria, pus, and adjuvants (**PURGE**)

3. Decompress abdominal compartment syndrome (**DECOMPRESS**)

4. Control both repair and purge (**QUALITY CONTROL**)

Standard operative management deals with the first and the second principle. The third and fourth principle are possible only with more advanced operative techniques such as staged abdominal repair (STAR).

Principle 1: Source Control (Occlusion of infectious leak)

Any suppurative peritonitis results from a focus from which infective material leaks into the abdominal cavity and subsequently spreads to the entire organism. Normally the infectious focus is a hollow viscus such as the intestinal tract that contains bacteria as part of the physiologic bowel flora. The leaking perforation must be **repaired**. This may be accomplished by suture closure, resection, or exteriorization. The repair varies with the disease and anatomical location (e.g. duodenal leaks cannot be exteriorized).

Less commonly, pathological accumulations of bacteria in normally sterile organs or spaces (abscesses, empyemata) may perforate and cause peritonitis. Examples are biliary and urinary tract infections with an empyema within the renal pelvis and ureters, the gallbladder and bile ducts, and surgically created blind bowel loops. An abscess or empyema must be drained or removed surgically. Antibiotic therapy alone is less likely to sterilize abscesses or empyemata.

Principle 2: Evacuate pus and adjuvants (PURGE)

Infectious peritoneal fluid, pus, fibrin, necrotic tissue and adjuvants either contain pathogenic bacteria or promote their growth. Pathological peritoneal fluid may be serous, fibrinous, bilious, purulent or even feculent and should be removed. This was recognized early in the development of surgical techniques. Fowler's position was meant to decrease flow of toxic peritoneal fluid to the thoracic lymphatic vessels to reduce systemic toxemia [1,2]. At the dawn of modern surgery a left-sided cervical lymhaticostomy was performed for the same reason [3]. Polk's controlled trial did not show radical peritoneal debridement to be beneficial [4]. It suggested that debridement should not be too radical to prevent intestinal fistula formation and excessive bleeding. Blood itself represents an adjuvant of infection [5,6]. All irrigation techniques should help to accomplish proper purging of the abdominal cavity. No fluid should be left within the abdomen to avoid suspending local defense such as macrophages in the fluid and diminishing their effectiveness. Local antiseptics are toxic to the peritoneum. Local antibiotics are ineffective, because concentrations to effectively kill bacteria are not sustained for sufficient long periods after abdominal washouts.

Principle 3: Decompress abdominal compartment syndrome

The peritoneum and its submesothelial loose connective tissue may absorb more than 10 Liters of inflammatory edema. Additionally, coexistent ileus my contribute to the increase in intra-abdominal pressure that impairs cardiovascular, pulmonary, renal and hepatic functions, venous return as well as splanchnic and abdominal wall blood flow and oxygenation [7]. The standard operation does not address this issue, since the abdominal fascia is closed, often under extreme tension using retention sutures. The abdominal compartment syndrome, however, can be avoided with the open abdomen technique or with staged abdominal repair (STAR).

Principle 4: Quality Control of repairs and purge

With the standard operation, there is no effective way of controlling whether an anastomosis heals, bowel segments remain viable or new purulence has formed within the abdominal cavity. These complications remain hidden following standard management for long periods until overt clinical symptoms are present. Notably, the surgeons' biases toward his own complications may hinder early diagnoses of postoperative surgical complications. It is a better idea to plan re-explorations when postoperative problems are suspected to ensure optimal healing, to diagnose bowel wall necroses early, and evacuate newly formed pus at early stages. [8-13]. This means that the abdominal cavity needs to be re explored after 24 hours. Bacteria grow fast after irrigation of the abdominal cavity, and within 24 hours numbers of bacteria are the same as before irrigation [14].

2. STANDARD OPERATION

The golden standard of operatively managing Intra-abdominal infections follows principles established during the first two decades of this century. Kirschner [3], in 1926, defined the classic therapeutic strategy as

1. Source Control in one single operation

2. Antibacterial treatment with drugs

3. Support of functional impairment

The operation's purpose is to eliminate or eradicate or control the infectious source (PRINCIPLE 1), and to evacuate purulent and necrotic material from the abdominal cavity by cleaning out bacteria and bacterial toxins and by debridement of necrotic tissue (PRINCIPLE 2).

This therapeutic strategy has become the standard operative management of intra-abdominal infections. Overall mortality was reduced from 90% in the 19th century, when treatment was non-operative, to about 40% in 1926, when the principles mentioned above became widely accepted [3]. The progress was remarkable, and concerns about PRINCIPLE 3 became an issue only in the 7th to 8th decade of the 20th century when no further decrease of mortality rates was seen and when the pathophysiology of intra-abdominal infections was better understood.

3. NEWER OPERATIVE METHODS

3.1. Historical Development

The era of new operative concepts started in 1975 with the dissertation of Pujol, a young physician from Paris University [15]. He concluded that intra-abdominal infections should be treated as any surgical infection ("ubi pus, ibi evacua." and ".....tota cutis super pus excidenda est.") [16]. And, thus, the abdomen should be left open. Subsequently, a series of authors published studies in which the abdomen was left open and treated as an open wound, but data-are inconclusive [17-36]. These studies were generally uncontrolled and did not stratify severity of disease, making comparison to other methods impossible. All studies, however, claim to have used the newer approaches for patients who were extremely sick with an extremely poor prognosis and who would otherwise have been abandoned. One may conclude that the mortality rates reported would have been higher in this selection of worst peritonitis cases if they would have been treated by standard therapy.

Huge incisional hernias complicated the simple open abdomen technique. Intestinal fistulae formed in up to 40% of the cases representing another severe complication. Fistulae probably form because the distended and inflamed intestines, when exposed to atmospheric pressure, are more likely to release the increased intraluminal pressure by perforation.

In recent years, many papers have been published propagating a variety of other new operative approaches for the treatment of diffuse suppurative peritonitis Most papers, as mentioned, are anecdotal, making it difficult to assess whether the new methods represent any therapeutic improvement (Table 1) [17-36]. In a few papers, patients have been stratified to allow for comparison of results [9,37,38]. These comparisons, however, even when done under more controlled conditions, are difficult to interpret because

Table 1
Mortality Reported With Various Forms Of Abdominostomy And Control Groups Respectively

Technique	Studies	Patients	Died	
	(n)	(n)	(n)	Ratio
Open Abdominostomy	37	869	362	41,7 %
Control group: Standard OP.		195	76	39,1 %
Mesh Abdominostomy	12	439	171	38,9 %
No control group	0	—	—	—
STAR Abdominostomy or (Mesh Abdominostomy combined with Planned relaparotomy)	11	385	108	28,1 %
Control group: Standard OP.	95	43	44,2 %	38,2 %

methods vary from center to center and from strategy to strategy. For that purpose, the International Society of Surgery asked several experts in the field to convene at the International Surgical Week 1993 in Hong Kong to clarify terminology [13]. Four basically different methods have emerged. These new operative management conceptions for intra-abdominal infections include:

1. Open abdomen/Abdominostomy (OPA)

2. Covered Abdominostomy (COLA)

3. Planned relaparotomy (PR)

4. Staged Abdominal Repair (STAR)

The new approaches address the THIRD THERAPEUTIC PRINCIPLE (to neutralize increased intra-abdominal pressure) and the FOURTH THERAPEUTIC PRINCIPLE "to perform a quality control on both, repair and purge" as a new feature of operative management (see table 2). With the addition of THIRD and FOURTH THERAPEUTIC PRINCIPLE, better results were expected. Figure 1 shows the differences bet-

Table 2
Fraction of the four Operative Principles accomplished by Various Operative Strategies for Intra-abdominal Infection

Operative Principles	1 Repair	2 Purge	3 Decompress	4 Control
Standard Operation	yes	yes	no	no
Open Abdomen (OPA)	yes	yes	yes	no
Covered Abdominostomy (COLA)	yes	yes	yes	no
Planned Relaparotomy (PR)	yes	yes	no	yes
Staged Abdominal. Repair (STAR)	yes	yes	yes	yes

ween results following standard operative management, open abdomen/Abdominostomy and STAR comparing groups with the similar risk factors. The adjustment for patient risk factors provides a more meaningful comparison and shows improved mortality only for patients in the STAR group.

3.2. Open abdomen/Open Abdominostomy (OPA)

Mainly French surgeons have used this method. The abdominal cavity is left open following laparotomy [17-36,38-42]. An important advantage of this method is that it counteracts deleterious rising of intra-abdominal pressure induced by inflammation and edema of the peritoneum and ileus. Intestines, however, perforate easily because augmented intraluminal pressure is missing its physiological counteraction by the intact abdominal wall. An additional disadvantage is that, definitive closure of the abdomi-

nal wall becomes impossible, and huge incisional hernias are the inevitable consequence and require secondary repair in most cases. More controlled comparison to standard operative management however, does not demonstrate any improvement in mortality (see table 1 and figure 1). Some surgeons combine the open-abdomen method with continuous post-operative abdominal lavage or planned relaparotomies.

3.3. Covered Abdominostomy (COLA)

Excessive fistula formation was recognized early and already in 1979 some authors propagated coverage of the exposed bowel, using a variety of materials such as plastic foam or meshes of various materials. These methods, however, consistently resulted in big incisional hernias and have been abandoned. Levy et al., however, continue to advocate the method and reports good results. They do not suture the fascia, but cover the

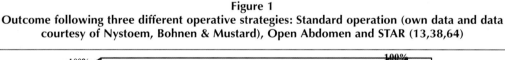

Figure 1
Outcome following three different operative strategies: Standard operation (own data and data courtesy of Nystoem, Bohnen & Mustard), Open Abdomen and STAR (13,38,64)

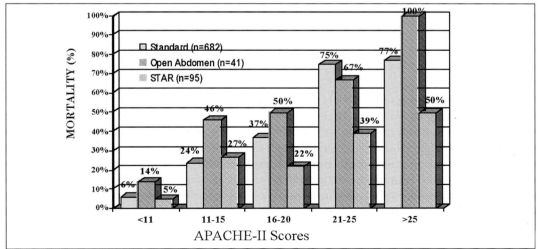

intestines by suturing the skin. If there is too much skin tension, lateral abdominal relaxing incisions provide release [27,43]. True comparisons to other methods, however, are missing and the mortality of 439 non-stratified patients of 12 studies was 39% (see table 1).

3.4. Planned relaparotomy (PR)

Another development of the leaving the abdomen open techniques was the addition of relaparotomies [27,43]. This approach involves multiple planned reoperations following the index operation either in the operating room or in the intensive care unit. Re-explorations were rather on demand than planned and usually too late with intervals ranging from 48-96 hours and more. Publications of this method are often not very clear as to the timing of re exploration. Mortality may be lower with planned shorter interval between two subsequent abdominal explorations [14].

3.5. STAR forerunner operations

Others who focused upon relaparotomy rather than open abdominal drainage [9,10,12,37,44-55] have taken a different approach. Relaparotomies were done in the operating room under optimal conditions, and the interval between the operations was fixed at 24-48 hours. The rationale for these operations were that planned re explorations enabled early diagnosis of complications, avoidance of problems seen with drains, and effective irrigation of the abdomen. The negative experience with continuous post-operative lavage boosted the development of these planned relaparotomy techniques, which were published under various names such as etappenlavage, staged operative repair, scheduled reoperations, scheduled relaparotomy, and second look operations, etc. Initially, retention sutures were used for temporary abdominal closure [15].

Later, when surgeons realized that the necrotic marks in the abdominal wall left by retention suture plates were caused by increased intra-abdominal pressure they started appreciating the importance of the abdominal compartment syndrome. New closure techniques were developed. The negative effects of increased intra-abdominal pressure were compensated for by bridging the gap between the separated fascial edges with devices including a Marlex mesh with a zipper [49,51,54] or the artificial bur [9, 55].

During the development of the new operative strategy, the name changed from scheduled lavage, which emphasized the scheduled cleansing event, to staged abdominal repair (STAR), which emphasized the continuous gentle repair required to cure the severely infected and injured intra-abdominal tissue [37,56].

Also, the STAR strategy unified the previous concepts of OPA, COLA or PR that had contributed to the confusion in terminology. The end of a STAR series, however, mandates suture closure of the abdominal fascia, thus avoiding hernia formation (Table 2). The new STAR operation is the only strategy that allows for adhering to all four principles of operative therapy for diffuse suppurative peritonitis. Conceptually it is one operation done in multiple steps, not multiple operations, a significant detail when obtaining consent form the patient or its family. OPA and COLA represent evolutionary temporary side tracts into dead ends in the evolution of more advanced operative strategies.

3.5.1. Increased intra-abdominal pressure

Classically, the goal of operative management has been to solve the problem with a single operation and to conclude the operation with definitive primary closure of the abdomen. In some cases, however, massive peritoneal edema develops and re-approximation of the abdominal wall fascia is possible only under enormous tension on suture lines. Tension promotes further perfusion deficits and consequently inhibits proper healing and antibacterial defense. Furthermore, closure in such circumstances leads to increased intra-abdominal pressure, pushes the diaphragm into the chest restricting ventilation, thereby promoting development of basal atelectasis and increasing the risk of pneumonia. All these events reduce the oxygen supply to tissue when higher supply is required mismatching supply and demand until the vicious circle closes in total tissue hypoxia. Purely perfused and eventually necrotic tissue is an excellent nutrient, feeding further bacterial growth.

Elevated intra-abdominal pressure, as mentioned above, also negatively influences cardiovascular, pulmonary, hepatic, and renal function (Table 3). The kidney does not tolerate too much external pressure in peritonitis, because in most instances it has been damaged from reduced perfusion due to hypovolemia. Under these conditions the filtration pressure is low and further increase of extra renal pressure will add to the deleterious effects of the disease on renal function. Reduction of pathologically increased intra-abdominal pressure reverses these effects [7].

Table 3
Impact of abdominal compartment syndrome: physiological consequences of elevated intra-abdominal pressure

	Increased	Decreased
mean blood pressure	-	-
heart rate	+	-
pulmonary capillary wedge pressure	+	-
peak airway pressure	+	-
central venous pressure	+	-
thoracic/pleural pressure	+	-
Inferior vena cava pressure	+	-
renal vein pressure	+	-
systemic vascular resistance	+	-
cardiac output	-	+
venous return	-	+
visceral blood flow	-	+
renal blood flow	-	+
glomerular filtration rate	-	+
abdominal wall compliance	-	+

3.5.2. *Temporary abdominal closure devices*

Early in the development of planned rela-parotomies, various techniques have been used to close the abdomen temporarily. To ease planned abdominal reentries, reten-tion sutures [47,50] and later a simple zip-per [37,44,50,56], was used to quickly ap-proximate the fascia between operations performed at intervals of 24 to 48 hours. This concept of planned relaparotomies la-ter merged with the open abdomen techni-que when the need for a tension-free abdo-minal wound became evident. To cover the "open abdomen" various materials have been used such as polyurethane foam, pol-yamide, polypropylene and polyglycolic acid meshes, a combination of a Marlex mesh with a zipper [37,56] and a slide fas-tener (Ethizip) [9]. The new concept of STAR uses the artificial burr [9] (Figure 2) because it is the only device that allows for gradual re-approximation of the fascial ed-ges without resuturing.

4. STAR

STAR is a one abdominal operation perfor-med in multiple steps (abdominal reentries) planned either before or during the first ab-dominal entry. The first abdominal entry is called INDEX STAR. Subsequent abdominal entries (STAR #2, #3, #4. etc) are performed at 24-hour intervals exclusively in the ope-rating room, never in the intensive care unit. The rationale for additional abdominal entries is not only to provide optimal staged conditions for a good primary surgical job but also to check the results of repair such as anastomotic healing e.g. the abdomen should be closed definitively only when sa-tisfactory healing is observed, the abdomen is clean, and the inflammatory edema has

disappeared to allow for fascial reunifica-tion by standard suture techniques.

The operative technique is outlined in the algorithm of Figure 3. Upon recognition of an intra-abdominal problem that is difficult to manage with a single operation, the de-cision to proceed with STAR is made. The decision to use STAR never can be made after the first abdominal entry. STAR, then, implies a commitment before or during the first abdominal exploration for multiple ab-dominal reentries done at 24-hour inter-vals. The wound with the bur in place ne-eds to be covered with the hypobaric wound shield (see below) to collect fluid losses for measurement and replacement of protein losses and to prevent further bacte-rial contamination. Systemic antibiotics with full activity against facultative and

Figure 2
Artificial Burr in place in a patient with diffuse peritonitis. The hook sheet (left side) overlaps the loop sheet (sutured to the right side). There is increased intra-abdominal pressure of 34 mmHg. The massive peritoneal edema pushes the bur closure outwards

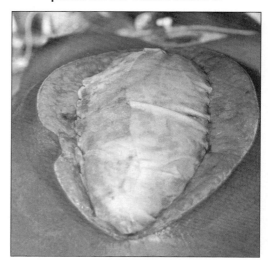

Figure 3
Algorithm of STAR Technique

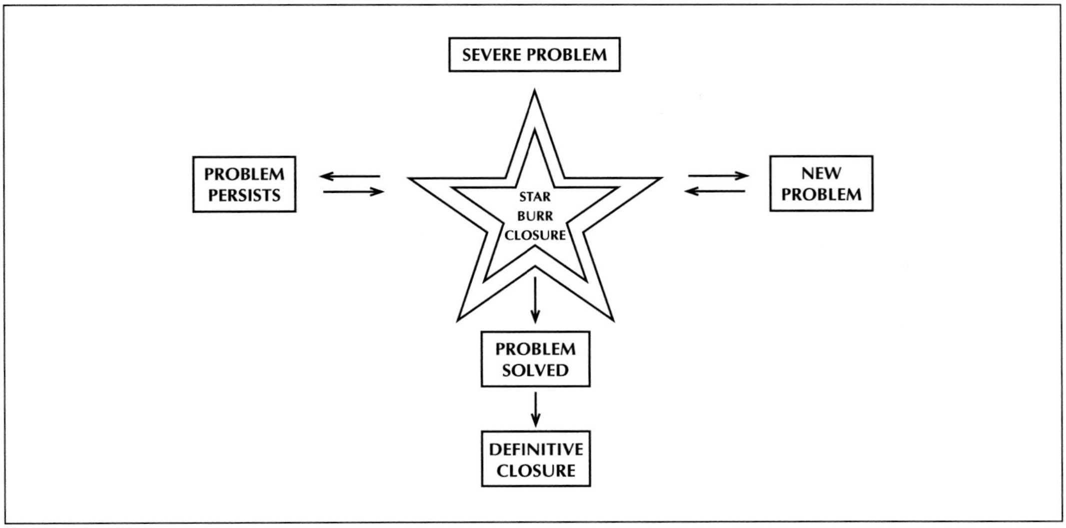

obligate anaerobic bacteria (particularly *E. coli* and *B. fragilis*) are integral part of the STAR procedure and reduce bacterial counts within the abdomen quickly (Figure 4) [57,58]. Star fails if the open abdominal wound is not protected and severe fascial necrosis may result. In addition to the regular antibiotic dosing, a separate antibiotic dose must be given 30 minutes prior to every abdominal entry to prevent additional bacteriema from operative manipulation of infected tissues.

4.1. Index star

A median or transverse incision is made as would be done for the standard operation. The infectious focus is removed or closed, the cavity debrided, and the abdomen may be irrigated with up to 10 liters of Ringer's lactate solution.

The purpose of the index STAR is to eliminate most of the bacteria and toxic pro-

ducts from the abdominal cavity and eliminate the leak (Source control). This measure may be life saving and should always have priority, even in septic shock. Surgical technique has to be extremely gentle and expeditious to avoid further trauma related incitement of the inflammatory response from sepsis [59,60]. If the patients conditions does not allow for extensive repair, temporary source control is a good option. Necrotic bowel segments may be resected and the blind loops of bowel stapled off. The formation of anastomoses can be deferred to the next days when the patient's condition has improved. Drains are not placed circumventing drain related complications.

The abdominal cavity can be temporally closed using new devices such as a zipper with larger seams (Ethizip) [9], a Marlex mesh with a zipper [37,56] or the artificial burr [9, 55] (Figure 5). The artificial bur or STAR Patch is the most practicable device

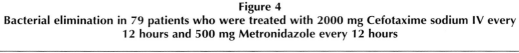

Figure 4
Bacterial elimination in 79 patients who were treated with 2000 mg Cefotaxime sodium IV every 12 hours and 500 mg Metronidazole every 12 hours

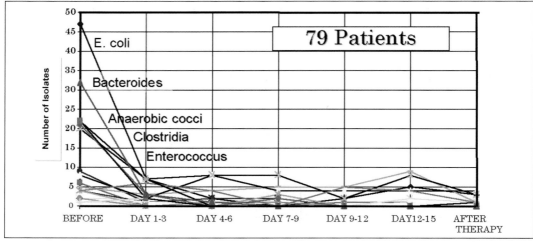

and consists of two bur sheets that stick to-gether at fascial strength. They can, howe-ver, be easily pealed of and reentry into the abdomen is simple and a matter of minu-tes. Initially both sheets are sutured to the incised edges of the abdominal wall FAS-CIA - not skin –using standard running-loo-ped nylon e.g. (figure 2 and 6). As perito-neal edema decreases, the edges may be trimmed off to gradually re approximate the fascia. Upon completion the burr is re-moved and the fascia can always be resu-tured as if only one operation had been performed.

The artificial burr has been approved for clinical use by the European and US he-alth authorities (FDA) and can be obtai-ned from HIDIH SURGICAL, Schloßstasse 13, D-55444 Dörrebach, Germany FAX: 049 6 724 8310 (www.hidih.com) or in the US from STARSURGICAL, Burlington, Wisconsin. 1-888-609-2470, (www.star-surgical.com).

4.2.1. *Hypobaric Wound shield*

The hypobaric wound shield protects the wound from bacterial contamination bet-ween abdominal entries when the patient is outside of the operating room. It also ap-plies negative pressure to the wound, which permits collection of peritoneal fluid and continuous suction of excessive com-partmentalized inflammatory cytokines such as Tumor Necrosis Factor. Details are given in section 4.5.4. and figures 7 and 8. Also protein losses and other factors can be measured to guide possible replacement of losses.

4.2. **Subsequent STARs**

At subsequent operations anastomoses may be sutured. If bleeding is a problem, packing until the next operation is a thera-peutic option. Complications such as he-matomas, necrotic tissue, leaking anasto-moses are diagnosed early and treated in a

Figure 5
Various devices that have been used for covered Abdominostomy and planned relaparotomy: upper left: Retention sutures. Note the pressure marks underneath the plates from increased intra-abdominal pressure. Upper right: Commercially available zipper, Lower left: The Ethizip closure which often opens spontaneously when the patient is moved in the ICU bed. That kind of accidental opening leads to external contamination of the abdomen. Lower left: 4 Meshes sutured to cover that abdominal aperture. Various material have been used this way : Vicryl, Dexon, Marlex, Gortex, vinyl, silicon etc. The use of these meshes is tedious and often expensive

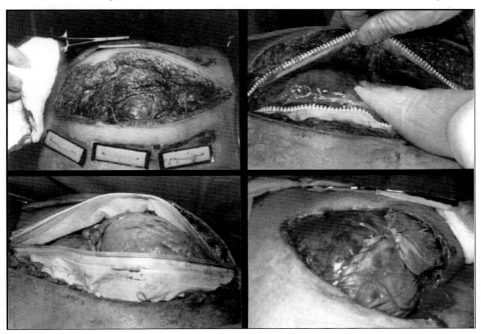

timely fashion. Leaks can be resutured. Contrary to the current teaching, they all heal and I have never seen a persistent bowel leak with STAR. Anastomoses heal better because perfusion is not compromised by increased intra abdominal pressure. Colostomies can be avoided in favor of anastomoses and are only necessary, when the rectum was extirpated. If a problem that was recognized at the first operation persists or if new problems are encountered, such as sudden necrotic area of the bowel close to an anastomosis, further STAR's are planned (Figure 3).

4.3. Final closure

Once all problems are solved, the artificial burr can be removed and the abdominal cavity closed definitively (Figure 9, 10). This may be done with a running O-loop nylon suture. If more than 5 abdominal entries or so have been performed, primary closure of the skin is possible (Figure 10) because most cases have generated sufficient granulation tissue. Good granulations in the abdominal wound indicate established host defense and contaminating bacteria have no chance to multiply when expo-

Figure 6
Insertion technique for the Artificial Bur (STAR-Patch)
A) Suturing the "LOOP SHEET' to the left fascial edge;
B) Suturing the "HOOK SHEET to the opposite fascial edge;
C) The abdominal gap is temporarily bridged with the artificial bur
(Further Information about the artificial bur go to www.hidih.com or www.starsurgical.com

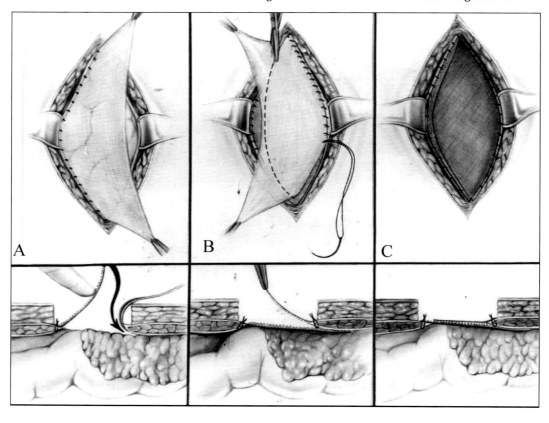

sed to massive numbers of macrophages in granulations.

Wound healing following 117 STARs was uncomplicated in 78% of patients. Fascial dehiscence developed in 7.8% [9]. The average number of operations performed is depicted in Figure 11. The decision to finally close is based on experience, and the factors listed in Table 4 may serve as guidelines.

4.4. Artificial Burr

The scientific name of the device that has been used in the literature is "Artificial Bur (Figures 2,6,7,8 and 9) The mechanism of adhesion has been copied from nature and is similar to the adhering mechanism of the fruit of certain plants of the genus *Arctium* (*Arctium lappa, Arctium tomentosum,* etc.). Common terms for these plants are burr,

Figure 7
Hypobaric Wound Shield placed on top of the Artificial Bur. Note the drain, which is placed within the gauze to suck off peritoneal fluid with an external suctioning pump. A self-adhesive plastic drape is placed on top of the dressing also covering 10 to 20 cm of abdominal wall skin to seal the wound. The prevent leakage along the drain tube a plastic mesentery is formed down to the skin

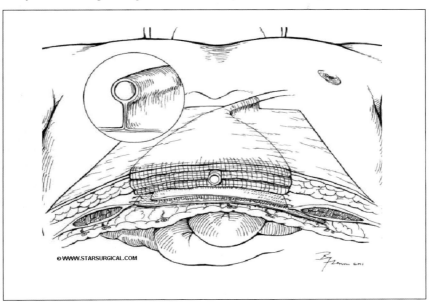

Figure 8
Hypobaric Wound Shield covering the artificial bur shown in figure 2. In this case an iodine coated plastic drape was used explaining the yellowish color. Note the negative pressure of the dressing and the drain tube contours underneath the plastic drape

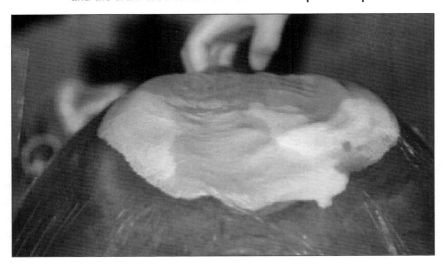

Figure 9
Gradual approximation of the fascial edges by trimming the bur shorter. This can be done until final fascial closure is possible. There is no need to replace the bur

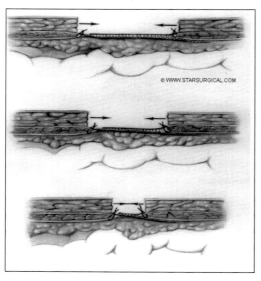

Figure 10
Skin closure in a patient with diffuse peritonitis and massive abdominal compartment syndrome 5 days following the last of 7 STAR abdominal entries. There was primary wound healing

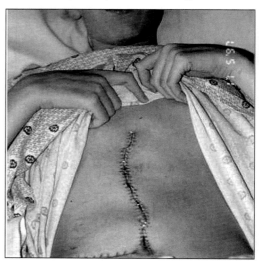

burdock breech, sticktight, and cocklebur. The tensile strength of the bur exceeds that of a normal fascia (Figure 12) (65). Adverse reactions have not been observed. In some cases of preexisting fascial necroses sutures have pulled out of the fascia. Debridement of the fascia and resuturing of the bur sheet resolves such problem. If, in rare cases, more the six abdominal reentries are necessary, one may consider replacing the bur.

4.5. Detailed description of operative technique

4.5.1. General

The artificial burr for temporary abdominal closure [bur] can be utilized in longitudinal and transverse incisions. A midline incision from the xyphoid process of the sternum to

the symphysis pubis is the incision of choice. The skin is incised with a scalpel, subcutaneous tissue including fascia are also separated using a scalpel or electrocautery. The peritoneum (mesothelial lining) is cautiously opened and transected using a pair of scissors as in any laparotomy. Care must be taken not to injure any of the contents of the abdominal cavity, particularly the large and small bowel.

Subsequent steps are dictated by the underlying pathology and follows general rules of abdominal surgery. Particular care must be taken to handle tissue gently, avoid mass ligatures, and perform meticulous hemostasis. In any case, an antibiotic such as imipenem/cilastatin or a third generation cephalosporin combined with metronidazole should be administered 30 minutes before opening the abdomen to

Figure 11
Number of STAR abdominal entries matched with number of patients. In most cases four abdominal entries were sufficient for cure.

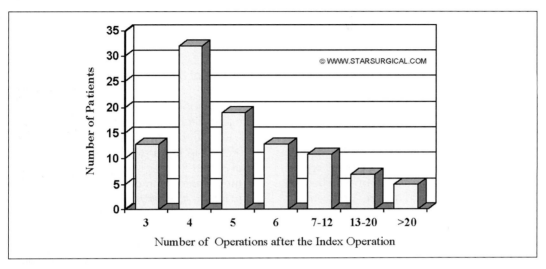

guarantee sufficient antibacterial tissue levels during operative manipulations. Following operative management of pathology, the abdomen may than be temporarily closed utilizing the bur. The first abdominal entry of a series is called index STAR, subsequent abdominal entries are numbered consecutively: STAR #2, STAR#3 etc.

4.5.2. Suturing Technique for the Burr

At the completion of operative management of intra-abdominal pathology, the omentum is directed to the lower abdomen to cover the large and small bowel. Then a lap sponge, an 18" x 18" cm laparotomy gauze cloth (LAP)[1] is used to cover the content of the abdominal cavity. On top of the

Table 4
When to Close the Abdomen definitively

Abdominal Pressure less than 20 mmHg when fascia are approximated
Score predicted mortality < 20%
No persistent bowel leak
Bowel continuity established
No healing problem expected
Debridement sufficient
Intra-abdominal pressure < 15-20 mmHg when fasciae are re-approximated

sponge, a so-called Fish plastic protector (FISH)[2] is used as a temporary protective coverage of the intra-abdominal structures while suturing the fascia. At this point, the wound edges on the left and the right sides are usually separated from 10 to 30 cm with the bowel and other abdominal structures somewhat protruding through the incisional opening.

Now the artificial burr is removed from the sterile packaging and both the fuzzy sheet as well as the hook sheet is identified. The fuzzy sheet consists of soft material representing loops. The backside of the sheet is reinforced with soft material. Both sheets should be of sufficient size to cover the entire abdominal opening. They are not trimmed at this point.

Insertion of Loop Sheet (Figure 6 a)

The left upper corner of the loop sheet (loops facing outward) is now sutured to the right upper fascia of the incisional opening, in close vicinity to the xyphoid process of the sternum. This is done with a looped suture material such as #1or #0 nylon[3]. Passing the needle through the loop following the first stitch fastening the burr sheet corner to the fascia. Following this, the left edge of the loop sheet is sutured to the right fascia all the way down the abdominal wall into the public area of the incision. The suturing technique is simple running suture, suturing the material to the fascia only. Subcutaneous fat and skin is not included in any stitch. The distance between two stitches, should be 1-2cm longitudinally and transversely at least 1.0 cm away from the fascial edge. Inclusion of muscle should be avoided if possible. Once the loop sheet is attached to the right side fascia from the most proximal to the most caudal point, the loops should face outward and the reinfor-

ced soft back side of the sheet should face toward omentum and bowel or other intra-abdominal organs. The entire sheet is then pushed underneath the left abdominal wall between the abdominal wall and intra-abdominal structures.

Insertion of hook sheet (Figure 6 b)

Now the hook side is prepared for insertion. The first stitch is placed to the upper end of the left sided fascia close to the xyphoid and close to the first stitch for attaching the loop sheet. Suturing technique is the same as the technique practiced on the right side, utilizing a #1or #0 looped nylon suture. The hook sheet is then attached to the left side of the fascia utilizing a simple running suture technique. The hook of the hook sheet should face inward, the reinforcement of the hook sheet facing outward. The last stitch and the knot is performed in the distal or lower corner of the fascia close to the last stitch of the loop sheet and tied.

4.5.3. *Establishing temporary closure of the abdomen* (Figure 6 c, 2, 7 and 8)

After attaching both sheets to opposing fascial edges the hook sheet is gently pressed onto the loop sheet that is covering the abdominal content. Excessive material is trimmed off the hook sheet to fit the sheet size to the wound size. To trim off the hook sheet to the correct size, scissors are used to cut the sheet at the level of the right fascia. Now the hook sheet and loop sheet are separated again. The hook sheet is pulled laterally and the loop sheet is also removed from the left side of the abdominal cavity and pulled laterally to the right side. The Fish[2] as well as LAPS[1] are removed and the loop sheet is reinserted again between the left side of the abdominal wall and intra-abdominal structures without having protective material (FISH and LAPS) underneath it. The loop sheet usually does not need to be trimmed off. It can be done easily, however, if necessary.

Once the loop sheet is inserted underneath the opposing fascia, the hook sheet is pulled toward the right side exerting some tension on the fascia and pressing hooks into the loops of the loop sheet. This establishes temporary abdominal closure. The intraabdominal pressure should not exceed 10-15 mm Hg after closure and there is sufficient tension on the fasciae to prevent their retraction.

4.5.4. Hypobaric Wound Shield
(Figure 7 and 8)

Now gauze such as Kerlix[3] is utilized to cover the hook sheet and subcutaneous tissue up to the level of the skin. A suction drain is imbedded into Kerlix gauze. Following this, a plastic drape is applied to the skin to cover the entire abdominal wall and the wound, leaving a tunnel with a mesentery for the drain. This seals the abdominal cavity and keeps it sterile. The area of the skin covered by the plastic drape should cover a distance of 20 cm from any edge of the abdominal wound. Once this plastic drape seals off the abdominal cavity a section of 10 cm water is applied to the suction drain to collect abdominal fluid or measurement of protein losses and other factors for possible replacement.

4.5.5. Intensive care unit

Between operations the patient remains in the intensive care unit to monitor vital signs including intra-abdominal pressure, cardiopulmonary, renal and hepatic function, and to permit sufficient nutrition, oxygen supply

and replacement of losses. The patient is usually sedated and requires mechanical ventilation for sufficient oxygenation of tissues for optimal healing.

4.5.6. Interval between two STAR's
and fascial re-approximation

The interval between two operations of a series of planned abdominal re-entries or staged abdominal repairs should not exceed 36 hours after the ending of the previous abdominal entry. It is important to definitively close the abdomen as early as possible when most of the peritoneal edema has disappeared. This process can be aided by forced diuresis as the pathology is surgically controlled (Source control complete). With every abdominal reentry the fascial edges should be pulled together to decrease the gap between the fascias (Figure 9).

4.5.7. Re-opening of the artificial burr

Approximately twenty-four hours after the index STAR, the second STAR is performed. For this purpose the patient is brought into the operating room and general anesthesia is induced if necessary. Subsequently, the Steri-drape[4] is peeled off the abdominal wound and the abdominal wall. Similarly, the Kerlex gauze[5], including the drain are removed and the patient's skin and the wound is prepped with betadine or hexachlorophene or other approved disinfectants/antiseptics. Prepping includes the skin around the abdominal wall opening and the outer surface of the artificial burr. It is done before all operations. Following this, sterile drapes are placed around the operating field and the instruments positioned as done with other laparotomies.

To open the abdomen, the hook sheet is peeled off the loop sheet by pulling it perpendicular off the loop sheet and toward the left side. Then a LAP[1] is placed into the wound and the hook sheet pressed into the LAP. Both the LAP with the hook sheet are pulled away from the wound toward the left side and bent over the wound edges. Then the loop sheet is removed from underneath the left sided fascia of the abdominal wall, similarly pulled over to the right side and bent over on top of the abdominal wall wound.

Now the abdominal wound is open and ready for inspection, debridement, irrigation, and necessary repair. At the end of the procedure the abdomen is closed the same way as it was closed at the index STAR: The loop sheet is inserted underneath the left side of the fascia of the abdominal wall to cover all abdominal structures of the wound. Then the LAP sheet is removed from the hook sheet and the hooks are inserted onto the loops of the loop sheet by exerting some tension on the fascia. Intra-abdominal pressure should be between 5-10 mm Hg. This can be measured transvesically. Following closure of the artificial burr, the HYPOBARIC WOUND SHIELD is placed (Figure 7 and 8): Kerlex[3] gauze is applied on top on the wound to cover the hook sheet and subcutaneous tissue up to the level of the skin. A suction drain is imbedded into Kerlix[4] gauze. Following this a plastic Steri-drape[5] is applied to the skin to cover the entire abdominal wall and the wound, leaving a tunnel with a mesentery for the drain. This seals the abdominal cavity and keeps it sterile. The area of the skin covered by the plastic drape should cover a distance of 20 cm from any edge of the abdominal wound. Once this plastic drape seals off the abdominal cavity a section of 10cm water is applied to the suction drain to collect abdominal fluid or measurement of protein losses and other factors for possible replacement. At the end of the procedure, the patient is brought from the Operating Room back to the Intensive Care Unit.

4.5.8. *Final closure of the abdominal wound* (Figures 9 and 10)

The abdominal cavity can be closed once the problem within the abdominal cavity is solved, healing is most likely to continue without further complication, and intra-abdominal pressure is less than 15-20 mm Hg with the fascial edges approximated. The bur sheets are removed by taking out the running sutures between bur and abdominal wall fascia. The hook sheet is first removed from the left side and then the loop sheet from the right side. Subsequent to this, the fascia is closed either by running suture technique using a looped #1 Maxon[6] or PDS[7] suture material or by the technique, which ever is the preference of the surgeon. The abdominal cavity is closed the same way as after a classical laparotomy. Before suturing the fascia, it is a good idea to have an abdominal X-ray done to identify missed laps or other unintended items are left within the abdominal cavity.

4.5.9. *Skin closure* (Figure 10)

After five STAR procedures there is usually sufficient granulation tissue to allow for skin closure with minimal risk for wound infection. If there is insufficient granulation tissue it is better to leave the subcutaneous tissue and the skin open and wait with the final skin closure until good granulation tissue has formed.

All procedures require application of a single dose prophylactic antibiotic, usually the antibiotic that is used for treating the underlying infection. The additional dose should be given 30 minutes prior to the laparotomy or relaparotomy.

4.5.9. Instruments and materials

[1]**LAP** = A sponge gauze measuring 18" x 18". Official name is laparotomy sponge. The manufacturer is Medical Action, 150 Motor Park Way, #204; Hauppaugae, New York 11788-5108; Tel: 1-800-645-7042; Fax: 1-516-231-4600.

[2]**FISH** = A sterile-radiopaque plastic product that is called the Glassman Viscera Retainer. The large size is used. Produced by Adept-Med International; 5040 Robert J. Mathews Pkwy; El Dorado Hills, CA 95762.

[3]**O-LOOP NYLON** =Nylon suture, Tradename Ethilon, black monofilament 150cm or 60in. suture of size 0 (3.5 metric) and looped on a _ circle taper CT needle. Produced by Ethicon Inc. Special order # D-4734.

[4]**STERIDRAPE** = Ioban-2; 90cm x 80cm. The manufacturer is 3M; Catalog #6651. Order from: Baxter Allegiance Valuelink; 3651 Birchwood Drive; Waukegan, IL 60085; Tel: 1-800-477-0811; Fax 708-578-2163; Sales Rep: Dale Micelspurger.

[5]**O LOOP MAXON** = Synthetic suture of monofilament polyglyconate, Tradename O Maxon 75cm of 30in suture of size 0 (1.5 metric) and looped on a _ circle taper T60 needle. Produced by Davis & Geck Product #3641-63.

[6]**KERLIX** = 6 ply-4.5in x 4.1 yd (11.4cm x 370cm) stretched. 1 roll supplied by Kendall, Order #6730. Kendall Health Care Products Company, Division of Kendall Company, Mansfield, MA 02048. Product information 1-800-962-9888.

ARTIFICIAL BUR supplied in the US by STAR-SURGICAL, 7781 Lakeview Drive, Burlington, Wisconsin 53105. Product information 1-888-609-2470 and for Europe, and other countries go to. for information.

4.6. Patients that would benefit form STAR

Initially, STAR was reserved for advanced stages of disease with sepsis and multi-system organ failure. Indications to perform STAR are listed in Table 5. Dramatic recoveries have been observed in patients with advanced suppurative peritonitis. On the other hand we also treated quite successfully patients with local problems not associated with high mortality.

General problems requiring STAR include dead bowel, pancreatic and other intra-abdominal necroses, transplant pancreatitis, huge incisional hernias with bowel fistulas and any conditions with increased intra-abdominal pressure following trauma and lengthy operations.

4.6.1. Suppurative Peritonitis

Diffuse suppurative peritonitis whether from spontaneous perforation or a leaking anastomosis or suture line that requires multiple debridements, is a good indication to perform the STAR procedure. Also when it is not possible to perform a primary anastomosis because of septic shock and circulatory breakdown, or excessive peritoneal edema STAR gives the opportunity for delayed repair and helps to avoid the abdominal compartment syndrome.

4.6.2. Infected pancreatic necrosis

In patients with pancreatic necrosis, debridement could be performed in a staged fashion and stopped when associated with too much local bleeding - to be continued the next day following packing of the bleeding infectious pancreatic and peri-pancreatic tissue. Removal of packs debrides necrotic tissue around the pancreas quite nicely. Once the majority of necroses are replaces by granulation tissue, it is safe to place a large round latex drain tube into the pancreas bed and remove the bur to close fascia to fascia. Recently we demonstrated very good results in transplant pancreatitis (66).

4.6.3. Dead bowel

Patients with dead bowel may benefit from STAR: The first operation would be done for resection of the dead bowel and the second or third for anastomosis when there was enough evidence of no further decay of bowel ends. It has been observed that anastomoses could be sutured in the presence of peritonitis and the healing could be observed and corrected during subsequent STAR procedures.

4.6.4. STAR and Apache stratification and outcome

Statistical analysis of patients with diffuse peritonitis stratified by APACHE-II [61-63]

compared favorably to huge patient populations who underwent standard operative management when adjusting for prognostic factors with a logistic model (Figure 13). Initially we thought that only patients with scores above 10 would benefit from STAR (Figure 1) [37]. The logistic model, after adjusting for risk factors, however, showed a significant difference between STAR and NON-STAR patients for all risk groups [64]. The most striking 20 to 40% improvements of mortality rates, however, are achieved in patients with APACHE scores from 10 to 20. These patients may be the best candidates for STAR.

4.6.5. Prospective Studies

No institution was able to carry out a prospective controlled trial to prove superiority of one procedure. Once the new method was introduced, ethics committees and surgeons considered the enrollment of patients in the non-STAR group an ethical problem because of the impression that STAR was

Table 5
When is STAR INDICATED?

STAR may be indicated in diffuse suppurative peritonitis, infected pancreatic necrosis, intestinal ischemia and trauma, when one or more of the following factors is present:

- Critical patient condition precluding definitive repair
- Excessive peritoneal and parietal edema (increased intra-abdominal pressure)
- Impossibility to eliminate or to control the source of infection
- Incomplete debridement of necrotic tissue
- Uncertainty as to viability of bowel
- Anastomosis and/or other repair needs re-inspection
- Uncontrolled bleeding (the need for 'packing')

Further indications for STAR are increased intra-abdominal pressure over 20 mm Hg, transplant pancreatitis, ruptured abdominal aneurysm, lengthy operations with peritoneal edema, certain organ transplant operations and complex abdominal operation when optimal postoperative perfusion of intra-abdominal tissue is desired.

Figure 13
Tensile strength of the artificial bur: It requires 57 pounds to disrupt 5 square cm of bur. The adhering surface in clinical practice is usually 40 x 10 cm = 400 square cm e.g.. 4560 pounds (or about 2 metric tons) are required to disrupt the bur closure.

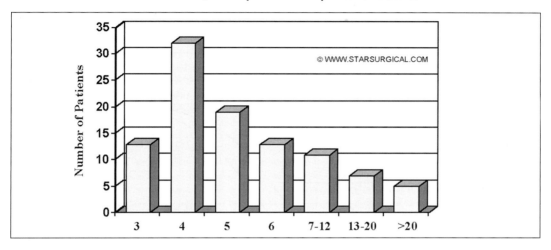

doing so much better. Additionally only 15% of all patients with diffuse peritonitis qualify for staged abdominal repair that means that for one single institution less than 20 patients are available per year, an insufficient number to plan a single institutional study. Multi-institutional studies are extremely difficult to form in disease with a myriad of different conditions and risk factors. After having tried for 15 years to conduct a prospective randomized trial, comparing STAR with the standard operation or other advanced procedures we must realize that this may never be possible. The anecdotal evidence, however, may be sufficiently convincing to recommend STAR for the sickest 15% of our patients with intra-abdominal infection.

5. SUMMARY

To improve mortality of intra-abdominal infections, since 1975, many surgeons world-wide have been extending the classical single-stage operative approach, and a variety of procedures have been introduced for similar if not the same type of operative strategy. Names such as open abdomen, abdominostomy, semi-open technique, planned relaparotomy, relaparotomy on demand, programmed laparotomy, programmed relaparotomy, four-quadrant lavage, scheduled reoperations, scheduled repeated laparotomy, etappenlavage, second-look strategy, abdominostomy, semi-open abdominostomy, staged operative repair, staged abdominal repair, etc., have been used. This study clarifies what these procedures have in common and what differentiates them from the standard operation.

Kirschner's definition for standard operation has been used to explore differences among the extended operative procedures. Papers since 1975 on operative management have been analyzed for classification purposes in

Figure 12
Comparing mortality rates of standard operation with mortality rates of the STAR procedure when adjusting for risk factors using the APACHE-II scoring system. The difference is significant p> 0.018). The lower curve represent the mortality associated with the STAR procedure, the upper curve that of the standard operation with relaparotomy on demand. Extrapolation of patients with an APACHE-II score of 20 yields a mortality improvement form 56 % for the standard operation to 34 % for STAR, an improvement of 22%

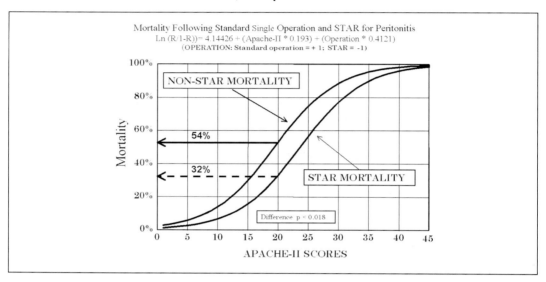

terms of risk factor stratification, origin and etiology of infection, number of operations, timing of reoperations, place of reoperations (operating room vs. ICU), interval between operations, devices to bridge the fascial gap, final closure technique, complications, and mortality.

All procedures can be classified into three concepts: open abdomen (OPA), covered abdominostomy (COLA), and staged abdominal repair (STAR). The complications of OPA are hernias and fistulae; of COLA, hernias and rare fistulae; and after STAR, the hernia rate is acceptable and fistulae are rare. Although there is no prospective, randomized trial, data suggest that mortality is lowest following staged abdominal repair.

REFERENCES

1. Costain WA: Lymphaticostomy in peritonitis. Surg Gynecol Obstet 1923;36:365

2. Fowler GR: Diffuse septic peritonitis, with special reference to a new method of treatment, namely the eleevated head and trunk posture, to facilitate drainage into the pelvis: With a report of nine consecutive cases of recovery. Med Rec 1900;57:617

3. Kirschner M: Die Behandlung der akuten eitrigen freien Bauchfellentzuendung. Langenb Arch Chir 1926;142:53-267.

4. Polk HC, Fry DE: Radical peritoneal debridement for established peritonitis. Ann Surg 1980;192:350-355.

5. Hau T, Lee JT, Simmons RL: Mechanisms of the adjuvant effect of hemoglobin in expe-

rimental peritonitis: IV. The adjuvant effect of hemoglobin in granulocytopenic rats. Surgery 1981;89:187-191.

6. Schein M, Wittmann DH, Aprahamian C, et al: Abdominal compartment syndrome. The physiological and clinical consequences of elevated intra-abdominal pressure. J Am Coll Surg 1995;180;745-753

7. Wittmann DH and Iskander GA. The Compartment Syndrome of the abdominal cavity; A State-of-the-Art Review. J Intensive Care Medicine 2000 201-220

8. Muhrer KH, Grimm B, Wagner KH, et al: Serum-Endotoxin-Spiegel wahrend des Verlaufs der offenen Peritonitisbehandlung. Chirurg 1985;56:789-797.

9. Wittmann DH, Aprahamian C, Bergstein JM: Etappenlavage, advanced diffuse peritonitis managed by planned multiple laparotomies utilizing zippers, slide fastener, and velcro analogue for temporary abdominal closure. World J Surg 1990;14:218-226.

10. Wittmann DH, Teichmann W: Therapy for pathogenic bacteria in diffuse peritonitis by scheduled relaparotomies. Langenb Arch Chir 1985;366:629

11. Morris J, Eddy T, Rutherford E, et al: The staged celiotomy for trauma. Ann Surg 1993;217:576-585.

12. Hedderich GS, Wexler M, McLean AP, et al: The Septic Abdomen: Open Management with Marlex Mesh with a Zipper.. Surgery 1986;99:4399.

13. Wittmann DH, Schein M, Nyström PO: Open Packing Abdominostomy in the septic abdomen; in Ruedi (ed): State of the Art of Surgery 1991/92. Chur, International Society of Surgery, 1992, pp 30-34.

14. Edmiston CE, Goheen MP, Kornhall S, et al: Fecal Peritonitis: Microbial Adherence to Serosal Mesothelium and Resistance to Peritoneal Lavage. World J Surg 1990;14:176-183.

15. Pujol JP, Complete: These de Medicine, Paris, U.E.R. X. Bichat. Paris, 1975.

16. Bohnen JMA, Mustard R: A critical look at scheduled relaparotomy for secondary bacterial peritonitis.. Surg Gyencol Obstet 1992;172 (Supp):25-29.

17. Anderson ED, Mandelbaum DM, Ellison EC, et al: Open packing of the peritoneal cavity in generalized bacterial peritonitis. Am J Surg 1983;145:131-134.

18. Bradley SJ, Jurkovich GJ: Controlled open drainage of severe intraabdominal sepsis. Arch Surg 1985;120:629

19. Broome A, Hansson L, Lundgren F, et al: Open treatment of abdominal septic catastrophies. World J Surg 1983;7:792-796.

20. Bytka PF, Khotinian VF, Brynze GV, et al: Open treatment of postoperative peritonitis. (Unknown Journal!) 1986;136:38-42.

21. Champault G, Magnier M, Psalmon F, et al: L'evisceration controlle dans le traitement des peritonites graves. Chirurgie 1979; 105:866-869.

22. Champault G, Magnier M, Psalmon F, et al: L'éviscération: élément thérapeutique des péritonites. La Nouvelle Presse Médicale 1979; 8:1349-1350,.

23. Duff JH, Moffat J: Abdominal sepsis managed by leaving abdomen open. Surgery 1981; 90:774-778.

24. Dupre A, Frere G, Guignier M, et al: Evisceration therapeutique controlee lors des peritonites dites depasses. Nouvelle Presse Med 1979;40:3257-3258.

25. Egiazarian VT, Nekrasov LP, Iakovenko AI, et al: Laparostomy in diffuse suppurative peritonitis. (Unknown Journal!) 1986;136:50-52.

26. Fagniez PL: La prevention des lesions intestinales lors de eviscerations. Nouv Presse Med 1978;7:1117

27 Hannoun L, Levy E, Flageul G, et al: Anatomical and physiological basis of parietal treatment of severe peritonitis and evisceration. Anat Clin 1984;5:235-243.

28. Hollender LF, Bur F, Schwenk D, et al: Das offengelassene abdomen. Technik, indikation, resultate. Chirurg 1983;54:316-319.

29. Ivatury RR, Nallathambi M, Rao PM, et al: Open management of the septic abdomen: Therapeutic and prognostic considerations based on APACHE II. Crit Care Med 1989;17:511-517.

30. Kinney EV, Polk HC: Open treatment of peritonitis: an argument against. Adv Surg 1987;21:19-28.

31. Maetani S, Tobe T: Open peritoneal drainage as effective treatment of advanced peritonitis. Surgery 1981;90:804-809.

32. Mastboom WJB, Kuypers HHC, Schoots FJ, et al: Small-bowel perforation complicating the open treatment of generalized peritonitis. Arch Surg 1989;124:689-692.

33. Mughal MM, Bancewicz J, Irving MH: "Laparostomy": A technique for the management of intractable intra-abdominal sepsis. Br J Surg 1986;73:253-259.

34. Neidhardt JH, Kraft F, Morin A, et al: Le traitement "aX` ventre ouverT" de certaines peX'ritonites et infections parieX'tales abdominales graves: etudes et technique. Chirurgie 1979;Verify:272-274.

35. Schein M, Saadia R, Jamieson JR, et al: The "sandwich technique" in the management of the open abdomen. Br J Surg 1986;73:369-370.

36. Stone HH, Strom PR, Mullins RJ: Pancreatic abscess management by subtotal resection and packing. World J Surg 1984;8:340-345.

37. Aprahamian C, Wittmann DH, Bergstein JM, et al: Gastrointestinal Complications; in Mattox (ed): Complications of trauma. New York, Churchill Livingstone, 1993, pp 465-480.

38. Schein M: Planned reoperations and open management in critical intra-abdominal infections: prospective experience in 52 cases. World J Surg 1991;15:537-545.

39. Meyer-Burg J, Arbeiter G: Der abdominelle Lymphkreislauf. Badeb-Badeb, Köln, New York, Verlag Gerhard Witzrock, 1977.

40. Greenfield CL, Walshaw R: Open peritoneal drainage for treatment of contaminated peritoneal cavity and septic peritonitis in dogs and cats: 24 cases (1980-1986). J Am Vet Med Assoc 1987;191:100-105.

41. Vasquez JMT, Speare OR: Gravity drainage in the treatment of patients with near fatal recurrent intra-abdominal sepsis. Military Med 1983;148:597-599.

42. Walsh GF, Chiasson P, Heddrich GS, et al: The Open Abdomen: the Marlex Mesh and Zipper Technique: a method of managing intraperitoneal infection. Surg Clin North Am 1988;68:25-40.

43. Levy E: Principles of surgery for diffuse peritonitis. Management of the abdominal wall. (In French). Ann Chir 1985;39:547-553.

44. Leguit P: Zip-closure of the abdomen. Neth J Surg 1982;34:40-41.

45. Kern E, Klaue P, Arbogast R: Programmierte Peritoneal-Lavage bei diffuser Peritontis. Chirurg 1983;54:306-310.

46. Penninckx FM, Kerremans RPJ, Lauwers PM: Lavin P (ed): Die chirurgische Behandlung der Peritonitis. Stuttgart, 1983, pp 103-105.

47. Penninckx FM, Kerremans RPJ, Lauwers PM: Planned relaparotomies in the surgical treatment of severe generalized peritonitis from intestinal origin. World J Surg 1983;7:762-766.

48. Hadjiminas D, Cheadle W, Spain D, et al: Antibiotic overkill of trauma victims.. Am J Surg 1994;168:288-290.

49. Heddrich GS, Wexler MJ, McLean AP, et al: The septic abdomen: open management with Marlex mesh with a zipper. Surgery 1986;99:399-408.

50. Teichmann W, Wittmann DH, Andreone A: Scheduled reoperations (Etappenlavage) for

diffuse peritonitis. Arch Surg 1986;121:147-152.

51. Garcia-Sabrido JL, Tallado JM, Christou NV, et al: Treatment of severe intra-abdominal sepsis and/or necrotic foci by an "open-abdomen" approach. Arch Surg 1988;123:152-156.

52. Hoffmann R, Largiader F: Problem beim definitiven Abdominalverschluss nach "Reissverschluss" und nach "left open abdomen". Helv Chir Acta 1990;57:47-50.

53. Penninckx FM, Kerremans RPJ, Filez L, et al: Planned relaparotomies for advanced, established peritonitis from colonic origin. (Unknown Journal!) 1990;90:269-274.

54. Bose SM, Kalra M, Sandhu NPS: Open management of septic abdomen by marlex mesh zipper. Aust NZ J Surg 1991;61:385-388.

55. Wittmann DH, Aprahamian C, Bergstein JM, et al: A burr-like device to facilitate temporary abdominal closure in planned multiple laparotomies. Eur J Surg 1993;159:75-79

56. Walsh GF, Chiasson P, Hedderich F, et al: The Open Abdomen: A Marlex Mesh and Zipper Technique: A Method of Managing Intraperitoneal Infection.. Surg Clin of Nor Amer 1988;(68)1:25

57. Aprahamian C, Schein M, Wittmann DH: Bacterial elimination in intra-abdominal infections treateded by staged abdominal repair STAR... Diagn Microbiol Infect Dis 1995;22:183-186

58. Wittmann DH, Bergstein JM, Frantzides CT: Calculated empiric antimicrobial therapy fot mixed surgical infections. Infection 1991;19 (Suppl6):345-350.

59. Wittmann DH: Intra-abdominal infections: pathophysiology and treatment, New York:Marcel-Dekker Publisher, 1990.

60. Wittmann DH, Walker AP, Condon RE: Peritonitis, intra-abdominal infection, and intra-abdominal abscess; in Schwartz SI, Shires GT, Spencer FC (eds): Principles of Surgery. New York, McGrawHill, 1993, pp 1449-1484.

61. Knaus WA, Draper EA, Wagner DP, et al: APACHE II: A severity of disease classification system. Crit Care Med 1985;13:818-829.

62. Nyström PO, Bax R, Dellinger EP, et al: Proposed Definitions for Diagnosis, Severity Scoring, Stratification, and Outcome for Trials on Intraabdominal Infection. World Journal of Surgery 1990;14:148-158.

63. Wong DT, Knaus WA: Predicting outcome in critical care: the current status of the APACHE prognostic scoring system. Can J Anaesth 1991;38:374-383.

64. Wittmann DH, Bansal N, Bergstein JM, et al: Staged abdominal repair compares favorable to conventional operative therapy for intra-andominal infections when adjusting for prognistic factors with a logistic model. Theor Surg 1994;9:201-207. (now Europ J. Surgery)

65. Wittmann DH, Aprahamian C, Bergstein JM, et al. A burr-like device to facilitate temporary abdominal closure in planned multiple laparotomies. Eur J Surg 1993; 159:75-79.

66. Wittmann DH. Newer methods of operative therapy for peritonitis. In Nyhus LM, Baker RJ, Fischer JE., eds. Mastery of Surgery. Boston: Little, Brown and Company, 1996

67. D. P. Slakey, C. P. Johnson, D. J. Cziperle, A. M. Roza, D. H. Wittmann, DH, D. W. Gray, J. A. Roake, J. Britton, P. J. Morris, and M. B. Adams. Management of severe pancreatitis in renal transplant recipients. Annals of Surgery 225 (2):217-222, 1997.

Therapeutic Challenges of Tertiary Peritonitis

Emilia Cercenado PhD and Fernando García-Garrote, PhD

1. TERTIARY PERITONITIS

The term tertiary peritonitis refers to superinfection of the peritoneal cavity, which usually occurs in a seriously ill patient after initial treatment for secondary peritonitis [46, 65]. After contamination of the peritoneal cavity with micro-organisms from the gastrointestinal tract, peritonitis will resolve in most patients who are treated with appropriate surgical and antimicrobial therapy. In those cases where the micro-organisms remain in the peritoneum, the infection may be contained and an intra-abdominal abscess may form. In some cases in which the residual infection cannot be contained, persistent generalized peritonitis (tertiary peritonitis) may develop. This process is generally accompanied by signs of unresolved sepsis, hypercatabolism, hemodynamic instability, and multiple organ dysfunction. Tertiary peritonitis probably represents a form of superinfection that is an indicator of more serious underlying host immunosuppression and physiological derangement. These patients are unable to compartmentalize and clear the initial infection, or subsequently develop a superinfection of the entire peritoneal cavity. When host defenses and antimicrobial therapy fail, resistant organisms overgrow (usually Gram-negative bacilli or fungi). Successful treatment of intra-abdominal sepsis entails the removal of the source of infection, eradication of residual bacteria and metabolic and hemodynamic support to counteract the physiological alterations that occur during sepsis. Although the primary mode of therapy for the vast majority of patients who develop intra-abdominal sepsis consists of surgical intervention to remove the source of peritoneal contamination, antimicrobial agents play a critical role in eradication of intraperitoneal pathogens; however, most clinical studies reviewing cases of severe intra-abdominal sepsis (i.e., intra-abdominal infection with concomitant systemic sepsis) report mortality greater than 15% [4, 16, 48, 69]. These patients frequently develop progressive multiple systems organ failure and, ultimately death results [28, 30, 32]. This overall clinical situation suggests a generalized failure of host defenses which is difficult to reverse using a standard surgical approach. Moreover, usually patients have been a long time in the hospital and have a poor prognosis despite a correct antimicrobial therapy [60].

2. ETIOLOGY

The spectrum of organisms associated with tertiary peritonitis differs from that associated with secondary peritonitis. Recovery of organisms may be altered by the use of pre-operative antimicrobial therapy, with more sensitive organisms inhibited and more resistant organisms over-represented. The microbiologic profile of patients who develop tertiary peritonitis is characterized by multi-resistant organisms that are insensitive to initial antimicrobial therapy [61]. It is unclear whether these organisms reach the peritoneum by translocation across the bowel wall or as a result of antimicrobial selective pressure at the time of the initial insult. Bacterial translocation may be promoted by intestinal ischemia, endotoxemia, malnutrition and heavy overgrowth of organisms under antimicrobial selective pressure. The common micro-organisms isolated from patients with secondary peritonitis, *Escherichia coli*, and *Bacteroides fragilis* are only occasionally found in these patients. The bacteria causing tertiary peritonitis have been classically considered innocuous colonizers rather than true pathogens; however, the fact that bacterial species such as *Staphylococcus epidermidis* and *Candida* species are true invasive pathogens in this disease rather than merely colonizing bacteria is clearly demonstrated by their ability to invade and become blood-borne. It is, therefore, likely that a relatively immuno-compromised host appears to contribute to their pathogenicity. Prevention of this situation by timely surgical intervention, appropriate antibiotics and, possibly, innovative techniques such as selective digestive de-contamination [36] or enhancing the integrity of the mucosal barrier [38, 39], may improve survival in this high-risk patient population. Micro-organisms isolated in ter-

tiary peritonitis belong to two types. In some cases there are very pathogenic bacteria which are resistant to many antimicrobials, like *Pseudomonas* species or multiresistant *Enterobacter* species. The other group includes micro-organisms resistant to initial therapy but of low pathogenicity in non-im-munosupressed patients, like coagulase negative *Staphylococcus*, *Enterococcus* species and *Candida* species. In severely ill patients the micro-organisms more frequently isolated are *Candida* species, *Enterococcus* species, *Pseudomonas* species and *Staphylococcus epidermidis*. Gram-negative micro-organisms are less frequently isolated. [65].

In one study [46, 66], the bacteriological spectrum of peritonitis in severely ill patients (APACHE II score, ≥ 15) was studied. Even though these patients were thought to have new-onset acute secondary peritonitis, 38% had monomicrobial infections; the dominant organisms were *Candida* species (isolated from 41% of patients), *Enterococcus* species (31%), *Enterobacter* species (21%) and *Staphylococcus epidermidis* (21%), while *E. coli* and *Bacteroides* species accounted for only 17% and 7%, respectively, of isolates. The authors conclude that antimicrobial selection pressure may have played a role in changing the spectrum of organisms seen. However, one-half of these patients received therapy with antimicrobial agents for ≤ 1 day before surgery. In a study of the micro-organisms isolated from patients in intensive care units who were dying of persistent peritonitis and multiple organ dysfunction syndrome (MODS) [61], a similar spectrum of isolates was found: a reduced frequency of *E. coli* (24% of patients) and *B. fragilis* (12%) and an increased frequency of fungi or yeast (72%), *S. epidermidis* (64%), *Pseudomonas* species (48%), *Enterobacter* species (32%) and *En-*

terococcus species (32%). While both of these studies were limited by a small sample size, they illustrate the need for further study of the bacteriological spectrum of peritonitis in severely ill patients.

Micro-organisms isolated in patients with tertiary peritonitis are difficult to eradicate even by use of appropriate antimicrobial therapy. Although there have been no convincing demonstrations that antimicrobial therapy in these patients improves survival, it is still recommended because treatment may prevent dissemination beyond the peritoneal cavity [21, 61].

3. ANTIMICROBIAL THERAPY

Table 1 summarizes the microbiology and treatment of tertiary peritonitis.

3.1. Antibacterial therapy

It has been considered that antimicrobial therapy is mandatory for the treatment of tertiary peritonitis because host defenses are inadequate to clear the infection [65].

However, Wittmann et al. consider that antimicrobial agents are of no help and that may contribute to the peritoneal superinfection with yeast or other pathogens [76].

Treatment of tertiary peritonitis should be based on culture and susceptibility results. In contrast to secondary peritonitis, the organisms responsible for tertiary peritonitis are frequently known with certainty. When microorganisms are cultured in this setting, it is prudent to have the micro-organisms subjected to comprehensive susceptibility testing. In vitro data, especially antimicrobial susceptibility testing, are predictive of the in vivo response of infecting bacteria to particular antibacterial agents.

On the other hand, the use of anti-infective agents may result in the development of bacterial resistance. This can take the form of initially susceptible isolates becoming resistant during treatment or the appearance of other organisms resistant to the antimicrobial agents used. Individual patients may develop extra-abdominal nosocomial infections with resistant organisms [5]. Treatment with two agents differing in their mechanism of action probably is advisable for re-

Table 1
Microbiology and treatment of tertiary peritonitis

Microbiology	First line[a]	Second line
Enterococci	Ampicillin	Vancomycin
Staphylococci	Cefazolin	Vancomycin
P. aeruginosa	b-lactam + aminoglycoside	Carbapenem
Enterobacter spp	Fourth-generation cephalosporin	Carbapenem
Candida spp	Amphotericin B 0.5-0.7 mg/kg ± flucytosine[b]	Fluconazole 400 mg

a) Depending on the in vitro susceptibility data.
[b] Flucytosine dose is 75-100 mg/kg/d in 2-4 divided doses with dosage adjustments.

sistant organisms. Ideally, the agent or agents chosen would not have demonstrated cross-resistance with the agent or agents that were employed as empiric therapy. Pragmatically, however, the choice of appropriate antimicrobial agents is often severely limited owing to the broad resistance patterns of the offending micro-organisms. Treatment must be individualized, depending on previous culture reports and local antimicrobial susceptibility patterns.

3.1.1. *Enterococcus spp*

The role of *Enterococcus* species in intra-abdominal sepsis has long been controversial; however, the isolation of enterococci is a predictor of treatment failure in complicated intraabdominal infections [9]. In cases of experimental or clinical peritonitis in which enterococci are present, successful therapy has been achieved by use of antimicrobial agents lacking enterococcal activity [52, 2]. However, enterococcal bacteremia with intra-abdominal sepsis has been associated with a poor outcome [26, 19]. Recently, *Enterococcus* have emerged as leading nosocomial pathogens [12]. *Enterococcus* species are important pathogens in tertiary peritonitis when more susceptible organisms have been eradicated by antimicrobial therapy. Along with their increasing incidence, *Enterococcus*, a micro-organism that is intrinsically resistant to multiple antimicrobials, has also adquired resistance to other antimicrobial agents [27, 50, 54, 55, 59, 64] and strains resistant to multiple or all available agents used to treat enterococcal infections have been identified [12, 54, 47]. In addition many strains are usually tolerant. Reported risk factors for serious enterococcal infections include urinary tract instrumentation, malignancy, renal failure, diabetes, burns and major surgery [1, 26,

29, 35, 44, 68]. Prior antimicrobial therapy, especially with cephalosporins or aminoglycosides, has been described as a risk factor for 48%-63% of patients with enterococcal infections [6, 29, 37].

It is not known who would be likely to benefit from early therapy with anti-enterococcal agents. It would be reasonable to use such therapy in patients hospitalized long term, with persistent or recurrent intra-abdominal sepsis and possibly those who are immunodepressed, such as transplant and burn patients [18]. Although these are the patients who seem most likely to develop enterococcal infections, the efficacy of early therapy has not been evaluated. Nathens et al. suggested that enterococcal bacteremia or the recovery of enterococci as the sole micro-organism from a residual or recurrent infection represents an indication for antienterococcal therapy. Since enterococci are essentially opportunistic micro-organisms, they suggest that antienterococcal therapy must be included in the initial management of immunocompromised patients. [51].

In general monotherapy with ampicillin or vancomycin is enough and it is not necessary use it in association with aminoglycosides except in severe infections. In the context of tertiary peritonitis, the use of vancomycin as the empirical first-line agent has been suggested as it also covers methicillin-resistant staphylococci because patient prognosis is poor from the outset and because antimicrobial failure would be expected to be even more detrimental than in secondary peritonitis. However, if enterococci is the only micro-organism isolated and is susceptible to ampicillin, this antimicrobial must be the first choice agent. The need for combinations as therapy for intra-abdominal infections has not been clearly established, however, it has been recommended in life-threatening intra-abdominal sepsis with *Enterococcus* species isolated in pure culture or a predominance of Gram-positive cocci in chains on gram staining of a peritoneal exudate [46].

In these severe infections it is necessary to obtain a bactericidal effect, by associating a cell wall inhibitor (penicillins or glycopeptides) with an inhibitor or the proteic synthesis (aminoglycosides). When aminoglycosides can not be used, high doses of ampicillin (>12 g/d) or a prolonged course of vancomycin therapy may be tried [34, 55]. The more resistant species isolated is *Enterococcus faecium*, however, the species more frequently isolated is *E. faecalis*. High rates of resistance to ampicillin, vancomycin and high level resistance to aminoglycosides (which precludes a synergistic bactericidal effect when associated with a cell wall inhibitor) have been described in different clinical settings. When the isolates are susceptible to ampicillin, this must be considered the drug of choice. Alternatively penicillin G or ureidopenicillins (mezlocillin or piperacillin) can be used. In the case of resistance to penicillins (which implies also resistance to carbapenems), glycopeptides must be used. The combination of amoxicillin plus clavulanic acid is effective in beta-lactamase producing strains, although they are very infrequent. In multiresistant strains it is necessary to know the in vitro susceptibility to other antimicrobials. Rifampin, fosfomycin, chloramphenicol, tetracyclines, sparfloxacin, clinafloxacin and nitrofurantoin have a variable in vitro activity against many isolates. Quinupristin/dalfopristin can be active against some *E. faecium* resistant strains. It may be necessary to use unproven therapies for infections due to multiresistant strains of *Enterococcus* species.

3.1.2. *Staphylococcus epidermidis and other coagulase-negative staphylococci*

The role of coagulase-negative staphylococci in tertiary peritonitis has also been controversial. However, in relatively immunocompromised hosts appropiate antibiotics may improve survival. These microorganisms are frequently multiresistant and there are few therapeutic alternatives. The rate of methicillin resistance among coagulase-negative staphylococci can be very high and usually it is associated with resistance to aminoglycosides, macrolides and fluoroquinolones. In one prevalence study performed in 1996, the rate of methicillin-resistance among coagulase-negative staphylococci was 50,7% [14]. In cases in which coagulase-negative staphylococci are methicicllin-susceptible, cloxacillin or cefazolin is the treatment of choice. In the case of resistance to methicillin it is necessary to know the in vitro susceptibility to other antimicrobials, however, in most cases these isoltaes are multiresistant and vancomycin is the only alternative, since the emergence of coagulase-negative staphylococci with diminished susceptibility to teicoplanin has also been reported [13].

3.1.3. *Pseudomonas aeruginosa*

Since *Pseudomonas aeruginosa* is intrinsically resistant to multiple antimicrobials and also has the ability to easily acquire new mechanisms of resistance, it is necessary to know the in vitro susceptibility to antimicrobials in order to make the appropiate choice for treatment [43, 58].

Aminoglycosides, fluoroquinolones, ticarcillin, piperacillin, piperacillin-tazobactam, cephalosporins like ceftazidime and cefepime, carbapenems like imipenem and Meropenem present, in general, good activity against most strains of *P. aeruginosa*. However, resistance to all these antimicrobials has been described and this is a cause of clinical concern. Superinfection by resistant *P. aeruginosa* has been cited as a cause of antibiotic failure in comparative studies of antimicrobial therapy in intra-abdominal sepsis [33, 77]. In order to overcome resistance, the use of synergistic antibiotic combinations is commonly used. For this approach a combination of an aminoglycoside (e.g. tobramycin) with a b-lactam (e.g. piperacillin, ceftazidime) has been used [31].

3.1.4. Enterobacter spp

As with the micro-organisms mentioned above multiresistant *Enterobacter* spp can be isolated in tertiary peritonitis as a consequence of antibiotic failure. Prior antibiotic therapy selects for multiresistant strains but third-generation cephalosporin use in particular selects for multiresistance among *Enterobacter* spp [15]. Treatment of these isolates must be individualized according to the in vitro susceptibility data. Aminoglycosides, fluoroquinolones, piperacillin, piperacillin-tazobactam, cefepime, imipenem and meropenem are, in general, active against *Enterobacter* with multiresistance to third-generation cephalosporins. No advance for combination therapy, as regards to the emergence of resistance has been demostrated in the case of severe infections due to *Enterobacter* spp [20]. In a study of *Enterobacter cloacae* infections, even with combination therapy with an aminoglycoside and third-generation cephalosporin, resistance to all beta-lactams, except the carbapenems, developed in nearly 50% of all patients investigated [24].

In summary, the spectrum of drugs effective against highly resistant enterobacteriaceae, nonfermenting Gram-negative aerobes and enterococci, leads to the choice of carboxypenicillins or ureidopenicillins with a beta-lactamase inhibitor or carbapenems. The inclusion of an aminoglycoside in the antibiotic regimen may be particularly justifiable when there is a major risk that *P. aeruginosa* or *Enterobacter* species are present at the infection site. The new cephalosporins are inactive against enterococci and might contribute to the emergence of these pathogens during therapy. Methicillin-resistant staphylococci and *E. faecium* appear to be emerging pathogens. The high incidence of these bacteria might justify the use of vancomycin for initial therapy in combination with aminoglycosides in some settings. However, the indiscriminate administration of vancomycin might result in the rapid emergence of vancomycin-resistant enterococci and/or staphylococci. With the exception of imipenem/cilastatin and meropenem, monotherapy is not recommended for severely ill patients [46, 57]. The duration of antimicrobial therapy will depend on the severity of infection, the clinical response and the return of the leukocyte count to normal. A retrospective review of 2,186 patients with intra-abdominal infections (1,419 patients) and other surgical infections confirmed the validity of fever and leukocytosis as markers for persistent or recurrent sepsis [72].

3.1.5. Antifungal therapy

Fungi are increasingly identified from cultures obtained during intra-abdominal infection. This is probably due to an increasing awareness of fungi as important pathogens as well as to an actual increase in infections due to the use of powerful broad-spectrum antibacterial agents and patient populations that are composed of an increasing proportion of immunincompetent patients. When these organisms are isolated later in the course of intra-abdominal infection or as an initial sole isolate, their presence within the abdominal cavity is indicative of relative immunincompetence of the host. Although there has been some degree of controversy about the extent to which fungi are pathogenic, the weight of experimental and clinical evidence strongly suggests an important role of fungi during peritonitis as both independent pathogens and as copathogens during bacterial infection [65].

Candida infection has been increasingly recognized as a cause of death late in the course of intra-abdominal sepsis. It may occur as monomicrobial peritonitis, as part of polymicrobial peritonitis, as an abscess [40] or as disseminated candidiasis [67].

The view of *Candida albicans* as a pathogen has changed from an opportunistic organism that resulted from antibiotic treatment and not requiring specific therapy, to a serious nosocomial pathogen requiring aggressive treatment. Although it is frequently difficult to differentiate colonization from invasive infection, it is now clear that deep mycoses require systemic, antifungal therapy because they are associated with high mortality. Although operative drainage of abscesses and the control of sources of contamination remain the most important interventions in peritonitis, treatment with antijungal agents remains a necessary adjunct. It is now clear that a certain percentage of these critically ill patients will be or become infected with *C. albicans* or other fungi and that they will require specific therapy. The difficulty will come in learning to predict which patients are at significantly high risk to warrant empirical

antifungal treatment. Antimicrobial therapy is the most frequently identified risk factor for candidal infection [3, 42, 70]. Alteration of the normal flora by antimicrobial therapy promotes the adherence of *Candida* to the intestinal mucosa, which creates a favorable environment for colonization and overgrowth [41]. The risk of invasive disease increases with heavy colonization [10]. Translocation of *Candida* across the intact intestinal mucosa has been demonstrated experimentally in animals [73]. Damage to the gut mucosa by local disease with perforation or physiological disruption of the mucosal barrier due to hypotension increases the risk of translocation. Additional risk factors for invasive candidal infection include diabetes, malnutrition, hyperalimentation, T cell defects, neoplasia and multiple abdominal surgeries [25].

When *Candida* is the sole isolate associated with clinical peritonitis, or *Candida* is isolated from cultures of both peritoneal fluid and blood, or candidal invasion is identified on histological examination of tissues, antifungal therapy is essential. Blood cultures are of poor predictive value in identifying patients with invasive disease, as cultures of blood from 50% of patients with documented invasive disease are not positive [56]. In many cases, the need for antifungal therapy is not so clear-cut. The decision to administer potentially toxic therapy requires a careful assessment of the risk factors. When *Candida* is identified as one of the multiple organisms contaminating the peritoneum after perforation of a viscus and its successful repair, antifungal treatment is generally not required [11, 62]. A polymicrobic abscess from which *Candida* is isolated also may not require specific antifungal therapy [62]. When *Candida* is isolated in large numbers in the presence of polymicrobial peritonitis or increasingly heavy growth of *Candida* is demonstrated in serial specimens, specific treatment is advised, particularly when host defenses are impaired [11]. When multiple risk factors exist, empirical antifungal therapy should be considered for the septic patient who is not responding to antibacterial therapy and does not have a drainable abscess. Isolation of *Candida* from the peritoneum of patients with acute pancreatitis also probably warrants specific therapy, as these patients are more likely to have invasive disease than simple contamination [11].

The BSAC (British Society for Antimicrobial Chemotherapy) set up a working party to develop recommendations for management in the absence of controlled trials [7]. These recommendations focus on the role of the microbiology laboratory, management strategies, the respective roles of amphotericin B, flucytosine and fluconazole and long-term maintenance therapy. The indications for initiation of therapy are given special consideration. According to these recommendations therapy is appropriate in those cases with positive cultures for *Candida* from a deep collection or as a heavy growth from a drain with clinical features of sepsis. A combination of peritoneal lavage without resorting to another laparotomy (for which there is little supportive data) and amphotericin B, with or without flucytosine, is appropriate. The first line recommendation for *Candida* peritonitis consists of amphotericin B 0.5-0.7 mg/kg ± flucytosine (75-100 mg/kg/d in 2-4 divided doses with dosage adjustments depending on renal function and/or serum concentrations). As a second line choice, fluconazole 400 mg is recommended.

Delay in the therapy is associated with a mortality rate between 70% and 100% [13, 45, 62, 71]. Inadequate dosing also has been associated with failure of antifungal therapy and death. We recommend a mini-mum 7- to 10-day treatment course of amphotericin B at a dose of 0.3 to 0.5 mg/kg/day once a significant intra-abdominal candidal infection has been identified.

The azoles (fluconazole and itraconazole) are less toxic alternative agents for therapy. Fluconazole is effective in vitro against *Candida* species and in vivo in animal models. Preliminary reports indicate that fluconazole has good clinical efficacy and minimal toxicity [53]. A clinical trial [42] of fluconazole therapy (300 mg daily) in conjunction with daily relaparotomies and lavage for patients with histologically proven invasive candidal peritonitis, reported that fungal peritonitis was controlled in all patients and that no deaths were due to candidal infection; however, 50% of patients died of severe underlying disorders. To our knowledge, controlled trials of fluconazole vs. amphotericin B for the treatment of candidal peritonitis have not yet been reported; however, there is evidence that fluconazole is less effective than amphotericin B in animal models of disseminated disease [10] and failures of treatment with fluconazole for invasive infections due to *Candida albicans* have been reported [22]. In addition, fluconazole's poor activity against *Candida krusei* and *Candida glabrata* is of concern [70, 75]. Fluconazole is more costly than amphotericin B but some of the costs may be offset for patients who may be candidates for oral outpatient therapy, which would allow for earlier discharge from the hospital.

Itraconazole is likely to be at least as effective as fluconazole in the treatment of intra-abdominal fungal infections but clinical data are not yet available.

Although the relative lack of toxicity is appealing, it has not been demonstrated that fluconazole is equivalent in efficacy to amphotericin B for the treatment of intra-abdominal fungal infections and we believe that the high mortality of intra-abdominal sepsis demands the use of the most efficacious agent available. For these reasons, we consider amphotericin B to be the drug of choice in intra-abdominal or systemic candidal infections and reserve the use of fluconazole in intra-abdominal sepsis for those fungi that are demonstrated to be resistant to amphotericin B or for use as long-term oral therapy subsequent to initial treatment with amphotericin B.

The duration of therapy for all forms of deep candidosis is uncertain. A larger total dose and longer duration of amphotericin B therapy are associated with lower mortality [23]. Rarely should therapy be for less than 4 weeks and in very ill patients it should be for longer (e.g. 8-10 weeks). The intensity of dosing can often be moderated after the 2 first 2 weeks of therapy. Maintenance therapy is only indicated occasionally for patients with serious candidal disease who are not immunocompromised. In almost all circumstances this relates to the persistent presence of foreign material infected with *Candida* which cannot be removed. Examples include Port-a-cath devices, vascular grafts, artificial joints and ventriculoperitoneal shunts, etc. In general, it is desirable to remove foreign material as it is extremely difficult to eradicate *Candida* infections without doing so but there are occasionally extenuating clinical circumstances which prohibit this course of action. In these circumstances lifelong therapy with antifungal agents may be appropriate. At present, the only agent appropriate for this use given its low toxicity and oral bioavailability is fluconazole. There are no data avilable as to the dose but 100-200 mg daily is probably appropriate. If the organism involved is re-sistant to fluconazole (*C. krusei* or *C. glabrata*) intermittent amphotericin B, with or without, flucytosine, is one choice; ketoconazole or itraconazole 400 mg/day may be useful depending on susceptibility testing [8]. No choice is ideal because of the requirement for monitoring for toxicity or serum concentrations and, in the case of amphotericin B, problems of cumulative toxicity and those associated with intravenous access including bacteremia. There are insufficient data to support the use of itraconazole for deep *Candida* infections even though it is effective for mucosal candidosis. In circumstances where currently available oral therapy is inadequate, early consideration of experimental therapy is appropriate. Isolates obtained from patients should also be monitored for the development of resistance [8].

In the surgical and intensive care unit, setting limited data suggest that modification of two aspects of care might reduce the incidence of serious candidal infection. Prevention is one important aspect to be considered. The number of antibiotic classes prescribed increases the risk of candidemia [23, 74], thus, reducing antibiotic prescription and more closely targeted therapy would probably have some impact on reducing candidemia and deep candidal infections. It is not known if the duration of antibiotic therapy is important, although this appears likely. In practice, therefore, a judicious approach to antibiotic prescribing in these patients is appropriate. The other factor likely to reduce candida infections is good compliance with infection control practices to reduce hospital staff transmision of *Candida*. Factors associated with earlier diagnosis and improved support and treatment such as CT, PCD, intensive care and appropriate antimicrobial therapy may be responsible for improved outcome [17, 63].

In summary, life threatening *Candida* infections are increased in frequency and importance, mortality remains high and inadequate data exist concerning the most appropriate management strategies, the antifungal agent of choice, the dose of that antifungal agent and the merit or otherwise of combination and/or sequential therapy. More antifungal agents will be marketed in the next decade generating additional uncertainty as to their place in clinical management and more multicenter trial work will be essential to address these questions.

4. CONCLUSIONS

The emergence of resistant strains is a major problem in post-operative peritonitis involving Gram-negative and Gram-positive strains. The ideal therapeutic regimen for these high-risk patients remains to be determined but empirical therapy directed against highly resistant Gram-negative strains and resistant Gram-positive cocci and fungi must be considered.[49]. If one or more micro-organisms isolated at the initial intervention is not susceptible to the antibiotics provided, a change of antimicrobial agents to provide such coverage is indicated, according to the in vitro susceptibility data. However, rarely will a change in antibiotics affect resolution of persistent or recurrent abdominal sepsis. In the case of candidiasis, early antifungal therapy started at the time of reoperation, might be proposed.

REFERENCES

1. Barie PS, Christou NV, Dellinger EP, Rout WR, Stone HH, Waymack JP. Pathogenicity of the enterococcus in surgical infections. Ann Surg 1990; 212: 155-159.

2. Barlett JG, Onderdonk AB, Louie T, Kasper DL. Gorbach SL. A review. Lessons from an animal model of intra-abdominal sepsis. Arch Surg 1978; 113: 853-857.

3. Bayer AS, Bluenkrantz MJ, Montgomerie JZ, Galpin LB. *Candida* peritonitis: Report of 22 cases and review of the English literature. Am J Med 1976; 61: 832-840.

4. Bohnen J, Boulanger M, Meakins JL, et al. Prognosis in generalized peritonitis: Relation to cause and risk factors. Arch Surg 1983; 118: 285-290.

5. Bohnen JMA, Solomkin JS, Dellinger EP, Bjornson HS, Page CP. Guidelines for clinical care: Anti-infective agents for intra-abdominal infection. Arch Surg 1992; 127: 83-89.

6. Boulanger JM, Ford-Jones EL, Matlow AG. Enterococal bacteremia in a paedriatic institution: a four year review. Rev Infect Dis 1991; 13: 847-856.

7. British Society for Antimicrobial Chemotherapy Working Party. Management of deep *Candida* infection in surgical and intensive care unit patients. Int Care Med 1994; 20: 522-528.

8. British Society for Antimicrobial Chemotherapy Working Party on Fungal Infection. Laboratory monitoring of antifungal chemotherapy. Lancet 1991; 357: 1577-1580.

9. Burnett RJ, Haverstock DC, Dellinger EP. Definition of the role of *Enterococcus* in intra-abdomonal infection: analysis of a prospective randomized trial. Surgery 1995; 118: 716-723.

10. Burchard KW. Fungal sepsis. Infect Dis Clin North Am 1992; 6: 677-692.

11. Calandra T, Bille J, Schneider R, Mosimann F, Francioli P. Clinical significance of *Candida* isolated from peritoneum in surgical patients. Lancet 1989; 2: 1437-1440.

12. CDC. Nosocomial enterococci resistant vancomycin United States. 1989-1993. MMWR 1993; 42: 597-599.

13. Cercenado E, García-Leoni ME, Díaz MD, Sánchez-Carrillo C, Catalán P, Bernaldo de Quirós JCL, Bouza E. Emergence of teicoplanin-resistant coagulase-negative staphylococci. J. Clin. Microbiol. 1996; 34: 1765-1768.

14. Cercenado E, Sánchez-Carrillo C, Alcalá L, Bouza E, and Grupo de Trabajo para el estudio de Estafilococos. Situación actual de la resistencia de *Staphylococcus* en España. Cuarto estudio nacional (1996). Rev. Clin. Esp. 1997; 197 (Monográfico 2): 18-24.

15. Chow JW, Fine MJ, Shlaes DM, et al. *Enterobacter* bacteremia: clinical features and emergence of antibiotic resistance during therapy. Ann. Intern. Med 1991; 115: 585-590.

16. Dellinger EP, Wertz MJ, Meakins JL, et al: Surgical infection stratification system for intra-abdominal infection: Multicenter trial. Arch Surg 1985; 120: 21-29.

17. Deveney CW, Lurie K, Deveney KE. Improved treatment of intra-abdominal abscess: A result of improved localization, drainage and patient care not technique. Surg Gynecol Obstet 1991; 123: 1126-1130.

18. Dougherty SH. Antimicrobial culture and susceptibility testing has little value for routine management of secondary bacterial peritonitis. Clin Infect Dis 1997; 25 (Suppl 2):S258-S261.

19. Dougherty SH, Flohr AB, Simmons RL. "Breakthrough" enterococcal septicemia in surgical patients: 19 cases and review of the literature. Arch Surg 1983; 118: 232-238.

20. Drusano GL. Infection in the intensive care unit: beta-lactamase-mdiated resistance among *Enterobacteriaceae* and optimal antimicrobial dosing. Clin. Infect. Dis. 1998; 27 (Suppl 1): S111-S116.

21. Dunn DL. The role of of infection and use of antimicrobial agents during multiple system organ failure. *In* Deitch EA (ed). Multiple organ failure: Pathophysiology and basic concepts of therapy. New York. Thieme Medical Publishers, 1990, p 150.

22. Evans TG, Mayer J, Cohen s, Classen D, carroll K. Fluconazole failure in the treatment of invasive mycoses. J Infect Dis 1991; 164: 1232-1235.

23. Fraser VJ, Jones M, Dunkel J, Storfer S, Medoff G, Dunagan WC. Candidemia in a tertiary care hospital: epidemiology, risk factors, apredictors of mortality. Clin Infect Dis 1992; 15: 414-421.

24. Fussle R, Biscoping J, Behr R, Sziegoleit A. Development of resistance by Enterobacter cloacae during therapy of pulmonary infections in intensive care patients. Clin Invest 1994; 72: 1015-1019.

25. Gaines JD, Remington JS. Disseminated candidiasis in the surgical patient. Surgery 1972; 72: 730-736.

26. Garrison RN, Fry DE, Berberich S, Polk HC. Enterococcal bacteremia: Clinical implications and determinants of death. Ann Surg 1982; 196: 43-47.

27. Gordon S, Swenson JM, Hill, BC et al. Antimicrobial susceptibility patterns of common and unusual species of enterococci causing infections in the United States. J Clin Microbiol 1992; 30: 2373-2378.

28. Greenman RL, Scein RMH, Martin MA, et al. A controlled clinical trial of E5 murine monoclonal IgM antibody to endotoxin in the treatment of Gram-negative sepsis. JAMA 1991; 266: 1097-1102.

29. Gullberg RM, Homman SR, Phair JP. Enterococal bacteremia: anlysis of 75 episodes. Rev Infect Dis 1989; 11: 74-85.

30. Hackford AW, Tally FP, Reinhold RB et al. prospective study comparing imipenem-cilastatin with clindamycin and gentamicin for the treatment of serious surgical infections. Arch Surg 1988; 123: 322-326.

31. Hancock REW. Resistance mechanisms in Pseudomonas aeruginosa and other nonfermentative Gram-negative bacteria. Clin Infec Dis 1998; 27 (Suppl 1): S93-S99.

32. Hau T, Ahrenholz DH, Simmons RL. Secondary bacterial peritonitis. The biological ba-

sis of treatment. Curr Probl Surg 1979; 16: 1-65.

33. Heseltine PNR, Yellin AE, Appleman MD, et al. Perforated and gangrenous appendicitis: An analysis of antibiotic failure. J Infect Dis 1983; 148: 322-329.

34. Herman DJ, Gerding DN. Screening and treatment of infections caused by resistant enterococci. Antimicrob Agents Chemother 1991; 35: 215-219.

35. Hoge CW, Adams J, Buchanan B, Sears SD. Enterococcal bacteremia to treat or not to treat, a repraisal. Rev infect Dis 1991; 13: 600-605.

36. Huizinga WKJ, Baker LW, Kadwa H et al. Management of severe intra-abdominal sepsis: Single agent antibiotic therapy with cefotetan versus combination therapy with ampicillin, gentamicin and metronidazole. Br J Surg 1988; 75: 1134-1138.

37. Huycke MM, Spiegel CA, Gilmore MS. Bacteremia caused by hemolytic high-level gentamicin-resistant Enterococcus faecalis. Antimicrob Agents Chemother 1991; 35: 1626-1634.

38. Inthorn D, Muhlbayer D, Hartl WH. Ticarcillin/clavulanate in the treatment of severe peritonitis. J Antimcrob Chemother 1989: 24 (Suppl B): S141-S146.

39. Jones RC, Thal ER Jonhson NA et al. Evaluation of antibiotic therapy following penetrating abdominal trauma. Ann Surg 1985; 291: 576-585.

40. Keiser P, Keay S. Candidal pancreatic abscess: report of two cases and review. Clin Infect Dis 1992; 14: 884-888.

41. Kennedy MJ, Volz PA. Ecology of Candida albicans gut colonization: inhibition of candida adhesion, colonization and dissemination from the gastrointestinal tract by bacterial antagonism. Infect Inmun 1985; 49: 654-663.

42. Kujath P, Lerch K, DammrichJ. Fluconazole monitoring in Candida peritonitis based on histological control. Mycoses 1990; 33: 441-448.

43. Lagast H, Meunier-Carpentier F, Klastersky J. Treatment of Gram-negative bacilliary septicemia with cefoperazone. Eur J Clin Microbiol 1983; 2: 554-558.

44. Maki DG, Agger WA. Enterococcal bacteremia clinical features, the risk of endocarditis and management. Medicine (Baltimore) 1988; 67: 248-269.

45. Marsh PK, Tally FP, Kellum J, Callow A, Gorbach SL. Candida infection in surgical patients. Am Surg 1983; 198: 42-47.

46. McClean KL, Sheehan GJ, Harding GKM. Intra-abdominal infection: A review. Clin Infec Dis 1994; 19: 100-106.

47. McDonnell RW, Sweeney HM, Cohen S. Conjugational transfer of gentamicin resistance plasmids intra- and interspecifically in Staphylococcus aureus and Staphylococcus epidermidis. Antimicrob Agents Chemother 1983; 23: 151-160.

48. Meakins JL, Solomkin JS, Allo MD, et al. A proposed classification of intra-abdominal infections. Arch Surg 1984; 119: 1372.

49. Montravers P, Gauzit C, Muller JP, Marmuse A, Fichelle A, Desmonts JM. Emergence of antibiotic-resistant bacteria in cases of peritonitis after intra-abdominal surgery affects the efficacy of empirical antimicrobial therapy. Clin Infect Dis 1996; 23: 486-494.

50. Murray BE. New aspects of antimicrobial resistamce and the resulting therapeutic dilemmans. J Infec Dis 1991; 163: 1185-1194.

51. Nathens AB, rotstein OD. Antimicrobial therapy for intra-abdominal infection. Am J Surg 1996; 172(suppl 6A):1S-6S.

52. Nicole LE, Harding GKM, Louie TJ, Thompson MJ, Blanchard RJ. Cefoxitin plus tobramycin and clindamycin plus tobramycin: A prospective randomized comparison in the therapy of mixed aerobic/anaerobic infections. Arch Surg 1986; 121: 891-896.

53. Nolla-Salas J, Leon C, Torres-Rodriguez JM, Martin E, Sitges-Serra A. Treatment of candidemia in critically ill surgical patients with intravenous fluconazole. Clin Infect Dis 1992; 14: 952-954.

54. Patterson JE, Wanger A, Zscheck KK, Zervos MJ, Murray BE. Molecular epidemiology of beta-lactamase-producing enterococci. Antimicrob Agents Chemother 1990; 34: 302-305.

55. Patterson JE, Colodny SM, Zervos MJ. Serious infection due to betalactamase-producing *Streptococcus faecalis* with high level resistance to gentamicin. J Infect Dis 1988; 158: 1144-1145.

56. Perfect JR. Antifungal therapy and its use in surgical treatment. Surg Gynecol Obstet 1990; 171(suppl): 41-48.

57. Pitkin D, Shikh W, Wilson S et al. Comparison of the activity of meropenem with that other agents in the treatment of intraabdominal, obstetric/gynecologic and skin and soft tissue infections. Clin Infect Dis 1995; 20(suppl 2): S372-375.

58. Reyes MP, Brow VJ, Lerner AM. Treatment of patients with *Pseudomonas* endocarditis with high dose aminoglycoside and carbenicillin therapy. Medicine 1978; 57: 57-67.

59. Rhinehart E, Smith NE, Wennerstern C et al. Rapid dissemination of beta-lactamase-producing aminoglycoside-resistant *Enterococcus faecalis* among patients and staff on an infant-toddler surgical ward. N England J Med 1990; 323: 1814-1818.

60. Rotstein OD, Meakins JI. Diagnostic and therapeutic challenges of intra-abdominal infections. World J Surg 1990; 14: 159-166.

61. Rotstein OD, Pruett TL, Simmons RL. Microbiologic features and treatment of persistent peritonitis in patients in the intensice care unit. Can J Surg 1986; 29: 247-250.

62. Rutledge R, mandel SR, Wild RE. *Candida* species insignificant contaminat or pathogenic species. Am Surg 1986; 52: 299-302.

63. Saini S, Kellum JM, O`Leary MP, et al. Improved localization and survival in patients with intra-abdominal abscesses. Am J Surg 1983; 145: 136-142.

64. Sapico FL, Canawati HN, Ginunas VJ et al. Enterococci highly resistant to penicillin and ampicillin: an emerging clinical problem. J Clin Microbiol 1989; 27: 2091-2095.

65. Sawyer MD, Dunn DL. Antimicrobial therapy of intra-abdominal sepsis.Infect Dis Clin North Am 1992; 6: 545-570.

66. Sawyer RG, Rosenlof LK, Adams RB, May AK, Spengler MD, Pruett TL. Perotinitis in the 1990s: Changing pathogens and changing strategies in the critically ill. Am Surg 1992: 58: 82-87.

67. Sawyer RG, Reid B, Adams MD et al. The role of *Candida albicans* in the pathogenesis of experimental fungal/bacterial peritonitis and abscess formation. Am Surg 1995; 61: 726-731.

68. Shales DM, Levy J, Wolinsky E. Enterococcal bacteremia without endocarditis. Arch Inter Med 1981; 141: 578-581.

69. Solomkin JS, Dellinger EP, Christou NV et al. Results of a multicenter trial comparing imepenem/cilastatin to tobramycin/clindamycin for intra-abdominal infections. Ann Surg 1990; 212: 581-591.

70. Solomkin JS, Flohr AB, Quie PG, Simmons RL. The role of *Candida* in intraperitoneal infections. Surgery 1980; 88: 524-530.

71. Solomkin JS, Flohr A, Simmons RL. *Candida* infectons in surgical patients: dose requeriments and toxicity of amphotericin B. Ann Surg 1982; 195: 177-185.

72. Stone HH, Bourneuf AA, Stinson LD. Reliability of criteria for predicting persistent of recurrent sepsis. Arch Surg 1985; 120: 17-20.

73. Stone HH, Kolb LD, Currie CA, Geheber CE, Cuzzell JZ. *Candida* sepsis: pathogenesis and principles of treatment. Ann Surg 1974; 179: 697-711.

74. Wey SB, Mori M, Pfaller MA, Woolson RF, Wenzel RP. Hospital-acquire candidemia. The attributable mortality and excess length of stay. Arch Intern Med 198; 148: 2642-2645.

75. Wingard JR, Merz WG, Rinaldi MG, Jonhson TR, Karp JE, Saral R. Increase in *Candida krusei* infection among patients with bone marrow transplantation and neutropenia treated prophylactically with fluco-nazole. N Engl J Med 1991; 325: 1274-1277.

76. Wittmann DH, Schein M, Condon RE. Managenent of secondary peritonitis. Ann Surg 1996; 224: 10-18.

77. Yellin AE, Heseltine PNR, Berne TV et al. The role of *Pseudomonas* species in patients treated with ampicillin and sulbactam for gangrenous and perforated appendicitis. Surg Gynecol Obstet 1985; 161: 303.

Intra-abdominal Infections Originated in Solid Organs

Eduard H. Farthmann, Rudolf Häring and Ulrich Schöffel

1. INTRODUCTION

Whether infections confined to solid abdominal organs (liver, pancreas, spleen) should be classified as intra-abdominal infections may be debatable. From the anatomical point of view, the parenchyma of those encapsulated organs are lying extraperitonealy. Since, however, those capsules are in close contact to the peritoneal cavity and its peritoneal lining, respective infections might well be classified as intra-abdominal for several reasons. Firstly, the clinical presentation of an abdominal solid organ infection (even if not yet leading to peritonitis) will not differ substantially from other localized intra-abdominal infections, e.g. from an intra-abdominal abscess. Secondly and even more important, the close contact of the infectious focus to the peritoneal surface will in many cases eventually result in localized or even diffuse peritonitis. Thirdly, penetration into the peritoneal cavity of infectious processes of the hepatobiliary or the pancreatic system, or more rarely of the spleen are major causes of secondary (bacterial) peritonitis. Moreover, necrotic areas of these organ systems may well lead to inflammatory reactions of the peritoneum with subsequent bacterial peritonitis if these lesions are becoming secondarily infected by ascending (liver and pancreas) or translocating bacteria from the intestinal tract.

In the following sections, infections of the hepato-biliary system, the pancreas and the spleen will be discussed separately since the clinical presentations as well as the therapeutic consequences show considerable differences.

2. BACTERIAL ABSCESSES OF THE LIVER AND SPLEEN

The liver and the spleen, with their cell mass, represent the main part of the reticuloendothelial system. One of their most important functions is to defeat an infection by clearing the blood stream of micro-organisms and by activating the immune system. On the other hand the structure and function of these organs can be altered by systemic infections through bacteria, viruses, fungi and parasites. This chapter will concentrate on the problems of bacterial infections of the liver and splenic parenchyma leading to bacterial abscesses which require regularly a surgical consultation.

2.1. Bacterial Abscesses of the Liver

2.1.1. Epidemiology

Hepatic abscesses have been recognized since the time of Hippocrates but the understanding of their nature, bacteriology, diagnosis and treatment is an emerging process of this century. Pyogenic hepatic abscesses are a rare but highly lethal condition.

The incidence of hepatic abscesses has been estimated from autopsy and hospital admission data and seems to be relatively constant during this century. Pyogenic liver abscesses occur in 0.29%-1.47% of large autopsy series [13, 48, 49] and are responsible for 0.007%-0.01% of hospital admissions [38, 43, 44, 48] in western countries. The true incidence of this entity is not known [44]. The same group observed a significant increase of the incidence of hepatic abscesses over the two time periods between 1952-1973 and 1973-1993 [24]. In the last period there were 20 cases of pyogenic hepatic abscesses per 100,000 hospital admissions. This increase reflects the development of modern imaging techniques such as ultrasound and CT. Most hepatic abscesses are nowadays diagnosed during hospital admission, the post mortem diagnosis by autopsy having decreased [1, 20, 32].

The male to female ratio is nearly equal with a slight predominance of the male gender and has remained relatively constant over time. Patients with hepatic abscesses are becoming older. The mean age of the patients shifted from the 4th decade at the beginning of this century, to the 5th decade with a peak incidence in the 6th and 7th decade today.

The size of pyogenic liver abscesses varies. In most reports the mean diameter is between 6-7 cm. Hepatic abscesses may be single or multiple. The percentage of multiple abscesses varies in large series between 30% and 70%. The right lobe of the liver is more frequently involved than the left, 60% to 70% of pyogenic abscesses being located in the right lobe, 10% to 15% in the left lobe and 20% to 30% bilaterally [7, 11, 35, 38].

2.1.2. Pathogenesis

The formation of a pyogenic liver abscess requires several conditions to be met. First, the liver parenchyma must be seeded with bacteria from an infectious focus elsewhere in the body. The possible routes of infection are via the biliary tree, via the portal vein, via the systemic circulation through hepatic artery or per continuitatem through infections of adjacent organs of the gastrointestinal tract or of the peritoneal cavity.

In healthy subjects transient bacteremia is usually controlled by the phagocytic capacity of the reticuloendothelial Kupffer cells, if the quantitative amount of these organisms does not exceed their capacity. Secondly, therefore, a compromise of the liver resistance and immune function is usually necessary for the formation of a pyogenic liver abscess. In the immunocompromised patient the bacterial inoculum can overwhelm the Kupffer cells leading to an abscess.

One can differentiate between a local compromise due to intrinsinc liver disease like cirrhosis, primary or secondary liver tumor or damaged liver parenchyma following trauma. The systemic immunocompromised state occurs in patients with systemic malignancy, human immunodefficiency virus infection, transplantion or systemic chemo- or immunosuppressive therapy. Diabetes mellitus is also a frequent underlying disease in patients with pyogenic hepatic abscess, the incidence varying between 8%-40% [8, 24, 35, 38]. Poorly controlled diabetes mellitus is the main condition associated with gas-forming pyogenic liver abscesses. It is hypothesized that an infection with gas-forming pathogens, high local tissue glucose levels for fermentation and an impairment of local tissue perfusion are contributive factors which deteriorate the ability to remove gas [9].

The spectrum of underlying etiology of hepatic abscesses has changed markedly during this century. In the preantibiotic era hepatic infections were mainly attributed to infections within the portal system. In 1938 Ochsner [43] ascribed 34% of all hepatic abscesses to appendicitis.

Today the most dominant etiologic factor for pyogenic liver abscesses are diseases of the biliary system (Table 1). Most abscesses result from ascending cholangitis secondary to acute extrahepatic biliary tract obstruction. They are mostly associated with common duct stones, malignant tumor or, less frequently with benign strictures of the bile ducts. With unrelieved obstruction the increasing pressure within the intrahepatic bile ducts leads to destruction of the hepatic parenchyma and to abscess formation. This results characteristically in multiple, small bilateral pyogenic abscesses [33].

In recent times more aggressive operative or nonoperative approaches to the management of hepatobiliary or pancreatic neoplasms resulted in an increase in pyogenic hepatic abscesses after biliary tract procedures such as hepatic resection, biliary-enteric anastomosis or palliative stenting of the biliary tree. The pathogenesis of hepatic abscesses in this group of patients is very of-ten multifactorial and not simply the result of recurrent obstruction. The clinical presentation in these cases is less dramatic and the abscesses are often solitary [33].

Pylethrombosis or pylephlebitis as a complication of intra-abdominal sepsis are rare instances in the era of antibiotics [16]. But the gastrointestinal tract still remains an important source of the formation of liver abscesses. Chronic inflammatory bowel disease [21, 53], sigmoid diverticulitis or malignant tumors of the gastrointestinal tract are not uncommonly associated with hepatic abscesses. A liver abscess may even be a warning indicator of silent colonic cancer [52]. Furthermore, all abscesses of the peritoneal cavity can lead to a hepatic abscess. However, appendicitis or perityphlitic abscess are nowadays very uncommon causes.

An important pathophysiological mechanism of abscess formation in the liver is the translocation of viable bacteria through the mucosa barrier to the mesenteric lymph nodes, eventually reaching the portal venous blood stream. Most of these abscesses are located in the right lobe of the liver. This phenomenon is attributed to the streaming effect of mesenteric blood flow within the portal vein because the effluent of the superior mesenteric vein preferentially flows to the right lobe of the liver [35]. Today, 20% of hepatic abscesses are secondary to an infection in the drainage area of the portal vein (Table 1).

Another 15% of hepatic abscesses occur in patients with systemic bacteremia from infections such as bacterial endocarditis, pneumonia, osteomyelitis etc. via the arterial blood supply of the liver. Their rate has remained relatively constant during this century. These abscesses are typically multiple and located in both lobes of the liver.

Table 1
Etiology of Pyogenic Liver Abscess

biliary tree	ascending cholangitis following obstruction by stones, tumor, stricture	35%
portal vein	IBD, diverticulitis, appendicitis, peritonitis GI-tract carcinoma	20%
hepatic artery	all infections associated with bacteremia	15%
primary hepatic	trauma tumor, ischemia	5% 5%
direct extension	infections of adjacent organs	5%
cryptogenic	unknown source of infection	15%

Only a small number of hepatic abscesses arise from direct extension of neighboring organs into the liver parenchyma. Examples are empyema of the gallbladder, pancreatic abscess or penetrating peptic ulcer or gastric carcinoma. Also only 5%-10% of hepatic abscesses originate in a primary hepatic lesion such as benign or malignant tumor, ischemic necrosis or traumatic tissue damage. But the incidence will most likely increase with the increasing frequency of palliative ligation of branches of the hepatic artery or chemoembolisation via the hepatic artery in the treatment of primary or secondary malignant lesions in the liver [3, 24, 32].

Cryptogenic abscesses occur in 15%-20% of patients. It is suggested that patients with cryptogenic liver abscesses have an underlying defect in their reticuloendothelial system's ability to clear opsonized particles from the systemic circulation [39]. Others suggested that cryptogenic abscesses may develop from small areas of intrahepatic thromboembolism or infarction that become infected secondarily by anaerobic organisms present in portal blood [29]. The most likely pathogenesis of cryptogenic abscess is multifactorial. The incidence of cryptogenic abscesses depends on the thoroughness of the diagnostic workup [12]. Therefore, whenever the etiology of a hepatic abscess is unknown at the time of therapy, a thorough search for the source of infection must be undertaken as soon as the condition of the patient has improved [42]. In some instances dental disease can be detected as an etiological factor of cryptogenic hepatic abscesses [14].

2.1.3. Clinical Presentation

The clinical signs and symptoms associated with pyogenic hepatic abscesses represent the local or systemic result of infection and are commonly non-specific (Table 2). Fever is the predominant symptom of hepatic abscesses. Its character may be intermittent, remittent or continous but 10%-30% of pa-

Table 2
Signs and Symptoms of Pyogenic Liver Abscess

Symptoms		Signs	
fever	85%	tenderness	54%
chills	45%	hepatomegaly	40%
abdominal pain	60%	jaundice	30%
anorexia/malaise	48%	ascites	5%
nausea	35%	rales, pleural effusion	15%
weight loss	38%	acute abdomen	8%
other	25%	other	15%

tients are afebrile. Nearly half of the patients develop chills and most of them experience abdominal pain. Nausea, vomiting, anorexia, malaise and weight loss are also frequent symptoms of pyogenic liver abscesses, whereas diarrhea, night sweats, pruritus or dyspnea are reported only occasionally.

The physical findings present in patients with pyogenic hepatic abscess are non-specific. The most prominent sign, is local tenderness in the right upper quadrant of the abdomen along with hepatomegaly in nearly 40% of patients. Jaundice is detectable in 20%-30% of patients and is most often associated with biliary tract disease. Thoracic signs like rales, pleural effusions are noted in 10%-18% of cases. Ascites and mental status disturbances are rare and represent an advanced critical illness. Complications of hepatic abscesses due to perforation of the abscess into neighboring structures such as the pleural cavity, the lung parenchyma, the peritoneal cavity, the abdominall wall, the hepatic veins or the pericardium are rare and occur in less than 10% of reported series.

2.1.4. Diagnosis of Liver Abscesses

The results of laboratory investigations in patients with hepatic abscesses reflect the systemic infection and the impairment of hepatic function. Abnormal laboratory data are found in over two thirds of patients. Leukocytosis >10,000 WBC/mm is common and is observed in 80%-90%, often accompanied by anemia [7, 11, 21, 24-25, 35]. The hepatic dysfunction is reflected by elevations of bilirubin, alkaline phosphatase, serum glutamic oxaloacetic transaminase, hypalbuminemia and prolonged prothrombin time. In multiple uni- or multivariate analyses of prognostic factors for pyogenic hepatic abscesses leukocytosis > 20,000 WBC/mm, anemia < 11g/dl, hyperbilirubinemia, hypoalbuminemia and prolonged activated prothrombin time were associated with poor prognosis [11, 8, 30, 40]. These laboratory data could not predict mortality, however, unless they became markedly abnormal [30].

Because of the non-specific symptoms and laboratory constellation, the diagnosis of a pyogenic hepatic abscess can seldom be made on clinical grounds alone. Eventually, the less dramatic and indolent course of the disease over weeks, may draw the attention of the physician away from the liver to a disease process elsewhere. Therefore, the clinician must have a high level of suspicion to establish the diagnosis. Until the 1970`s the diagnostic workup could only be done with chest and plain abdominal roentgenograms or liver scanning. Since then, ultrasound and computed tomographic technology has been improved and is now the most important imaging technique for evaluation of pyogenic liver abscesses.

Indirect signs for pyogenic abscesses in the roentgenogram of the chest are the elevation of the right diaphragm, pleural effusions, right lower lobe atelectasis or infiltration. They occurr in half of the patients, whereas abnormalities on plain abdominal films, such as hepatomegaly or gas within the abscess, are less frequently reported.

The most important progress to avoid delay of diagnosis was made after the introduction of radionuclide scanning techniques in the 1960`s. The antemortem diagnosis of hepatic abscess increased from 19% to 78%. The mortality rate decreased conclusively [1, 29]. The technetium sulfur colloid (^{oo}Tc) or gallium citrate (^{oo}Ga) liver scans are useful in definig location, size and number of liver abscesses. Pyogenic lesions are detected with an accuracy in the range of 70%-95% [35]. A decreased accuracy has been reported for multiple, small lesions < 2cm. The differentiation between malignant or pyogenic lesions is not always possible. Therefore, the specifity of liver scans for pyogenic abscess in one study was only 14% [25].

A further refinement of the diagnosis was reached after the introduction of ultrasound and CT. Moreover, they created the possibility of performing simultaneously guided aspiration or drainage of the abscess cavity. Ultrasound is simple, inexpensive and has a sensitivity in the range between 80% to 94% [6, 7, 25, 50, 51]. It has the disadvantage that multiple small lesions < 2cm, ocu-

rring often as a consequence of ascending cholangitis, are not always detectable. In addition its usefullness can be limited by obesity and the location of the abscesses in the dome of the liver. In these situations CT is superior in detecting pyogenic liver abscesses. Therefore, the sensitivity of CT is in the range of 94%-100% [7, 24, 50, 51]. Both imaging techniques are useful also in the follow-up for assessing the results of therapy.

It is essential for planning the treatment to know the etiology of the abscess. Therefore, endoscopic techniques like gastroscopy, ERCP and colonoscopy are extremely helpful to detect the source of infection. ERC is especially necessary when a biliary origin of the abscess is suspected. This technique allows not only to establish the diagnosis of a biliary obstruction but also gives the opportunity to simultaneously reestablish biliary flow and to decompress the bile ducts by papillotomy or by intubation of the bile ducts with endoprotheses, stents or nasobiliary tubes. If an ERC is impossible because of technical difficulties like partial gastric resection or local tumor growth percutaneous transhepatic cholangiography and drainage (PTC/D) it is a valuable diagnostic alternative to confirm a biliary originated liver abscess and to decompress the biliary tree.

2.1.5. Bacteriology

Virtually all known pathological micro-organisms have been detected in cultures of hepatic abscesses. In recent times anaerobe bacteria and fungi are detected with increasing frequency [7, 24, 32]. Nearly 50% of positive abscess cultures show polymicrobial growth of organisms [7, 21, 38, 50], while 10%-20% of abscess cultures are still

Table 3
Bacteriology of Hepatic Abscesses

Organisms	%
Gram-Positive Aerobes	23.4
Staphylococci	7.1
Streptococci	17.5
Enterococci	10.8
Gram-Negative Aerobes	61.1
Klebsiella	39.9
E.coli	29.9
Pseudomonas	5.9
Proteus	5.8
Others	10.9
Anaerobes	15.5
Bacteroides	10.9
Fusobacterium	3.6
Clostridia	2.0
Others	6.9
Mixed Infections	39.4
Sterile Cultures	15.9

represents 1208 isolates from 798 patients [7, 9, 11, 20-22, 25, 38, 46, 50-51]

sterile. On the other hand, multiple-resistant bacteria and mixed bacterial and fungal infections are more often detected. This reflects the wide use of broad spectrum antibiotics before getting a pus collection for culture, especially in patients with indwelling biliary stents for treatment or prevention of recurrent cholangitis [24].

Most of detected bacteria are enteric organisms (Table 3). The predominant species are Gram negative organisms in 60% of positive cultures, especially Klebsiella and E. coli. Gram positive organisms are detected in nearly 25% of cases with streptococci, enterococci and staphylococci as most common bacteria. Anaerobe infections could be demonstrated in 15%-20% of cases with Bacteroides species as predominant organisms. No clear relationship between the pathogenesis of the abscess and its bacteriology can be drawn from the microbiological data. Also, there exists no correlation between the bacteriology and the extent of hepatic abscesses, whereas fungal abscesses are most often mutiple and small [7, 32].

2.1.6. Treatment

The prognosis of undiagnosed or untreated pyogenic abscesses of the liver is poor and the course nearly always fatal. Until the seventies a combination of open surgical drainage and systemic antibiotic therapy was

Table 4
Therapeutic Modalities

antibiotics alone
closed aspiration + antibiotics
percutaneous drainage + antibiotics
open surgical drainage + antibiotics
liver resection + antibiotics

generally recommended as treatment for pyogenic liver abscess. After the introduction of modern imaging techniques, less invasive procedures became possible, such as CT or ultrasound guided percutaneous aspiration and drainage. As a consequence, many reports have been published in recent times which document the success of these treatment strategies. This led to graded treatment recommendations considering the characteristics of the abscess and the condition of the patients. The feasible treatment modalities for pyogenic hepatic abscesses are listed in table 4.

2.1.6.1. Antibiotic Therapy

Antibiotic therapy is very important and should be started once the diagnosis of a pyogenic abscess of the liver is suspected or has been established. The antibiotic regimen chosen for treatment can be deduced from the knowledge of the common spectrum of organisms most often detected in bacterial abscesses of the liver. As stated earlier, there are three main groups of bacteria, singly or in combination, which have been detected in liver abscesses: (1) Gram negative aerobe enterobacteria (e.g. Klebsiella, E. coli, Pseudomonas), (2) Gram positive aerobes (e.g. Staphylococci, Strepto-

cocci, Enterococci) and (3) anaerobic bacteria (e.g. Bacteroides species, Clostridia). Therefore, until bacteria have been isolated and their sensivity has been established, a broad spectrum antibiotic coverage is necessary. This treatment regimen should consist of a combination of ampicillin, an aminoglycoside and clindamycin or metronidazole or a suitable beta lactam broad spectrum antibiotic with a satisfactory anaerobic spectrum, such as imipenem/cilastatin, Meropenem, piperacillin/Tazobactam, ampicillin/sulbactam or cefoxitin, especially in patients with impaired renal function instead of an aminoglycoside. Independently, aspirates of the abscess for culture should be taken as soon as possible and the therapeutic regimen be adjusted to the culture results with regard to the spectrum of organisms and their sensitivity to antibiotics.

There exists limited experience only of successful antibiotic therapy alone for the treatment of pyogenic liver abscesses [23, 31, 41]. Most series report an unacceptable high mortality rate for antibiotic therapy alone [9, 24, 25, 36, 38, 47]. The reason for failure of antibiotic therapy alone may be that bactericidal concentrations are not achieved within the abscess cavity. Therefore, the attempt of solitary antibiotic therapy may only be undertaken in a careful selected group of patients. For example, patients with diffuse small, multiple pyogenic abscesses of biliary origin, accompanying suppurative cholangitis are candidates for antibiotic therapy alone, provided that a decompression of the biliary tree has been achieved [20, 33, 46]. Children are also candidates for initial conservative treatment of liver abscesses. Moore [41] reported successful non-operative management and healing of pyogenic liver abscesses in 37% of 124 children aged less than 14 years.

On the contrary most of amebic liver abscesses are cured with amebicides without intervention. The first line amebicide is metronidazole. With the presumptive diagnosis of amebic liver abscess, a combination of antibiotics of metronidazole, aminoglycoside and penicillin should be initiated to provide appropriate antibiotic coverage in the case of erroneous diagnosis of amebic liver abscees [16].

Most authors recommend a prolonged course of antibiotic treatment over 6 weeks for pyogenic hepatic abscess [16, 45] but these recommendations are not based on clear clinical or microbiological data. Therefore, the duration of antibiotic therapy should be based on clinical evidence of the resolution of infection, radiological resolution of the abscess and the general condition of the patient [6]. The decision to stop the antibiotic coverage may be undertaken when the patient is afebrile, asymptomatic and without leukocytosis [50].

2.1.6.2. Closed Aspiration and Antibiotics

Sonographically guided needle aspiration of pyogenic hepatic abscesses was first reported by McFadzean [37] in 1953. 14 patients who had pyogenic abscesses could be cured with needle aspiration followed by injection of antibiotics into the abscess cavity. However, this method has not gained widespread popularity. Aspiration is considered to be a method for diagnosing hepatic abscesses and to obtain pus collections for culture [23, 27]. There are numerous reports of acceptable treatment results of closed aspiration [2, 4, 15, 19, 50]. The largest experience was reported by an Italian group [19]. They performed an average of 2,2 needle aspirations per pyogenic liver abscess in 115 patients. After ultrasonic guided puncture of the hepatic lesions with needles of varying calibers (16-22 gauge), the abscess cavity was evacuated, followed by lavage with saline solution and instillation of antibiotics, followed by systemic antibiotic therapy. With this technique a resolution of symptoms and hepatic lesions was achieved without mortality in 98% of patients with pyogenic hepatic abscess. These results could be confirmed by others with success rates between 79%-96% and acceptable mortality rates below 10% [2, 4, 15, 50]. The advantages of this method compared to percutaneous or open surgical drainage are less discomfort for the patients, simpler patient care and low costs [19]. But whether the combination of percutaneous aspiration and systemic antibiotical treatment without drainage is an appropriate therapy, remains a controversial issue [24].

In other reports percutaneous aspiration and systemic antibiotic therapy were associated with low success rates between 10% to 70%, high recurrence rates and a mortality above 10% [10, 34, 47]. Controlled trials of closed aspiration versus percutaneous drainage are locking. The criteria for percutaneous aspiration are not well defined, therefore, the decision to drain or aspirate the abscess is in most cases made empirically by the treating physician [50]. Dondelinger [15] proposed that patients in the younger age group, less than 40 years old, who are not debilitated, not critically ill and who are without evident causal disease, can undergo closed aspiration in combination with antibiotic therapy. In summary, closed aspiration may be applicable to carefully selected patients with the philosophy behing to have a low threshold to perform a drainage procedure if signs of infection persist or the condition of the patient deteriorates [24].

2.1.6.3. Percutaneous Drainage

With the advent of modern imaging techniques of the liver, more refined methods to assess the location, size and number of pyogenic hepatic abscesses have become possible. Since then, many reports of successful percutaneous treatment of hepatic abscesses have been published. The literature reviews of this era state a success rate of 78% to 85%, associated with a mortality rate between 3% to 6% [15, 18, 54].

As a consequence US or CT-guided percutaneous drainage of liver abscesses has gained wide acceptance. In most current series these positive results could be confirmed [5, 10, 11, 17, 22, 24, 28, 46, 50, 51]. Successful percutaneous treatment was achieved in 90% of solitary hepatic abscesses and in 73% of multiple abscesses [15]. Percutaneous drainage has also proven to be effective in patients with hepatic abscesses of biliary origin and persistent communication of the biliary tree with the abscess cavity, on the condition that the biliary obstruction could be managed [28].

Therefore, if no contraindications are present, percutaneous drainage is nowadays the initial standard procedure in the treatment of pyogenic liver abscess. Contraindications or absence of a safe route of drainage, ascites, multiple small hepatic abscesses, abscess perforation, and underlying disease which require surgical treatment. But primary percutaneous drainage may be beneficial because of a temporizing effect for stabilization of a critically ill patient. After that, elective surgery for the underlying disease has been shown to be possible without mortality or significant morbidity [42].

The technique of percutaneous drainage involves exact localisation of the abscesses by ultrasound or CT and planning the drainage route to avoid injury to the bowel, gallbladder or pleura. It is advantegous to choose a route for the catheter passing through a wide bridge of liver parenchyma to avoid the risk of peritoneal spillage of infected material.

A skin incision is made under local anesthesia and a sleeve needle is inserted. After aspiration of pus, a guide wire is placed in the abscess cavity and over the guide wire the access is dilated. Hereafter, a pigtail catheter of appropriate diameter is introduced over the guide wire. The caliber of the drainage must be adapted to the viscosity of the drained fluid. For most pyogenic abscesses Ch. 8-14 catheters are adequate [18].

Percutaneous drainage of abscesses following infected hematomas or tumor necrosis is not easily feasable because these lesions often contain particulate matter. Therefore, abscesses that contain debris frequently require open surgical drainage [38, 42].

After correct placing of one or multiple drainage catheters, when there exist more than one abscess, irrigation or lavage are not generally required. Moreover, such a maneuver can lead to extrahepatic spillage of infected material. That is why contrast sonograms should not be performed before complete drainage of the abscess cavity has been obtained. The drainage catheter should be rinsed through, regularly to prevent obstruction [15]. The instillation of antibiotics into the abscess cavity is not recommended.

Possible complications of percutaneous drainage, comprise hemorrhage, injury to the bowel, gallbladder or bile ducts, intraperitoneal or intrapleural spillage of purulent material and dislodgement of catheters. Clinically significant complications are rare but the hospital stay of patients is often prolonged because critically ill patients are selected for percutaneous drainage [5, 15].

Efficient percutaneous drainage usually leads to rapid improvement of the patient`s general condition. When there is no clinical change 48-72 hours after introducing a percutaneous drainage catheter or the condition of the patient deterioriates, failure of percutaneous drainage must be considered and radiological reassessment is necessary. The potential causes for failure of percutaneous drainage are listed in table 5. One can differentiate between failure because of techniqual reasons, abscess characteristics or the condition of the patient and the underlying disease. When failure is proven, a new attempt may be useful by repeated percutaneous drainage, especially if there is dislodgement of the catheter, the choosen caliber of the catheter is to small or there are more hepatic abscesses. In most cases of failure, however, open surgical drainage is required.

The decision to stop percutaneous drainage may be made when secretion is reduced,

Table 5
Causes for Failure of Percutaneous Drainage

Technical Reasons	hemorrhage iatrogenic injury of adjacent organs peritoneal or pleural contamination insufficient calibre of the catheter catheter dislodgement premature catheter removal
Abscess Characteristics	viscous fluid, sequestration multiloculated abscesses multiple abscesses biliary fistula unrecognised abscess
Condition of the Patient	persistent source of sepsis immunocompromised patient multiple organ failure
	debilitated patient (post-operative, cirrhosis, diabetes, malnutrition, progressive cancer)

culture results of drainage contents are sterile, the abscess cavity is collapsed and there are no more signs of infection.

2.1.6.4. Operative Treatment

Under the impression of the high mortality of pyogenic hepatic abscesses, Ochsner and associates [43] formulated the principles of surgical drainage in 1938. They stated: "only that type of drainage which completely avoids the slightest possibility of contamination of a virgin pleural or peritoneal surface should be employed. This surgical principle is an absolute desideratum". Therefore, extraserous drainage of hepatic abscesses was regarded as standard in the treatment of liver abscesses in former times.

The exact route for an extra- or retroperitoneal access depends on the location of the abscess. Anterior abscesses can be reached through a subcostal incision, whereas for posteriorly located abscesses in the right lobe of the liver, a posterior retroperitoneal incision through the bed of the 12th rib is suitable. Abscesses located high on the dome of the liver can be managed by a trans-

pleural, transdiaphragmatic access. Abscesses best suitable for an extraserous surgical drainage are those with dense local adhesions between the abscess wall and peritoneum. Disadvantages of the extraserous approach are the limited exposure. Particularly multiple or small abscesses may be overlooked and are not amenable to this approach. The detection and, or therapy of an intra-abdominal source of infection is also impossible by extraserous drainage.

For these reasons and because of the relative safety of the transperitoneal approach with appropriate antibiotic coverage and peritoneal lavage, open transperitoneal surgical drainage is nowadays favoured. Despite the establishment of percutaneous drainage techniques there are still clear indications for initial or secondary open surgical drainage (Table 6). In most cases there exists an underlying disease or intra-abdominal source of infection which requires surgery or percutaneous drainage has failed to improve or cure the patient. Complications of the abscess, like rupture into the peritoneal cavity or complications of primary percutaneous drainage are rare indications for open surgical drainage. Also

Table 6
Indications for Surgical Treatment

underlying disease requires surgery
failed percutaneous drainage
complications of the abscess (rupture)
complications of percutaneous drainage
percutaneous drainage technically impossible
suspected malignancy
destruction of liver parenchyma

seldom is an abscess not technically amenable for percutaneous drainage because of its location. The need to rule out malignancy or severe destruction of liver parenchyma may occasionally be an indication for surgery.

Open surgical drainage is effective in the treatment of pyogenic liver abscesses, with reported success rates between 75 to 100 per cent [5, 10, 11, 20, 22, 24, 25, 47, 51] and mortality rates between 0 to 19 per cent [7, 10, 11, 20, 22, 25, 51]. There are no randomized controlled studies, comparing the treatment results of open surgery with percutaneous drainage. Also not permissible for favouring one of both treatment modalities, is the comparison of the hitherto presented cure and mortality rates because of the variability of patient populations. Therefore, percutaneous and surgical drainage are not considered competitive but rather complementary procedures. The relative merits of each must be weighed for the individual patient and the selection of one or both treatment techniques should be based on a careful assessment of each patient [17, 24].

Partial liver resection is the exception in the treatment of pyogenic hepatic abscesses.

Indications for a segmental resection or lobectomy are suspected or proven malignancy, the destruction of liver parenchyma, multiple abscesses confined to segments or one lobe of the liver which does not resolve after conservative treatment and thick-walled non-collapsing abscesses after failure of percutaneous or surgical drainage. In these situations hepatic resection is successful with low mortality, provided that the condition of the patient is stable and the amount of normal liver parenchyma is sufficient [10, 25, 26, 48].

2.1.7. Prognosis

77% of patients in the series Ochsner [43] collected in 1938 died. This figure did not change significantly even after introduction of antibiotics. The first step in improving the prognosis of pyogenic hepatic abscesses was the advent of radionuclide scanning techniques because the rate of postmortem diagnoses significantly decreased [1, 29]. However, in the collected series of pyogenic liver abscesses for the time period between 1950 to 1980 the mortality rate of the patients was still 46% [35]. Only after further improvements in the imaging techni-

Table 7
Risk Factors for Mortality in Patients with Hepatic Abscesses
(Multivariate Analysis)

Malignancy	Leukocytosis > 14,000-20,000
Age > 60 years	Anemia
high APACHE II score	elevated Bilirubin
Sepsis	low Albumin
Pleural effusions	elevated Serum Creatinine

(adapted from 8, 30, 40)

ques, could better treatment results be achieved. Nowadays, some series report mortality rates below 10% [15, 17, 19, 50]. In most recent series the mortality ranges between 10 to 20 per cent [7, 10, 11, 16, 22, 25, 47, 51]. The reasons for this continued high mortality include the failure to establish the diagnosis, overseen multiple small abscesses, failure of percutaneous or surgical drainage, failure to control the source of sepsis or the presence of immunosuppression, immunodeficiency or progressive cancer.

To define the patients at risk for a fatal outcome, several studies investigated potential risk factors using univariate or multivariate logistic regression analysis [8, 11, 30, 40, 44]. The risk factors identified included old age, female gender, multiple abscesses, polymicrobial culture results, complications of abscess, gas forming abscesses, concomitant malignancies, high APACHE II scores and a battery of laboratory disturbances, such as leukocytosis, low hemoglobin levels, high concentrations of serum urea nitrogen, serum creatinine and serum bilirubin, elevated activated partial thromboplastin time and low levels of serum albumin. The factors listed in table 7 were all in one or more of these studies associated with poor outcome after multivariate regression analysis. In general they reflect the systemic effects of hepatic abscesses with sepsis and multiple organ failure and not local extension of the disease. Therefore, the prognosis of hepatic abscesses depends mainly on the time between the start of disease and the introduction of an appropriate treatment regimen and on concomitant diseases. The treatment modality, whether aspiration, percutaneous drainage or surgical drainage, when initiated in time, is of lesser importance for outcome.

2.2. Pyogenic Splenic Abscesses

2.2.1. Epidemiology and Pathogenesis

Splenic abscess is a rare clinical condition with a reported incidence of 0.14% to 0.70% in autopsy series [58,71]. The true incidence is not known most as of the reported cases in the literature are simply case reports. Therefore, it is difficult to draw clear statistical conclusions but it seems that the incidence of splenic abscess cases is rising [59].

Most splenic abscesses occur in conjunction with systemic infections. The spleen serves as an efficient filter of blood borne organisms because of its microarchitecture and blood supply. Nevertheless a splenic abscess remains an infrequent finding. This is due to the phagocytic activity and immune competence of the spleen, which resist the development of local infections. Therefore, a compromise of the blood supply, destruction of the architecture of the splenic parenchyma or a suppressed immune function is needed for establishing an abscess.

The patients at risk for development of splenic abscesses can be classified into four groups according to the pathogenesis of splenic infection [59,65] (Table 8). The first group includes those patients with a pyogenic focus elsewhere in the body and apparently normal spleens. The splenic suppuration arises following primary hematogenous seeding. The septic focus reported most frequently is bacterial endocarditis [68]. Additional related conditions include diabetes mellitus, alcoholism, drug abuse or an immunocompromised state following disease or treatment of disease with steroid or chemotherapeutic agents [61,63,66,73]. The second group comprises patients with a variety of hematological disorders like hemo-

Table 8
Groups at Risk for the Development of Splenic Abscess

I	systemic infection, immunocompromised patient, normal spleen
II	systemic infection, hematologic disease, splenomegaly
III	splenic trauma, damaged splenic tissue
IV	direct, contiguous extension of local infection

globinopathies and hematological malignancy associated with an enlargement of the spleen. In these patients repeated splenic infarcts are common [59,65,77]. The infarcted areas provide ideal foci in which bacteria following bacteremia may deposite and proliferate [74]. Splenic abscesses have also been described after therapeutic embolization of the splenic artery [79]. Nearly two thirds of patients with splenic abscess may be classified into one or both these groups [55,73,80]. Splenic abcesses are reported in an increasing frequency, especially in children and most of then are associated with hematologic disease, mainly leukemia [69].

10% to 15% of patients belong to the third group of splenic abscesses following blunt splenic trauma, managed nonoperatively or by splenorrhaphy [76,78,80,85]. The fourth category in the pathogenesis of splenic suppuration is that of local spread of infection arising from direct, contiguous extension of an infectious complication, usually originated in the colon, kidney, pancreas or stomach. It is the least common cause of splenic abscess in nearly 10% of cases [77,83].

Most splenic abscesses are solitary but multiple abscesses occur in 40% of cases and are more common in immunosuppressed patients, whereas the great majority of patients with endocarditis develop solitary splenic abscesses [73].

2.2.2. *Clinical Presentation*

The most predominant symptom of patients with splenic abscess is fever in 90% of cases along with other symptoms of systemic infection like chills or malaise. Two thirds of patients experience abdominal pain in the left upper abdominal quadrant radiating to the left shoulder or show left abdominal tenderness. An enlarged palpable spleen exists in one third of patients. Left chest signs, like rales and pleural effusion may also be present [59,65,73]. In summary the possibility of a splenic abscess should be considered in patients presenting the triad of fever, sepsis and left upper abdominal pain [77].

2.2.3. *Diagnosis of Splenic Abscesses*

Optimal results and low mortality in the management of splenic abscesses depend on prompt diagnosis. Plain abdominal and chest roentgenograms are non-specific for splenic abscesses but abnormal findings on roentgenograms of the chest, such as elevated left hemidiaphragm, left pleural effusion and left basilar pulmonary infiltrates, are noted in more than 80% of patients [59,73].

In earlier times the most useful diagnostic tests were technetium-99m liver and spleen scan or gallium scanning with a sensitivity of 70% to 75% [72,73]. These radiological techniques have been replaced by ultrasonography and computed tomography. Ultrasound is slightly less effective in the diagnosis of splenic abscess than are CT scans, especially in patients with multiple small abscesses [65,73]. The best diagnostic technique is CT scan with a high sensitivity and specifity of more than 90%. The lesion usually presents as an irregular low density area with or without rim enhancement and sometimes intrasplenic gas formation. Additionaly, CT scans give better anatomical information about the perisplenic area and contiguous organs [65,73,83-84]. Computed tomography and ultrasound facilitated the diagnosis of splenic abscesses and allowed an earlier effective treatment, reducing the mortality of splenic abscesses [57,61].

2.2.4. Bacteriology

The recovered organisms cultured from splenic abscesses are predominantly Gram positive or negative aerobes (60%-70%) and more often various species of staphylococci, streptococci, E.coli and Salmonella [55,65,73]. Anaerobe infections were detected in 12% to 18% of cases but in 10% to 20% the cultures are sterile. This is due to ineffective culture techniques, especially for anaerobe organisms or the effect of previously started antibiotic treatment.

In recent times fungal infections are detected with increasing frequency, with Candida species as the most often cultured organism [67,73]. In general, the organisms growing from abscess culture depend on the source of infection and the underlying disease. For example, nearly all splenic abscesses in drug addicts are caused by staphylococcus aureus [63], whereas immunosuppressed patients are more likely to have fungal infections, mixed infections and multilocular abscesses [66,73].

2.2.5. Treatment

Splenic abscess is nearly always fatal when undiagnosed [74,80]. The reported mortality rates of splenic abscesses in earlier series is given between 40% to 100% [64,72,80]. This high mortality rate associated with splenic abscesses has been attributed to the delay of clinical diagnosis and surgical treatment. In nearly 40% of patients in these reports, the diagnosis was established by autopsy. The patients died because of persistent sepsis with multiple organ failure or complications such as rupture of the abscess into the peritoneal cavity and the consequences of peritonitis.

Therefore, early diagnosis is the key to reduce mortality. This was achieved after introduction of modern imaging techniques like CT scan and ultrasonography. After the diagnosis of a splenic abscess has been established a combination of broad-spectrum antibiotics and splenectomy remains the treatment of choice [18]. With this regimen the mortality rates were reduced below 10% [55,59,73,77,81]. Nowadays, the mortality of patients with splenic abscess depends on factors such as underlying disease, duration of infection and concomitant diseases.

In recent times conservative treatment strategies of splenic preservation have gained importance because of the awareness of the short and long-term risks of splenectomy, i.e. overwhelming postsplenectomy infection (OPSI), especially in children below 4 years or in patients with immunodeficiency and cancers [60,70]. Treatment modalities, therefore, comprise antibiotic or antifungal therapy alone, CT- or ultrasound guided percutaneous drainage or partial splenectomy [56].

Patients cured with antibiotic therapy alone are the exception. This approach may be justified in cases of multiple small splenic abscesses in otherwise healthy children, on condition that careful clinical and ultrasound observation of these patients is guaranteed to detect deterioriation of the patient early [62]. This is also true for immunocompromised patients with disseminated fungal infections and multiple small splenic abscesses. In these cases an attempt with broad spectrum antibiotics and systemic antifungal therapy may be undertaken [67,73] but the criteria for this approach are not clearly defined. Therefore, early splenectomy is recommended if the condition of the patients fails to respond to conservative treatment [66,81].

There are numerous reports in the literature of percutaneous drainage of splenic abscesses. This approach is recommended in selected groups of patients. Candidates for CT-guided percutaneous drainage are patients who carry a high risk of splenectomy because of age, previous operations or underlying disease. The abscess best qualified for percutaneous drainage is unilocular with a discrete wall and thin fluid contents without septation [61,65]. If these criteria are met more than 90% of abscesses can be cured by percutaneous drainage and systemic antibiotic treatment without significant mortality or morbidity [57,65]. The overall success rate of percutaneous drainage is given as 75% if complex or multilocular abscesses are included [73,75,84]. If percutaneous drainage fails in curing the abscess, percutaneous drainage may hve a beneficial temporizing effect because the patient at risk is more stable and better capable of withstanding surgical treatment [82].

Possible complications of percutaneous abscess drainage include hemorrhage, injury of contiguous organs, intra-abdominal or intra-pleural leakage of purulent material or the dislodgement of the catheter but they are unusual [65]. Relative contraindications for percutaneous drainage, therefore, are small, multiple abscesses, septated abscesses, the presence of abdominal conditions in contiguous organs requiring surgery, a bleeding diathesis, the presence of ascites or splenic abscesses that would not be accessible percutaneously without crossing the pleural cavity [61,65]. An absolute contraindication for percutaneous drainage is the rupture of the abscess into the free peritoneal cavity. In these cases and when percutaneous has drainage failed, early splenectomy is warranted. Most patients can be cured nowadays with this stepwise treatment approach.

3. ACUTE CHOLECYSTITIS AND CHOLANGITIS

3.1. Pathogenesis of Acute Cholecystitis

In 85 to 95 per cent of patients acute cholecystitis follows obstruction of the cystic duct by gallstones. The consequences of obstruction are chemical damage of the gallbladder mucosa and compromised capillary blood flow within the gallbladder wall. The chemical inflammation is caused by the concentrated bile acids and the breakdown of cell membrane phospholipids by the action of phospholipase A, which is released from damaged mucosal epithelium [165]. When gallstones are present, the gallbladder mucosa reacts with increased secretion of fluid and mucus, mediated by prostaglandins and leukotrienes. In the case of obstruction this continued secretion leads to an increased intraluminal pressure and dilatation of the gallbladder wall [94]. When the intraluminal pressure exceeds capillary blood flow, gangrene of the gallbladder wall will ensue [86].

The bile of gallbladder and bile ducts is usually sterile [93]. Bacteria are not important for the formation of gallstones. The exception are brown pigmented gall stones. They are the result of bile duct stasis and chronic anaerobic infection of the bile with associated hydrolysis of biliary lipids and bilirubin conjugates, which results in the precipitation of several insoluble organic calcium salts [91]. Therefore, acute cholecystitis is primary a sterile inflammation, followed secondarily by invasion of bacteria and bacterial overgrowth.

Patients at risk for acute cholecystitis are those at risk for the development of gallstones (Table 9). Most patients who harbour gallstones are asymptomatic. Two thirds of these patients will remain asymptomatic lifelong, whereas only 2% will develop mild symptoms of stones per year [99,106]. In symptomatic patients there is a risk for the development of acute cholecystitis of 10% over 10 years, corresponding to an annual rate of 1% [99,106,142].

In 5 to 15 per cent of patients with acute cholecystitis no stones are detectable. Acalculous cholecystitis is usually a serious complication of major surgery and critical illness and is observed with increasing frequency [88,110,162]. Acalculous cholecystitis was observed after emergency surgery for ruptured abdominal aortic aneurysms [163] or complicated open heart surgery [164]. It occurs also after major trauma and severe burns [101,103,141]. But the development of acute acalculous cholecystitis is not limited to injured or postoperative patients. It may also result from abdominal vasculitis, hypotension, use of vasoactive substances, application of antibiotics, hepatic artery embolisation or follows bone marrow transplantation [117,151,161,168-169]. Acalculous cholecystitis may be the result of primary or secondary infection of the gallbladder with bacteria or fungi following systemic infections, such as typhoid fever, gastrointestinal infections, urinary tract infections, or pneumonia [98,112,119]. Acute acalculous cholecystitis is a known manifestation of the acquired immune deficiency syndrome (AIDS), caused by infections with cytomegalovirus and cryptosporidia [120,179]. It is the most common indication for celiotomy in patients with AIDS [126]. Acute acalculous cholecystitis may also follow obstruction of the cystic duct due to a compression by metastasis of solid tumors or lymphomas in the porta hepatis.

Compared with calculous cholecystitis, there is most likely no difference in the pathogenesis of acute acalculous cholecystitis. The most important conditions to be met are bile stasis and ischemia. But there are seve-

Table 9
Risk Factors for the Formation of Gallstones

Female gender	Obesity	Crohn`s disease
Pregnancy	Diet	Intestinal bypass surgery
Age over 40 years	Hemolytic anemia	Genetic factors

Table 10
Different Features in Acute and Emphysematous Cholecystitis

Feature	Acute	Emphysematous
Male gender	30%	70%
Diabetes	10%	30%
Acalculous	10%	30%
Chlostridia	<5%	50%
Perforation	4%	20%
Mortality	4%	15%

adapted from Mentzer

ral interrelated risk factors in critically ill patients. Bile stasis may result from postoperative fasting condition and total parenteral nutrition [115,154,159]. Motility disorders of the gastrointestinal tract, medications, e.g. opioid analgesics, catecholamines and mechanical ventilation with positive end-expiratory pressure (PEEP), may lead to bile stasis [103,113,154]. The other important factor in the pathogenesis is ischemia of the gallbladder. This may be caused by clinical low flow states following hypovolemic or cardiac shock, cardiac insufficiency, visceral ischemia or multiple organ failure [88,161,163,170]. Warren [177] demonstrated that gallbladders with calculous cholecystitis were associated with arterial dilatation and extensive venous filling, whereas those with acalculous cholecystitis showed multiple arterial occlusions and minimal to absent venous filling.

The course of acute cholecystitis may be edematous, gangrenous, empyematous or emphysematous. If complicated by perforation it leads to pericholecystic abscess, generalised peritonitis or formation of a cholecysto-enteric fistula. Perforation is found in 2% of patients undergoing chole-

cystectomy and 10% of patients treated conservatively [153]. The mortality of acute, complicated cholecystitis in elderly, immunocompromised or diabetic patients varies between 15% to 50% [100,165].

Emphysematous cholecystitis is an uncommon variant of acute cholecystitis. It is characterised by the demonstration of gas on plain film radiogram, ultrasound or CT scan in the lumen or wall of the gallbladder or the biliary ducts. Emphysematous cholecystitis is caused by gas-forming bacteria, such as anaerobe Chlostridia, Gram negative E.coli or Klebsiella. Diabetes mellitus is a common underlying disease. The course of emphysematous cholecystitis is, however more dramatic. Perforation of the gallbladder occurs in 20% of cases, associated with a mortality of 15% [145]. The different features of normal acute cholecystitis and emphysematous cholecystitis are summarised in Table 10.

3.2. Pathogenesis of Acute Cholangitis

The main pathophysiological mechanism for the development of acute cholangitis is

Table 11
Etiology of Acute Cholangitis

Choledocholithiasis	Chronic pancreatitis
Benign biliary stricture	Mirizzi-syndrome
Malignant biliary tree obstruction	Choledochal cysts, Caroli`s disease
Stricture of biliary-enteric anastomosis	Duodenal diverticulum

obstruction of the common bile duct due to a variety of diseases (Table 11), followed by secondary bacterial overgrowth. In earlier times the most common causes of acute cholangitis were choledocholithiasis and benign strictures of the biliary tree [90,107]. In recent times, the causes for acute cholangitis shifted toward malignant strictures [133]. This reflect the increasing use of long-term biliary stents or endoprotheses in the treatment of malignant biliary obstruction.

In healthy people bacterial overgrowth is prevented by mechanical and immunological defense mechanisms within the biliary tract. They comprise the competent sphincter of Oddi, undisturbed bile flow to the lumen of the gut, the composition of biliary mucus and bile salts, the tight junctions between hepatocytes, the function of the RES, especially the Kupffer cells and immunoglobulines secreted in the biliary mucous [130,172].

Bacterial overgrowth in acute cholangitis may develop by ascending bacteria from the duodenum via the papilla, by hematogenous seeding or as a consequence of bacterial translocation across the intestinal mucosal barrier to mesenteric lymph nodes, reaching the bile via portal venous blood [125]. In the case of obstruction a circulus vitiosus is started. As a consequence of obstruction bile flow, secretion of bile salts, bi-

le mucous and immunoglobulines are reduced or inhibited. This leads to an imbalance of the bacterial flora in the gut with overgrowth of Gram negative bacteria. The result is increased translocation of bacteria and endotoxin. The endotoxinemia increases again the permeability of the mucosa barrier and additionally the function of the RES and phagocytic Kupffer cells is impaired [97,121].

The spincter of Oddi may also be disrupted by stents or papillotomy. Continued obstruction results in increasing intraductal pressure, which exceeds the secretory pressure of the liver. Tight junctions between hepatocytes are disrupted and cholangiovenous or cholangiolymphatic reflux of infected bile arises [95,138,171]. The consequence may be bacteremia or endotoxinemia resulting in generalised sepsis and multiple organ failure or hepatic abscesses.

Acute cholangitis or cholecystitis may also be caused by percutaneous or endoscopic manipulations of the biliary tree for diagnostic or therapeutic reasons by introducing the bacteria from the outside [87,132,148].

3.3. Clinical Presentation

The most prominent clinical presentation of acute cholecystitis is abdominal pain located in the right upper quadrant of the abdomen or near the epigastrium with radiation to the right shoulder, when the peritoneum becomes inflamed. The pain character is not colicky and with ongoing inflammation of increasing intensity, usually associated with nausea and vomiting. Two thirds of patients have previous symptoms referable to the biliary tract in their anamnesis [165]. The onset of pain occurs typically after ingestion of a fatty meal. Fever is generally low with high temperatures indicating a complication of acute cholecyystitis.

The clinical examination shows muscular guarding and tenderness in the right upper quadrant of the abdomen. Point tenderness over the gallbladder that leads to inspiratory arrest during deep inhalation, is a positive Murphy`s sign. In approximately 20 percent of cases a palpable mass in the right upper abdomen is present, whereas a rigid abdomen suggests a complication of cholecystitis, such as gangrene or perforation.

The laboratory evaluation in acute cholecystitis usually demonstrates slight elevations of white blood cell counts (up to 15,000/mm°) and mildly elevated bilirubin, alkaline phosphatase and transaminase concentrations. Bilirubin levels over 4 mg/dl suggest associated choledocholithiasis and a rapid rise in bilirubin of more than 5 to 6 mg/dl in a day is suspicious for perforation of the gallbladder [165,170].

The classical symptoms of acute cholangitis are right upper quadrant abdominal pain, jaundice and fever (Charcot`s triad). However, only 50 to 70 per cent present with all of these symptoms [90,107,133]. Over 90 percent of patients have fever (> 38°C), while nearly 70 per cent have jaundice. Pain is reported less frequently in 42 percent of patients, whereas in former times jaundice and abdominal pain were the predominant

symptoms. This change has been attributed to the shift of etiology of acute cholangitis with increasing incidence of patients with malignant obstruction and indwelling stents [48]. The most severe form of acute cholangitis, so called acute suppurative septic, or toxic cholangitis with fever, jaundice, abdominal pain and additional mental disturbancy or lethargy and shock is presented by 5 to 15 percent of patients [90,107,133, 158].

Most patients with acute cholangitis show a combination of leukocytosis, hyperbilirubinemia and elevations of alkaline phosphatase, AST and ALT by labarotory evaluation. The hyperbilirubinemia is usually moderate but patients with malignant obstruction generally have higher bilirubin concentrations than do patients with benign obstruction [174].

3.4. Radiological Evaluation

Plain abdominal radiograms are frequently obtained in patients with acute right upper quadrant abdominal pain but they rarely confirm the diagnosis of acute cholecystitis. Signs attributable to biliary tract disease include the presence of calcified stones or the evidence of gas within the biliary tract [165]. The most useful test for patients with suspected acute cholecystitis is ultrasound. Sonographic signs of acute cholecystitis are listed in table 12.

A positive sonographic Murphy sign is only present when the point of maximum tenderness corresponds to the sonographically localised gallbladder. Ralls reported this sign to be positive in 99% of patients with acute cholecystitis and in combination with gallstones the positive predictive value amounted to 95% [155]. In critically ill pa-

Table 12
Sonographic Signs of Acute Cholecystitis

Positive sonographic Murphy sign	Distension of the gallbladder
Gallstones	Presence of intramural gas
Thickening of gallbladder wall > 3mm	Sonolucent intramural layer (halo)
Sludge	Pericholecystic fluid

tients with acute acalculous cholecystitis this sign can not be elicited because of relaxation for mechanical ventilation.

In patients with gangrenous cholecystitis the sonographic Murphy sign is of limited value with a prevalence of only 33% [167]. In gangrenous cholecystitis marked irregularities of the gallbladder wall and intraluminal membranes could be detected in 58% of patients [118]. Thickening of the gallbladder wall of more than 3 mm is a reliable diagnostic criteria for acute cholecystitis [96] but does not correlate directly with the severity of gallbladder disease or pathological findings [160]. False positive examinations may occur in other conditions unrelated to gallbladder disease, such as hepatitis, hypoalbuminemia, ascites, congestive heart failure and nephrotic syndrome [119].

Sludge within the gallbladder is recognised increasingly as a cause of biliary pathology [119,152] and may be associated with acute acalculous cholecystitis. But very often sludge is the result of prolonged fasting or parenteral hyperalimentation. Other sonographic signs indicative of acute cholecystitis are distension of the gallbladder, a sonolucent intramural layer or "halo" that represents intramural edema or the presence of intramural or intraluminal gas, in emphysematous cholecystitis. The presence of pericholecystic fluid in combination with one or more of the above mentioned signs

is highly indicative of for gallbladder perforation. Summary ultrasound is the most useful diagnostic test for the evaluation of the gallbladder in suspected acute cholecystitis because of its high sensitivity (90-95%) and specifity (94-98%) [139].

Radionuclide scanning with technetium labeled isotopes (HIDA) is also a useful test for acute cholecystitis. The isotopes are rapidly secreted by hepatocytes into bile canaliculi and visualise the biliary tract and are concentrated in the gallbladder over a period of 1 to 4 hours. The diagnosis of acute cholecystitis is established when a gallbladder image does not appear within 4 hours. The sensitivity of this test is above 90% but the specifity is lower than ultrasound [102]. False positive results may be obtained in patients with alcohol abuse, acute pancreatitis, carcinoma of the gallbladder or in patients receiving total parenteral nutrition.

Computed tomography scans are no more helpful in establishing the diagnosis of acute cholecystitis than ultrasound. Indirect signs of acute cholecystitis are thickening of the gallbladder wall, local edema or pericholecystic fluid. The diagnosis can be established with comparable accuracy by CT or ultrasound.

The diagnosis of acute cholangitis is usually suspected on the basis of the history and clinical presentation. The initial test to establish the diagnosis is ultrasonography, with emphasis on examination of the liver for bile duct size, hepatic massesand tumor and cysts of the extrahepatic biliary tract, the gallbladder and the pancreas. Ultrasound or CT may reveal dilated common or intrahepatic ducts, a common or intrahepatic duct stone, a biliary or pancreatic tumor, liver abscess or liver atrophy. The next step to clarify the etiology is cholangiography by the percutaneous transhepatic or endoscopic route. Endoscopic retrograde cholangiography (ERC) is favoured because it offers a simultaneous treatment approach, such as sphincterotomy, stone extraction, stenting or decompression of the biliary tract with naso-biliary catheter drainage. Percutaneous transhepatic cholangiography or drainage (PTC/D) are more useful when the cause of obstruction is located more proximally in the biliary tract or intrahepatic. The proximal end of the lesion may be defined more exactly. However, both imaging procedures carry the risk of aggravating the symptoms of acute cholangitis and entail a morbidity of 1 to 7 percent and mortality of 0,25 percent [133]. Therefore cholangiography should be avoided unless decompression of the biliary tract is achieved at the same time or the patient has stabilised [133,147].

3.5. Bacteriology

The gallbladder and bile ducts of humans are usually sterile [93]. Bacteria may gain entry to the biliary tree by ascending from the duodenum, by hematogenous seeding, by translocating through the mucosal barrier of the gut or they are introduced by percutaneous manipulations, such as T-tube cholangiography or percutaneous drainage. In most cases the recovered organisms, therefore, are of enteric origin. In acute cholecystitis positive bile cultures are obtained in 40 to 60 percent [128,173]. The most commonly detected bacteria are Gram negative E.coli, Klebsiella species, Gram positive enterococci and less frequent anaerobes, such as Clostridia and Bacteroides species. In recent times more resistant Gram negative organisms, such as Pseudomonas and Enterobacter species, and polymicrobial infections have been detected with increasing frequency. This phenomenon reflects the shift of etiology of acute cholangitis toward patients with malignant obstruction and indwelling tubes [173]. In critically ill, immunocompromised patients acalculous cholecystitis from Candida species may be seen [98].

3.6. Treatment

The initial management of patients with either acute cholecystitis or acute cholangitis comprises nasogastric decompression, intravenous hydration, correction of electrolyte imbalances and parenteral antibiotics. The antibiotics chosen must cover Gram negative bacteria, most commonly E. coli and Klebsiella and in recent times with increasing frequency Pseudomonas and Enterobacter species, as well as enterococci and anaerobes. Antibiotics for the treatment of acute biliary tract infections must fulfill some more essential conditions. Sufficiently active concentrations in bile must be achieved, even when jaundice is present and bile must not develop antagonistic activity against antibiotics. Suitable antibiotics for acute biliary tract infections are broad spectrum penicillins, a combination of an aminoglycoside with penicillin, second or third generation cephalosporins or beta-lactam antibiotics, such as imipenem/cilastatin/ and piperacillin/Tazobactam

[128,131,149,174]. Antibiotic therapy should be started before the results of culture of bile have been obtained but may be changed according to culture results and the course of the disease.

3.6.1. Acute Cholecystitis

Many cases of acute cholecystitis resolve spontaneously resulting in chronic cholecystitis. However, the mainstay of therapy for calculous or acalculous cholecystitis is cholecystectomy. 10 to 20 percent of all cholecystectomies are indicated because of acute cholecystitis. In recent times several trends in surgery for acute cholecystitis have been observed. The patients with acute cholecystitis are significantly older with a higher proportion of males and diabetics. There is also an increase in accompanying common bile duct stones, acalculous cholecystitis and gangrenous cholecystitis [109,135,157].

The relative merits of the timing of operation, i.e. early (within 1 to 4 days of onset of symptoms) versus interval cholecystectomy (after more than 6 weeks) have been discussed and are controversial. On the basis of several randomised trials [116,124,140,150] early cholecystectomy is favoured. Early operation has the advantage of easier dissection of the gallbladder, prevents complications of cholecystitis such as empyema or perforation, shortens hospital stay and patients return sooner to work without increasing morbidity or mortality.

At the beginning of the era of laparoscopic cholecystectomy, acute cholecystitis was regarded as a contraindication for the laparoscopic approach. Greater experience with laparoscopic techniques and improvement of instruments have led many centers to attempt laparoscopic cholecystectomy in patients with acute cholecystitis. The published reports confirm that laparoscopic cholecystectomy for acute cholecystitis is safe, cost effective and successful, incluiding in the elderly as well and offers the patients the benefits of the laparoscopic approach, such as fewer post-operative complaints, shorter hospital stay, quick return to normal activities and aesthetic benefits [92,104,123,136-137,146,156,175,180].

Mortality and morbidity did not increase as compared to open cholecystectomy for acute cholecystitis but laparoscopic cholecystectomy has significantly higher rates of conversion to open cholecystectomy, longer operation times and increased morbidity rates compared with elective laparoscopic cholecystectomy. The aforementioned studies reported conversion rates between 7% to 35% which is almost three times that reported for chronic cholecystitis [89]. The factors contributing to conversion are difficulties in grasping the gallbladder, multiple tears in the gallbladder and inability to identify anatomical structures or to separate the gallbladder from liver bed or inflammatory masses [156]. Elderly patients, patients with a prolonged interval from onset of symptoms to operation and those with evidence of severe inflammation are at risk for conversion to open cholecystectomy [92,122,134,136,156]. Therefore, early operation between 48 to 96 hours after the onset of symptoms is strongly recommended for laparoscopic cholecystectomy in acute cholecystitis.

Conversion of a laparoscopic approach to open cholecystectomy ensures the safety of the procedure because most bile duct injuries occur in patients with acute cholecystitis. The true incidence of bile duct injuries is certainly higher than that reported by experienced centers. As for open cholecystectomy, intraoperative cholangiography is recommended for laparoscopic cholecystectomy. The merit of this procedure is the recognition of a bile duct injury that can be immediately repaired and not the prevention of injury [156].

The mortality rate for cholecystectomy of 3.4% in acute cholecystitis is ten fold higher than that of chronic cholecystitis [108,143,165]. The mortality increases to 10% in elderly patients [100,109]. One reason for this increased mortality is the high incidence of associated common duct stones in more than 30% of older patients requiring exploration of the common duct, compared to an incidence of 10% in the younger age group [109]. In patients with critical illness, septic shock, severe concomitant diseases or complications of cholecystitis, the mortality is between 6% to 30% [105,162,165].

For those critically ill patients considered not to be able to undergo emergency cholecystectomy, open or percutaneous cholecystostomy may be a lifesaving alternative [88,144,176]. The procedure is a temporizing measure in calculous cholecystitis. The catheter should remain in place until cholecystectomy follows. In the majority of patients with acute acalculous cholecystitis it may be the definitive therapy, provided that a normal cholangiogram with free flow of bile into the duodenum is obtained [144,166,176].

The main advantages of percutaneous cholecystostomy are bedside applicability and the use of local anesthesia. Puncture of the gallbladder is guided by ultrasonography. The gallbladder is entered through the liver bed to prevent leakage of bile and a pigtail catheter is introduced over a guide wire. The catheter position is confirmed roentgenographically and the catheter is placed at gravity drainage. Bile may be aspirated for culture.

Intravenous antibiotic therapy is started before the procedure. If percutaneous drainage is successful, rapid improvement of the condition of the patient is to be expected. When patients fail to improve an erroneous diagnosis of acute acalculous cholecystitis may be the cause. Perforated peptic ulcer, pancreatic abscess, pneumonia and pericarditis have all been discovered after failure of percutaneous cholecystostomy [178]. Therefore, an operation should be performed without delay in patients who fail to improve after percutaneous drainage. Also all patients with generalised peritonitis must be explored operatively because gallbladder perforation is likely [88].

The mortality rates for percutaneous cholecystostomy vary between 0% to over 50% [88,144,166,176] but it is difficult to compare mortality rates in the different series because the patient groups are small and different with regard to risk factors and severity of disease.

3.6.2. Acute Cholangitis

Patients with acute cholangitis represent a wide spectrum of illness. Most patients respond to supportive and antibiotic therapy. However 5 to 23 per cent of patients present the most severe form, acute suppurative or toxic cholangitis [90,130]. These patients will require intensive care management and urgent decompression of the obstructed biliary tract [133]. This can be achieved by endoscopic, percutaneous or surgical measures.

Table 13
Independent Risk Factors Predicting Mortality In Acute Cholangitis

Acute renal failure
Liver abscess
Cirrhosis
High malignant stricture
Percutaneous transhepatic cholangiography
Female gender
Age > 50 years

from Gigot et al

In former times only surgical decompression of the biliary tract was applicable but the mortality for emergency surgery in acute toxic cholangitis is high, up to 40% [90]. Nowadays, surgical decompression for acute cholangitis is only indicated when endoscopic and percutaneous attempts fail or these drainage procedures are not available. The best operation to be performed in these instances is a choledochotomy and insertion of a T-tube. The underlying disease or lesion can be managed later when the condition of the patient has improved.

Percutaneous or endoscopic procedures also carry a high risk of mortality and morbidity in toxic cholangitis [111,114,129,131]. In suppurative cholangitis spill-over of bacteria into the systemic circulation and bleeding can occur. Other complications are bile leakage, retroduodenal perforation and pancreatitis. In the emergency situation, endoscopic decompression of the biliary tree either by placing a naso-biliary drainage catheter or by inserting an endoprothesis, if possible without sphincterotomy or image intensification, is recommended [147]. In most cases patients improve and endotoxemia aborts [127]. After improvement, defi-

nitive endoscopic procedures, such as sphincterotomy, extraction of stones, or insertion of stents, may be undertaken with low morbidity and mortality.

For patients with mild to moderate cholangitis due to choledocholithiasis, simultaneous endoscopic cholangiography, sphincterotomy and stone extraction is recommended. In patients with a history of a biliary-enteric anastomosis or central perihilar located obstruction, percutaneous transhepatic drainage is the preferred route for decompression.

Prognosis of acute cholangitis depends on several factors. Gigot [107] found seven independent risk factors after multivariate analysis predictive for mortality (Table 13). When given proportional weight a scoring system could be obtained. Mortality was 1.8 percent with less than 7 points while those with over 7 points had a mortality of 49 percent. The patients at high risk for mortality could be detected with a sensitivity of 81% and a specifity of 92% and a positive predictive value of 91.5%. However, mortality also depends on the underlying etiology of acute cholangitis. The patients with the worst prognosis and highest mortality are those with malignant obstruction [174].

4. PANCREATIC INFECTIONS

4.1. Introduction

In contrast to sterile inflammatory lesions of the pancreas and some viral infections (mainly in immuno-compromised patients) primary bacterial infections of normal pancreatic tissue are extremely rare events and may be virtually non-existent in the clinical setting.

From experimental findings it has been concluded that autodigestion of the pancreas and hence pancreatitis, may be the consequence of the action of proteolytic enzymes derived from bacteria [181]. However, although bacteria are present in the bile of most patients with common bile duct stones, evidence for a role of bacteria in the etiology of biliary pancreatitis is lacking. A post-mortem analysis did not reveal bacteria in pancreatic ducts of patients who had died from acute pancreatitis [182]. On the other hand, pancreatic enzymes may well digest bacteria and thus may prevent their detection.

Major pancreatic bacterial infections almost always result from secondary infection of pancreatic lesions such as pancreatic or peripancreatic necroses, pancreatic pseudocysts and, very rarely, pancreatic cysts. Pancreatic necrosis and most pancreatic pseudocysts, are usually as a consequence of episodes of acute pancreatitis.

Pathological findings in acute pancreatitis range from mild edema to extensive pancreatic and peripancreatic necrosis. Clinically, the spectrum extends from mild, self

Table 14
Definitions According to the Atlanta Classification System (3)

- **Severe acute pancreatitis:**
  acute inflammatory process, with variable involvement of other regional tissues, associated with organ failure and/or local complications, such as necrosis, pseudocyst, or abscess.

- **Actue fluid collections:**
  occur early in the course of acute pancreatitis, are located in or near the pancreas, and always lack a wall of granulation or fibrous tissue. Bacteria are variably present.

- **Pancreatic necrosis:**
  diffuse or local area(s) of nonviable pancreatic parenchyma, which is typically associated with peripancreatic fat necrosis. *Infected* pancreatic necrosis is characterized by the presence of micro-organisms.

- **Acute pseudocyst:**
  collection of pancreatic juice enclosed by a wall of fibrous or granulation tissue. The presence of bacteria may indicate contamination.

- **Pancreatic abcess:**
  circumscribed intra-abdominal collection of pus, containing little or no pancreatic necrosis.

limiting symptoms to fulminant illness that may rapidly lead to multiple organ failure and death. Varying etiologies and numerous complications which occasionally occur at the very beginning of the process may additionally influence the variability of the disease. Agreement on precise definitions is lacking and attempts have recently been made to introduce some uniformity into this field [183] (Table 14). The clinically based Atlanta Classification System does not refer to pancreatic morphology as did earlier attempts to classify acute inflammatory disorders of the pancreas. In spite of some obvious short-comings which are inherent in most products of consensus conferences, the adherence to this terminology may be clinically useful and indeed may facilitate comparison of interinstitutional data.

Pancreatic or peripancreatic necroses, peripancreatic fluid collections and pancreatic pseudocysts are the lesions usually prone to secondary infection.

Pancreatic abscesses, there fore, may either result from loculated infected necrosis, from infection of an acute pseudocyst or from loculization of an infected fluid accumulation. For the purpose of therapeutic strategy, pancreatic necroses, infected fluid accumulations and pancreatic abscesses often are considered separately. However, it must be kept in mind that these definitions describe different aspects of local complications of severe acute pancreatitis rather than true pathological entities [183,184].

4.2. Pathogenesis

Acute pancreatitis may be initiated by a number of factors, including obstruction or overextension of the pancreatic duct, exposure to ethanol and other toxins, hyper-triglyceridemia, hypercalcemia, hyperstimulation of the gland or trauma.

Irrespective of the etiology, ectopic protease activation with resultant autodigestion of pancreatic or peripancreatic tissue, has been suggested as the main pathogenetic mechanism of acute pancreatitis. The formation of trypsin by enzymatic cleavage of trypsinogen is believed to initiate a cascade-like activation of other zymogens. It has been shown experimentally that the magnitude of trypsinogen cleavage (measured as the concentration in plasma and ascites of trypsinogen activation peptides) correlates with histopathological alterations and the severity of the disease [185].

Erroneous co-localization of lysosomal enzymes with zymogen granules resulting in "autophagic granules", may result in intracellular premature activation of zymogens by hydrolases [186,187]. A loss of polarization with atypical basolateral exocytosis of proteases into the interstitial space, may also explain the onset of inflammatory reactions [188].

The critical step, however, in the transition of interstitial inflammation to interstitial necrosis or necrosis of the peripancreatic fatty tissue is still ill defined. However, it has been suggested that pancreatic ischemia plays a role [189].

Pancreatic necrosis usually involves destruction of small intralobular or interlobular ducts. Leaking pancreatic juice thus reaches the necrotic area where, following activation, it will contribute to its enlargement. In most cases peripancreatic fatty tissue will become digested as well and in some cases detectable necrosis seems to be restricted to peripancreatic tissue. Whether this, however, necessarily predicts a more benign course or a lower probability of subsequent infection is not yet clear.

It has been concluded from large series that necrotizing pancreatitis develops in about 15%- 20% of all episodes of acute pancreatitis [190-193]. However, there is no general agreement whether interstitial edematous pancreatitis, as classified according to pathomorphological criteria, indeed represents a form of the disease pathophysiologically different from necrotizing pancreatitis [194] or whether the term necrotizing pancreatitis simply encompasses severe forms with larger areas of detectable necrosis [183].

The pathomorphological changes in acute pancreatitis may well represent a continuum with interstititial edema and minimal fatty tissue necrosis at one end and large confluent areas of pancreatic and peripancreatic necrosis and hemorrhage at the other.

Usually, the extent of the disease seems to be determined in the early phase allowing for clinical classification during the first few days. Occasionally, however, some forms of radiologically diagnosed interstitial edematous pancreatitis, develop considerable necrosis several days later, in spite of the obvious absence of persistent etiological factors. In an autopsy analysis of 405 cases it has been shown that necrosis was present in every fatal case [195].

4.2.1. *Infected pancreatic necrosis*

Dependent on duration of the disease, infection will eventually occur in 30% to more than 80% of patients with sterile necrosis [190,193,196-200]; (Figure 1). Secondary infection of pancreatic necrosis is believed to account for 80% of all deaths from acute pancreatitis. However, there is still conside-

Figure 1
Development of Invectious Complications

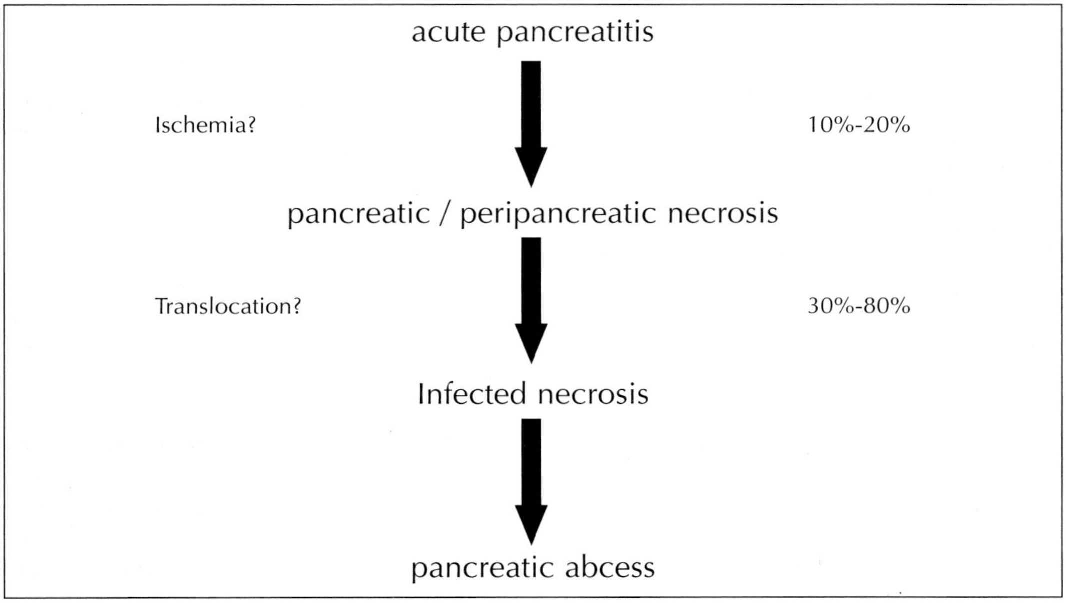

acute pancreatitis

Ischemia?   10%-20%

pancreatic / peripancreatic necrosis

Translocation?   30%-80%

Infected necrosis

pancreatic abcess

Table 15
Routes of Infection of Pancreatic Necrosis

Acsending via pancreatic ducts	Translocation into portal venous system
Translocation via mesenteric lymphatics	Transmural translocation and direct invasion

rable controversy as to whether infection of pancreatic necrosis per se results in higher mortality rates [193,197,200-205]; whether the extent of the necrosis or its anatomical site influence the prognosis [206]; or whether the extent of the necrosis [190] or the degree of the inflammatory response determine the risk of secondary infection.

Depending upon the timing of percutaneous fine needle aspiration or an operative procedure, infection rates increase from 25% in patients operated upon very early [190] to more than 80% in patients operated on after three to four weeks [193,196-198].

A large body of evidence derived from both bacteriological findings in patients and animal studies suggests that the gut is the principal source of infection. Bacteria isolated from infected necrosis are almost exclusively members of the enteric flora. Gram-negative aerobes, Gram-positive aerobes and, to a lesser extent, anaerobes and fungi are usually grown from fine needle aspirates or intraoperative samples [184]. Earlier data have shown that monoinfection was more often detected than poly-bacterial infections and that Enterobacteriaceae still outnumber other species. However, common experience suggests that Gram-positive rods such as Staphylococcus aureus and Candida species are now becoming more frequently found [207].

The exact route of infection as well as the therapeutic implications are less clear. Basi-

cally, infection may result from bacterial ascendence via the pancreatic duct, from translocating bacteria which may reach extraintestinal tissue after passage through draining lymphatic vessels via the thoracic duct and the systemic circulation; from translocation into the portal venous system; or from direct transmural migration to the intraperitoneal or retroperitoneal spaces (Table 15). Each possibility seems to be supported by experimental findings [208-219]. In the human situation, the route of infection is not yet clear. Intestinal bacterial overgrowth with diminished colonization resistance, however, may play an important role as well as an enhanced intestinal permeability [220]. Mucosal ischemia, decreased gut motility and suppression of gut-specific immune function may all contribute to translocation-induced infection of extraintestinal sites [221,222], even if the role of systemic immunodepression seems less clear [223-225].

4.2.2. Acute fluid collections

The accumulation of fluid in or near the pancreas is a common finding in acute pancreatitis. The acute inflammatory response invariably leads to some degree of tissue edema with accompanying exudate. This may be localized in the narrow pancreatic interstitium or may collect in the peripancreatic region where the soft fatty tissue is no major barrier against its spread into the retroperitoneal spaces of the bilateral pericolic compartments, the mesenteries, the

Table 16
Peripancreatic Fluid Collections

Inflammatory exudate
Liquefied tissue necrosis
Leaking pancreatic juice
Loculated exudate in the lesser sac
Pancreatogenic ascites

perirenal spaces and, along the major vessels, even up into the mediastinum and down into the pelvis.

This exudate usually contains considerable amounts of pancreatic enzymes and may be almost exclusively composed of pancreatic fluid. To what extent liquification of necrosis contributes to these fluid collections and which role can be attributed to a ductal blow-out can rarely be defined in the individual case.

The close contact between the ventral surface of the pancreas and the lesser sac explains the concomitant occurrence of detectable fluid in the omental bursa and sometimes even in the free abdominal cavity. This pancreatogenic ascites may also contain variable amounts of activated enzymes depending upon the permeability of the peritoneal barrier or its disruption by the retroperitoneal process. The resulting diffuse peritonitis primarily represents a so-called chemical peritonitis.

The volume of the peripancreatic fluid as well as the extent of its spread seems to reflect the severity of the inflammatory process [226]. This relation, however, is certainly not linear and may be influenced by the composition of the fluid, the extension of peripancreatic necrosis, hydration and

other individual factors. Fluid accumulations of up to ten liters may be encountered (Table 16).

Apparently, more than half of these collections resolve spontaneously within several weeks [227,228], if the pancreatic duct lesion has closed spontaneously, if the inflammatory response decreases and if the fluid does not become secondarily infected. Other factors are as yet ill defined. If infection of pancreatic or peripancreatic necrosis occurs the respective fluid accumulations may also contain bacteria.

In mild pancreatitis, where necroses are absent or confined to small focal areas of fatty tissue, fluid accumulations may be detected as well. However, resolution then is even more common and contamination or infection are certainly the exception.

4.2.3. *Acute pseudocysts*

Progressing or persisting fluid collections eventually will become localized by a defined wall of granulation or fibrous tissue. Pathomorphologically, the presence of such a wall distinguishes an acute pseudocyst from acute fluid collections. Whilst in earlier definitions the term pseudocyst also encompassed fluid accumulations loculated by fibrinous or necrotic walls and thus has

Figure 2
Possible Developments of Local Complications

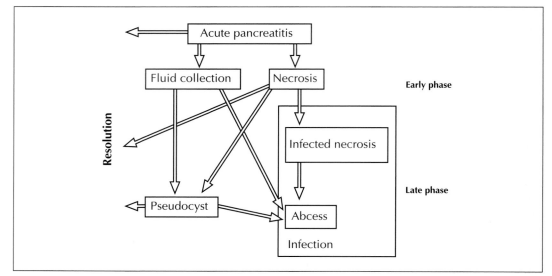

been used early in the course of pancreatitis, the newer definition refers to formations which may require four or more weeks from the onset of the disease to develop [227]. Pseudocysts not only represent encapsulated fluid collections but may also result from localization of necroses which then become liquefied (Figure 2). A communication with pancreatic ducts may be present.

4.2.4. Pancreatic abscess

Whether bacteria detected in pancreatic pseudocysts represent contamination rather than infection is debatable. If, however, the content of walled-off lesions contains micro-organisms and can be described as pus, there is broad consensus that this lesion should be termed pancreatic abscess. Thus, abscesses either result from loculated infected and liquefied necroses, from walled-off infected fluid collections or from secondary

infection of primarily sterile (or contaminated) pseudocysts (figure 2). The formation of a well defined wall of granulation or fibrous tissue again occurs late in the course of acute pancreatitis and may be detectable only after a period of four weeks or more.

Since pancreatic abscesses should not contain considerable amounts of necroses, the differentiation between localized infected necroses and pancreatic abscess sometimes may depend on rather subjective evaluation criteria. Bacteria grown from pancreatic abscesses usually resemble those found in infected necroses and there seems to be a somewhat larger rate of poly-microbial infections [202]. This, however, may be related to culture conditions and to a decreased anti-bacterial effect of pancreatic fluid in the abscesses.

Concerning the role of pancreatic lesions in the pathogenesis of intra-abdominal infections, infected necroses, infected fluid accumulations and pancreatic abscesses may all be considered as possible infectious foci.

4.3. Clinical Presentation

Irrespective of the etiology, acute pancreatitis usually has a rapid onset. Upper abdominal pain radiating into the back in a typical belt-like fashion is the predominant complaint. Corresponding to the variety of possible pathomorphological alterations, the abdominal findings on physical examination range from mild tenderness to obvious rebound. Distension, nausea, vomiting and hypoactive or absent bowel sounds are frequently found. Systemic signs of local inflammation such as fever and leukocytosis are often present but unspecific. Most often, pancreatic enzyme levels (amylase, lipase, elastase) are elevated in blood and urine. However, there is no clear correlation between their concentration and the magnitude of pancreatic injury.

A severe form of pancreatitis must be considered if failure to improve within 24 to 48 hours is associated with a palpable epigastric mass or if ecchymoses are detectable in the flank (Grey-Turner sign) or periumbilically (Cullen's sign).

The early response, elicited by the pancreatic inflammation and by the systemic reaction to the release of activated enzymes, vasoactive factors and toxic substances from the inflamed pancreas may result in a shock-like state. Fluid sequestration with subsequent hypovolemia is an additional factor and may be associated with increasing signs of multiple organ dysfunction. However, during this early phase, there are no clinical prognostic signs for the develop-

ment of or are indicative of the presence of infectious complications.

In assessing the severity of acute pancreatitis various attempts have been made to identify prognostic criteria using laboratory [229-232] or clinical parameters [233] or combinations of both [196,234-236]. It seems obvious that severity-dependent pathophysiological changes are reflected by defined constellations of laboratory parameters. However, not every individual patient with more than three Ranson's signs or an APACHE II score of more than 15 suffers from severe pancreatitis [193,230,237]. Hence these scores are useful mainly for identifying groups of patients who may be at increased risk from their acute illness.

A large variety of inflammatory parameters in the plasma, on the other hand, may reflect a systemic inflammatory response syndrome (SIRS) which is clearly related to the severity of the disease [46,50,58].

The degree of such a systemic inflammatory response, again, is not predictive for pancreatic infections during this early phase. Thus failure to respond to initial treatment within a few days, the presence of severe SIRS and the clinical finding of peritonitis only suggest severe pancreatitis with a high probability of the presence of major necrosis.

When etiologic factors -, if detectable -, have been dealt with adequately, in many patients spontaneous resolution of pancreatic inflammation can be expected under appropriate therapy. This is usually associated with a relief of symptoms and gradual normalization of clinical findings and laboratory data.

If however, the systemic inflammatory response persists beyond the first week or re-

Figure 3
Clinical Course of Severe Acute Pancreatitis

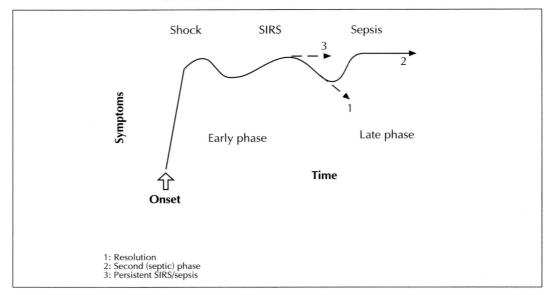

1: Resolution
2: Second (septic) phase
3: Persistent SIRS/sepsis

curs after a period of apparent amelioration, then the existence of an infectious focus has to be considered (Figure 3).

In the individual situation it is almost impossible to differentiate clinically between a prolonged systemic inflammatory response as a consequence of the presence of sterile necroses and a septic response due to secondary infection of local complications such as pancreatic or peripancreatic necrosis, fluid accumulations or acute pseudocysts.

Moreover, since infectious and non-infectious complications may occur simultaneously, the clinical presentation may become even more confounding during the later stages. Generally, infected necroses and accumulations of infected fluid present earlier in the course of pancreatitis than pancreatic abscesses which either result after several

weeks from liquefied necrosis, from loculization of infected fluid or from secondary infections of acute pseudocysts. The presence of a defined wall around pancreatic abscesses may explain the often mitigated clinical presentation.

Other complications such as retroperitoneal or intra-abdominal bleeding, pancreatic or colonic fistulization or necrosis of the large bowel wall, all of which are more common during the later course, may aggravate the clinical picture or initiate intra-abdominal infection under otherwise sterile conditions.

4.4. Diagnosis of infectious complications

When clinical symptoms and elevated serum levels of pancreatic enzymes are suggestive of acute pancreatitis, history may give hints as to etiology and recurrences. If biliary pancreatitis is suspected, ultrasonography and endoscopic retrograde cholangio-pancreatography (ERCP) are primary diagnostic procedures followed by endoscopic sphincterotomy (ES) in case of prepapillary impacted common bile duct stones.

With laboratory parameters being notoriously unreliable, further diagnosis is based mainly on visualization by imaging procedures. Plain films of the chest and abdomen are of little help but may reveal pleural effusions, free abdominal air or ileus as signs of local complications.

Most questions, however, regarding the extent of pathomorphological alterations, such as the presence of local complications and the quantity of peripancreatic fluid require contrast enhanced computed tomography [239,240]. Recent experiences with magnetic resonance imaging (MIR) seem promising. There are, however, as yet no data available comparing its diagnostic value to the gold standard of contrast-enhanced CT.

The clinical course of patients with normal findings on CT is usually benign [61]. Radiographic enhancement of the pancreas following contrast injection is generally interpreted as evidence of tissue perfusion and viability [2422463]. Non-enhancement may indicate tissue necrosis but also may indicate reduced perfusion only. As to the detection of necrotic areas, overall accuracy rates of more than 90% have been achieved [193,238,239]. Further findings may include diffuse or segmental enlargement of the pancreas, irregularity of the tissue borders with diffuse inflammatory infiltrations of the peripancreatic fatty tissue and other retroperitoneal spaces and acute fluid collection confined to the retroperito-

neum, extending into the lesser sac or even into the peritoneal cavity.

There is generally no need for an emergency CT scan. In the very early phase radiological signs may be indifferent or even misleading. Two or three days after the onset of an acute episode, CT findings become highly specific for the presence of local complications. Fluid collections and larger areas of pancreatic or peripancreatic necrosis seem predictive of the development of later infectious complications. It has been reckoned that non-enhancement in this phase is followed by secondary infection in up to three out of four patients.

With the relatively rare exception of radiologically detectable gas bubbles in the peripancreatic or pancreatic tissues [192], CT findings cannot differentiate between infected and non-infected fluid or necrosis in the earlier stages.

Contrast-enhanced CT scans are also essential parts of the follow-up and may reveal further spread of inflammatory or liquefying processes in the retroperitoneum, alterations in the extent of fluid accumulations, reappearing of tissue enhancement or late complications such as walled-off liquid processes. Again, the differentiation between pseudocysts and abscesses is not reliable by imaging procedures.

Since, however, the differentiation between infected and non-infected complications has major implications on surgical treatment, percutaneous fine needle aspiration (FNA) with bacteriological evaluation is the mainstay of the diagnostic follow-up [198,244]. This can be performed either by sonographic or computer tomographic guidance. Safe access routes may not always be evident but even punctures across hollow viscera seem to give reliable results. Accuracy rates of up to 100% if bowel penetration had been avoided have been reported [193].

As to the timing of aspiration, most authors agree that it should be performed immediately if signs of a systemic inflammatory response coincide with CT findings of pancreatic or peripancreatic necrosis or loculated fluid [193,196-198]. FNA does not appear justified in clinically improving cases. If a FNA culture yields a negative result reaspiration is recommended after a couple of days if clinical symptoms persist or even increase.

Depending upon surgical strategy and the expected time of secondary infection the first FNA may be delayed until the second or third week. Even in the presence of pancreatic ascites FNA should be directed to the pancreatic region.

When, during the later course, pseudocysts or abscesses are detected by the visualization of defined, well-perfused walls, FNA again may confirm the respective diagnosis. Without clinical signs of sepsis, however, a wait-and-see policy will be appropriate. Regression or resolution then suggest the presence of non-infected pseudocysts.

4.5. Therapy

Basically therapeutic interventions may be considered for several purposes: amelioration of the clinical course, treatment of complications and prevention of recurrencies. While operative treatment is mostly directed against etiological factors (e.g. biliary pancreatitis) or focuses on complications, the conservative approach attempts to influence the clinical course of acute pancreatitis.

4.5.1. General treatment

Attempts to influence pathogenetic mechanisms right at the beginning of an acute episode have failed. Neither protease inhibition [245,246] nor the reduction of pancreatic secretory activity by somatostatin or its analogue [247-249] have proven beneficial in clinical trials. Experimantally, the development of pancreatic necrosis seems to be preventable by isovolumic hemodilution [250,251]. The results of larger clinical trials, however, are still lacking.

Thus symptomatic therapy is based on the correction of hemodynamic disturbances by adequate volume replacement; on effective analgesia while avoiding the effects of opioids on the sphincter of Oddi and on support of organ function if necessary.

Since the rationale of laying the pancreas at rest by the removal of gastric contents is no longer supported [252-254], the use of naso-gastric tubes can be restricted to patients with severely disturbed intestinal motility. The effect of secretory stimulation by enteral nutrition, however, has to be weighed against the possibility of enhanced bacterial translocation under total parenteral nutrition. Long naso-jejunal tubes or percutaneous jejunostony are options when the acute phase of pancreatic inflammation has resolved.

There is growing evidence that early antibiotic prophylaxis may be of benefit in patients with severe acute pancreatitis. Most respective comments suggest that antibiotic treatment may prevent translocation or colonization and thus eventually secondary infectious complications [255]. The idea seems intriguing. After earlier failures, the first clinical trial reporting benefit from prophylactic antibiotic therapy was published in

1993 [256]. Patients who received imipenem for 14 days developed less secondary infections of pancreatic necrosis. Mortality rates, however, were not significantly influenced. From this result it may be concluded that infection of pancreatic necroses does not invariably enhance the severity of the disease. Since infected necroses have been associated with higher mortality rates [190], patients with more severe disease may be at higher risk of secondary infection.

Two randomized studies in patients with alcoholic pancreatitis also suggest positive effects of prophylactic treatment with intravenous cephalosporins [257,258]. A randomized multicenter trial of selective decontamination of the digestive tract (SDD) plus iv Cefotaxime has shown a significant reduction of Gram-negative pancreatic infections and of late mortality (if adjusted for severity grading) in the treatment group [259]. Since antibiotics systemically given may efficiently inhibit translocation, contamination and eventual infection, the necessity of SDD may be questioned. Nevertheless, SDD seems to work, at least in the experimental setting [260].

Taken together, there is indeed some evidence that antibiotic treatment is able to prevent secondary infection and may, to a lesser extent, influence mortality. Questions as to which treatment, when, for how long and in which patient, must be addressed in further studies. Whether antibiotics exert their supposed effect in the bowel lumen, on the routes of translocation or -, less probably -, in the area of necrosis must remain open. Moreover, possible effects of prolonged antibiotic treatment on intestinal bacterial overgrowth and subsequent translocation of more resistant pathogens have also to be considered.

4.5.2. Operative treatment of acute pancreatitis

Once the diagnosis of acute pancreatitis has been established and an impacted concrement at the ampulla of Vater removed by the endoscopic approach, operative treatment will concentrate on local complications and the prevention of recurrences. Since early interventions for clearance of the papilla of Vater and the bile duct without obvious obstruction do not seem to alter the clinical course of biliary pancreatitis [261,262], biliary surgery may be delayed until recuperation.

4.5.2.1. Infected necrosis

Irrespective of some casuistic reports on conservative treatment of pancreatic infections, there is broad consensus that secondary bacterial infection is an absolute indication for surgical treatment. In the absence of FNA-results, however, there are little other objective data on which the indication may be based. A "strong suspicion of infection" will lead many surgeons to consider operative intervention. However, there is considerable controversy whether this may be based on progressive deterioration in a patient with SIRS [263]; non-response to intensive medical treatment within several days [197,264]; or the clinical findings of peritonitis [265].

It seems questionable at least, whether patients with non-infected necrosis benefit from any operative intervention. While in earlier studies "necrosis" alone was accepted as an indication for operative therapy [200,202], more recently it has been shown that sterile necrosis can safely be managed conservatively even if organ failure develops [193]. Moreover, the rationale for removing sterile necrosis to prevent systemic effects or secondary infection is not supported by clinical or experimental data [205,265-268].

At present, we would suggest basing a strong suspicion of infection on hard criteria such as the CT-finding of pancreatic necrosis with extraluminal gas inclusions. Whether sterile necrosis of more than 50 per cent of the gland, necrosis with hemodynamic instability or multiple organ failure or necrosis with relentless downhill clinical course in an early stage should be considered as further indications remains to be established.

It should be kept in mind that the later the operative intervention is performed the better the necrotic tissue will be demarcated. Thus, in the absence of proven infection, a "wait-and-see" policy appears certainly warranted in a non-septic patient. On the other hand, whether an operation may be delayed in a stable patient with FNA-proven infection remains an open question.

The decision to intervene is closely related to the choice of the therapeutic approach. Once the diagnosis of infected pancreatic and peripancreatic necrosis has been established, percutaneous procedures do not

seem advisable. Nor is there any evidence to support simple operative drainage for infected necrosis. Peritoneal lavage has lost its place in the therapeutic repertoire [269,270]. Formal resections were suggested, favored and abandoned in the seventies. At present, pancreatic/peripancreatic debridement is the standard procedure, either performed through the gastrocolic ligament, through the transverse mesocolon or via the retroperitoneal routes from the flanks.

The extent of necrosis may require additional measures. Thorough debridement and gravity drainage are sufficient for small, well-delineated processes, while in cases with more extensive necroses, postoperative continuous closed lavage of the lesser sac or staged reinterventions every 24 to 48 hours seem advisable [196,236,264,271]. If both colonic flexures have to be taken down to allow wide exploration of the retrocollic spaces and if there is poor differentiation of viable from non-viable tissue, open packing procedures may be considered, with secondary closure of the abdominal wound once the retroperitoneal necrosis has been eliminated and replaced by granulation tissue [193,263,272].

Table 17
Operative Therapy of Pancreatic Necrosis

Débridement and closed drainage/lavage*		
Mortality:	7*%-44%	Pemberton 86, Beger 88*, Nicholson 88*, Teerenhovi 89, Larvin 89, Pederzoli 90*, Harris 95*, Farkas 96*
Reexploration:	17*%-78%	Rattner 92, Broughan 94, Harris 95, Farkas 96*
Débridement and open treatment		
Mortality:	11%-33*%	Pemberton 86, Bradley 87, Gracia-Sabrido 88, Stanten 90, Bradley 91+93, Doglietto 94, Harris 95

Table 18
Comparison of Operative Strategies Following Necrosectomy

	Closed	Open
No. of series	9	10
Mortality	7%-44%	11%-33%
Mobidity	60%-87%	45%-90%
Pancreatic fistula	10%-22%	18%-48%
Gastrointestinal fistula	1%-48%	4%-36%

Review of the literature 1980-1996.

With all of these procedures excellent results have been reported during the last few years, with overall mortality rates of between 10% and 40% in patients with infected necrosis [191,196,197,271,273] (Table 17). It should be noted, however, that the necrotizing process may continue after early primary debridement, thus perhaps explaining the less favorable results reported in some series treated with one-stage necrosectomy and simple gravity drainage [267,280].

Comparing the results after necrosectomy followed by closed drainage with or without continuous lavage and the open packing approach, no clear advantage of either procedure becomes apparent (Table 18). Such comparisons, however, are certainly biased since there are no prospective randomized studies available. The wide range in outcome variables may be related to site-specific therapeutic regimens, to small patient numbers or to ill-comparable populations. Additionally, attempts to gauge objectively the severity of disease were inconsistently reported.

4.5.2.2. Infected fluid collections

If acute fluid collections are associated with overt pancreatic or peripancreatic necroses,

any secondary infection will rapidly spread across the respective compartments. Thus treatment has to be directed against the infected necrosis. If, however, fluid collections result from ductal blow-out, secondary infection will occur more rarely and may be adequately treated by simple drainage. This can well be achieved by the percutaneous approach. Further therapeutic interventions will be directed towards a reduction of the sequelae of the ductal lesion by improving pancreatic drainage. In addition to endoscopic papillotomy, endoscopic implantation of a pancreatic duct stent may be optional [281].

In cases with ductal pathologies and adequate external drainage, an external pancreatic fistula will result which may need secondary internal drainage. This usually will be performed after a waiting period of some four to six weeks. Infected fluid which does not completely resolve will eventually become walled-off by fibrous or granulation tissue and then has to be classified as a pancreatic abscess.

4.5.2.3. Pancreatic abscess

Pancreatic abscesses usually occur late in the course of acute pancreatitis, commonly

Table 19
Local Complications of Acute Pancreatitis

Necrosis	Fistula (pancreatic/intestinal)
Infected necrosis	Colonic necrosis
Acute pseudocyst	Bleeding
Abscess	Pleural/bronchial involvement

beyond the third week after the onset of symptoms. They are easily detectable by contrast-enhanced computed tomography and diagnostic percutaneous aspiration and are associated with a lower mortality than infected pancreatic necrosis [197]. Once the diagnosis is established, the indication for intervention is given.

Percutaneous drainage which may be curative after infection of pseudocysts or localized fluid often serves as a temporizing measure only if the abscess has resulted from infected necrosis [282-284]. Since in persistent septic cases non-liquefied necrotic material is common wide surgical exploration, debridement and drainage should be performed. Because subsequent necrosis is not to be expected in these late complications, simple sump or gravity drainage, sometimes combined with continuous or intermittent irrigation, may be adequate if the process is well-delineated and if debridement can be performed completely. Soft, wide-bore drainage tubes should be placed in every abscess cavity and should be brought out as far as posteriorly possible. Drainage through the bed of the resected 11th or 12th rib may be helpful. With these strategies, repeat operations may be avoided in almost half of the patients.

The alternative procedure, which should be considered in less well-delineated and more extended processes where radical debridement has its limitations, is necrosectomy and open packing. Redebridement will be necessary every two to four days until the cavity has reduced in size and its walls are covered with granulation tissue. Using this procedure mortality rates of 0% -20% have been published [197,263,272,285]. In evaluating study results and comparing mortality rates, it must be kept in mind that abscesses resulting from infection of pseudocysts carry a more favorable prognosis [274,286] than abscesses secondary to infection of pancreatic necroses.

4.5.2.4. Other complications

Regarding local complications (Table 19), pancreatic and gastrointestinal fistulae are common before and after the initial operation. They may be caused by either ischemic, enzymatic or iatrogenic injury. While most pancreatic fistulae may resolve spontaneously, a considerable part of gastrointestinal fistulae may eventually require operative intervention for either control or direct repair [287]: if adequately drained and well walled-off, fistulae will not significantly affect survival [197,287,288].

Spontaneous necrosis of the transverse colon with frank perforation is not a rare event in severe acute pancreatitis and certainly requires prompt resection, unless interenteric or enterocutaneous fistulae are already present providing protection against diffuse intra-abdominal infection [289,290].

Major bleeding, finally, is a life-threatening complication which may be difficult to control. It may be a consequence of enzymatic degradation of vessel walls, of denudation and subsequent erosion of vessels during debridement or of direct injury. Transaortic catheter-embolization of the damaged vessel or the insertion of a vascular stent to bridge an aneurysmatic segment may be alternatives to a direct operative approach.

REFERENCES

1. Altemeier WA, Schowengerdt CG, Whiteley DH: Abscesses of the liver: surgical considerations. Arch Surg 1970, 101, 258.

2. Baek SY, Lee MG, Cho KS, Lee SC, Sung KB, Auh YH: Therapeutic percutaneous aspiration of hepatic abscesses: effectiveness in 25 patients. AJR 1993, 160, 799-802.

3. De Baere T, Rocha, Amenabar JM, Lagrange C, Ducreux M, Rougier P, Elias D, Lasser P, Patriarche C: Liver abscess formation after local treatment of liver tumors. Hepatology 1996, 23, 1436-1440.

4. Berger LA, Osborne DR: Treatment of pyogenic liver abscess by percutaneous needle aspiration. Lancet 1982, i, 132-134.

5. Bertel CK, van Heerden JA, Sheedy II PF: Treatment of pyogenic hepatic abscesses. Arch Surg 1986, 121, 554-557.

6. Bowers ED, Robison DJ, Doberneck RC: Pyogenic liver abscess. World J Surg 1990, 14, 128-132.

7. Branum GD, Tyson GS, Branum MA, Meyers WC: Hepatic abscess: Changes in etiology, diagnosis and management. Ann Surg 1990,212, 655-662.

8. Chou FF, Sheen-Chen SM, Chen YS, Chen MC, Chen FC, Tai DI: Prognostic factors for pyogenic abscesses of the liver. J Am Coll Surg 1994, 179, 727-732.

9. Chou FF, Sheen-Chen SM, Chen YS, Lee TY: The comparison of clinical course and results of treatment between gas-forming and non-gas-forming pyogenic liver abscess. Arch Surg 1995, 130, 401-405.

10. Chou FF, Sheen-Chen SM, Chen YS, Chen MC: Single and multiple pyogenic liver abscesses: clinical course, etiology and results of treatment. World J Surg 1997, 21, 384-388.

11. Chu K, Fan S, Lai EC, Lo C, Wong J: Pyogenic liver abscess, an audit of experience over the past decade. Arch Surg 1996, 131, 148-152.

12. Cohen JL, Martin FM, Rossi RL, Schoetz jr DJ: Liver abscess: the need for complete gastrointestinal evaluation. Arch Surg 1989, 124, 561-564.

13. Collins AN: Abscess of the liver. Minn Med 1932, 15, 756.

14. Crippin JS, Wang KK: An unrecognized etiology for pyogenic hepatic abscesses in normal hosts: dental disease. Am J Gastroenterol 1992, 87, 1740-1743.

15. Dondelinger RF, Kurdziel JC, Gathy C: Percutaneous treatment of pyogenic liver abscess: a critical analysis of results. Cardiovasc Intervent Radiol 1990, 13, 174-182.

16. Donovan AJ, Yellin AE, Ralls PW: Hepatic abscess. World J Surg 1991, 15, 162-169.

17. Farges O, Leese T, Bismuth H: Pyogenic liver abscess: an improvement in prognosis. Br J Surg 1988, 75, 862-865.

18. Gerzof SG, Johnson WC, Robbins AH, Nabseth DC: Intrahepatic pyogenic abscesses: treatment by percutaneous drainage. Am J Surg 1985, 149, 487-493.

19. Giorgio A, Tarantino L, Mariniello N, Francica G, Scala E, Amoroso P, Nuzzo A, Rizzatto G: Pyogenic liver abscesses: 13 years of experience in percutaneous needle aspiration with US guidance. Radiology 1995, 195, 122-124.

20. Gyorffy EJ, Frey CF, Silva J, McGahan J: Pyogenic liver abscess, diagnostic and therapeutic strategies. Ann Surg 1987, 206, 699-705.

21. Hansen N, Vargish T: Pyogenic hepatic abscess: a case for open drainage. Am Surg 1993, 59, 219-222.

22. Hashimoto L, Hermann R, Grundfest-Broniatowski S: Pyogenic hepatic abscess: results of current management. Am Surg 1995, 61, 407-411.

23. Herbert DA, Rothman J, Simmons F, Fogel DA, Wilson S, Ruskin J: Pyogenic liver abscess: successful non-surgical therapy. Lancet 1982, i, 134-136.

24. Huang CJ, Pitt HA, Lipsett PA, Osterman FA, Lillemoe KD, Cameron JL, Zuidema GD: Pyogenic hepatic abscess, changing trends over 42 years. Ann Surg 1996, 223, 600-607.

25. Klatchko BA, Schwartz SI: Diagnostic and therapeutic approaches to pyogenic abscess of the liver. Surg Gynecol Obstet 1989, 168, 332-336.

26. Knoop M, Kling N, Langrehr JM, Bechstein WO, Blumhardt G, Keck H, Neuhaus P: Gibt es noch eine Indikation zur Leberresektion bei Leberabszessen? Zentralbl Chir 1995, 120, 461-466.

27. Kuligowska E, Connors SK, Shapiro JH: Liver abscess: sonography in diagnosis and treatment. AJR 1982, 138, 253-257.

28. Lambiase RE, Deyoe L, Cronan JJ, Dorfman GS: Percutaneous drainage of 335 consecutive abscesses: results of primary drainage with 1-year follow-up. Radiology 1992, 184, 167-179.

29. Lee JF, Block GE: The changing clinical pattern of hepatic abscess. Arch Surg 1972, 104, 465.

30. Lee KT, Sheen PC, Chen JS, Ker CG: Pyogenic liver abscess: multivariate analysis of risk factors. World J Surg 1991, 15, 372-377.

31. Maher jr JA, Reynolds TB, Yellin AE: Successful medical treatment of pyogenic liver abscess. Gastroenterology 1979, 77, 618-622.

32. Marcus SG, Walsh TJ, Pizzo PA, Danforth jr DN: Hepatic abscess in cancer patients. Arch Surg 1993, 128, 1358-1364.

33. Matthews JB, Gertsch P, Baer HU, Blumgart LH: Hepatic abscess after biliary tract procedures. Surg Gynecol Obstet 1990, 170, 469-475.

34. Mc Corkell SJ, Niles NL: Pyogenic liver abscesses: another look at medical management. Lancet 1985, i, 803-806.

35. Mc Donald AP, Howard RJ: Pyogenic liver abscess. World J Surg 1980, 4, 369-380.

36. Mc Donald ML, Corey GR, Gallis HA, Durack DT: Single and multiple pyogenic liver abscess: natural history, diagnosis and treatment with emphasis on percutaneous drainage. Medicine 1984, 63, 291.

37. Mc Fadzean AJS, Chang KPS, Wong CC: Solitary pyogenic abscess treated by closed aspiration and antibiotics: fourteen consecutive cases with recovery. Br J Surg 1953, 41, 141-152.

38. Miedema BW, Dineen P: The diagnosis and treatment of pyogenic liver abscesses. Ann Surg 1984, 200, 328-334.

39. Minuk GY, Nicole LE, Sherman T: Cryptogenic abscess of the liver. Arch Surg 1987, 122, 906-908.

40. Mischinger HJ, Hauser H, Rabl H, Quehenberger F, Werkgartner G, Rubin R, Deu E: Pyogenic liver abscess: studies of therapy and analysis of risk factors. World J Surg 1994, 18, 852-858.

41. Moore SW, Millar AJW, Cywes S: Conservative initial treatment for liver abscess in children. Br J Surg 1994, 81, 872-74.

42. Nosher JL, Giudici M, Needell GS, Brolin RE: Elective one stage abdominal operations after percutaneous catheter drainage of pyogenic liver abscess. Am Surg 1993, 59, 658-663.

43. Ochsner A, De Bakey M, Murray S: Pyogenic abscess of the liver. An analysis of 47 cases with review of the literature. Am J Surg 1938, 40, 292-319.

44. Pitt HA, Zuidema GD: Factors influencing mortality in the treatment of pyogenic hepatic abscess. Surg Gynecol Obstet 1975, 140, 228-234.

45. Pitt HA: Surgical management of hepatic abscesses. World J Surg 1990, 14, 498-504.

46. Rintoul R, O`Riordain MG, Laurenson IF, Crosbie JL, Allan PL, Garden OJ: Changing management of pyogenic liver abscess. Br J Surg 1996, 83, 1215-1218.

47. Robert JH, Mirescu D, Ambrosetti P, Khoury G, Greenstein AJ, Rohner A: Critical review of the treatment of pyogenic hepatic abscess. Surg Gynecol Obstet 1992, 174, 97-102.

48. Rubin RH, Swartz MN, Malt R: Hepatic abscess: changes in clinical, bacteriological and therapeutic aspects. Am J Med 1974, 57, 601-610.

49. Sherman JD, Robbins SL: Changing trends in the casuistics of hepatic abscess. Am J Med 1960, 28, 943-950.

50. Stain SC, Yellin AE, Donovan AJ, Brien HW: Pyogenic liver abscess, modern treatment. Arch Surg 1991, 126, 991-996.

51. Swallow CJ, Rotstein OD: Management of pyogenic liver abscess in the era of computed tomography. Can J Surg 1990, 33, 355-362.

52. Teitz S, Guidetti-Sharon A, Manor H, Halevy A: Pyogenic liver abscess: warning indicator of silent colonic cancer. Dis Colon Rectum 1995, 38, 1220-1223.

53. Vakil N, Hayne G, Sharma A, Hardy D, Slutsky A: Liver abscess in Crohn's disease. Am J Gastroenterol 1994, 89, 1090-1095.

54. Wong KP: Percutaneous drainage of pyogenic liver abscesses. World J Surg 1990, 14, 492-497.

55. Alonso Cohen MA, Galera MJ, Ruiz M, Puig La Calle jr J, Rius X, Artigas V, Puig La Calle J: Splenic abscess. World J Surg 1990, 14, 513-517.

56. Battacharyya N, Ablin DS, Koloske AM: Stapeled partial splenectomy for splenic abscess in a child. J Pediatr Surg 1989, 24, 316-317.

57. Chou YH, Hsu CC, Tiu CM, Chang T: Splenic abscess: sonographic diagnosis and percutaneous drainage or aspiration. Gastrointest Radiol 1992, 17, 262-266.

58. Chulay JD, Lankerani MR: Splenic abscess. Am J Med 1976, 61, 513-522.

59. Chun CH, Raff MJ, Contreras L, Varghese R, Waterman N, Daffner R, Melo JC: Splenic abscess. Medicine 1980, 59, 50-65.

60. Cullingford G, Watkins D, Watts A, Mallon D: Severe late postsplenectomy infections. Br J Surg 1991, 78, 716.

61. Faught WE, Gilbertson JJ, Nelson EW: Splenic abscess: presentation, treatment options, and results. Am J Surg 1989, 158, 612-614.

62. Fernandes ET, Tavares PB, Garcette CB: Conservative management of splenic abscesses in childhood. J Pediatr Surg 1992, 27, 1578-1579.

63. Fry DE, Richardson JD, Flint LM: Occult splenic abscess: an unrecognized complication of heroin abuse. Surgery 1978, 84, 650-654.

64. Gadacz T., Way LW, Dunphy JE: Changing clinical spectrum of splenic abscesses. Am J Surg 1974, 128, 182-186.

65. Gleich S, Wolin DA, Herbsman H: A review of percutaneous drainage in splenic abscess. Surg Gynecol Obstet 1988, 167, 211-216.

66. Hatley RM, Donaldson JS, Raffensperger JG: Splenic microabscesses in the immuno-

compromised patient. J Pediatr Surg 1989, 24, 697-699.

67. Helton WS, Carrico CJ, Zaveruha PA, Schaller R: Diagnosis and treatment of splenic fungal abscesses in the immuno-suppressed patient. Arch Surg 1986, 121, 580-585.

68. Johnson JD, Raff MJ, Barnwell PA, Chun CH: Splenic abscess, complicating infectious endocarditis. Arch Intern Med 1983, 143, 906-912.

69. Keidl CM, Chusid MJ: Splenic abscess in childhood. Pediatr Infect Dis J 1989, 8, 368.

70. Konigswieser H: Incidence of serious infections after splenectomy in children. Progr Pediatr Surg 1985, 18, 173.

71. Lawhorne TW, Zuidema GD: Splenic abscess. Surgery, 1976, 79, 686-689.

72. Linos DA, Nagorney DM, McIlrath DC: Splenic abscess - the importance of early diagnosis. Mayo Clin Proc 1983, 58, 261-264.

73. Nelken N, Ignatius J, Skinner M, Christensen N: Changing clinical spectrum of splenic abscess. Am J Surg 1987, 154, 27-33.

74. Pickleman JR, Paloyan E, Block GE: The surgical significance of splenic abscess. Surgery 1970, 68, 287-293.

75. Quinn SF, van Sonnenberg E, Casola G, Wittich GR, Neff CC: Interventional radiology in the spleen. Radiology 1986, 161, 289-291.

76. Sands M, Page D, Brown RB: Splenic abscess following non-operative management of splenic rupture. J Pediatr Surg 1986, 21, 900-901.

77. Sarr MG, Zuidema GD: Splenic abscess-presentation, diagnosis, and treatment. Surgery 1982, 92, 480-485.

78. Shah MR, Cue'J, Boyd CM et al: Solitary splenic abscess: a new complication of splenic salvage treated by percutaneous drainage. J Trauma 1987, 27, 337-339.

79. Shah R, Mahour GH, Ford EG, Stanley P: Partial splenic embolization. An effective alternative to splenectomy for hypersplenism. Am Surg 1990, 56, 774-777.

80. Simson JNL: Solitary abscess of the spleen. Br J Surg 1980, 67, 106-110.

81. Smith MD jr, Nio M, Camel JE, Sato JK, Atkinson JB: Management of splenic abscess in immunocompromised children. J Pediatr Surg 1993, 28, 823-826.

82. van Sonnenberg E, Wing VW, Casola GV: Temporizing effect of percutaneous drainage of complicated abscesses in critically ill patients. AJR 1984, 142, 821-826.

83. Tikkakoski T, Siniluoto T, Paivansalo M, Taavitsainen M, Leppanen M, Dean K, Koivisto M, Suramo I: Splenic abscess. Imaging and intervention. Acta Radiologica 1992, 33, 561-565.

84. Van der Laan RT, Verbeeten B, Smits NJ, Lubbers MJ: Computed tomography in the diagnosis and treatment of solitary splenic abscess. J Comput Assist Tomogr 1989, 13, 71-74.

85. de Wit CW, Bode PJ, van Vugt AB: Splenic abscess following non-operative treatment of a splenic rupture caused by blunt abdominal trauma. Injury 1994, 25, 405-406.

86. Ahmad MM, Macon WL: Gangrene of the gallbladder. Am Surg 1983, 49, 155-158.

87. Ainley CC, Williams SJ, Smith AC et al: Gallbladder sepsis after stent insertion for bile duct obstruction: management by percutaneouscholecystostomy. Br J Surg 1991, 78, 961-963.

88. Barie PS, Fischer E: Acute acalculous cholecystitis. J Am Coll Surg 1995, 180, 232-244.

89. Bass EB, Pitt HA, Lillemoe KD: Cost-effectiveness of laparoscopic cholecystectomy versus open cholecystectomy. Am J Surg 1993, 165, 466-471.

90. Boey JH, Way LW: Acute cholangitis. Ann Surg 1980, 191, 264-270.

91. Carey MC: Pathogenesis of gallstones. Am J Surg 1993, 165, 410-419.

92. Cox MR, Wilson TG, Luck AJ, Jeans PL, Padbury A, Toouli J: Laparoscopic cholecystectomy for acute inflammation of the gallbladder. Ann Surg 1993, 218, 630-634.

93. Csendes A, Fernandez M, Uribe P: Bacteriology of the gallbladder bile in normal subjects. Am J Surg 1975, 129, 629-631.

94. Csendes A, Sepulveda A: Intraluminal gallbladder measurements in patients with chronic or acute cholecystitis. Am J Surg 1980, 139, 383-384.

95. Csendes A, Sepulveda A, Burdiles P: Common bile duct pressure in patients with common bile duct stones with or without acute suppurative cholangitis. Arch Surg 1988, 123, 697-699.

96. Deitch EA: Utility and accuracy of ultrasonically-measured gallbladder wall as a diagnostic criteria in biliary tract disease. Dig Did Sci 1981, 26, 686-693.

97. Diamond T, Dolan S, Thompson RLE, Rowlands BJ: Development and reversal of endotoxemia and endotoxin-related death in obstructive jaundice. Surgery 1990, 108, 370-375.

98. Diebel LN, Raafat AM, Dulchowsky SA, Brown WJ: Gallbladder and biliary tract candidiasis. Surgery 1996, 120, 760-765.

99. Diehl AK: Epidemiology and natural history of gallstone disease. Gastroenterol Clin North Am 1991, 20, 1-19.

100. Edlund G, Ljungdahl M: Acute cholecystitis in the elderly. Am J Surg 1990, 159, 414-416.

101. Fabian TC, Hickerson WL, Mangiante EC: Post-traumatic and post-operative acute cholecystitis. Am Surg 1986, 52, 188-192.

102. Fink-Bennett DD, Freitas JE, Ripley SD, Bree RL: The sensitivity of hepatobiliary imaging and real-time ultrasonography in the detection of acute cholecystitis. Arch Surg 1985, 120, 904-906.

103. Flancbaum L, Majerus TC, Cox EF: Acute post-traumatic acalculous cholecystitis. Am J Surg 1985, 150, 252-256.

104. Flowers JL, Bailey RW, Scovill WA, Zucker KA: The Baltimore experience with laparoscopic management of acute cholecystitis. Am J Surg 1991, 161, 388-392.

105. Frazee RC, Nagorney DM, Mucha jr P: Acute acalculous cholecystitis. Mayo Clin Proc 1989, 64, 163-167.

106. Friedman GD: Natural history of asymptomatic and symptomatic gallstones. Am J Surg 1993, 165, 399-404.

107. Gigot JF, Leese T, Dereme T, Coutinho J, Castaing D, Bismuth H: Acute cholangitis: multivariate analysis of risk factors. Ann Surg 1989, 209, 435-438.

108. Glenn F: Acute cholecystitis. Surg Gynecol Obstet 1976, 143, 56-60.

109. Glenn F: Surgical management of acute cholecystitis in patients 65 years of age or older. Ann Surg 1981, 193, 56-59.

110. Glenn F, Becker CG: Acute acalculous cholecystitis: an increasing entity. Ann Surg 1982, 195, 131-136.

111. Gogel HK, Runyon BA, Volpicelli NA: Acute suppurative obstructive cholangitis due to stones: treatment by urgent endoscopic sphincterotomy. Gastrointest Endosc 1987, 33, 210-213.

112. Hiatt JR, Kobayashi MR, Doty JE, Ramming KD: Acalculous candida cholecystitis: a complication of critical surgical illness. Am J Surg 1991, 57, 825-829.

113. Howard RJ: Acute acalculous cholecystitis. Am J Surg 1981, 141, 194-198.

114. Huang SM, Yu SC, Tsang YM, Wei TC, Hsu SC, Chen KM: Complication of percutaneous transhepatic cholangiography and its drainage. J Clin Gastroenterol 1989, 96, 446-452.

115. Hwang TL, Chen MF: Percutaneous gallbladder drainage for acute acalculous cho-

lecystitis during total parenteral nutrition. Br J Surg 1992, 79, 237-238.

116. Järvinen HJ, Hästacka J: Early cholecystectomy for acute cholecystitis. Ann Surg 1980, 191, 501-505.

117. Jardines LA, O'Donnell MR, Johson DL et al: Acalculous cholecystitis in bone marrow transplant patients. Cancer 1993, 71, 354-358.

118. Jeffrey RB, Laing FC, Wong W, Callen PW: Gangrenous cholecystitis: diagnosis by ultrasound. Radiology 1983, 148, 219-221.

119. Jennings WC, Drabek GA, Miller KA: Significance of sludge and thickened wall in ultrasound evaluation of the gallbladder. Surg Gynecol Obstet 1992, 174, 394- 398.

120. Kavin H, Jonas RB, Chowdhury L, Kabins S: Acalculous cholecystitis and cytomegalovirus infection in the aquired immune deficiency syndrome. Ann Intern Med 1986, 104, 53-53.

121. Kimmings AN, van Deventer SJH, Obertop H, Rauws EA, Gouma DJ: Inflammatory and immunologic effects of obstructive jaundice: pathogenesis and treatment. J Am Coll Surg 1995, 181, 567-581.

122. Koo KP, Thirlby RC: Laparoscopic cholecystectomy in acute cholecystitis. What is the optimal timing for operation? Arch Surg 1996, 131, 540-545.

123. Kum CK, Goh JR, Tekant Y, Ngoi SS: Laparoscopic cholecystectomy for acute cholecystitis. Br J Surg 1994, 81, 1651-1654.

124. Lahtinen J, Alhava EM, Aukee S: Acute cholecystitis treated by early and delayed surgery. A controlled clinical trial. Scand J Gastroenterol 1978, 13, 673-678.

125. Lai ECS, Tam PC, Paterson IA, Ng MMT, Fan ST, Choi TK, Wong J: Emergency surgery for acute cholangitis: the high risk patients. Ann Surg 1990, 211, 55-59.

126. La Raja RD, Rotherberg RE, Odom JW, Mueller SC: The incidence of intra-abdo-

minal surgery in aquired immune deficiency syndrome: a statistical review of 904 patients. Surgery 1989, 105, 175-179.

127. Lau JYW, Chung SCS, Leung JWC, Ling TKW, Yung MY, Li AKC: Endoscopic drainage aborts endotoxaemia in acute cholangitis. Br J Surg 1996, 83, 181-184.

128. Lee W, Chang KJ, Lee CS, Chen KM: Surgery in cholangitis: bacteriology and choice of antibiotic Hepatogastroenterology 1992, 39, 347.

129. Leese T, Neoptolemos JR, Baker AR, Carr-Locke DL: Management of acute cholangitis and the impact of endoscopic sphincterotomy. Br J Surg 1986, 73, 988-992.

130. Leung JWC, Chung SCS, Sung JJY, Banez VP, Li AKC: Urgent endoscopic drainage for acute suppurative cholangitis. Lancet 1989, i, 1307-1309.

131. Leung JWC, Venezuela RR: Cholangiosepsis: endoscopic drainage and antibiotic therapy. Endoscopy 1991, 23, 220-223.

132. Lillemoe KD, Pitt HA, Kaufman SL, Cameron JL: Acute cholecystitis occuring as a complication of percutaneous transhepatic drainage. Surg Gynecol Obstet 1989, 168, 348-352.

133. Lipsett PA, Pitt PA: Acute cholangitis. Surg Clin North Am 1990, 70, 1297-1312.

134. Liu CL, Fan ST, Lai ECS, Lo CM, Chu KM: Factors affecting conversion of laparoscopic cholecystectomy to open surgery. Arch Surg 1996, 131, 98-101.

135. Lo CM, Lai ECS, Fan ST, Liu CL, Wong J: Laparoscopic cholecystectomy for acute cholecystitis in the elderly. World J Surg 1996, 20, 983-987.

136. Lo CM, Liu CL, Lai ECS, Fan ST, Wong J: Early versus delayed laparoscopic cholecystectomy for treatment of acute cholecystitis. Ann Surg 1996, 223, 37-42.

137. Lujan JA, Parilla P, Robles R, Torralba JA, Ayllon JG, Liron R, Sanchez-Bueno F: La-

paroscopic cholecystectomy in the treatment of acute cholecystitis. J Am Coll Surg 1995, 181, 75-77.

138. Lygidakis NJ, Brummelkamp WH: The significance of intrabiliary pressure in acute cholangitis. Syrg Gynecol Obstet 1985, 161, 465-469.

139. Marton KI, Doubilet P: How to image the gallbladder in suspected cholecystitis? Ann Intern Med 1988, 109, 722.

140. Mc Arthur P, Cuschieri A, Sells RA, Shields R: Controlled clinical trial of early versus interval cholecystectomy. Br J Surg 1975, 62, 850-852.

141. Mc Dermott MW, Scudamore CH, Brileau LO, Snelling CFT, Kramer TA: Acalculous cholecystitis: it`s role as a complication of major burn injury. Can J Surg 1985, 28, 529-533.

142. Mc Sherry CK, Ferstenberg H, Calhoun WF, Lahman E, Virshup M: The natural history of diagnosed gallstone disease in symptomatic and asymptomatic patients. Ann Surg 1985, 202, 59-63.

143. Mc Sherry CK: Cholecystectomy: the gold standard. Am J Surg 1989, 158, 174-178.

144. Melin MM, Sarr MG, Bender CE, van Heerden JA: Percutaneous cholecystostomy: a valuable technique in high-risk patients with presumed acute cholecystitis. Br J Surg 1995, 82, 1274-1277.

145. Mentzer jr RM, Golden GT, Chandler JG, Horsley III JS: A comparative appraisal of emphysematous cholecystitis. Am J Surg 1975, 129, 10-15.

146. Miller RE, Kimmelstiel FM: Laparoscopic cholecystectomy for acute cholecystitis. Surg Endosc 1993, 7, 296-299.

147. Misra SP, Dwivedi M: Biliary endoprothesis as an alternative to endoscopic nasobiliary drainage in patients with acute cholangitis. Endoscopy 1996, 28, 746-749.

148. Motte S, Deviere J, Dumonceau JM, Serruys E, Thys JP, Cremer H: Risk factors for septicemia following endoscopic biliary stenting. Gastroenterology 1991, 101, 1374-1381.

149. Muller EL, Pitt HA, Thompson jr HE, Doty JE, Mann LL, Manchester B: Antibiotics in infections of the biliary tract. Surg Gynecol Obstet 1987, 165, 285-291.

150. Norrby S, Herlin P, Holmin T, Sjödahl R, Tagesson C: Early or delayed cholecystectomy in acute cholecystitis? A clinical trial. Br J Surg 1983, 70, 163-165.

151. Parry SW, Pelias ME, Browder W: Acalculous hypersensitivity cholecystitis: hypothesis of a new clinicopathologic entity. Surgery 1988, 104, 911-916.

152. Ohara N, Schaefer J: Clinical significance of biliary sludge. J Clin Gastroenterol 1990, 12, 291-294.

153. Ong CL, Wong TH, Rauff A: Acute gallbladder perforation - a dilemma in early diagnosis. Gut 1991, 32, 956-958.

154. Orlando R, Gleason E, Drezner AD: Acute acalculous cholecystitis in the critically ill patient. Am J Surg 1983, 145, 472-476.

155. Ralls PW, Colletti PM, Lapin SA: Real-time sonography in suspected acute cholecystitis. Radiology 1985, 155, 767-771.

156. Rattner DW, Ferguson C, Warshaw AL: Factors associated with successful laparoscopic cholecystectomy for acute cholecystitis. Ann Surg 1993, 217, 233-236.

157. Reiss R, Nudelman I, Gutman C, Deutsch A: Changing trends in surgery for acute cholecystitis. World J Surg 1990, 14, 567-571.

158. Reynolds BM, Dargan EL: Acute obstructive cholangitis, a distinct clinical syndrome. Ann Surg 1959, 150, 299-303.

159. Roslyn JJ, Pitt HA, Mann L, Fonkalsrud EW, Den Besten L: Parenteral nutrition induced gallbladder disease: a reason for early cholecystectomy. Am J Surg 1984, 148, 58-63.

160. Sariego J, Matsumoto T, Kerstein M: Significance of wall thickness in gallbladder disease. Arch Surg 1992, 127, 1216-1218.

161. Savoca PE, Longo WE, Pasternak B, Gusberg RJ: Does visceral ischemia play a role in the pathogenesis of acute acalculous cholecystitis? J Clin Gastroenterol 1990, 12, 33-36.

162. Savoca PE, Longo WE, Zucker KA, McMillen MM, Modlin IM: The increasing prevalence of acalculous cholecystitis in outpatients: results of a 7-year study. Ann Surg 1990, 211, 433-437.

163. Scher KS, Sarap D, Jaggers RL: Acute acalculous cholecystitis complicating aortic aneurysm repair. Surg Gynecol Obstet 1986, 163, 475-478.

164. Sessions SL, Scoma RS, Sheik FA, Mc Geehin WH, Smink jr RD: Acute acalculous cholecystitis following open heart surgery. Am Surg 1993, 59, 74-77.

165. Sharp KW: Acute cholecystitis. Surg Clin North Am 1988, 68, 269-279.

166. Shirai Y, Tsukada K, Kawaguchi H, Ohtani T, Muto T, Hatakeyama K: Percutaneous transhepatic cholecystostomy for acute cholecystitis. Br J Surg 1993, 80, 1440-1442.

167. Simeone JF, Brink JA, Mueller PR: The sonographic diagnosis of acute gangrenous cholecystitis: importance of the Murphy sign. Am J Roentgenol 1989, 152, 289-290.

168. Simmons RK, Sinanan MN, Coldwell MD: Gangrenous cholecystitis as a complication of hepatic artery embolisation: Surgery 1992, 112, 106-110.

169. Smith JP, Bodai BI: Empyema of the gallbladder - potential consequence of medical intensive care. Crit Care Med 1982, 10, 451-452.

170. Stevens PE, Harrison NA, Ramford DJ: Acute acalculous cholecystitis in acute renal failure. Intensive Care Med 1988, 14, 411.

171. Stewart L, Pellegrini CA, Way LW: Cholangiovenous reflux pathways as defined by corrosin casting and scanning electron microscopy. Am J Surg 1988, 155, 23-28.

172. Sung JY, Costerton JW, Shaffer EA: Defense system in the biliary tract against bacterial infection. Dig Dis Sci 1992, 37, 689.

173. Thompson jr JE, Bennion RS, Doty JE, Muller EL, Pitt HA: Predictive factors for bactibilia in acute cholecystitis: indications for therapy. Arch Surg 1990, 125, 261-264.

174. Thompson jr JE, Pitt HA, Doty JE, Coleman J, Irving C: Broad spectrum penicillin as an adequate therapy for acute cholangitis. Surg Gynecol Obstet 1990, 171, 275-282.

175. Unger SW, Rosenbaum G, Unger HM, Edelman DS: A comparison of laparoscopic and open treatment of acute cholecystitis. Surg Endosc 1993, 7, 408-411.

176. Vauthey JN, Lerut J, Martini M, Becker C, Gertsch P, Blumgart LH: Indications and limitations of percutaneous cholecystostomy for acute cholecystitis. Surg Gynecol Obstet 1993, 176, 49-54.

177. Warren BL: Small vessel occlusion in acute acalculous cholecystitis. Surgery 1992, 111, 163-168.

178. Werbel GB, Nahrwold DL, Joehl RJ, Vogelzang RL, Rege RV: Percutaneous cholecystostomy in the diagnosis and treatment of acute cholecystitis in the high- risk patient. Arch Surg 1989, 124, 782-786.

179. Wind P, Chevallier JM, Jones D, Frileux P, Cugnenc PH: Cholecystectomy for cholecystitis in patients with aquired immune deficiency syndrome. Am J Surg 1994, 168, 244-246.

180. Zucker KA, Flowers JL, Bailey RW, Graham SM, Buell J, Imbembo AL: Laparoscopic management of acute cholecystitis. Am J Surg 1993, 165, 508- 514.

181. Keynes WM: A non-pancreatic source of the proteolytic enzyme amidase and bacteriology in experimental pancreatitis. Ann. Surg 1980, 191:187-199.

182. Foulis A K: Histological evidence of initiating factors in acute necrotizing pancreatitis in man. J. Clin. Pathol. 1980, 33:1125-1131.

183. Bradley III E L: A clinically based classification system for acute pancreatitis. Arch. Surg. 1993, 128:581-584.

184. Frileux P, Parc Y: Pancreatic infections. Eur. J. Surg. 1996, Suppl., 576:53-55.

185. Schmidt J, Fernandez-del Castillo C, Rattner DW, Lewandrowski K, Compton CC, Warshaw AL: Trypsinogen activation peptides in experimental pancreatitis in the rat. Prognostic implications and histopathologic correlates. Gastroenterology 1992, 103:1009-1016.

186. Steinberg W, Tenner S: Acute pancreatitis. N. Engl. J. Med. 1994, 330:1198-1210.

187. Watanabe O, Baccino FM, Steer ML, Meldolesi J: Supramaximal cerulein stimulation and ultrastructure of rat pancreatic acinar cell: early morphological changes during development of experimental pancreatitis. Am. J. Physiol. 1984, 246:G457.

188. Warshaw AL: Damage prevention versus damage control in acute pancreatitis. Gastroenterology 1993, 104:1216-1219.

189. Klar E, Rattner DW, Compton C, Stanford G, Chernow B, Warshaw AL: Adverse effect of therapeutic vasoconstrictors in experimental pancreatitis. Ann Surg 1991, 214:168-174.

190. Beger, HG, Bittner R, Block S, Büchler M: Bacterial contamination of pancreatic necrosis. Gastroenterology 91, 1986, 433-438.

191. Beger HG, Büchler M, Bittner W, Oettinger W, Block, S, Nevalainen T: Necrosectomy and post-operative local lavage in patients with necrotizing pancreatitis: Results of a prospective clinical trial. World J. Surg. 12, 1982, 255-262.

192. Balthazar EJ, Robinson DL, Megibow A J, Ranson JHC: Acute pancreatitis: Value of CT in establishing prognosis. Radiology 1990, 174: 331-336.

193. Bradley III EL, Allen K: A prospective longitudinal study of observation versus surgical intervention in the management of necrotizing pancreatitis. Am. J. Surg. 1991, 19-25.

194. Beger HG: Surgery in acute pancreatitis. Hepato-Gastroenterology 1991, 38:92-96.

195. Renner IG, Savage III WT, Pantoja JL, Renner VJ: Death due to acute pancreatitis: a retrospective analysis of 405 autopsy cases. Dig. Dis. Sci. 30, 1985, 1005-1018.

196. Larvin M, Chalmers AG, Robionson PJ, McMahon M J: Debridement and closed cavity irrigation for the treatment of pancreatic necrosis. Br. J. Surg, 76, 1989, 465-471.

197. Stanten R, Frey CF: Comprehensive management of acute necrotizing pancreatitis and pancreatic abscess. Arch. Surg. 1990, 125: 1269-1275.

198. Gerzof SG, Banks, PA, Robbins, AH et al: Early diagnosis of pancreatic infection by computed tomography-guided aspiration. Gastroenterology 1987, 93:1315-1320.

199. Widdison AL, Karanjia ND: Pancreatic infection complicating acute pancreatitis. Br. J. Surg. 1993, 80:148-154.

200. Rattner DW, Legermate DA, Lee MJ, Mueller PR, Warshaw AL: Early surgical debridement of symptomatic pancreatic necrosis is beneficial irrespective of infection. Am. J. Surg., 1992, 163, 105-110.

201. Machado MCC, Bacchella T, Moneiro da Cunha JE et al: Surgical treatment of pancreatic necrosis. Dig. Dis. Sci 1986, 31:25 S.

202. Bittner R, Block S, Büchler M, Beger HG: Pancreatic abscess and infected pancreatic necrosis: differential local septic complications in acute pancreatitis. Dig. Dis. Sci. 1987, 32, 1082-1087.

203. Pederzoli P, Bassi C, Elio A, Corra S, Nifosi F, Benetti G: The infected necrosis is a prognostic factor in necrotizing pancreatitis. Gastroenterology 1989, 96:A387.

204. D'Egidio A, Schein M: Surgical strategies in the treatment of pancreatic necrosis and infection. Br. J. Surg. 1991, 78:133-137.

205. Howard TJ, Wiebke EA, Mogavero G et al: Classification and treatment of local septic complications in acute pancreatitis. Am. J. Surg. 1995, 170:44-50.

206. Kemppainen E, Sainio V, Haapiainen R, Kivisaari L, Kivilaakso E, Puolakkainen P: Early localization of necrosis by contrast-enhanced computed tomography can predict outcome in severe acute pancreatitis. Br. J. Surg. 1996, 83:924-929.

207. Farkas G, Marton J, Mandi Y, Szederkenyi E: Surgical strategy and management of infected pancreatic necrosis. Br. J. Surg. 1996, 83:930-933.

208. Dickson AP, Foulis AK, Imrie CW: Histology and bacteriology of closed duodenal loop models of experimental acute pancreatitis in the rat. Digestion 1986, 34:15-31.

209. Gianotti L, Munda R, Alexander JW, Tchervenkov JI, Babcock GF: Bacterial translocation: a potential source for infection in acute pancreatitis. Pancreas 1993, 8:551-558.

210. Widdison AL, Karanjia ND, Reber HA: Routes of spread of pathogens to the pancreas in a feline model of acute pancreatitis. Gut 1994, 35:1306-1310.

211. Widdison AL, Alvarez C, Chang YB, Karanjia ND, Reber HA: Sources of pancreatic pathogens in acute pancreatitis in cats. Pancreas 1994, 9:536-541.

212. Runkel NF, Moody FG, Smith GS, Rodriguez LF, LaRocco MT, Miller TA: The role of the gut in the development of sepsis in acute pancreatitis. J. Surg. Res. 1991, 51:18-23.

213. Mainous M, Tso P, Berg RD, Deitch EA: Studies of the route, magnitude and time course of bacterial translocation in a model of systemic inflammation. Arch. Surg. 1991, 126:33-37.

214. Medich DS, Lee TK, Melhem MF, Rowe MI, Schraut WH, Lee KKW: Pathogenesis of pancreatic sepsis. Am. J. Surg. 1993, 165:46-50.

215. Tarpila E, Nyström PO, Franzen L, Ihse I: Bacterial translocation during acute pancreatitis in the rat. Eur. J. Res. 1993, 159:109-113.

216. Runkel NSF, Rodriguez LF, Moody FG: Mechanisms of sepsis in acute pancreatitis in opossums. Am. J. Surg. 1995, 169:227-232.

217. Foitzik T, Fernandez-del Castillo C, Ferraro MJ, Mithöfer K, Rattner DW, Warshaw AL: Pathogenesis and prevention of early pancreatic infection in experimental acute necrotizing pancreatitis. Ann. Surg. 1995, 222:179-185.

218. Wang X, Andersson R, Soltesz V, Leveau P, Ihse I: Gut origin sepsis, macrophage function and oxygen extraction associated with acute pancreatitis in the rat. World J. Surg. 1996, 20:299-308.

219. Rao R, Prinz RA, Kazantsev GB et al: Effects of granulocyte colony-stimulating factor in severe pancreatitis. Surgery 1996, 119:657-663.

220. Berg R, Wommack E, Deitch EA: Immunosuppression and intestinal bacterial overgrowth synergistically promote bacterial translocation from the GI tract. Arch. Surg. 1988, 123:1359-1364.

221. McFadden DW: Organ failure and multiple organ system failure in acute pancreatitis. Pancreas 1991, 6 (Suppl 1):37-43.

222. Andersson R, Wang XD, Ihse I: The influence of abdominal sepsis on acute pancreatitis in rats. Pancreas 1995, 11: 365-373.

223. Curley PJ, McMahon MJ, Lancaster F et al: Reduction in circulating levels of CD4-positive lymphocytes in acute pancreatitis: relationship to endotoxin, Interleukin 6 and disease severity. Br. J. Surg. 1993, 80:1312-1315.

224. Larvin M, Alexander DJ, Switala SF, McMahon MJ: Impaired mononuclear phagocyte function in patients with severe acute pancreatitis: evidence from studies of plasma clearance of trypsin and monocyte phagocytosis. Dig Dis Sci 1993, 38:18-27.

225. Widdison AL, Cunningham S: Immune function early in acute pancreatitis. Br. J. Surg. 1996, 83:633-636.

226. Beger HG, Krautzberger W, Bittner R, Block S, Büchler M: Results of surgical treatment of necrotizing pancreatitis. World J. SURG. 1985, 9:972-979.

227. Bradley III EL, Gonzalez AC, Clements JL (jr): Acute pancreatic pseudocysts: incidence and implications. Ann. Surg. 1976, 184:734-737.

228. Siegelman SS, Copeland BE, Saba GP, Cameron JL, Sanders RC: CT of fluid collections associated with pancreatitis. AJR 1980, 134:1121-1132.

229. Wilson C, Heads A, Shenkin A, Imrie CW: C-reactive protein, antiproteases and complement factors as objective markers of severity in acute pancreatitis. Br. J. Surg. 1989, 76:177-181.

230. Schöffel U, Lausen M, Gross V, Heinisch A, Lay L, Schölmerich J, Farthmann EH: Monitoring of septic complications in acute pancreatitis. Surg. Res. Comm. 1990, 7:329-334.

231. Imrie CW, Benjamin IS, Ferguson JC, McKay AJ, Mackenzie I, O'Neill J, Blumgart LH: A single-center double-blind trial of Trasylol therapy in primary acute pancreatitis. Br. J. Surg. 1978, 65: 337-341.

232. Gross V, Schölmerich F, Leser HG et al: Granulocyte elastase in assessment of severity of acute pancreatitis. Dig. Dis. Sci. 1990, 35: 97-105.

233. Bank S: Chronic pancreatitis: clinical features and medical management. Am. J. Gastroent. 1986, 81:153-167.

234. Ranson JHC, Rifkind KM, Roses DF, Fink SD, Eng K, Spencer FC: Prognostic signs and the role of operative management in acute pancreatitis. Surg. Gyn. Obstet. 1974, 139:69-81.

235. Wilson C, Heath I, Imrie CW: Prediction of outcome in acute pancreatitis: a comparative study of APACHE II, clinical assessment and multiple factor scoring systems. Br. J. Surg. 1990, 77:1260-1264.

236. Sarr MG, Nagorney DM, Mucha P jr, Farnett MB, Johnson CD: Acute necrotizing pancreatitis: management by planned, staged pancreatic necrosectomy/debridement and delayed primary wound closure over drains. Br. J. Surg. 1991, 78: 576-581.

237. Ranson JHC: Etiological and prognostic factors in human acute pancreatitis: a review. Am. J. Gastroent. 1982, 77: 633-638.

238. Block S, Maier W, Bittner R, Büchler M, Malfertheiner P, Beger HG: Identification of pancreas necrosis in severe acute pancreatitis: imaging procedures versus clinical staging. Gut 1986, 27:1035-1042.

239. Clavien PA, Hauser H, Meyer P, Rohner A: Value of contrast-enhanced computerized tomography in the early diagnosis and prognosis of acute pancreatitis. Am. J. Surg. 1988, 155:457-466.

240. Larvin M, Chalmer AG, McMahon MJ: A technique of dynamic CT angiography for the precise identification of pancreatic necrosis. Gastroenterology 1988, 94:251-256.

241. Silverstein W, Isikoff MB, Hill MC, Barkin J: Diagnostic imaging of acute pancreatitis: prospective study using CT and sonography. AJR 1981, 137:497-502.

242. Bradley III EL, Murphy F, Ferguson C: Prediction of pancreatic necrosis by dynamic

pancreatography. Ann. Surg. 1989, 210:495-503.

243. Nuutinen P, Kivisaari L, Schroeder T: Contrast-enhanced computed tomography and microangiography of the pancreas in acute human hemorrhagic/necrotizing pancreatitis. Pancreas 1988, 3:53-60.

244. Hiatt JR, Fink AS, King W: Percutaneous aspiration of peripancreatic fluid collections: a safe method to detect infection. Surgery 1987, 101:523-530.

245. Büchler M, Malfertheiner P, Uhl W et al: Gabexate mesilate in human acute pancreatitis. Gastroenterology 1993, 104:1165-1170.

246. Valderrama R, Perez-Mateo M, Navarro S et al: Multicenter double-blind trial of gabexate mesilate(FOY) in unselected patients with acute pancreatitis. Digestion 1992, 51:65-70.

247. Choi TK, Mok F, Zhan WH, Fan ST, Lai EC, Wong J: Somatostatin in the treatment of acute pancreatitis: a prospective randomized controlled trial. Gut 1989, 30:223-227.

248. D'Amico D, Favia G, Biasiato R et al: The use of Somatostatin in acute pancreatitis - results of a multicenter trial. Hepatogastroenterology 1990, 37:92-98.

249. Gjorup I, Roikjaer O, Andersen B et al: A double blind multicenter trial of Somatostatin in the treatment of acute pancreatitis. Surg. Gynecol. Obstet. 1992, 175:397-400.

250. Klar E, Mall G, Messmer K, Herfarth C, Rattner DW, Warshaw AL: Improvement of impaired pancreatic microcirculation by isovolemic hemodilution protects pancreatic morphology in acute biliary pancreatitis. Surg. Gynecol. Obstet. 1993, 176:144-150.

251. Schmidt J, Fernandez-del Castillo C, Rattner DW, Lewandrowski KB, Messmer K, Warshaw AL: Hyperoncotic ultrahigh molecular weight dextran solutions reduce trypsinogen activation, prevent acinar necrosis and lower mortality in rodent pancreatitis. Am. J. Surg. 1993, 165:40-44.

252. Levant JA, Secrist DM, Resin H, Sturdevant RAL, Guth PH: Nasogastric suction in the treatment of alcoholic pancreatitis: a controlled study. JAMA 1974, 229:51-52.

253. Loiudice TA, Lang JF, Mehta H, Banta L: Treatment of acute alcoholic pancreatitis: the roles of cimetidine and nasogastric suction. Am. J. Gastroenterol. 1984, 79:553-558.

254. Naeije R, Salingret E, Clumeck N, De Troyer A, Devis G: Is nasogastric suction necessary in acute pancreatitis? BMJ 1978, 2:659-660.

255. Johnson CD: Antibiotic prophylaxis in severe acute pancreatitis. Br. J. Surg. 1996, 83:883-884.

256. Pederzoli P, Bassi C, Vesentini S, Campedelli A: A randomized multicenter trial of antibiotic prophylaxis of septic complications in acute necrotizing pancreatitis with Imipenem. Surg. Gynecol. Obstet. 1993, 176:480-483.

257. Sainio V, Kemppainen E, Puolakkainen P et al: Early antibiotic treatment in acute necrotizing pancreatitis. Lancet 1995, 346:663-667.

258. Delcenserie R, Yzet T, Ducroix JP: Prophylactic antibiotics in treatment of severe acute alcoholic pancreatitis. Pancreas 1996, 13:198-201.

259. Luiten EJT, Hop WCJ, Lange JF, Bruining HA: Controlled clinical trial of selective decontamination for the treatment of severe acute pancreatitis. Ann. Surg. 1995, 222:57-65.

260. Gianotti L, Munda R, Gennari R, Pyles T, Alexander JW: Effect of different regimens of gut decontamination on bacterial translocation and mortality in experimental acute pancreatitis. Eur. J. Surg. 1995, 161:85-92.

261. Fan ST, Lai ECS, Mok FPT, Lo CM, Zheng SS, Wong J: Early treatment of acute biliary pancreatitis by endoscopic papillotomy. N. ENGL. J. MED. 1993, 328:228-232.

262. Fölsch UR, Nitsche R, Lüdtke R et al: Early ERCP and papillotomy compared with conservative treatment for acute biliary pancreatitis. N. ENGL. J. MED. 1997, 336:237-242.

263. Bradley III EL: Management of infected pancreatic necrosis by open drainage. Ann. Surg. 1987, 206:542-550.

264. Beger HG, Büchler M, Bittner R, Block S, Nevalainen T, Roscher R: Necrosectomy and post-operative local lavage in necrotizing pancreatitis. Br. J. Surg. 1988, 75:207-212 .

265. Teerenhovi O, Nordback I, Isolauri J: Influence of pancreatic resection on systemic complications in acute necrotizing pancreatitis. Br. J. Surg. 1988, 75:793-795.

266. Aldridge MC, Ornstein M, Glazer G, Dudley HAF: Pancreatic resection for severe acute pancreatitis. Br. J. Surg 1985, 72:796-800.

267. Smadja C, Bismuth H: Pancreatic debridement in acute necrotizing pancreatitis: an obsolete procedure? Br. J. Surg. 1986, 73:408-410.

268. Kelly TR, Wagner DS: Gallstone pancreatitis: a prospective randomized trial of the timing of surgery. Surgery 1988, 104:600-605.

269. Ihsel, Evander A, Holmberg JT, Gustafson I: Influence of peritoneal lavage on objective prognostic signs in acute pancreatitis. Ann. Surg. 1986. 204:122-127.

270. Mayer AD, McMahon MJ, Corfield AP et al: Controlled clinical trial of peritoneal lavage for the treatment of severe acute pancreatitis. NEJM 1985, 312:399-404.

271. Teerenhovi O, Nordback I, Eskola J: High volume lesser sac lavage in acute necrotizing pancreatitis. Br. J. Surg. 1989, 76:370-373.

272. Pemberton JH, Becker JM, Dozois RR, Nagorney DM, Jestrup, D, Remine WH: Controlled open lesser sac drainage for pancreatic abscess. Ann. Surg. 1986, 203:600-604.

273. Ranson JHC: The role of surgery in the management of acute pancreatitis. Ann. Surg. 1990, 211:382-393.

274. Nicholson ML, Mortensen NJ, Espiner HJ: Pancreatic abscess: results of prolonged irrigation of the pancreatic bed after surgery. Br. J. Surg. 1988, 75:88-91.

275. Doglietto GB, Gui D, Pacelli F et al: Open versus closed treatment of secondary pancreatic infections. Arch. Surg. 1994, 129:689-693.

276. Broughan TA, Hermann RE, Hardesty IJ, Paranandi L: Fascial closure in the management of infected pancreatic necrosis. Am. Surg. 1994, 60:309-312.

277. Pederzoli P, Bassi C, Vesentini S et al: Retroperitoneal and peritoneal drainage and lavage in the treatment of severe necrotizing pancreatitis. Surg. Gynecol. Obstet. 1990, 170:197-203.

278. Garcia-Sabrido JL, Tellado JM, Christou NV, Polo JR, Valdecantos E: Treatment of severe intra-abdominal sepsis and/or necrotic foci by an "open-abdomen" approach: zipper and zipper-mesh techniques. Arch. Surg. 1988, 123:152-156.

279. Harris JA, Jury RP, Catto J, Glover JL: Closed drainage versus open packing of infected pancreatic necrosis. Am. Surg: 1995, 61:612-618.

280. Allardyce DB: Incidence of necrotizing pancreatitis and factors related to mortality. Am. J. Surg. 1987, 154:295-299.

281. Traverso LW: Discussion to: Stanten R, Frey CF: Comprehensive management of acute necrotizing pancreatitis and pancreatic abscess. Arch. Surg. 1990, 125:1274.

282. Gerzof SG, Johnson WC, Robbins AH, Spechler SJ, Nebseth DC: Percutaneous drainage of infected pancreatic pseudocysts. Arch Surg 1984, 119:888-893.

283. Rotman N, Matieu D, Anglade MC, Fagniez PL: Failure of percutaneous drainage of pancreatic abscesses complicating severe acute pancreatitis. Surg. Gynecol. Obstet. 1992, 174:141-144.

284. Lee MJ, Rattner DW, Legemate DA et al: Acute complicated pancreatitis: redefining the role of interventional radiology. Radiology 1992, 183:171-174.

285. Stone HH, Strom PR, Mullins RJ: Pancreatic abscess management by subtotal resection and packing. World J. Surg. 1984, 8:340-345.

286. Stricker PD, Hunt DR: Surgical aspects of pancreatic abscess. Br. J. Surg. 1986, 73:644-646.

287. Tsiotos GG, Smith CD, Sarr MG: Incidence and management of pancreatic and enteric fistulas after surgical management of severe necrotizing pancreatitis. Arch. Surg. 1995, 13:48-52.

288. Doberneck RC: Intestinal fistula complicating necrotizing pancreatitis. Am. J. Surg. 1989, 76:362-367.

289. Bouilot JL, Alexandre JH, Vuong NP: Colonic involvement in acute necrotizing pancreatitis: results of surgical treatment. World J. Surg. 1989, 13:84-87.

290. Aldridge MC, Francis ND, Glazer G, Dudley HAF: Colonic complications of severe acute pancreatitis. Br. J. Surg. 1989, 76:362-367.

Specific Approaches to Intra-abdominal Infections in Liver Transplant Recipients

Faouzi Saliba, Jina Krissat and Henri Bismuth

1. INTRODUCTION

Liver transplantation (LT) has become an accepted therapy for end stage liver disease. Despite improvements in surgical technique and immunosuppressive regimen, infection remains the most serious complication occurring after LT. Although much attention was focused on viral recurrence infection following LT, bacterial infections remain the major cause of morbidity and mortality in these patients. In previous studies from the University of Pittsburgh, infections were reported in 81% to 83% of the liver transplant recipients with a mean of 1.85 to 2.8 episodes of infection per patient [1,2]. We and other centers reported infections in 47% to 75% of the patients with a mean of 0.8 to 2.5 episodes of infection per patient [3-6] with an incidence of major infections ranged between 57% to 67%.

Intra-abdominal infection (IAI) and bacteremia constitute the most frequent type of bacterial infections following LT. Studies of IAI in non-transplant recipients have yielded a mortality that ranged from 3.5% to more than 60% [7]. After LT, mortality is as-

sociated with infection in more than 70% of the patients. The liver transplant recipient is a prime candidate for bacterial infection given the direct exposure of the biliary tract and graft to endogenous gastrointestinal flora. The risk of translocation of bacteria and endotoxins is enhanced due to increased intestinal permeability engendered by the surgical procedure. The necessity for administration of corticosteroids and other immunosuppressive agents to induce and maintain graft tolerance is another major determinant of infection. Distinctly, the high rate of infection in the liver transplant patient is directly related to the technical aspects of liver transplantation.

2. GENERAL AND OPERATIVE ASPECTS OF LIVER TRANSPLANTATION

2.1. Surgical technique

Hepatic allografts were harvested using a rapid perfusion technique [8]. LT was performed using a standard manner. In patients who tolerate intraoperative supra-hepatic veina cava (IVC) cross-clamping test for a period of at least 2 minutes, LT was performed without the use of a veino-venous by-pass (VVB). Those patients who, despite adequate volume resucitation, develop hemodynamic instability with IVC cross-clamping test, underwent LT with the support of VVB during the anhepatic phase.

The liver graft was then revascularized by sequential completion of the supra-hepatic and infra-hepatic caval anastomosis. Patients who underwent a total hepatectomy with preservation of the caval flow, had an end-to-side caval anastomosis. Prior to completing the portal vein anastomosis, the liver graft was flushed via the portal vein with cold 4% serum albumin solution. The arterial anastomosis was carried out in an end-to-end fashion and was usually performed between the donor celiac axis and the recipient vessel, at the level of the bifurcation of the common hepatic artery. Reconstruction of the biliary tract consisted of a choledocho-choledochostomy with primary anastomosis of the donor to the recipient's common bile duct with or without a T-tube, or a choledocho-jejunostomy with anastomosis of the biliary duct to a Roux-en-Y jejunal loop. Usually, three large-bore closed suction drains were placed, one in the right supra-hepatic area and 2 in the right and left infra-hilar regions.

2.2. Immunosuppression

The type of immunosuppressive basic regimen changed during the history of the program. From our experience, eight hundred and thirty three patients (96%) received a triple drug immunosuppressive basic regimen: ciclosporine was initiated post-operatively at 1 mg/kg/day and rapidly increased to 6 mg/kg/day, by the third post-operative

day; ciclosporine was adjusted to maintain monoclonal blood levels initially in the 450 to 650 ng/ml range and subsequently between 250 and 450ng/ml. Methylprednisolone was administered at the dose of 10 mg/kg at day 0, 5 mg/kg at day 1, then rapidly reduced to 0.3 mg/kg/day by day 8. Azathioprine was given at 2 mg/kg/day. One hundred and twenty six patients (14%) received prior to the ciclosporine regimen a course of 10 to 14 days of rabbit antilymphocyte globulin due to acute perioperative renal failure. More recently, thirty nine patients were treated with a combination of Tacrolimus and steroids as a part of the European multicenter tacrolimus trial. Tacrolimus was initiated post-operatively at 0,3 mg/kg/day by the naso-gastric tube until they were able to take oral medications. Steroids were given at 10 mg/Kg/day at day 0, then 20 mg daily.

Rejection episodes were treated with one to three boluses of 1000 mg of methylprednisolone followed by a 10-day course of ALG or OKT3 monoclonal antibodies for episodes of rejection refractory to steroid treatment.

2.3. Postoperative care

Antibioprophylaxis consisted of the administration of an Ureidopenicillin during 48 to 72 hours. Those patients who had prior to transplantation previous episodes of infections received a 7 to 10 day course of antibiotherapy adapted to previous cultured micro-organisms. Patients were maintained on elective ventilation for 6 to 36 hours, until they were normothermic hemodynamically stable with satisfactory blood gases and urinary output. Parenteral nutritional support was instituted at an early stage in patients who had clinical signs of denutrition prior to transplantation. Abdominal drains, urinary catheters, intraveinous and intra-arterial cannulae were removed as soon as possible to minimize risk of retrograde contamination and infection. Abdominal doppler-ultrasonography was routinely performed each day of the first week to confirm vascular anastomosis patency and to detect perihepatic ascitic fluid or blood collections. If there was any doubt of vascular patency, then an angiography was performed to assess the diagnosis in time for corrective surgery. In the presence of fever, puncture of collections under ultrasound guidance for culture was performed; and if there was evidence of sepsis a drainage and if necessary a laparotomy was carried out. The biliary T-tube remained on free drainage for 14 days, then a T-tube cholangiogram was performed and if there was no evidence of leakage or obstruction, the tube was clamped. The T-tube was removed after 3 months. Liver biopsies were done only when clinically or biochemically indicated. Cultures of blood, urine, tracheal aspirates and abdominal drainage were done routinely twice a week in the Intensive care unit and once a week in the hospital ward as well if fever occurred. A bronchial fibroscopy with distal bronchial aspiration and broncho-alveolar lavage cultures were done if clinical and radiological signs of pneumopathy were present.

3. DEFINITIONS

• Bacteremia was defined by the isolation of bacteria in at least one blood culture; for Staphylococcus epidermidis, 2 blood cultures were required.

• IAI were stratified into wound or parietal infections, peritoneal collections (blood, biliary or others), ascitic fluid infections

and peritonitis. Proof of infection necessitated either intraoperative findings and cultures, positive percutaneous ultrasound-guided cultures or heavy growth bacteria in peritoneal liquid drainage.

• Cholangitis required the presence of fever, an elevation of liver enzymes and evidence of cholangitis on the cholangiogram or liver biopsy, together with the isolation of the same micro-organism from both the bile and blood.

4. TIME OCCURRENCE OF BACTERIAL INFECTION

The results of LT have regulary improved over the past decade and data available from both the PITT-UNOS and the European Liver Transplant Registry [9, 10] indicate that the actuarial one-year survival exceeds 70% (figure 1). But analysis of the causes of death indicates that infection still remains the main cause of mortality and morbidity. Forty-two to 89% of the deaths in liver transplant recipients have been associated with infection [1- 5]. In our serie (table 1), mortality was due to infection or sepsis in 89 of the 279 patients (32%). Bacterial infection was responsible death in 29% (82 patients) and accounted for nearly half of the major infections. Micro-organisms involved with bacteremias are resumed in table 2. Fifty six percent of the patients had their first episode of infection within the first two weeks after liver transplantation (Figure 2). The most common sources of bacteremias were IAI (31%), whereas 20% were catheter related, 16% were secondary to pulmonary infections, 2% were due to urinary infections and 31% were of unknown origin. IAI are the most frequent source of bacteremia in liver transplant recipients. In our study as in other reports,

Figure 1
Ten Years Actuarial Patient Survival after Liver Transplantation
(1000 liver transplantations/872 patients)

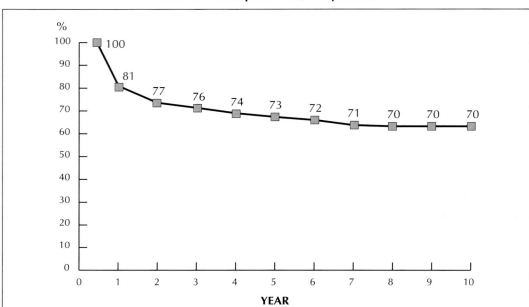

one-third of the origin of bacteremias were related to IAI [1]. Paya et al reported an incidence of IAI of 24.5% diagnosed in 53 patients, whereas 46% of the IAI were associated with bacteremia [3]. Recently, Singh et al found a 24% incidence of bacterial infections with a lower frequency of IAI (7%) and only 14% of the IAI being associated with bacteremia [7].

5. ETIOLOGY OF IAI

IAI were often related to the technical aspects of liver transplantation. The persistence of perihepatic fluid collection or the occurrence of perihepatic hematomas related to the difficulty of the surgery and to coagulation disorders mainly in patients with se-

vere portal hypertension and were very frequent in the early post-operative period. These collections are rarely infected at the time of surgery and frequently were later superinfected. The main micro-organism involved in IAI was Staphylococcus aureus (66%). Abdominal infection usually occurred in the early posto-perative period and is related to vascular anastomosis thrombosis, biliary complications, superficial or deep wound infection, the presence of perihepatic hematomas due to coagulopathy, thrombocytopenia and portal hypertension and to persistent collections of ascitic fluid in the peritoneal cavity. Peritonitis due to rupture of an abdominal viscus, rarely occur. The diagnosis of IAI in these patients is sometimes difficult because of the problem of differentiating between colinization and

Table 1
Causes of death after Liver Transplantation (279 deaths / 872 liver transplantations)

	1 month	2 months	3 months	> 3 months	> 12 months
Operative	11	0	0	0	0
Decerebration	16	1	0	0	0
Primary Non Function	1	0	0	0	0
Cerebral Hemorrhage	4	1	1	0	1
Sepsis	**34**	**14**	**7**	**17**	**17**
Multiple Organ Failure	10	6	1	6	2
Cardiac Disease	4	0	2	3	5
Hyper Acute Rejection	1	0	0	0	0
Chronic Rejection	0	0	0	5	8
Viral Recurrence	0	0	0	3	11
Cancer Recurrence	0	0	0	16	33
Lymphoma	0	0	1	1	3
De Novo Malignancy	0	0	0	4	6
Other	2	2	2	5	12
Total	**83**	**24**	**14**	**60**	**98**

* Decerebration: in patients transplanted for fulminant hepatitis

tissue invasion. Strict surveillance using abdominal ultrasound and CT scan of the abdominal cavity and guided ultrasound puncture of collection or hematomas for cultures are mandatory in patients with fever or hyperleucocytosis. Agressive therapeutic measures using drainage or laparotomy together with an appropriate antibiotherapy should be rapidly installed to avoid fatal progression to septic shock and multiple organ failure.

Many reports in non-transplant recipients [11,12,13] have reported mortality in IAI ranged between 40% to 60%. In our serie, operative mortality for IAI was 17% (table 3). Despite of increasingly effective antimicrobial drugs, IAI remains a life-threatening complication after surgery, indicating the importance of immunological host defense failure following surgical complications. Recent clinical and experimental reports sheds new light to explain IAI [14,15,16]. The concept of gut-origin sepsis contends that several mechanisms causing a failure of the intestinal barrier and leading to translocation of bacteria and endotoxin contribute to the septic state and/or IAI in critically ill patients who have undergone surgery [17,18,19]. In addition to the primary insults enhancing translocation, contributory iatrogenic factors such as systemic antibiotics, prolonged non-enteral nutrition and blood transfusion, predominate [20,21]. The

Table 2
Microorganisms involved with Bacteremia (1066 Positive Blood Cultures in 389 Patients)

BACTERIA	Number of positive blood cultures (%)
GRAM POSITIVE	**737 (69.1%)**
Staphylococcus aureus	420 (39%)
Staphylococcus epidermidis	228 (21%)
Enterococcus	77 (7%)
Other Streptococcus	9
Listeria monocytogenes	3
GRAM NEGATIVE	**320 (30%)**
E. Coli	81 (7.6%)
Pseudomonas aeruginosa	71 (6.6%)
Stenotrophomonas maltophilia	13 (1.2%)
Acinetobacter	48 (4.5%)
Enterobacter cloacae	44 (4.1%)
Klebsiella pneumoniae	40 (3.7%)
Klebsiella oxytoca	9
Serratia marcescens	9
Citrobacter freundii	3
Proteus mirabilis	2
ANAEROBES	**9 (0.9%)**
Bacteroides fragilis	6
Clostridium difficile	3

process of organ transplantation alters the various intrinsic defense mechanisms in a variety of ways [22,23]. Surgical trauma associated with organ transplantation has a direct effect on barrier disruption. Moreover, the concomitant use of antibiotics and antirejection drugs (steroids) also impairs the natural defense mechanisms of the gastro-intestinal tract by altering the rate and type of secretions such as gastric acid, mucus and bile. These same agents also alter the fine balance that exists between the various components of the endogenous flora, leading to alterations within it, that allow one or another organism to predominate, or new organisms to take hold and induce disease symptoms. Immunosuppressive regimens used to prevent liver graft rejection would enhance infection by impairing hu-

moral antibody responsiveness and altering T-cell-mediated immunity [24,25]. Despite the careful use of drugs, it is often difficult to achieve a balance between maintaining an adequate immunosuppressive therapy for graft tolerance and the risk of infection because of lack of true markers for monitoring host defense mechanisms. Therefore, bacterial infection, septicemia and multiple organ failure remains the most common causes of morbidity and early mortality after liver transplantation [26, 27]. In the setting of LT several studies have addressed the role of the endotoxin portion of the Gram-negative bacterial cell wall and the subsequent cascade of cytokines in these complications [28,29]. Other studies have focused on sources of early endotoxemia occurring in the recipient, such as major intraoperati-

Table 3
Laparotomy for intra-abdominal infection after Liver Transplantation (172 / 872 patients)

Indication	Number of patients	Day* of occurrence (mean ± SD)	Deaths in patients (Day*: mean + ±D)	
Infected Collection	49	50 ± 103	0	
Infected Haematoma	20	19 ± 22	6	(33 ± 45)
Infected Ascitis	38	9 ± 8	10	(139 ± 167)
Abscess	20	76 ± 147	5	(152 ± 126)
Peritonitis	28	31 ± 47	9	(48 ± 38)
Wound Infection	19	23 ± 23	0	

Day*: day after liver transplantation

ve gastrointestinal manipulation, the anhepatic phase, portal occlusion, ischemia-reperfusion phenomenon of both the graft and the gut upon portal unclamping [30,31,32]. New experimental and clinical studies have showed that endotoxin and its effects can be transferred from the liver graft donor to the recipient [33,34,35] Yokoyama et al [36] reported that one third of the donors had measurable levels of endotoxin. Fukushima et al [37] found that translocation is commonly noted in brain-dead donors. Liver ischemia and reperfusion contribute to a decrease resistance to endotoxinemia [38]. The reperfusion of the liver graft after a phase of cold ischemia, combined with the stress of surgery in a hostile immunological environment could trigger an amplified tissue response. The liver itself has been found to be the special infectious risk factor [39,40,41]. In the early post-operative period, ischemia, partial or complete hepatic devascularization, biliary obstruction and rejection were frequently accompanied by systemic infections. At a later time, febrile and other manifestations of systemic infection were found in the majority of cases to be related to biliary complications.

Biliary complications in liver transplantation remain the biggest group of surgical complication in our serie (15%) and was responsible for almost half of IAI (table 4). Earlier, biliary anastomosis was called the (Achille's heel of LT). The rate of biliary complications reported in the literature range from 5.5% to 30% [42,43]. Many factors were incriminated in the occurrence of biliary complications. Inadequate blood supply or ischemic damage of the bile ducts, local infection, graft rejection (which has been shown to reduce the hepatic artery blood flow and might also contribute to ischemic damage of the biliary tree in the case of delayed treatment or steroid-resistance), changes in bile secretion, drug toxicity and operative techniques [44- 47]. A surgical approach for treatment is intentionnally chosen for most of the patients. Percutaneous desobstruction and/or dilatation was essentially left for non-anastomotic strictures and for stenosis which appears at an early stage. Biliary repair was the most frequent surgical procedure chosen. Retransplantation was performed in patients in whom vascular complications and/or rejection were associated to hepatic failure. Our post-operative protocol consisted of Doppler ultrasound

Figure 2
Date of occurence of Bacteremia after Liver Transplantation
1066 Positive blood Cultures/389 patients

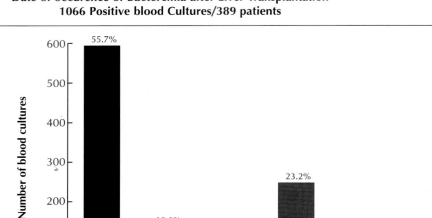

scanning, which detects early vascular problems. The best treatment of biliary complication, however, remains their avoidance by a careful dissection along the common bile duct during donor and recipient hepatectomy, adequate hepatic arterial reconstruction and a short ischemia time.

6. CONCLUSION

An awareness of surgical complications which may follow liver transplantation, enables the preparation of a careful approach to the post-operative stage of patient management. In addition to a better understanding of the basic events that characterize infection after LT, recent advances in diagnostic approach and in establishing the therapeutic principles for septic conditions, have led to considerable improvements in the results. There must be close surveillance after LT for surgical complications and IAI. Because bacteremias are so often the first signal of evolving diseases, single minded determination is necessary to clearly explain their causation, particulary if positive blood cultures persist in multiple samples. The use of Doppler ultra-sonography, cholangiograms, needle biopsies, scans and serial liver function tests allows for an earlier diagnosis and permit an adequate therapy at an early stage before impairements occurr. However, LT offers to over fifty percent of patients, the chance of a full rehabilitation from life-threatening disease and the prospect of a normal life style and full time employment.

Table 4
Surgical Procedures for Biliary Complications

	Strictures (n = 100)	Bile peritonitis (n = 26)	Bile fistulas (n = 8)
Biliary repair	55	0	0
Percutaneous drainage	45	15	6
Surgical drainage	0	5	2
Laparoscopic drainage	0	6	0
Retransplantation	14	0	0

REFERENCES

1. Kusne S, Dummer JS, Singh N et al. Infections after liver transplantation: an analysis of 101 consecutive cases. Medicine 1988; 67 (2): 132-143.

2. Dummer JS, Hardy A, Poorsattar A, Ho M. Early Infections in kidney, heart and liver transplant recipients on cyclosporin. Transplantation 1983; 36(3): 259-67.

3. Paya CV, Hermans PE, Washington JA, Smith TF, Anhalt JP, Wiesner RH, Krom RA. Incidence, distribution and outcome of episodes of infection in 100 orthotopic liver transplantations. Mayo Clin Proc 1989; 64 (5): 555-64.

4. Colonna JO, Winston DJ, Brill JE, Goldstein LI, Hoff MP, Hiatt JR, Quinones-Baldrich W, Ramming KP, Busuttil RW. Infectious complications in liver transplantation. Arch Surg 1988; 123 (3): 360-4.

5. Mora NP, Gonwa TA, Goldstein RM, Husberg BS, Klinmalm GB. Risk of post-operative infection after liver transplantation: an univariate and stepwise logistic regression analysis of risk factors in 150 consecutive patients. Clin Transplant 1992; 46: 443.

6. Saliba F, Ephraim R, Mathieu D, Samuel D, Richet H, Castaing D, Bismuth H. Risk factors for bacterial infection after liver transplantation.Transplant Proc 1994; 26,1: 266.

7. Singh N, Gayowski T, Wagener M, Yu VL. Infectious complications in liver transplant recipients on tacrolimus: prospective analysis of 88 consecutive liver transplants. Transplantation 1994; 774-78.

8. Starzl TE, Hakala T, Rosenthal JT. A flexible procedure of multiple organ procurement. Surg Gynecol Obstet 1984; 158: 223-25.

9. Belle SH, Beringer KC, Murphy JB, Detre KM. The Pitt -UNOS liver transplant registry In: Terasaki PI, Cecka JM, eds. Clinical Transplants. Los Angeles: UCLA tissue typing laboratories 1992: 17-32

10. Bismuth H, Castaing D. The European Liver Transplant Registry, eds. Paris: Paul Brousse Hospital, June 1997.

11. Meakins JL, Solomkin JS, Allo MD, Dellinger EP et al. A proposed classification of intra-abdominal infections. Arch Surg 1984; 119: 1372-78.

12. Bohnen JMA, Boulanger M, Meakins JL et al. Prognosis in general peritonitis: relation to cause and risk factors. Arch Surg 1983; 118: 285- 90.

13. Pitcher WD, Musher DM: Critical importance of early diagnosis and treatment of intra-abdominal infections. Arch Surg 1982; 117: 328-33.

14. Goris RJA, Boekholtz WKF, Van Bebber IPT et al. Multiple-organ failure and sepsis without bacteria. An experimental model. Arch

Surg 1986; 121: 897- 901

15. Steiberg S, Flynn W, Kelley K et al. Deve-
    lopment of a bacterial-independent model
    of the multiple organ failure syndrome. Arch
    Surg 1989; 124: 1390-5.

16. Muhvich KH, Myers RAM, Marzella L. Ef-
    fects of hyperbaric oxygenation combined
    with antimicrobial agents and surgery in a
    rat model of intra-abdominal infection. J In-
    fect Dis 1990; 157: 1058-61.

17. Saadia R, Schein M, MacFarlane C, Boffard
    KD. Gut barrier function and the surgeon.
    Br J Surg 1990; 77: 487-92

18. Deitch EA.The role of intestinal barrier fai-
    lure and bacterial translocation in the deve-
    lopment of systemic infection and multiple
    oragn failure. Arch Surg 1990; 125: 403-4

19. Marshall J, Sweeney D. Microbial infection
    and the septic response in critical surgical
    illness. Arch Surg 1990; 125: 17-23.

20. Bounous G. The intestinal factor in multiple
    organ failure and shock. Surgery 1990; 107:
    118- 19.

21. Naetani S, Nishikawa T, Tobe T, Hirakawa
    A. Role of blood transfusion in organ failure
    following major abdominal surgery. Ann
    Surg 1986; 203: 275-81

22. Yolken RH, Bishop CA, Townsend TR, Bol-
    yard TR et al. Infectious gastroenteritis in
    bone-marrow transplant recipients. N Engl J
    Med 1982; 306: 1010-12

23. Van Thiel DH. Gastrointestinal and liver
    complications. In Toledo-Pereyra LH, eds.
    Complications of organ transplantation
    1987: 169-85

24. Starzl TE, Iwatsuki S, Shaw BW et al. Immu-
    nosuppression and other non-surgical fac-
    tors in the improved results of liver trans-
    plantation. Semin Liver Dis 1985; 5: 334-43

25. Hofflin JM, Potasman I; Baldwin JC et al. In-
    fectious complications in heart transplant
    recipients receiving cyclosporin and corti-
    costeroids. Ann Intern Med 1987; 106: 209-
    16

26. Cuervas-Mons V, Martinez AJ, Dekker A,
    Starzl TE, Van Thiel DHJ. Adult liver trans-
    plantation: an analysis of the early causes of
    death in 40 consecutive cases. Hepatology
    1986; 6: 495-501

27. Park GR, Gomez-Arnau J, Lindop MJ, Klinck
    JR, Williams R, Calne RY. Mortality during
    intensive care after orthotopic liver trans-
    plantation. Anaesthesia 1989; 44: 959-63

28. Andus T, Bauer J, Gerok W. Effects of cyto-
    kines on the liver. Hepatology 1991; 13:
    364-75

29. Doi F, Goya T, Torisu M. Potential role of
    hepatic macrophages in neutrophil-media-
    ted liver injury in rats with sepsis. Hepato-
    logy 1993; 17: 1086-94

30. Olcay I, Kitahama A, Miller RH et al. Reti-
    culoendothelial dysfunction and endotoxe-
    mia following portal vein occlusion. Surgery
    1974; 75: 64-70

31. Shibayama Y. The relation of endotoxaemia
    to the cause of death and fatal hepatic da-
    mage following obstruction of the portal
    vein. J Pathol 1990; 160: 355-60

32. Shibayama Y. Role of endotoxaemia in the
    development of hepatic failure following
    hepatic artery occlusion. J Pathol 1990;
    161: 321-25

33. Gottesdiener KM. Transplanted infections:
    donor-to-host transmission with the allo-
    graft. Ann Int Med 1989; 110: 1001-16

34. Deitch EA, Berg R, Specian R. Endotoxin
    promotes the translocation of bacteria from
    the gut. Arch Surg 1987; 122: 185-90

35. Azoulay D, Astarcioglu I, Lemoine A et al.
    Effects of donor and recipients endotoxemia
    on TNF-(production and mortality in the rat
    model of syngenic orthotopic liver trans-
    plantatio).

36. Yokoyama I, Todo S, Miyata T, Selby R,
    Tzarkis AG, Starzl TE. Endotoxemia and hu-
    man liver transplantation. Transplant Proc
    1989; 21: 3833-41

37. Fukushima R, Gianotti L, Alexander JW. The primary site of bacterial translocation. Arch Surg 1994; 129: 53-58

38. Maessen JG, Greve JWM, Buurman WA. Increased sensitivity to endotoxemia by tissue necrosis. Surgery 1991; 109: 154-59

39. Brettschneider L, Tong JL, Boose DS et al. Specific bacteriological problems after orthotopic liver transplantation in dogs and pigs. Arch Surg 1968; 97: 313-22

40. Alican F, Hardy JD. Replantation of the liver. J Surg Res 1967; 7: 368-82. Transplantation 1995; 59: 825-29

41. Schröter GPJ, Hoelscher M, Putnam CW et al. Infections complicating orthotopic liver transplantation: a study emphasizing graft-related-septicemia. Arch Surg 1976; 111: 1337-47

42. Bismuth H, Castaing D, Gugenheim J et al. Roux-en-Y-hepaticojejunostomy: a safe procedure for biliary anastomosis in liver transplantation. Transplant Proc 1987; 19: 2413-15.

43. Bechstein WO, Blumhardt G, Ringe B, et al. Surgical complications in 200 consecutive liver transplants. Transplant Proc 1987; 5: 3830-31

44. Ringe B, Oldhafer K, Bunzendahl H et al. Analysis of biliary complications following orthotopic liver transplantation. Transplant Proc 1989; 21: 2472-76

45. Colonna JO, Shaked A, Gomes AS et al. Biliary strictures complicating liver transplantation. Ann Surg 1992; 216: 344-52

46. Northover JMA, Terblanche J. A new look at the arterial supply of the bile duct in man and its surgical implications. Br J Surg 1979; 66: 379-84

47. Scotté M, Dousset B, Calmus Y et al. The influence of cold ischemia time on biliary complications following liver transplantation. J Hepatol 1994; 21: 340-46

Common Intra-abdominal Infections in Aids Patients

Fernando E. Kafie, MD, Michael Budd, BS and Russell Williams, MD

1. INTRODUCTION

As the number of patients with acquired immunodeficiency syndrome (AIDS) steadily climbs, so has the need for surgical consultations. It has become increasingly important that physicians be aware of the specific abdominal and gastrointestinal diseases which develop in patients with AIDS. Approximately 50% of AIDS patients develop gastrointestinal manifestations during the course of their illness [1]. Gastrointestinal symptoms in AIDS patients are frequently non-specific, presenting diagnostic and management difficulties. In this population, symptoms from non-surgical disorders frequently overlap with those from true surgical emergencies, making patient selection for operative intervention difficult and requiring the surgeon to investigate rigorously.

As of October 31, 1995, a total of 501,310 patients with AIDS have been reported to the CDC by state and territorial health departments; 311,381 (62%) have died.[2] Of the cumulative AIDS cases, 247,741 (49%) were reported from 1993 - October 1995. The proportion of AIDS cases among females increased from 8% (1988-1987) to 18%

(1993 - Oct. 1995). The proportion of cases among whites decreased from 60% to 43%, while the proportion among African Americans and Hispanics increased from 25% to 38% and 14% to 18%, respectively [2]. The proportion of cases among persons who reported injecting-drug use and heterosexual transmission increased from 17% (1981-1987) to 27% (1993-Oct. 1995) and 3% to 10%, respectively.

However, cases among homosexual men decreased from 64% to 45% [2]. Finally, during 1993 - Oct. 1995, the largest number of cases (86,462) were reported from the South, which also accounted for the largest proportionate increase of reported cases (31%) [2].

Although these statistics are somewhat overwhelming, it is only a minority of patients with HIV infection who will need operative intervention. A study by LaRaja et al. showed that of 904 patients with a diagnosis of AIDS admitted to the Cabrini Medical Center in New York over a 3-year period, only 36 (4.2%) of the patients required an operation [3]. In addition, recent reviews [4] have described decreased morbidity and mortality rates compared to initial reports. Davidson et al [5] documented an 11% operative mortality rate after emergency laparotomy in 28 AIDS patients. Also, Diettrich[6] and co-workers described a 13% mortality rate for emergency operations and 2% for elective procedures. These values reflect the improved antiretroviral and antimicrobial therapies for opportunistic infections which have extended the period of good health in HIV infected patients and allowing AIDS patients to better tolerate surgical procedures.

The surgeon should be prepared to evaluate increasing numbers of patients with AIDS and abdominal pain. In a study by Barone et al.[7], 12% of hospitalized AIDS patients had abdominal pain warranting surgical consultation. A study from the John Hopkins University School of Medicine showed that 16% of emergency room presentations among HIV patients were for abdominal pain or other gastrointestinal complaints [3]. Many surgical consultations range from minor procedures for vascular access or lymph node biopsies to diagnosis of opportunistic diseases or neoplasm's. These less invasive procedures are considered elective and are tolerated well by all immunocompromised patients [5].

Four distinct disease processes, cytomegalovirus (CMV), Kaposi's sarcoma, non-Hodgkin's lymphoma and mycobacterial infection, account for the majority of intra-abdominal processes that may require surgical intervention. These can include enterocolitis, appendicitis, obstructive jaundice due to sclerosing cholangitis, obstruction of the gastrointestinal tract, cholecystitis and spontaneous bacterial peritonitis (SBP). When there is no clear indication for surgical intervention, abdominal and pelvic computed tomography (CT) is the investigation of choice for an elusive diagnosis. Some other

helpful investigative methods that may be performed as indicated include endoscopy, aspiration biopsy, abdominal ultrasound, standard radiographic series, barium radiography and endoscopic retrograde cholangiopancreatography (ERCP). Intraabdominal disease processes occurring in the HIV infected population can vary remarkably. Infected patients can not only develop typical surgical problems seen in immunocompetent individuals (appendicitis, cholecystitis, diverticulitis, etc.) but also often develop atypical pathological processes necessitating surgery as a result of opportunistic infection or neoplasm. It can be difficult distinguishing these disease processes, many of which are treated without surgery, from the more classic causes of acute abdomen. This inability to easily clarify abdominal disease processes, along with the reluctance of many surgeons to operate in HIV infected patients, has led to delays in surgical exploration and treatment until a more advanced stage of the disease.

2. DETERMINATION OF THE DEGREE OF IMMUNOSUPPRESSION

The CD4+ lymphocyte count or the CD4+ /CD8+ ratio, correlates with progression of the HIV disease. The risk of developing AIDS with a CD4+ lymphocyte count less than 300 has been shown to be 10-fold greater than for patients who have a CD4+ cell count greater than 500. In general, the CD4+ lymphocytes decrease by approximately 10% per year after the HIV infection has been identified serologically [7].

Patients with a CD4+ lymphocyte count greater than 500 per cubic milliliter, generally do not have significant immunosuppression [7]. On the other hand, if the CD4 lymphocyte count is less than 200, patients are usually given antimicrobial prophylaxis to prevent contracting PCP pneumonia for which they are otherwise at great risk. A ratio of CD4+/CD8+ cells less than 0.3 places the patient at high risk for opportunistic infections compared to a patient whose CD4+/CD8+ ratio is greater than 0.6.

3. Abdominal diseases in HIV-infected adult

Intraabdominal diseases account for the majority of morbidity and mortality encountered by the general surgeon when dealing with AIDS patients. Diseases of the liver, gallbladder, and bile ducts have been described with increasing frequency among patients with AIDS [8]. Many reports have described AIDS-associated "cholangiopathy" with abnormalities of both the intrahepatic and/or extrahepatic bile ducts.[9] The etiology of AIDS cholangiopathy is uncertain.

3.1. Acalculous Cholecystitis

Although acalculous cholecystitis typically has a non-infectious etiology, opportunistic pathogens play an important role in cholecystitis occurring in patients infected with the human immunodeficiency virus (HIV) [10]. The presence of right upper quadrant pain and fever in HIV-positive individuals warrants consideration for infectious acute acalculous cholecystitis caused by cytomegalovirus (CMV) [8] a common pathogen in immunocompromised hosts.

Patients presenting with acalculous cholecystitis secondary to CMV usually present with right upper quadrant pain and tenderness. Fever, weight loss and Murphy's sign are common. In all cases jaundice ia either absent or not mentioned.[8]

The usual sonographic findings in CMV cholecystitis include extensive gallbladder wall thickening or ulceration [11]. Marked sonographic abnormalities are often associated with astonishingly mild symptoms and signs. A HIDA scan usually reveals a non-visualized gallbladder and is a sensitive test for CMV cholecystitis. However, a negative HIDA scan should not delay operative intervention.

Pathoanatomy of the gallbladder establishes the diagnosis of CMV acalculous cholecystitis. There are consistent patterns of transmural inflammation and edema in gallbladders infected with CMV, often greater than 1.0 cm. Diffuse gallbladder wall inflammation is the principal pathological process as opposed to obstruction-related mural inflammation or ischemia progressing to transmural gangrene, as seen with calculous gallbladder disease. Specimens exhibite CMV intranuclear inclusion bodies in epithelial endothelial or stromal cells. A proposed mechanism of this intense gallbladder inflammation is CMV-induced vasculitis [12]. Focal mucosal necrosis and ulceration are common findings. In contrast to calculous cholecystitis, it is not known whether CMV cholecystitis will progress to perforation and its attendant high morbidity.

Evidence is accumulating in favor of CMV as a pathogen in biliary disease of the immunocompromised [10]. Recent support of an etiologic role for CMV in neonatal hepatitis demonstrates the affinity of the virus for human bile duct epithelium [13]. During acute CMV viremia, significant cholestasis occurs with no mechanical biliary obstruction [14]. Cholestasis also occurs in AIDS patients with documented CMV end stage organ disease [15]. Bile cultures devoid of bacteria support the pathogenic role of CMV in cholecystitis.

Figure 1
ERCP. Arrow points to papillary stenosis

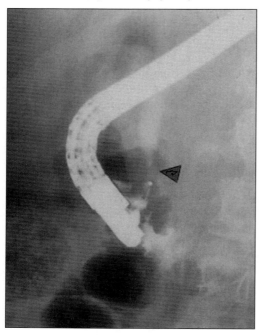

Patients treated with intravenous antibiotics have recurring symptoms and respond poorly. Cardiovascular compromise, septicemia, prolonged fasting, or multiorgan failure are surprisingly uncommon. In contrast to more common forms of acute acalculous cholecystitis [16], leukocytosis and hyperbilirubinemia are uncommon and liver function tests may be normal or reflect mild cholestasis [17]. The total leukocyte count is an unreliable indicator being normal or decreased despite severe gallbladder inflammation and local peritonitis. Morbidity and mortality for cholecystectomy in AIDS patients with CMV cholecystitis are surprisingly low despite markedly diminished cellular immunocompetence as evidenced by reduced CD4:CD8 lymphocyte ratios.

Cytomegaloviral cholecystitis may be a manifestation of reactivated latent infection [15] or impending disseminated CMV disease. After cholecystectomy, diligent surveillance for disseminated CMV infection should be undertaken. Serum titers for detecting anti-CMV IgG and IgM antibodies are drawn in acute and convalescent phases.

In AIDS patients, a distinctive variety of biliary tract disease occurs independent of cholecystitis and may present either as an isolated phenomenon or arise months after cholecystectomy as the cause of recurrent right upper quadrant abdominal pain, fever and cholestatic liver function abnormalities [16]. This HIV-associated disease has been called "papillary stenosis/sclerosing cholangitis" (PS/SC) [14,18] because of cholangiographic mucosal irregularities similar to primary sclerosing cholangitis [17]. AIDS patients with systemic CMV have a 3-11 per cent probability of developing PS/SC, with or without cholecystitis [14].

Although its presentation is similar to cholecystitis, this clinical syndrome represents a separate pathologic entity, seemingly attributable to CMV or cryptosporidium.[10] Following cholecystectomy, if symptoms resembling cholecystitis recur or a patient develops chronically abnormal liver function tests, biliary tree abnormalities may be detected by ultrasound, computed tomography or ERCP (Figure 1). Endoscopic papillary biopsy and sphincterotomy are appropriate interventions with PS, endoscopic dilation may be necessary for sclerotic bile ducts.[10] Papilla biopsy has been used to diagnose cholangitis due to CMV and cryptosporidium.

3.2. Papillary Stenosis

Multiple pathogens and malignancies have been described within the ampulla and bile ducts of patients undergoing endoscopic retrograde cholangiopancreatography sphincterotomy. They include Kaposi's sarcoma, cytomegalovirus, cryptosporidium, Mycobacterium avium complex and more recently microsporidia [19, 20]. There have been four specific patterns of AIDS cholangiopathy: papillary stenosis, sclerosing cholangitis, long extrahepatic bile duct strictures and papillary stenosis with sclerosing cholangitis.

For patients with distal common bile duct obstruction due to papillary stenosis of any etiology, endoscopic sphincterotomy appears to be a promising modality, given the hope of providing immediate relief of extrahepatic bile duct obstruction with the potential relief of biliary symptoms. Sphincterotomy provides long-term pain relief in the majority of patients but does not alter the intrahepatic progression of disease nor its biochemical abnormality.

Several studies have noted improvement in abdominal pain following ERCP sphincterotomy for AIDS-associated cholangiopathy. Benhamou et al [21] noted "rapid and lasting disappearance of pain" in all 20 patients treated, while Bouche et al [22] reported pain relief in 13 of 15 patients undergoing sphincterotomy. Neither study reported the duration of follow-up, nor attempted to quantify the severity of pain before or following sphincterotomy.

Despite sustained improvement in biliary-type pain, there was no change in mean serum alkaline phosphatase levels during the course of follow-up. While it is difficult to assess the overall impact of ERCP sphincterotomy on patient care, there is a reliable, reproducible and sustained improvement in biliary-type pain in patients undergoing ERCP sphincterotomy for AIDS-associated papillary stenosis. While the procedure is not without risks, ERCP sphincterotomy is a worthwhile undertaking for patients suffering from AIDS-associated papillary stenosis.

3.3. Cholangitis

During their illness, nearly all HIV-infected patients have symptoms suggestive of the presence of liver or biliary disease or both. Liver diseases are by far the most frequent but a few isolated cases [23,24] and a small series of AIDS-related cholangitis have been reported [19-22, 26].

The location of cholangiogram abnormalities can be established as follows: diffuse AIDS-related cholangitis, isolated intrahepatic cholangitis and isolated extrahepatic cholangitis. Papillary stenosis was encountered in 60% of the patients.

Usually, AIDS-related cholangitis is a late complication of AIDS. The diagnosis is based on four major clinical signs: jaundice, fever, diarrhea and abdominal pain. Biological cholestasis is frequent and occurred in 53% of our patients. Bile-duct dilation or wall thickening on abdominal ultrasonography are suggestive of the diagnosis. ERCP makes differential diagnosis possible, excluding other etiologies of biliary-tract dilatation in AIDS patients such as bile-duct lymphoma or choledocholithiasis.

3.4. Gastrointestinal diseases

3.4.1. *Mycobacterium avium intracellulare*

Disseminated Mycobacterium avium intracellulare (MAI) is one of the most commonly encountered opportunistic infections in the AIDS population. MAI is a slow growing, non-photochromogenic acid-fast bacillus and although ubiquitous, it uncommonly produces clinical disease other than pulmonary infections superimposed on pre-existing lung disease. Extrapulmonary infection from MAI is rare even in immunocompromised groups other than AIDS patients [26,27].

Bacteremia is common, and AIDS patients with disseminated MAI often complain of severe abdominal pain and systemic symptoms including fever, night sweats and weight loss. Among AIDS patients with a specific infectious cause for diarrhea, MAI is the most common offending pathogen and can be isolated in at least 25% of cases [26].

The duodenum and small bowel are the predominant site of gastrointestinal tract involvement with this disease. Both radiographically and pathologically, MAI enteritis can closely resemble Whipple disease and thus has been referred to as pseudo-Whipple disease. A barium small bowel series commonly reveals irregular, thick and undulating folds with fine nodularity as well as mild dilatation of the small bowel. Hypersecretion with segmentation and flocculation of barium frequently is observed and aphthous ulcers are demonstrated occasionally. The small bowel findings result from inflammation and edema and thus are often non-specific. In addition to other opportunistic infections such as cryptosporidiosis and isosporiosis, the differential diagnosis must also include bowel infections seen in the general homosexual population such as Giardia and Strongyloides, lymphoma and edema due to hypoprotenemia.

Extensive bulky mesenteric and retroperitoneal adenopathy is characteristically seen in addition to dilation of the small bowel, wall thickening and prominent nodular mucosal folds. Splenomegaly is seen in virtually every proven case as well as hepatomegaly. The findings of multiple low density necrotic areas within the nodes, favors a diagnosis of MAI over lymphoma but may be even more commonly seen with Mycobacterium tuberculosis infection [28,29].

3.4.2. Mycobacterium tuberculosis

Immunosuppressed patients, including those with AIDS, are particularly susceptible to tuberculosis infection, the incidence of which is as high as 67% in intravenous drug users with AIDS worldwide. The incidence of tuberculosis across all AIDS patients in the United States is estimated at 10%. AIDS patients also have an unusually high rate of disseminated and extrapulmonary tuberculosis, approaching 72% [30]. Gastrointestinal tuberculosis can result from ingestion, extension from the lymphatic system, or hematogenous dissemination, although the latter is probably most important in the AIDS patient [31].

Tuberculosis of the gastrointestinal tract involves the ileocecal area in 90% of cases. Patients often present with abdominal pain, chronic diarrhea, fever and a right lower quadrant mass. The tuberculin test is frequently negative in AIDS patients, reflecting cellular anergy and there is a tendency for these patients not to form granulomas [32]. The typical radiological findings include a thickened ileocecal valve with a widened aperture, submucosal nodules and frequent ulceration [33]. In advanced stages of the disease, the terminal ileum may be fibrotic with a rigid ileocecal valve and a markedly deformed and retracted cecum. In differentiating this radiographic appearance from

Crohn's disease, it is important to note that in the latter, the cecum usually is not involved and the ileocecal valve is competent.[34]

The characteristic CT findings of tuberculosis include 1) prominent and asymmetric thickening of the cecum with a predominance of the medial wall; 2) a possible central mass in the ileocecal valve with entrapment of the terminal ileum; and 3) low density lymphadenopathy. Peritonitis can be manifest on CT scans by ascitic fluid that may be loculated or hyperdense.

The adenopathy classically described in association with tuberculosis involves the peripancreatic and mesenteric regions near the diseased intestinal segments.

3.4.3. Cryptosporidium

Cryptosporidium is a coccidial protozoan that, prior to the AIDS epidemic, was known to infect birds and other animals and cause a self-limited diarrheal illness in travelers and children exposed to infected animal feces. Cryptosporidium in the immunosuppressed AIDS patient causes severe abdominal cramping, prolonged cholera-like diarrhea and malabsorption. Severe dehydration with electrolyte imbalances, wasting and even death can ensue [35].

On barium enema mucosal fold thickening confined to the proximal small intestine may be seen. Spasm and irritability of the small intestine are often seen, with increased secretions throughout the small bowel.

Cryptosporidiosis is commonly manifest on abdominal CT by mural thickening of the proximal small bowel with luminal narrowing, mesenteric thickening and small mesenteric nodes [35].

3.4.4. Cytomegalovirus colitis

Approximately 90% of patients with AIDS will develop a clinically apparent CMV infection during their lifetime [36], making it the most common pathogen identified in the AIDS population. CMV is a member of the herpes group and can be found in almost every organ system of the patient with AIDS. It can manifest as retinitis, pneumonitis, pancreatitis, encephalitis, adrenalitis and inflammation of the whole gastrointestinal tract [37]. However, of those with CMV infection, approximately 30% will have CMV in the gastrointestinal tract.

Colitis is the most common gastrointestinal manifestation of CMV infection in patients with AIDS [38] and in approximately 25% of cases, it provides the basis for the initial clinical diagnosis of AIDS.[38] Early diagnosis and treatment are extremely important to avoid potentially fatal complications and to prevent CMV dissemination to distant sites, which occurs in 15% of untreated patients in 14 days [38]. CMV infects both epithelial and endothelial cells and fibroblasts. Vasculitis develops in the blood vessels of the submucosa, which leads to thrombosis. Extensive submucosal thrombosis produces mucosal ischemia, which is followed by bleeding, ulceration and eventually, transmural gangrene of the bowel wall. The perforations are typically punctate when viewed from the mucosal or serosal aspect of the bowel. Generalized peritonitis follows perforation. Massive bleeding or perforation may occur anywhere within the GI tract, although the colon and terminal ileum are the most frequent sites.

The characteristic CMV lesion is a sharply demarcated punctate ulcer covered by a fibrous exudate (Figure 2)[4] that may be up to 1-2 cm in diameter. The ulcer may clo-

Figure 2
CMV Mucosal Ulcer of the Stomach

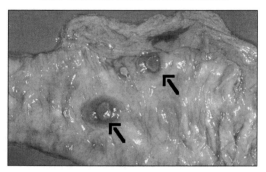

sely resemble those of regional enteritis or ulcerative colitis, the most common misdiagnosis. The disease marks a continuum from the most severe manifestations (massive bleeding or perforation of the bowel) to a less severe indolent illness (developing with mild vasculitis). Patients may present with a syndrome of abdominal pain (usually in the lower right abdomen), fever, hematochezia, diarrhea, weight loss and occasional bleeding from the bowel, particularly melena. The frequency of patients reported by Murray et al. who presented with these symptoms are as follows, 64% severe abdominal pain, 80% fever, 23% hematochezia, 70% had persistent diarrhea for 2 months with a mean of 7.5 liquid stools per day and 89% had weight loss (mean of 8.9 kg).

The diagnosis of CMV enteritis is made when characteristic fibrin-covered ulcers can be seen with endoscopy. For confirmation of this diagnosis, the margins of these ulcers may be biopsied and stained with hematoxylin and eosin to make the hallmark intranuclear inclusion bodies characteristic to CMV visible. In addition, the infected endothelial cells are often markedly swollen, with inclusion bodies also showing a perinuclear halo. The specimen can be cultivated for CMV but this analysis is not as accurate as a biopsy. Coinfection may also occur with one or more opportunistic agents such as Salmonella, Shigella, Compylobacteria, Clostridium difficile, Crytosporidium, Microsporidium, Entamoeba and Giardia [37]. As a result, the diagnosis of medical and surgical abdominal emergencies in patients with AIDS can be limited by the considerable overlap that exists in presenting signs and symptoms [38]. As a result, CT may provide the most comprehensive radiographic evaluation of patients with AIDS and non-specific abdominal pain. CT scans also avoid the risk of colonic perforation that is present with a barium enema [38]. Murray et al [40] reported that the most common CT feature of CMV colitis in their series was colonic wall thickening (92% of patients). In addition, mural thickening was apparent before direct measurement, as the mean maximal mural diameter was 5 times the normal thickness.[38] The mean mural thickness of 15 mm seen in CMV colitis is significantly greater than that seen in ulcerative colitis (7.8mm) and somewhat greater than seen in both Crohn's colitis (11-13mm) and pseudomembranous colitis (11mm) [38]. In contrast to ulcerated and pseudomembranous colitis, Murray et al. [40] reported, that mural thickening was circumferential in only 71% of their patients.

Extracolonic manifestations have included inflammatory stranding in the perirectal and pericolonic fat seen 23 patients (96%) of cases reported by Murray et al [38]. Although infiltration of pericolonic fat is useful in aiding diagnosis, infiltration of perirectal fat is seen in more than 90% of homosexual men [38], usually due to nonspecific proctitis, and is thus of little value in diagnosing CMV colitis. In addition, small bowel disease was reported in 42% of the patients, a useful feature in differentiating CMV disease from pseudomembranous colitis; where changes are confined to the colon.[38] Ascites was seen in 42% of the colitis cases reported by Murray et al. but it is rarely seen in either ulcerative or Crohn's colitis [39]. Lymphadenopathy is not a prominent feature of CMV colitis,[38] and when seen in association with ileocecal disease should prompt a search for Mycobacterium tuberculosis.

CMV enterocolitis is usually managed non-operatively with ganciclovir or foscarnet but there is a report that drug therapy alone is not sufficient to induce remission of CMV enterocolitis once severe inflammation with ulcers is seen [37]. Soderlund et al [41] reported that seven of their eight patients had been on CMV therapy from 5 days to 14 months (usually 2-3 weeks) prior to any operation without any effect. In addition, they also reported that although not curative of the CMV infection, surgical resection of macroscopically inflamed bowel in combination with anti-CMV therapy seems to offer good palliation and survival with a mean relapse-free survival of 14 months. They stress the importance of operating on localized but pronounced CMV enterocolitis at a relatively "early" stage, before acute bleeding or perforation enforces an emergency operation, with it's poor survival. Perioperative mortality rates after emergency operations for CMV colitis have been previously reported up to 71% [37].

However, peritonitis secondary to CMV enterocolitis with perforation or bleeding, is the most common cause of emergency abdominal surgery in AIDS patients. Colonic perforation patients frequently have minimal abdominal tenderness, no fever and a normal WBC count [38]. A CT scan which demonstrates pneumoperitoneum or abscess formation establishes the diagnosis of perforation and may expedite earlier surgical intervention in these patients [40]. In addition, impending perforation may first be suggested on the basis of CT detection of pneumatosis intestinalis [40]. Prior to an operation, the patient must be resuscitated and given broad spectrum antibiotics, as with any other patient with bowel perforation. Should there be evidence of another opportunistic infection, it is advisable to institute antimicrobial therapy specifically for that infection. At operation, the segment of the bowel bearing the perforation is resected [36]. Primary anastomosis is not recommended due to a high likelihood of anastomotic complications, particularly breakdown with recontamination of the peritoneal cavity by intestinal contents. Rather, the divided proximal bowel is exteriorized as an ileostomy or colostomy. With diffuse CMV gastroenteritis, other areas of the bowel are at risk of perforation, which appears more likely to evolve in the post-operative period. A stoma avoids possible complications from an anastomosis in the post-operative period and attention to post-operative nutritional support may help reduce post-operative complications and mortality.

CMV is the most common cause of intestinal perforation, which is often followed by a rapid demise of the patient despite surgical treatment. This is due not only to the development of overwhelming peritonitis in an immunocompromised state but also to the progression of associated opportunistic infections that lead to pulmonary complications and eventual multisystem organ failure. A lesser intensity of medical and surgical treatment may be administered in the knowledge that bowel perforation due to CMV is often a terminal event. Consideration of the patient's current health status, overall prognosis and individual wishes help to determine the treatment plan.

3.4.5. *Clostrydium difficile*

Clostrydium difficile, the etiological agent of pseudomembranous colitis, is not unique to the AIDS population but is nontheless prevalent in this group. The organism invades colonic mucosa as a superinfection, usually in the setting of recent antibiotic therapy. Pseudomembranous colitis is caused by an overgrowth of C. difficile, which releases an enterotoxin causing inflammation and consequent breakdown of the colonic mucosa. The inflammatory reaction produces small white or yellowish pseudomembranes on the surface of the colonic lining, which consist of mucous and inflammatory debris. Pseudomembranes become confluent as the disease progresses. Unlike its presentation in the immunocompetent host, pseudomembranous colitis often presents in the AIDS patient with acute abdominal pain and symptoms more suggestive of abdominal catastrophe or bowel perforation [42].

The classic CT appearance with pseudomembranous colitis is that of prominent and irregular bowel wall thickening (average wall thickness, 1.5 cm). Contrast material may be trapped between thickened haustral folds, producing a so-called accordion sign on CT [43]. Barium enema findings include thickened haustral folds, nodularity with numerous plaquelike lesions producing a shaggy wall contour, mucosal edema and dilation of the bowel lumen.[44] Bowel wall changes in pseudomembranous colitis are usually restricted to the colon, whereas cytomegalovirus frequently involves the terminal ileum in addition to the cecum.

3.4.6. *Typhlitis*

Typhlitis refers to an inflammatory necrotic process involving the cecum, appendix and/or terminal ileum. Described initially as a complication in leukemia and severe neutropenia, this condition has since been documented in patients with lymphoma, aplastic anemia, renal transplantation and AIDS. Typhlitis in the AIDS population may be caused by infection, or less commonly, lymphomatous infiltrates. Early diagnosis is critical, as the untreated disease can progress rapidly to transmural necrosis and perforation, with which there is a high mortality. Due to the risk of perforation, CT is preferred over fluoroscopic contrast-enhanced studies [45]. The CT findings in typhlitis include diffuse wall thickening, occasionally showing low attenuation intramural areas consistent with edema or necrosis; pneumatosis; pericolonic fluid and thickening of fascial planes [44].

3.4.7. *Proctitis*

Rectal and perirectal inflammatory disease are common in AIDS patients, identified in up to 82% of homosexual men [46]. Perirectal and perianal abscesses and fistulas frequently complicate proctitis and may rarely be manifested by acute abdominal pain. Neisseria gonorrhea is the most common offending organism in infectious proctitis, responsible for approximately 40% of cases, whereas Herpes simplex II ranks second in frequency and Chlamydia trachomatis third.

While barium enema may reveal rectal ulceration and spasm or widening of the presacral space, CT is generally a preferable examination for clinical management of proctitis. CT findings include rectal wall thickening and a hazy increased density in the perianal fat [47]. CT is also useful in distinguishing perirectal cellulitis from abscesses and in localizing complex abscesses prior to surgical drainage.

3.4.8. Gastritis

The stomach is the least frequently involved segment of the gastrointestinal tract by opportunistic infection, although AIDS patients with gastritis may present with a clinically acute picture, particularly in the setting of perforation. Gastric lesions tend to be found at the esophagogastric junction or in the gastric antrum and pylorus. Cytomegalovirus is the most common cause of AIDS-related gastritis, with cryptosporidiosis seen less often and gastric tuberculosis also reported [48].

3.5. Laboratory Tests as Determinants of Morbidity/Mortality

As expected, AIDS patients fared worse than those patients who were HIV positive. The more depressed immunity of AIDS patients, which has allowed for prior opportunistic infection or atypical neoplasm, portends a worse prognosis with poorer wound healing, more complications and a higher mortality.[6] Wexner et al [49] reported that those patients with lower total white blood counts had poorer wound healing. A study from Dallas showed a significantly higher morbidity after anorectal surgery in HIV/AIDS patients with T4 lymphocyte counts less than 200 [50]. These findings are disputed, however, by a report from St. Lukes-Roosevelt Hospital in New York that showed no significant correlation between wound healing and T4 counts [51].

The study of WBCs in HIV/AIDS patients undergoing abdominal surgery has frequently shown a lack of leukocytosis in the acute abdomen [52]. Attempts to correlate preoperative total and differential WBCs with outcome after abdominal surgery have thus far been unsuccessful [53].

Two factors that consistently affect outcome after surgery on HIV-infected patients are the classification of the patient as having AIDS and whether the surgery was emergent. Emergency surgery has a higher mortality rate than elective procedures in any cohort of patients. The AIDS patients also had a significantly longer post-procedure hospitalization.

Preoperative serum albumin levels are used to help predict outcome after surgery in many groups of patients, notably cirrhotics who need portosystemic shunts. This marker of overall nutritional status and general health, however, has not been investigated as enthusiastically as leukocyte counts in HIV patients undergoing surgery. In one study from Chicago, hypoalbuminemia (defined as serum albumin <2.5 g/L) combined with a history of opportunistic infection was associated with a shorter survival [6].

There is no question that HIV patients do better than those who have progressed to AIDS. In addition, it is apparent that total WBC is not a useful indicator of operative outcome. There is a trend in low versus high hematocrit values as a predictor of outcome. Total serum albumin is significant when comparing mortalities with non-appendectomy survivors.

3.6. Spontaneous Peritonitis

Spontaneous bacterial peritonitis (SBP) which most commonly occurs with cirrhotic liver disease and ascites may also present in the AIDS patients. Spontaneous peritonitis may be caused by opportunistic pathogens, including cytomegalovirus, Mycobacterium avium intracellulare (MAI), Mycobacterium tuberculosis, Cryptococcus neoformans, and Strongyloides [54,55].

SBP usually presents with an abrupt onset of fever and chills associated with abdominal rebound tenderness. These patients require a thorough investigation to rule out free perforation of the gut. A diagnostic paracentisis is performed and characteristically, with spontaneous peritonitis, the fluid will be cloudy on visual examination. The diagnosis of spontaneous peritonitis is confirmed by demonstration greater than 500 white blood cells per cubic millimeter, and/or greater than 250 polymorphonuclear cells per cubic millimeter on microscopic examination of the paracentesis fluid. A peripheral white blood cell count greater than 20,000 may also be found. The ascitic fluid is sent for Gram's stain, fungal stain, and aerobic and anaerobic bacterial, viral and fungal cultures.

Patients with alcoholic liver disease and spontaneous bacterial peritonitis are most commonly infected with Gram-negative bacilli. Less frequently pneumococci, or other Gram-positive bacteria may be present. Unless an organism is identified on Gram's stain, empiric treatment with ampicillin and an aminoglycoside, or cefotaxime should be instituted until culture results become available. The treatment for uncomplicated SBP is usually 10-14 days of antibiotics.

3.7. Acute Appendicitis

The incidence of acute appendicitis was slightly more than 10% of all those AIDS patients undergoing laparotomy for an acu-

te abdomen. This incidence appears to be very high, particularly in view of the fact that the number of people who have developed this disease has decreased so markedly within the past few decades. According to the National Center for Health Statistics there were 157.3 appendectomies per 100,000 people in 1971. In 1990, the rate was 96 per 100,000, or a decrease of 38.8% 56. However, the finding in the AIDS population is not unexpected when one considers the wide distribution of cytomegalovirus in the gastrointestinal tract and that it frequently targets the appendix and the small and large intestine.

Acute appendicitis may be quite difficult to diagnose in AIDS patients because many do not have the typical McBurneys syndrome. Abdominal pain with localization to the right lower quadrant, nausea and vomiting usually occurs but diarrhea, rather uncommon in infections of the appendix in the general population, is seen frequently in AIDS patients [56]. In addition, leukocytosis, a classical finding among non-AIDS patients, is absent in the majority of cases of acute appendicitis among those with AIDS [52,56].

Fever, too, is an inconstant finding in AIDS-appendicitis. Sonography [57] and CT scans might prove helpful in differentiating an acute appendix from enterocolitis or an intraperitoneal abscess. When the diagnosis is still not clear, laparoscopy may reveal the cecal and appendiceal region, thus leading to a more dependable diagnosis [52].

The difficulty in making an early precise diagnosis has led many physicians and surgeons to delay surgery for several days in suspected cases of appendicitis. Such delays are thought by many to be partly responsible for the large number of gangrenous and ruptured appendices found among this group of patients.

Differential diagnosis is complicated in AIDS-appendicitis by the knowledge that ileitis and ileocolitis are such common entities in the disease. The differentiation is of major importance because these latter diseases are most often treated medically, not surgically. Despite difficulties in diagnosis, on the basis of symptoms, the physical signs are often typical in appendicitis of AIDS origin. Tenderness with muscle spasm, rigidity and rebound in the right lower quadrant of the abdomen are present and if the appendix has ruptured, signs of localized or generalized peritonitis becomes evident.

When the diagnosis appears assured, surgery is indicated and appendectomy is performed in the usual manner. If localized collection of pus or peritonitis is found, drainage may be indicated. However, drainage should be avoided whenever possible in order to reduce the chances of contamination of those charged with post-operative care. Those patients who had suppurative lesions should receive post-operative antibiotics.

4. NEOPLASMS

The relationship between AIDS, Kaposi sarcoma and lymphoma has been extensively investigated and there is evidence suggesting that the severe cellular immune deficiency caused by the HIV, not only predisposes affected individuals to the many opportunistic infections characteristic of AIDS but also may place them at increased risk of contracting oncogenic viruses [44,58,59].

The clinical manifestations of both Kaposis sarcoma and AIDS-related lymphomas vary

Figure 3
Mucosal Kaposis Sarcoma

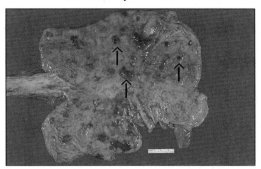

and are often difficult to distinguish from concurrent diseases. Severe abdominal pain, fever, weight loss and diarrhea or hematochesia are common complaints in AIDS patients, with or without a history of Kaposis sarcoma or lymphoma. These patients may present with an even more acute clinical picture when neoplasia is complicated by intussusception, obstruction, or perforation.

4.1. Kaposis Sarcoma

Kaposis sarcoma is one of the primary clinical manifestations of AIDS, occurring in 27% of all reported cases [27,60]. Approximately one half of homosexual men with AIDS will develop Kaposis sarcoma of the gastrointestinal tract. This incidence is significantly higher than that seen in other high-risk groups such as intravenous drug users. The gastrointestinal tract is the most common target organ after skin and nodes. Lesions are commonly multifocal and can involve the entire alimentary tract [44] (Figure 3).

The disease has long been endemic in Africa where at least four clinical subtypes are recognized: 1) a nodular form, which has an indolent and relatively benign coarse; 2) an aggressive form, which is more severe and often involves extensive cutaneous lesions as well as bone involvement; 3) a generalized form, which has disseminated cutaneous and visceral involvement and 4) a lymphadenopathic form, which affects children and younger adults and often spares the skin [27].

With Kaposis sarcoma, findings on barium contrast studies include nodularity, thickened folds, polypoidal lesions, plaques, umbilication and mass effect. Central umbilication or ulceration of nodules producing a so-called target or bull's eye appearance has been cited as a finding highly suggestive of Kaposis sarcoma, although this is not common [61]. There is a high incidence of duodenal as well as colorectal disease with Kaposi sarcoma [62]. The rectum tends to show the most severe form of involvement, with individual submucosal nodules coalescing and circumferentially infiltrating the rectal wall to produce an irregular and rigid narrowing of the rectum. This appearance has been described as mimicking Crohn's disease [61].

Initial reports of CT findings in AIDS-related Kaposi sarcoma emphasized the overlap between this disease and the lymphadenopathy syndrome [63]. Splenomegaly and mild retroperitoneal and mesenteric adenopathy are common to both.

Kaposi sarcoma lesions involving the intestine are usually submucosal in location and (Figure 3) have a characteristic violaceous appearance or endoscopy or colonoscopy. Two basic types of lesions are encountered at endoscopy of proven alimentary tract Kaposi sarcoma: 1) multiple small, flat hemorrhagic patches and 2) discrete, raised nodular, violaceous lesions that occasionally demonstrate central umbilications or superficial ulcerations. Because of their very characteristic endoscopic appearance, biopsies of these lesions are often considered unnecessary.

4.2. Lymphoma

It has been increasingly reported that AIDS patients are at increased risk of developing malignant non-Hodgkin lymphomas primarily involving the central nervous system and abdomen [64]. These lymphomas may precede the clinical onset of AIDS. AIDS patients with lymphoma frequently present with localizing signs and symptoms related to the abdomen, such as pain, a palpable mass, or gastrointestinal bleeding [65].

There are several unique manifestations of the disease within this subset of patients. There is a dramatic increase in extranodal involvement in AIDS-related lymphoma, including brain, bone marrow, abdominal viscera and cutaneous sites. AIDS-related non-Hodgkin lymphoma are very aggressive tumors and are reported to be of highly malignant histologic subtypes and to have both extensive adenopathy and multiorgan dissemination more commonly than non-Hodgkin lymphoma in the general population [66]. When compared to patients with non-Hodgkin lymphoma without AIDS, the response to treatment has been poor and there is a generally unfavorable prognosis.

Nevertheless, the poor outcome and higher mortality appear to be more dependent on the presence of concurrent infection or illness than on the histological subtype or extent of disease [27]. CT remains the study of choice for the detection and staging of both non-Hodgkin and Hodgkin lymphoma. CT enables accurate assessment of lymphoma involvement and can be used to plan appropriate therapy as well as follow-up response to therapy [67].

AIDS patients are more likely than is the general population to have gastrointestinal tract involvement by non-Hodgkin lymphoma. Although any portion of the gastrointestinal tract can be involved, gastric, distal ileal and rectal sites have been cited as the most common [64].

Associated lymphadenopathy and splenic or hepatic involvement is frequently seen in these cases. When bulky abdominal adenopathy is noted on CT in an AIDS patient, coexisting hepatic and splenic lesions favor lymphoma, whereas multiple low density necrotic areas within the nodes suggests the presence of MAL [27].

The stomach is the most frequent site of gastrointestinal lymphoma in both the general population and in AIDS patients [65]. The radiological appearance of gastric lymphomas are similar in both groups. Findings on barium radiography include an intraluminal fungating form, a polypoid form, an ulcerating form, an infiltrating form and diffuse enlargement of the gastric folds [68]. CT has been invaluable in the diagnosis of gastric lymphoma. CT usually demonstrates gastric wall thickening with a smoothly lobulated outer border that is clearly separable from surrounding viscera and associated lymphadenopathy that may extend below the renal hilum [67].

Gastric thickening may be circumferential or focal and eccentric. Associated ulceration is not uncommon [65]. In addition the gastric lumen may be nearly obliterated by extrinsic compression from large lymphomatous masses [67].

The small bowel is the second most frequent site of gastrointestinal involvement by AIDS-related lymphoma, with most occurring in the distal ileum. Obstructive symptoms are a common presentation, as is a palpable mass. Perforation and intussusception may complicate lymphoma of the small bowel. On barium radiography, the appearances of small bowel lymphoma include an aneurysmal form, an ulcerative form, a nodular/polypoid form, a constrictive form, a mesenteric form and a sprue form [68]. CT most commonly demonstrates one or more segments of circumferential or eccentric wall thickening. Associated excavated mesenteric masses also may be seen [65].

Lymphoma of the colon is uncommon but has been increasingly reported in the AIDS population [69]. Two main forms of colonic lymphomas have been described: a large polypoid mass and a diffuse form.

In an AIDS patient, MAI is the other important consideration in the differential diagnosis. Even when developing in the setting of AIDS, a colonic lymphoma manifest as a discrete mass may not be associated with abdominal adenopathy. When a solitary mass lesion is seen in the colon, CT findings can help distinguish primary lymphoma from adenocarcinoma. Cecal tumors that extend to involve the terminal ileum, tumors that are fairly well demarcated from the surrounding pericolonic fat and show no evidence of invasion or obstruction of neighboring viscera and tumors that perforate in the absence of desmoplastic reaction should suggest lymphoma, particularly in light of a clinical history of AIDS or risk factors for HIV infection [69].

The use of fine needle aspiration biopsy for accurate diagnosis and subtyping of non-Hodgkin lymphoma is controversial. Endoscopically guided biopsy of alimentary tract lesions has been fairly successful. Owing to its submucosal origin, however, lymphoma may be poorly visualized at endoscopy. Because proper chemotherapy often will depend on accurate histologic subtyping, surgical biopsy may still be needed in questionable cases [70].

5. ABDOMINAL DISEASES IN HIV-INFECTED CHILDREN

Approximately 5000 children in the United States have contracted AIDS from perinatal exposure [71]. Modes of transmission to infants include infected amniotic fluid, transplacental infection, exposure to infected maternal blood or body fluids and infected breast milk. Adolescent modes of infection are the same as for adults. Opportunistic infections of the upper and lower gastrointestinal tract, chronic non-specific diarrhea and wasting syndromes are among the most frequent complications seen in children with AIDS [72]. World wide, gastrointestinal infections are the leading cause of morbidity and mortality in HIV-infected children.

5.1. Lymphoma

Lymphoma should be included in the differential diagnosis of virtually any intra-abdominal mass in a patient with AIDS. The clinical presentation of children with AIDS-related lymphoma is different from that of adults in that they tend to have site-specific symptoms as opposed to the systemic B-type symptoms seen in adults [73]. Unlike adults, lymphoma is the most common AIDS-related neoplasm in the pediatric patient [73] but it is only a part of the many B-cell proliferative disorders associated with AIDS. The non-neoplastic syndromes include hypergammaglobulinemia, lymphocytic interstitial pneumonitis, diffuse infiltrative lymphocytosis and gut-associated lymphoid tissue. The neoplastic syndrome includes non-Hodgkin lymphoma with B-cell origin [73]. A distinguishing feature of AIDS in pediatric patients is the prominence of B-cell proliferative disorders, such as lymphocytic interstitial pneumonitis and gut-associated lymphoid tissue [75], with non-Hodgkin lymphoma being the most common AIDS-related neoplasm in children. In addition, Siskin et al [75] reported pediatric patients with non-Hodgkins lymphoma frequently presented with tumors in more than one anatomic site with the liver (78% of patients) as the most common site of involvement, followed by the spleen (55%), chest (55%), bone (44%) and kidneys (44%). Other sites included the brain, renal glands and parotid gland. The pathogenesis of these disorders has been shown to correlate with previous exposure to the Epstein-Barr virus [65]; this may relate to the known ability of the virus to stimulate a polyclonal

5.2. B-cell proliferation.

Approximately two-thirds of adult patients have intra-abdominal involvement with AIDS-related lymphoma but it has rarely been reported in pediatric patients [74]. However, Siskin et al [75] has recently reported 78% of their pediatric AIDS patients presented with intra-abdominal lymphoma involvement. This was slightly higher than the reported frequency in adults. In addition, 86% of patients with evidence of abdominal lymphoma had extranodal [75]. Radiological findings for intra-abdominal lymphoma in the pediatric population are similar to findings reported in the adult radiology literature [75]. The differential diagnosis for lesions found in the liver, spleen and kidneys in pediatric patients should include mycobacterial infection and rarely Kaposi sarcoma. Although primary lymphoma of bone is rare, secondary involvement is common in both Hodgkin and non-Hodgkin lymphoma [76]. The prevalence of secondary bone involvement in non-Hodgkins lymphoma is higher in children than in adults, with approximately 25% of pediatric patients with lymphoma having secondary bone lesions [75]. The common sites for bone involvement include the skull, pelvis and spine [77].

5.3. Diarrhea

Diarrhea occurs in approximately 20% to 40% of HIV-infected children [78] but frequently no enteric pathogen can be identified. As a result, many of the HIV-infected children may develop abdominal pain with malnutrition or growth failure. However, in the United States and Europe diarrheal gastrointestinal infections do not decrease longevity.

In the immunocompromised child, careful evaluation for an enteric infection should be attempted. The presence of blood or polymorphonuclear leukocytes in stool supports a diagnosis of colitis, whereas stools containing carbohydrate suggest malabsorption and enteritis [78]. The more common infections in the pediatric population that cause diarrhea are Cryptosporidium, Giardia lamblia, Candida albicans, Mycobacterium avium-intracellulare, Salmonella, Shigella, Campylobacter, CMV, Adenoviral and Rotavirus. The identification of a treatable pathogen as the cause of HIV related diarrheal disease in children with AIDS is the first step of the diagnostic approach to this population [78]. If no bacterial or parasitic pathogenic infection is found, detec-

tion of a viral cause of the diarrhea can result in effective treatment.

Determination of the degree of intestinal injury in the HIV-infected child with diarrhea from which no enteric pathogen can be found can be assessed by lactose breath and D-xylose absorption tests [78]. An abnormal lactose breath test in children should result in a lactose-free diet or exogenous lactase with meals containing lactose. Decreased D-xylos absorption suggests that the absorptive surface area of the intestine is diminished. In one study of HIV-infected children, patients with decreased d-xylos absorption had an increased chance of being infected with an enteric pathogen [79]. An esophagogastroduodenoscopy is also beneficial in defining the degree of intestinal injury by obtaining tissue to measure the activity of brush-border enzymes, often decreased in HIV-infected children [79]. These procedures to determine the degree of intestinal injury in the immunocompromised child with diarrhea, aid the clinician in decisions regarding specific enteral nutritional support or other therapy.

5.3.1. Viral

Rotavirus is the most common viral enteric pathogen in immunocompromised children. It causes chronic diarrhea and disseminated illness which can involve other organs such as the liver [80]. Diagnosis is made by enzyme-linked immunoassay on stool. The recommended therapy is supportive care but human serum immunoglobulin given internally also can be effective [81]. Adenovirus serotypes 40 and 41 are the most common sources of enteric infection in normal children. In the immune deficient child, adenovirus infection may result in fulminant hepatitis and gastrointestinal hemorrhage, often part of a disseminated adenoviral infection that can affect the lungs, bone marrow, heart and brain [82]. Supportive care is the most common therapy but human serum globulin and ribavirin are also potential therapeutic agents [72]. CMV can cause ulcerative lesions anywhere along the gastrointestinal tract. If the small intestine is involved, abdominal pain, vomiting, diarrhea, or gastrointestinal bleeding can occur [83]. Viral shedding can also occur in the intestine in children with or without active CMV making it difficult to prove CMV as the causative pathogen. Ganciclovir and, alternatively, foscarnet can be used to treat CMV-related gastrointestinal disease [72]. Both medications have been associated with bone marrow suppression [25]. Unlike adults, astrovirus, picobirnavirus and calicivirus have not been identified in HIV-infected children [72].

5.3.2. Bacterial

Although enteric bacteria are not a major cause of diarrhea in HIV-infected children living in the United States and Europe, almost half the bacteria isolated from the blood of HIV-positive children with bacteremia were enteric pathogens [84]. Although bacterial overgrowth has been reported to occur in HIV-infected children with diarrhea [85], the prevalence and significance of bacterial overgrowth in relation to diarrhea and malabsorption are not known [72]. Children with CD4 counts less than $50/mm^3$ are at increased risk for developing Mycobacterium avium-intracellulare, or Mycobacterium avium complex (MAC), infection involving the bone marrow, lungs, liver, mesenteric lymph nodes and/or gastrointestinal tract.[86] Abdominal pain and diarrhea are common presenting symptoms, usually experienced in conjunction with recurrent fe-

vers. At the present time, there is no effective treatment for MAC infection. However, azithromycin, clarithromycin, ethambutol, ciprofloxacin, amikacin, rifampin and clofazamine have been used individually or in combinations. Parenteral or, if possible, enteral nutritional support should be provided to children with MAC infection on the basis of quality-of-life parameters [72].

5.3.3. Protozoan

Although Isospora beli and Microsporida have been identified in HIV-infected adults, evaluation of tissue from HIV-infected children has failed to show these infections [72]. Sometimes Giardia infections are asymptomatic but can also cause watery diarrhea, bloating and abdominal pain. An effective therapeutic choice is the administration of metronidazole or furazolidone for 10 to 14 days. On the other hand, Cryptosporidium can severely compromise the nutritional status of arimmune deficient child by causing chronic secretory diarrhea. Cryptosporidium infects the small and large intestine but also can invade the mucosa of the gallbladder, bile ducts and pancreatic duct, resulting in cholangitis and/or pancreatitis [87]. There is no effective therapy to treat Cryptosporidium infections, although isolated reports with the use of hyperimmune bovine colostrum are promising.[88]

5.3.4 Fungal

The most common fungal infections in HIV-positive children are Candida or Histoplasma. The esophagus is the most common area for Candida albicans infection but other areas of the gastrointestinal tract can also be involved. In the immunocompromised child, disseminated candidiasis often develops if a central venous catheter is implanted, if parenteral nutrition or antibiotics are received, or oral thrush is present [89]. Fluconaxole is effective therapy for esophagitis, while amphotericin B is more frequently given for disseminated candidiasis.

5.3.5. Hepatomegaly

HIV-Positive children commonly experience hepatomegaly in conjunction with splenomegaly and abnormally increased transaminase levels but hepatocellular dysfunction, characterized by ascites, fulminanthepatic failure, prolonged clotting, hypoalbuminemia, hepatic fibrosis, or cirrhosis with portal hypertension, is rare.[90] Medications, nutritional factors or hepatotoxic pathogens frequently cause elevated transaminase levels. In the case of viral or drug induced hepatitis, transaminase levels are usually more than four times normal. In addition, increased alkaline phosphatase levels can be associated with MAC, hepatic Pneumocytis carinii, fungal infections of the liver, granulomatous hepatitis, cholangiopathy, or the obstruction of the extrahepatic bile duct. HIV-infected children seem to have more difficulty with chronic active hepatitis than do adults. Due to immunologically mediated hepatocellular injury of the hepatitis B virus, these differences could be attributed to the relative preservation of cellular immune function and higher numbers of CD4 lymphocytes in HIV-positive children than in adults.

5.4. Pancreatitis

Pancreatitis is common in the pediatric AIDS population with a reported incidence of 17% [91]. Miller et al. reported exposure to pentamidine isethionate, especially in conjunction with low CD4 T-lymphocyte counts (<100 cells/mm3), to be significantly associated with pancreatitis. In adults with HIV infection, pentamidine isethionate or tri-methoprim-sulfamethoxazole, administered for prophylaxis or therapy for P.Carinii pneumonia, has been associated with pancreatitis [91]. Pentamidine isethionate can be detected in serum samples obtained from patients as much as 1 year after the last dose of the drug [91]. Thus, discontinuing pentamidine isethionate with the onset of pancreatitis may not immediately alter the patient's clinical course. Administration of pentamidine isethionate in HIV-infected children with low CD4 T-lymphocyte counts should be carefully reconsidered because Miller et al [84] reported 62 % of their pediatric patients who were given pentamidine isethionate developed pancreatitis. Other medications that have been associated with pancreatitis in adults include sulfonamide-containing drugs, 2',3'-Dideoxyinosine (ddI) and 2',3'-Dideoxycytidine. Several opportunistic infections are also associated with the onset of pancreatitis, such as CMV, Cryptosporidium, pneumocystis carinii pneumonia and Mycobacterium avium intracellulare. Coinfection with CMV may be associated with a protracted course of pancreatitis [91].

Miller et al [84] reported clinical presenting symptoms of vomiting, abdominal distention and intolerance to feedings [91]. As a result, the presence of normal or minimally elevated amylase values should not exclude the diagnosis of pancreatitis. Thus, serum lipase levels should be measured in children with symptoms because levels 16.4 times the normal have been reported [91]. The true incidence of pancreatitis may be underestimated because gastrointestinal symptoms are prominent in HIV-infected children. In a series of 35 adult patients infected with HIV who were admitted consecutively to an intensive care unit, 46% had clinically unsuspected pancreatitis diagnosed by elevations of both serum amylase and lipase values [89]. Likewise, elevations in serum amylase values without increases in serum lipase values have been detected in the HIV population and may represent either salivary amylase or macroamylasemia [91]. Serum lipase activity should be measured routinely both in HIV-infected children with clinical symptoms of pancreatitis and in those with asymptomatic increases in serum amylase values [91]. Quick diagnosis is important because pancreatitis has been associated with a poor prognosis [91].

REFERENCES

1. Tanowitz HB, Simon D, Wittner M. Medical Management of AIDS Patients: Gastrointestinal Manifestations. Med Clin N AM 1992; 76:45-62

2. Centers for Disease Control and Prevention: Morbidity and Mortality Weekly Report Nov 24, 1995; 44:46

3. LaRaja RD, Rothenberg RE, Odom JW, et al: The incidence of intra-abdominal surgery in acquired immunodeficiency syndrome: A Statistical review of 904 patients. Surgery 105(No2, part 1): 175-179, 1989.

4. Lowy AM, Barie PS: Laparotomy in Patients Infected with Human Immunodeficiency Virus: Indications and Outcome. British Journal of Surgery 1994; 81: 942-945.

5. Davidson T, Allen-mersh TG, Miles AF et al: Emergency Laparotomy in Patients with Aids. Br J Surg 1991; 78: 924-6.

6. Diettrich NA Cacioppo JC, Kaplan G, Cohen SM. A Growing Spectrum of Surgical Disease in Patients with Human Immunodeficiency Virus/Acquired Immunodeficiency Syndrome. Experience with 120 Major Cases. Arch Surg 1991; 126: 860-6.

7. Barone JE, Gingold BS, Nelson TF et al. Abdominal Pain in Patients with Acquired Immune Deficiency syndrome. Ann Surg 204: 619-623, 1986.

8. Blumberg RS, Kelsey P, Perrone T et al. Cytomegalovirus and cryptosporidium-associated acalculous gangrenous cholecystitis. Am J Med. 1984;76:1118-1123.

9. Margulis SJ, Honig Cl, Soave R, et al. Biliary tract obstruction in the acquired immunodeficiency syndrome. Ann Intern Med. 1986;105:207-210.

10. Schneiderman DJ. Hepatobiliary abnormalities of AIDS. Gastroenterol Clin North Am 1988; 17:615-30.

11. Adolph MD, Bass SN, Lee SK et al. Cytomegaloviral Acalculous Cholecystitis in Acquired Immunodeficiency Syndrome Patients. The American Surgeon. 1993;59:679-84.

12. Burt AD, Scott G, Shiach CR, Isles CG. Acquired immunodeficiency syndrome in a patient with no known risk factors: A pathological study. J Clin Pathol 1984;37:471-4.

13. Finegold MJ, Carpenter RJ. Obliterative cholangitis due to cytomegalovirus: A possible precursor of paucity of intrahepatic bile ducts. Hum Patho 1982;13:662-5.

14. Jacobson MA, Cello JP, Sande MA. Cholestasis and disseminated cytomegalovirus disease in patients with the acquired immunodeficiency syndrome. Am J Med 1988;84:218-24.

15. Mintz L, Dreww L, Miner RC, Braff EH. Cytomegalovirus infections in homosexual men: An epidemiological study. Ann Intern Med 1983;99:326-9.

16. Fox MS, Wilk PJ, Weissmann HS, Freeman LM, Gliedman ML. Acute acalculous cholecystitis. Surg Gynecol Obstet 1984;159:13-6.

17. Dolmatch BL, Laing FC, Federle MP, Jeffrey RB, Cello J. AIDS-related cholangitis: Radio-

graphic findings in nine patients. Radiology 1987;163:313-6.

18. Schneiderman DJ, Cello JP, Laing FP. Papillary stenosis and sclerosing cholangitis in the acquired immunodeficiency syndrome. Ann Intern Med 1987;106:546-9.

19. Cello JP. Acquired immunodeficiency syndrome cholangiopathy: spectrum of disease. Am J Med. 1989;86:539-546.

20. Pol S, Romana C, Richard S et al. Microsporidia infection in patients with the human immunodeficiency virus and unexplained cholangitis. NEJM. 1993;328:95-99.

21. Benhamou Y, Caumes E, Gerosa Y et al. AIDS-related cholangiopathy: critical analysis of a prospective series of 26 patients. Dig Dis Sci. 1993;38:1113-1118.

22. Bouche H, Housset C, Dumont JL et al. AIDS-related cholangitis: diagnostic features and course in 15 patients. J Hepatol. 1993;17:34-39.

23. Guarda LA, Stein SA, Cleary KA, Ordonez NGH: human cryptosporidiosis in the acquired immunodeficiency syndrome. Arch Pathol Lab Med 1983, 107:562-566.

24. Roulot D, Valla D, Brun-Vezinet F et al.: Cholangitis in acquired immunodeficiency syndrome: report of two cases and review of the literature. Gut 1987, 28:1653-1660.

25. Teixidor HS, Godwin TA, Ramirez EA: Cryptosporidiosis of the biliary tract in AIDS. Radiology 1991, 180:51-56.

26. Farhi DC, Mason UG, Horsburgh CR: Pathologic findings in disseminated Mycobacterium avium-intracellulare infection. Am J Clin Pathol 85:67-72, 1986.

27. Nyberg DA, Federle MP, Jeffrey RB et al: Abdominal CT findings of disseminated Mycobacterium avium-intracellulare in AIDS. AJR 145:297-299, 1985.

28. Nyberg DA, Jeffrey RB, Federle MP et al. AIDS-related lymphomas: Evaluation by abdominal CT. Radiology 159:59-63, 1986.

29. Radin DR: Intraabdominal Mycobacterium tuberculosis vs. Mycobacterium avium intracellulare infections in patients with AIDS: Distinction based on CT findings. AJR 156:487-491, 1991.

30. Soriano E, Mallolas J, Gatell JM: Characteristics of tuberculosis in HIV-infected patients: A case-control study. AIDS 2:429-432, 1988.

31. Hulnick DH, Megibow AJ, Naidich DP et al: Abdominal tuberculosis: CT evaluation. Radiology 157:199-204, 1985.

32. Nakano H, Jaramillo E, Watanabe M et al: Intestinal tuberculosis: Findings on double-contrast barium enema. Gastrointest Radiol 17:108-114, 1992.

33. Bargallo N, Nicolau C, Luburich et al: Intestinal tuberculosis in AIDS. Gastrointest Radiol 17:115-118, 1992.

34. Thoeni RF, Margulis AR: Tuberculosis gastrointestinal. Semin Roentgenol 14:408-429, 1979.

35. Berk RN, Wall SD, McArdle CB et al: Cryptosporidiosis of the stomach and small intestine in patients with AIDS. AJR 143:549-554, 1984.

36. Goedert JJ, Biggar RJ, Melbye M et al.: Effect of T4 Count and Cofactors on the Incidence of AIDS in Homosexual Men Infected with Human Immunodeficiency Virus. JAMA 1987; 257(3): 331-334.

37. Lemp GF, Payne SF, Rutherford GW et al. Projections of AIDS morbidity and mortality in San Francisco. JAMA 1990;263:1497-501.13 Phair JP. Estimating Prognosis in HIV-1 Infection. Ann. Int. Med. 1993;118:742-4.

38. Sander RB, Russel JC, Jeffrey F. Laboratory Parameters as Predictors of Operative Outcome After Major Abdominal Surgery in AIDS- and HIV-Infected Patients. AM Surg, 1993 Nov, 59 (11):754-7.

39. Murray JG, Evans JS, Jeffrey BP, Hwlvorsen RA. Cytomegalovirus Colitis in AIDS: CT Features. AJR 1995;165:67-71.

41. Soderlund C, Goran BA, Lennart E et al. Surgical Treatment of Cytomegalovirus Enterocolitis in Severe Human Immunodeficiency Virus Infection. Dis Col Rectum 1994 Jan:63-72.

42. Kuhlman JE, Fishman EK: Acute abdominal disorders in AIDS: CT evaluation. Crit Rev Diagn Imaging 32: 229-237, 1991.

43. Fishman EK, Kavuru M, Jones B et al: CT evaluation of pseudomembranous colitis: A review of 26 cases. Radiology 180:57-60, 1991.

44. Jones BJ, Fishman EK: CT of the gut in the immunocompromised host. Radiol Clin North Am 27:763-771, 1989.

45. Wall SD, Jones B: Gastrointestinal tract in the immunocompromised host: Opportunistic infections and other complications. Radiology 185:327-335, 1992.

46. Smith PD: Gastrointestinal infections in AIDS. Ann Intern Med 116:63-77, 1992.

47. Megibow AJ, Balthazar EJ, Hulnick DH: Radiology of non-neoplastic gastrointestinal disorders in acquired immune deficiency syndrome. Semin Roentgenol 22:31-41, 1987.

48. Balthazar EJ, Megibow AJ, Hulnick DH: Cytomegalovirus esophagitis and gastritis in AIDS. AJR 144:1201-1204, 1985.

49. Wexner SD. Sexually Transmitted Diseases of the Colon, Rectum, and Anus. The Challenge of the Nineties. Dis Colon Rectum 1990;33:1048-62.

50. Moenning S, Huber P, Simonton C et al. Prediction of morbidity by T4 lymphocyte count in the HIV positive or AIDS anorectal outpatient. Dis Colon Rectum 1993 (in press).

51. Safavi A, Gottesman L, Dailey TH. Anorectal surgery in the HIV+ patient: Update. Dis Colon Rectum 1991;34:299.

52. Binderow SR, Shaked AA. Acute appendicitis in patients with AIDS/HIV infection. Am J Surg 1991;162:9.

53. Deziel DJ, Hyser MJ, Doolas A et al. Major abdominal operations in AIDS. Am Surg 1990;56:445.

54. Potter DA, Danforth DN, Macher AM et al: Evaluation of abdominal pain in the AIDS patient. Ann Surg 199:332-339, 1984.

55. Barnes P, Leedom JM, Radin DR et al: An unusual case of tuberculous peritonitis in a man with AIDS. West J Med 144:467-469, 1986.

56. Fauci AS, Macher Am, Longo DL et al: NIH Conference on AIDS: Epidemiologic, clinical, immunological and therapeutic consideration. Ann Int Med 100:92-106, 1984.

57. Jeffrey RB, Laing FC, Lewis FR: Acute appendicitis: high resolution real-time ultrasound findings. Radiol 163:11, 1987.

58. Ioachim HL, Cooper MC, Hellman GC: Lymphomas in men at high risk for acquired immunodeficiency syndrome (AIDS). Cancer 56:2831-2842, 1985.

59. Urba WS, Longo DL: Clinical spectrum of human retroviral induced diseases. Cancer Res 45:4637-4643, 1985.

60. Longo DL: Kaposi's sarcoma and other neoplasms. Ann Intern Med 100:92-106, 1984.

61. Rose HS, Balthazar EJ, Megibow AJ: Alimentary tract involvement in Kaposi's sarcoma: Radiographic and endoscopic findings in 25 homosexual men. AJR 139:661-666, 1982.

62. Wall SD, Ominsky S, Altman DF et al: Multifocal abnormalities of the gastrointestinal tract in AIDS. AJR 146:1-5, 1986.

63. Hill CA, Harle TS, Mansell PWA: The prodrome, Kaposi sarcoma and infections associated with acquired immunodeficiency syndrome: Radiologic findings in 39 patients. Radiology 149:393-399, 1983.

64. Haskal ZJ, Lindan CE, Goodman PC: Lymphoma in the immunocompromised patient. Radiol Clin North Am 28:885-899, 1990.

65. Radin DR, Esplin JA, Levine AM et al: AIDS-related non-Hodgkin's lymphoma: Abdomi-

nal CT findings in 112 patients. AJR 160:1133-1139, 1993.

66. Ziegler JL, Beckstead JA, Volberding PA et al: Non-Hodgkin's lymphoma in 90 homosexual men-relation to generalized lymphadenopathy and the acquired immunodeficiency syndrome. N Engl J Med 3111:565-570, 1984.

67. Fishman EK, Kuhlman JE, Jones RJ; CT of lymphoma: Spectrum of disease. Radiographics 11:647-669, 1991.

68. Dodd GD: Lymphoma of the hollow abdominal viscera. Radiol Clin North Am 28: 771-783, 1990.

69. Wyatt SH, Fishman EK, Hruban RH et al: CT of primary colonic lymphoma: Radiologic/pathologic correlation. Clin Imaging 18:131-141, 1994.

70. Jeffrey RB, Nyberg DA, Bottles D et al. Abdominal CT in Acquired Immunodeficiency Syndrome. AJR 1985;146:7-13.

71. Schwartz DL, So HB, Bungarz WR et al: A Case of Life-Threatening Gastrointestinal Hemorrhage in an Infant with AIDS. J Pediatr Surg 24:313,1989.

72. Jain A, Reif S, O'Neil K et al: Small Intestinal Bacterial Overgrowth and Protein-Losing Enteropathy in an Infant with AIDS. J Pediatr Gastroenterol Nutr 15:452,1992.

73. Grattan-Smith D, Harrison LF, Singleton EB. Radiology of AIDS in the Pediatric Patient. Curr Probl Diagn Radiol 1992; 21:79-109.

74. Rosenberg SA, Diamond HD, Taslowitz B et al. Lymphosarcoma: Review of 1269 Cases. Medicine 1961;40:31-84.

75. Grattan-Smith D, Harrison LF, Singleton EB. Radiology of AIDS in the Pediatric Patient. Curr Probl Diagn Radiol 1992; 21:79-109.

76. Pratt RD, Hatch R, Dankner WM et al: pediatric Human Immunodeficiency Virus Infection in a Low Seroprevalence Area. Pediart Infect Dis J 12: 304,1991.

77. Gilger MA, Matson DO, Conner ME et al: Extraintestinal Rotavirus Infections in Children with Immunodeficiency. J Pediatr 120:912,1992.

78. Bernstein LJ, Krieger BZ, Novick B et al: Bacterial Infection in the Acquired Immunodeficiency Syndrome of Children. Pediatr Infect Dis J 4:472,1985.

79. Young SA, Crocker DW. Burkitt's Lymphoma in a Child with AIDS. Pediatr Pathol 1991;11:115-122

80. Krilov LR, Rubin LG, Frogel M et al: Disseminated Adenovirus Infection With Hepatic Necrosis in Patients with Human Immunodeficiency Virus Infection and other Immunodeficiency States. Rev Infect Dis 12:303,1990.

81. Dagan R, Schwartz RH, Insel RA et al: Severe Diffuse adenovirus 7a pneumonia in a Child with Combined Immunodeficiency: Possible Therapeutic Effect of Human Serum Immunoglobulin Containing a Specific Neutralizing Antibody. Pediatr Infect Dis J 3:246,1984

82. Gudnason T, Belani KK, Balfour HH: Ganciclovir Treatment of Cytomegalovirus Disease in Immunocompromised Children. Pediatr Infect Dis J 8:436,1989.

83. Rustein RM, Cobb P, McGowan KL et al: Mycobacterium Avium Intracellulare Complex infection in HIV-infected Children. AIDS 7:507,1993.

84. Ungar BLP, Ward DJ, Fayer R et al: Cessation of Cryptosporidium-associated Diarrhea in an Acquired Immunodeficiency Syndrome Patient after Treatment with Hyperimmune Bovine Colostrum. Gastroenterology 98:486,1991.

85. Leibovitzz E, Rigaud M, Chandwani S et al: Disseminated Fungal infection in children infected with Human immunodeficiency Virus. Pediart Infect Dis J 10:888,1991.

86. Miller TL, Winter HS, Lynn M et al. Pancreatitis in Pediatric Human Immunodeficiency Virus Infection J of Pediatr:120 223,1992.

87. Zugar A, Wolf BZ, El-Sadir W, Simberkoff MS, Gahal JJ. Pentamidine-associated fatal Acute Pancreatitis. JAMA 1986;256:2383-5.

88. Mallory A, Kern F. Drug-induced pancreatitis: a Critical Review. Gastroenterology 1980;78:813-820.

89. Brivet F, Coffin B, Bedossa B et al. Pancreatic lesions in AIDS. Lancet 1987;2:570-1.

90. Siskin GP, Haller JO, Miller S, Sundaram R; Aids-Related Lymphoma: Radiologic Features in Pediatric Patients. Radiology 1995; 196: 63-66.

91. Greenberg RE, Bank S, Singer C: Macroamlylasemia in association with the Acquired Immunodeficiency Syndrome. Postgrad Med J 1987;63:677-9.

Pediatric Intra-abdominal Infections

Frazier W. Frantz, MD, and Moritz M. Ziegler, MD.

Intra-abdominal infections are characterized by a purulent exudate in the peritoneal cavity which results from an inflammatory response of the peritoneum to micro-organisms and their toxins. The two major manifestations of intra-abdominal infection are peritonitis, acute bacterial infection of the peritoneal cavity and abscess formation, in which infection has been localized into a collection of purulent material walled off from the remainder of the peritoneal cavity. An important subset of intra-abdominal infections is comprised of those cases where the infectious process is contained within a diseased organ or viscus and can be eradicated by surgical resection without the need for prolonged antibiotic therapy [1].

While the principles of management of pediatric intra-abdominal infections are similar to those in adults, particularly in adolescents, there are many unique aspects of these infections in pediatric or neonatal patients with regard to etiology, pathophysiology, microbiology and the role of an immature immune defense mechanism. The common causes of intra-abdominal infection in adults are trauma, appendicitis, perforated duodenal ulcer, perforated sigmoid colon (caused by diverticulitis, volvulus, or cancer), strangulation obstruction of the small intestine, necrotizing pancreatitis and post-operative peritonitis due to anastomotic disruption [2]. In children, the causes vary significantly depending upon the age of the child and the presence of underlying medical or congenital pathology. In neonates, for instance, the most common cause of intra-abdominal infection is necrotizing enterocolitis (NEC), whereas appendicitis is much more prevalent in older children and adolescents. Causes related to underlying medical/ congenital conditions include Hirschsprung's enterocolitis, Meckel's diverticulitis, cholangitis related to choledochal cyst or following portoenterostomy for biliary atresia and meconium peritonitis.

In this chapter, the classification and general management principles of pediatric intra-abdominal infections will be presented. These infections will be organized according to patient age at presentation and the site-specific nature of the intra-abdominal infection. Diagnostic and management recommendations will be outlined for these infections. Finally, special consideration will be given to intra-abdominal infections in immunocompromised pediatric patients (children with cancer, solid organ transplant recipients and children with HIV/AIDS) and patients with short gut syndrome.

1. PERITONITIS

Peritonitis can be classified into a primary or secondary form, the latter being far more common. Prognosis for both primary and secondary peritonitis in children is good, the mortality being less than 10%. In adults, a third form, tertiary peritonitis, is characterized by the persistence of diffuse intra-abdominal infection despite appropriate and timely antibiotic administration and surgical intervention for secondary peritonitis and is often associated with a fatal outcome [3].

1.1. Primary Peritonitis

Primary peritonitis is a diffuse bacterial peritoneal infection in which there is no obvious source for organism portal of entry (i.e., no evidence of viscus perforation). The settings in which this entity is encountered include: (1) spontaneous peritonitis in children (otherwise healthy), (2) spontaneous peritonitis associated with cirrhosis or the nephrotic syndrome and (3) peritonitis in patients on peritoneal dialysis[1]. Peritonitis is also among the intra-abdominal complications observed in patients with ventriculoperitoneal shunts and will be discussed in this section. One distinguishing feature of primary peritonitis is that it is typically a monomicrobial, aerobic infection. The presence of mixed flora or obligate anaerobes in peritoneal fluid cultures suggests secondary peritonitis and necessitates an investigation to rule out viscus perforation.

In children with primary peritonitis, an isolated distant infection may be present but it is not in obvious continuity with the perito-

neum. Bacteria may gain access to the peritoneal cavity via hematogenous, lymphatic (transdiaphragmatic from pneumonia), genital (ascending through fallopian tubes) or urinary tract routes. They may even enter via transmucosal migration in the intestinal tract [4].

Primary peritonitis accounts for 1 to 2 percent of all pediatric abdominal emergencies [5] and may be responsible for up to 15% of all cases of diffuse peritonitis [4]. The peak age incidence is 5 to 9 years. It is more commonly seen in girls than boys. The incidence of primary peritonitis in children appears to be decreasing as a result of the increased use of antibiotics for urinary tract and respiratory infections.

1.2. Spontaneous peritonitis in "normal" children

Primary peritonitis in otherwise healthy children is rarely diagnosed preoperatively. The clinical picture mimics secondary bacterial peritonitis with fever, nausea, vomiting and diffuse abdominal tenderness with evidence of peritoneal irritation on physical examination. Infants may present with manifestations of sepsis, including lethargy, poor feeding and hypothermia. With evidence of peritonitis, older children typically undergo urgent laparotomy for presumptive acute appendicitis. The ill nature of these children in association with high fever and significant leukocytosis that can be seen with primary peritonitis may even suggest perforated appendicitis as the preoperative diagnosis. Unfortunately, in this otherwise healthy population of children, there are no signs or symptoms specific for primary peritonitis.

At operation, cloudy fluid is found in the peritoneal cavity. The appendix is normal and no source for the peritonitis can be identified. The fluid should be sampled and sent for aerobic and anaerobic cultures and Gram stain. Intra-abdominal exploration should be thorough within the confines of a limited incision and should include inspection of the bowel, gall bladder, kidney and pelvic organs. The appendix should be removed. In the unusual case that an abscess is found, it should be drained. Post-operatively, broad spectrum antibiotics (appropriate examples include ampicillin/gentamicin/clindamycin or ampicillin/sulbactam and gentamicin) should be continued until Gram stain/culture results dictate a more specific antibiotic coverage. When primary peritonitis is suspected, blood, urine and vaginal cultures may also be helpful in identifying the offending micro-organism.

In this group of patients, the most common causative organisms are Gram-positive cocci (*Streptococcus pneumoniae* and group A streptococci). These organisms can be treated with intravenous penicillin G. Gram-negative infections may be seen in girls and are usually due to a vaginal portal of entry. The duration of antibiotic therapy for primary peritonitis in otherwise healthy children is not well-defined but it should probably continue for at least 5 days or until fever, leukocytosis, ileus and other abdominal symptoms subside.

1.3. Spontaneous peritonitis associated with cirrhosis or nephrotic syndrome

Certain disease states predispose children to primary peritonitis. Most notably, children with nephrotic syndrome or ascites due to cirrhosis appear to be at particularly high risk [2]. Immune deficiencies, systemic lupus erythematosus and carcinoma may also put patients at risk. Primary peritonitis

in these settings has been termed spontaneous bacterial peritonitis (SBP). The pathogenesis of this infection is unclear but defects in reticuloendothelial and neutrophil function, low serum and ascitic fluid levels of complement and impaired bacterial opsonization are felt to be partially responsible [6]. Intrahepatic shunting in children with severe liver disease may also play a role. The best predictor of the development of SBP in patients with cirrhosis is a low total protein concentration in the ascitic fluid (patients with levels ≤ 1 g/dl are ten times more likely to develop SBP).

Primary peritonitis should be considered when a child with these underlying diseases, particularly with known ascites, presents with fever, abdominal pain and leukocytosis. Unfortunately, primary peritonitis in this susceptible population may present in a more subtle fashion, requiring a high index of suspicion. Such infections are usually caused by a single organism of gut origin. Gram-negative enteric organisms, most commonly *E. Coli*, account for 60% to 80% of adult cases. In children, *S. pneumoniae*, *H. flu*, and *N. meningitides* may cause relatively higher percentages of cases [7].

In addition to such differences in causative microbiology, primary peritonitis in susceptible versus healthy children mandates a different diagnostic and therapeutic plan. Because of a higher operative risk associated with these patients, a more conservative approach is taken. The diagnosis of peritonitis can be made using paracentesis. Peritoneal fluid is examined for cell count, differential, pH, levels of lactate, glucose, protein, and lactic dehydrogenase as well as Gram stain and cultures. An incubation period for the cultures of 24 to 72 hours is necessary before the etiologic organism of the peritonitis can be diagnosed by microbiology. Thus, therapy is usually initiated on the basis of selected rapid test results. An elevated neutrophil count (>250/mm^3), a reduced pH (<7.35) and an elevated lactate level (>32 mg/dl) have been found to be highly predictive of the presence of peritonitis [8].

Once the diagnosis of peritonitis is made, it is important to determine whether the infection has arisen from perforation or inflammation of the GI tract (secondary peritonitis) or is spontaneous (primary peritonitis). Because it is difficult to distinguish these entities based on clinical findings, laboratory parameters can be used to help determine the need for further investigation. If the ascitic fluid analysis reveals a glucose level below 50 mg/dl, a lactic dehydrogenase level higher that the upper limit of the normal serum range and a protein concentration higher than 1 g/dl, the likelihood of a secondary peritonitis is increased. In this setting, plain abdominal X-rays and water-soluble gastrointestinal contrast studies should be done. Surgical intervention is indicated if: (1) free air is present on plain films, (2) leakage from the GI tract is evidenced on contrast studies, (3) the ascitic fluid culture yields a mixed aerobic-anaerobic flora or (4) the patient fails to improve after the initiation of medical therapy [2].

Definitive therapy for primary peritonitis in this patient group includes broad-spectrum coverage for Gram-negative enteric and Gram-positive bacteria. While the combination of an aminoglycoside and ampicillin would be an acceptable regimen, single agent therapy with cefotaxime has been reported to be equally effective and less toxic [9]. Antimicrobial therapy should be adjusted based upon final culture and sensitivity results. Paracentesis should be repeated 48 hours after initiating antibiotic therapy as a gauge for predicting response to therapy.

Failure of the ascitic fluid leukocyte count to fall or continued positive cultures on repeat paracentesis may indicate underlying secondary peritonitis and the need for surgical intervention.

The issues of duration of therapy and potential antibiotic prophylaxis against recurrence have not been extensively evaluated in pediatric patients. Historically, affected children in this susceptible population have been treated for 10 to 14 days, especially with their first episodes of peritonitis. In adults, several trials have documented the safety and efficacy of a five-day antibiotic course with regard to mortality, cure rate and recurrence rate [10,11]. While the role of antibiotic prophylaxis in preventing recurrent peritonitis in adults with liver disease has been studied in great detail, the value of prophylaxis in children is unclear. In adults, intestinal decontamination with oral, non-absorbable antibiotics has been proven effective in reducing SBP recurrence, especially in high risk patients with gastrointestinal hemorrhage or acute liver failure. The benefits of long-term prophylaxis with regard to improving survival, decreasing morbidity or reducing the number of hospital admissions are known, however, have not been demonstrated [12].

1.4. Peritonitis in patients on peritoneal dialysis

Peritonitis is the most common complication of peritoneal dialysis. The incidence of this complication has previously been reported as one episode per 12.4 patient-months [13]. The cause of these infections is unclear but breaks in technique while changing dialysis bags are suspected. Mortality and serious morbidity are unusual. At presentation, cloudy dialysate effluent is found and is usually associated with low grade fever, abdominal pain and tenderness. The dialysate fluid may dilute mediators of inflammation, however, signs and symptoms are variable. The dialysate is obtained for culture and sensitivities, Gram stain and cell count. Criteria for establishing the diagnosis of peritonitis include: (1) the presence of micro-organisms on Gram stain or culture, (2) cloudy fluid with inflammatory cells (leukocyte count >100/mm³ with at least 50 per cent neutrophils) and (3) signs and symptoms of peritoneal irritation [14]. Micro-organisms cultured from the peritoneal fluid typically are normal skin flora (*Staph. epidermidis*, *Staph. aureus*, and *Strep. viridans*). Gram-negative organisms (*E. coli* and *P. aeuroginosa*) account for less than 30 per cent of cases. Approximately 4 per cent of children undergoing peritoneal dialysis have developed infections due to *Candida* or other fungi.

Treatment for children on peritoneal dialysis who present with peritonitis begins immediately after obtaining adequate peritoneal cultures. Appropriate antibiotics are included in the dialysate and passes for 10 to 14 days. Heparin is usually added to the dialysate to prevent adhesion formation and the dwell time of the dialysate is shortened. Empiric antibiotic coverage for Gram-positive and Gram-negative organisms is initiated and the drugs chosen are eventually adjusted based on culture and sensitivity data. If clinical improvement does not occur after 7 to 10 days, the effluent should be recultured and a change in antibiotics considered [2]. While most children can be treated in the ambulatory setting, infants and children with severe symptomatology may require hospitalization and intravenous antibiotics.

Peritonitis that does not clear with antibiotics should be treated by catheter removal. The likelihood of such antibiotic-resistant peritonitis is especially high when virulent organisms, such as *Pseudomonas* species or *Candida*, are the causative organisms. With Candidal infections, occasional patients respond to intravenous amphotericin B therapy but, in general, catheter removal is recommended. Additional scenarios when peritoneal dialysis catheter removal is recommended include: (1) recurrent episodes of peritonitis caused by the same organism (suggesting that the catheter may be the source of infection) and (2) after laparotomy is required for fecal peritonitis [2].

The timing of peritoneal catheter replacement is dependent upon several factors including the causative organisms and the severity of peritonitis present at the time of catheter removal. If peritonitis is mild, a new dialysis catheter may be inserted at the same operation. To minimize the chance for bacterial seeding of the new catheter, intraoperative Gram stains can be used. For patients with purulent peritonitis, a delay of one week before new catheter insertion reduces the risk of recurrent infection [15]. Catheters removed for recurrent or fecal peritonitis should not be replaced for two to three weeks to allow the peritoneal inflammation to resolve [2].

While the treatment of peritonitis in children on peritoneal dialysis is generally straight-forward, special consideration is required in the management of patients whose peritoneal fluid cultures reveal multiple enteric organisms. Because of the possibility of underlying secondary peritonitis in these patients (for example, caused by catheter erosion into the bowel) further diagnostic studies and, potentially, surgical intervention may be indicated. CT scanning and water-soluble contrast studies may help to diagnose coincident appendicitis or a perforated viscus, respectively. In the absence of identifiable foci of infection based upon these diagnostic studies, conservative treatment with appropriate antibiotics is optimal and it is supported by data from adult studies [16]. This plan is continued as long as the patient shows clinical improvement on dialysis and the peritoneal effluent is sterilized by the antibiotic therapy. Persistent abdominal pain and failure to demonstrate clinical improvement would mandate surgical exploration. It should be understood that while this conservative approach may be useful in selected adults with primary peritonitis related to peritoneal dialysis, the experience in children is limited and the presence of multiple enteric organisms on peritoneal cultures in association with physical findings of generalized peritonitis may be sufficient to warrant early operative intervention in children with this illness.

1.5. Peritonitis and intra-abdominal complications related to ventriculoperitoneal shunts

Ventriculoperitoneal (VP) shunting is a widely accepted procedure for the management of hydrocephalus. Abdominal complications of VP shunts are reported to occur at a rate of 10 to 30 per cent and include viscus perforation by the abdominal portion of the shunt, peritonitis secondary to infected cerebrospinal fluid (CSF), massive accumulation of CSF ascites and loculated intraperitoneal CSF-collections or pseuodcysts (frequently infected) [17]. Viscus perforation by a VP shunt can but does not usually produce acute peritonitis. The catheter may gravitate transmurally into the bowel lumen over a prolonged period while being surrounded by fibrous encasement at the enterotomy without subsequent peritoneal irritation. The formation of CSF pseudocysts is related to chronic low-grade inflammatory responses

to the catheter itself, to infected CSF or to sterile xanthochromic CSF with fibrous encapsulation of the irritated area [17]. Pseudocysts are more common in the setting of shunt infection, peritoneal adhesions, prior abdominal surgeries, increased CSF protein content and multiple shunt revisions [18]. Pseudocysts may become quite large and present with evidence of gastrointestinal or genitourinary obstruction [17].

The presenting complaints in children with these shunt complications commonly include a constellation of abdominal symptoms (abdominal pain, distension and tenderness as well as a potential abdominal mass) and fever, although neurological symptoms may predominate. The child with a VP shunt who presents with an acute abdomen requires special consideration. Shunt infection can produce the picture of an acute abdomen [19]. The work-up includes a complete physical examination with special attention to neurological and abdominal findings and laboratory evaluation including blood count with differential and CSF for cell count, differential, Gram's stain, culture and sensitivity. Radiological studies should begin with an abdominal plain film to rule out obvious causes of an acute abdomen, to identify a mass or displacement of the bowel gas pattern and to verify intraperitoneal position of the shunt. If an abdominal mass is palpable, ultrasonography may confirm the diagnosis of an abdominal pseudocyst. CT scan can also confirm the presence of a pseudocyst and is particularly useful in evaluating other primary or associated intra-abdominal pathologies when a mass is not appreciated by examination or ultrasound. Shunt function can be assessed by injection of radionuclide material into the reservoir to confirm patency and pattern of drainage [17].

Appropriate operative therapy is dependent upon the preoperative diagnosis. The standard management of infected VP shunts entails shunt removal and external ventricular drainage in conjunction with systemic and intraventricular antibiotics. Shunt revision using intraperitoneal repositioning, intrapleural repositioning or conversion to ventriculovenous shunting may be considered once the infection has resolved [17]. The operative treatment of CSF pseudocysts is somewhat controversial. One treatment strategy is to assume that all pseudocysts are infected and to treat them as outlined above [18]. The second strategy employs selective management based upon CSF analysis and culture results. In the presence of infection, treatment consists of shunt removal, external drainage and antibiotics. In the absence of infection, single-step procedures have been used including intraperitoneal shunt repositioning or shunt conversion with or without aspiration, paracentesis or pseudocyst excision [17]. Laparoscopy has been successfully employed in single-stage VP shunt repositioning for uninfected CSF pseudocysts [20].

1.6. Secondary Peritonitis

Secondary bacterial peritonitis is an acute suppurative inflammation of the peritoneal cavity caused by intrinsic pathology of the abdominal viscera, trauma or operations involving the peritoneal contents. Secondary peritonitis usually refers to inflammation throughout the peritoneal cavity (typically caused by perforation of a hollow viscus or transmural necrosis of the GI tract) but localized inflammation can occur as well. Intraabdominal infection where the infectious process remains contained within a diseased organ or viscus is usually accompanied by localized peritonitis. The prognosis of patients with peritonitis depends on many factors, including patient age, source of infection, extent of infection, presence of other disease states or organ dysfunction, nutritional status and the applied therapy [21]. While treatment of focal intra-abdominal infections will be dictated by the specific organ or viscus involved, the principles of management of "generalized" bacterial peritonitis are uniform. These principles are very similar in both children and adults.

1.7. Diagnosis

The diagnosis of localized or generalized peritonitis is based on the patient's symptoms and physical examination. The predominant symptom is abdominal pain (initially most severe at the site of greatest inflammation), often accompanied by nausea, vomiting and anorexia. Fever is usually present in the early stages of peritonitis but subnormal temperature may be seen in infants or in advanced peritonitis with sepsis. While the physical examination will vary according to the cause and extent of peritonitis, abdominal tenderness is the hallmark. Spasm or involuntary rigidity ("guarding") of the abdominal wall muscles are further evidence of peritoneal irritation/inflammation. The diagnosis of peritonitis is straightforward in the majority of cases but signs of peritonitis may be greatly attenuated in certain patients, requiring a high index of suspicion. This group includes the neonate (especially preemies), patients taking steroids or immunosuppressive drugs, those recovering from intra-abdominal operations, those with head injury and altered states of consciousness due to toxic encephalopathy and paraplegic patients [21].

In general, laboratory and radiographic studies do not add much to the clinical diagnosis of peritonitis in patients presenting with clear symptoms and physical findings. In children of certain ages, particularly infants and young children, however, more value is placed on these ancillary studies because of the inability of the child to voice complaints or to cooperate with a controlled physical examination. The presence of leukocytosis with a shift to the left supports the clinical diagnosis of peritonitis. Leukopenia in a sick infant and child is worrisome for potential underlying sepsis. Evidence of metabolic acidosis on either an arterial blood gas or blood chemistry suggests sepsis with hypoperfusion or, potentially, ischemic intestine. Urinalysis is essential to rule out pyelonephritis and renal colic, both of which can mimic peritonitis. As in adults, serum amylase and lipase values are essential in patients suspected of having pancreatitis.

Radiographic studies are warranted when peritonitis is suspected but physical findings are equivocal or attenuated. In the pediatric population, these studies can be a vital element in helping to establish the diagnosis and in directing initial therapy. In premature neonates, for example, the findings of pneumatosis intestinalis or portal vein gas without free air will support the clinical suspicion of necrotizing enterocolitis and reassure the surgeon in continuing non-operative therapy. Except for the demonstration of free intra-abdominal air associated with bowel perforation, plain films of the abdomen may not be helpful in diagnosing peritonitis. Examples of findings that may suggest an underlying etiology for the patient's presentation include an appendicolith, nephrolithiasis, cholelithiasis, intraperitoneal calcifications (meconium peritonitis), and pneumatosis intestinalis, as mentioned above. Other special radiographic studies are often used to confirm the diagnosis of peri-

tonitis in certain settings. Ultrasound can be very useful in pediatric patients to evaluate right upper quadrant pain and lower abdominal/pelvic pain which may be related to cholecystitis and appendicitis/ovarian pathology, respectively. Water-soluble contrast studies of the gastrointestinal tract can be helpful in diagnosing intestinal anastomotic leaks in post-operative patients. Computed tomography (CT) is particularly useful in evaluating pediatric trauma patients who present with abdominal pain after blunt injury. In the absence of diffuse peritonitis or clinical instability, pediatric trauma patients with intraperitoneal fluid associated with solid organ injury are typically managed non-operatively. In those patients with intraperitoneal fluid and no evidence of liver or spleen injury, bowel injury is likely and laparoscopy/laparotomy may be warranted. CT examination may also be used in the pediatric patient who presents with a several day history of signs and symptoms suggestive of peritonitis but who has an equivocal abdominal exam or a palpable mass. CT may not only diagnose complicated appendicitis in this setting but may facilitate abscess drainage via CT-guidance. An additional benefit of CT over other imaging/diagnostic modalities is that it provides information regarding both intraperitoneal and retroperitoneal structures. This is particularly helpful in cases where retroperitoneal pathology (for example, pyelonephritis, retroperitoneal abscess or pancreatitis) can produce peritonitis.

It is important to point out that, despite the utilization of appropriate radiographic and laboratory studies, there are instances where the diagnosis of peritonitis remains unclear. Occasional cases of intra-abdominal infections (early appendicitis, for instance) may be associated with normal laboratory and radiographic studies. Regardless of ancillary test results, when the suspicion for peritonitis looms, based upon persistence of signs and symptoms or abnormal physical exam findings, the safest plan of action is operative intervention by laparotomy or laparoscopy to establish a diagnosis and begin treatment. The potential risks and complications of delaying appropriate operative therapy in the setting of underlying peritonitis significantly outweigh the potential morbidity associated with an uncomplicated surgical procedure, particularly in children.

1.8. Treatment

The primary treatment of secondary bacterial peritonitis is surgical. The major principles of management of patients with secondary peritonitis are (1) fluid resuscitation, (2) antibiotic administration and (3) operative control of the underlying pathological condition.[3] In general, patients with secondary peritonitis should be operated on as expeditiously as possible after undergoing appropriate preoperative preparation. The goal of preoperative resuscitation is to restore the patient's physiological state towards normal in order to ensure optimal tissue perfusion during the ensuing anesthesia and operation. This can usually be accomplished over the course of a few hours. In children and neonates who present late in the clincial course, especially when shock, acidosis and coagulopathy are present, however, preoperative preparation may take longer and may require ventilator support or vasopressor drugs.

All patients with peritonitis have some degree of hypovolemia secondary to large third-space fluid losses into the inflamed peritoneum, intestinal wall and bowel lumen. Sufficient volumes of crystalloid solu-

tion or blood should be administered to children to restore intravascular volume. Fluid boluses generally begin in the range of 20 cc/kg for crystalloid and 10 cc/kg for blood. The adequacy of resuscitation may be assessed by monitoring blood pressure, heart rate, peripheral perfusion/capillary refill and hourly urine output with a urinary catheter in place (target 0.5 to 1 cc/kg/hr). In the absence of cardiac or renal disease, children tolerate rapid volume infusion very well. In pediatric patients that present in shock with hypotension and/or metabolic acidosis, it may be necessary to administer vasoactive drugs (typically beginning with dopamine at a dose of 5 to 10 mcg/kg/min) or sodium bicarbonate to temporarily correct these abnormalities while intravascular volume is restored.

Parenteral antibiotic therapy should be initiated as soon as the diagnosis of secondary peritonitis is made, before operation and before peritoneal cultures can be obtained. Initial antibiotic therapy is empirical and should be directed against organisms normally recovered from the gastrointestinal tract. For patients with generalized peritonitis and those suspected of having a perforated viscus, this antimicrobial therapy should include an agent or combination of agents, that has activity against both aerobic (predominantly Gram-negative enteric organisms) and anaerobic bacteria. In children, the most frequently utilized regimen to treat severe intra-abdominal infections includes classic "triple-drug" therapy (ampicillin, an aminoglycoside and clindamycin or metronidazole) or combination therapy with either a third-generation cephalosporin or extended-spectrum penicillin and an aminoglycoside.

The duration of antibiotic treatment in children with secondary peritonitis is dependent upon several factors, including the immunocompetence of the patient (particularly important in neonates and in children with malignancy), the severity of the infection (infection localized within a diseased viscus versus a perforated viscus with peritoneal soilage and inflammation) and the patient's clinical response to initial operative and antibiotic therapy. In general, when antibiotic therapy is begun, a prospective time limit for treatment is set depending upon the nature of the infection. In perforated NEC or perforated appendicitis, for instance, this time would be 7 days. Objective criteria used to determine when to safely discontinue antibiotics without risking recurrent or residual infection include: (1) the patient is afebrile for 48 hours, (2) the leukocyte count is within normal limits and (3) the leukocyte band count is less than 3 percent [3]. In addition to these parameters, the patient should be improving clinically, as manifested by increased activity and mobility, return of gastrointestinal function and improved appetite.

In accordance with the recommendations of the Surgical Infection Society [22], there are several clinical circumstances in children representing "simple" intra-abdominal infections that do not require prolonged therapeutic post-operative antibiotics. These include uncomplicated acute appendicitis, cholecystitis and traumatic enteric perforations operated on within 12 hours of injury. The common feature of these infections is the minimal degree of peritoneal soilage and inflammatory response present at the time of laparotomy.[1]

The goals of operative management of secondary peritonitis are: (1) to eliminate the source of infection/contamination, (2) to reduce the bacterial inoculum and (3) to prevent recurrent or persistent sepsis. The operative technique used to control contamination depends upon the location and nature of the pathological condition in the gastrointestinal tract [2]. The management of these various pathological conditions will be detailed below. The general principles of operative therapy will be addressed here.

The choice of incision in children with peritonitis depends upon the age of the patient, the presumptive diagnosis and whether the patient has localized or diffuse peritoneal signs. In premature neonates, the presentation is typically diffuse peritonitis and the diagnosis is usually NEC. A transverse, supraumbilical incision allows access to the entire abdominal cavity, provides a place for a lower quadrant enterostomy, and allows for a 2-layer fascial closure. In young children who present with localized or diffuse peritonitis, appendicitis is usually the culprit. These patients can usually be approached via a transverse right lower quadrant incision although laparoscopy is a reasonable alternative when the diagnosis truly is in doubt. Laparoscopy not only allows visualization of the entire peritoneal cavity, it also provides a means to effect a focal treatment of various intra-abdominal infections. In the unusual event that the source of infection cannot be reached through an initial right lower quadrant approach, this incision can be extended across the midline or a separate incision can be made to address the pathology. In older children and adolescents, appendicitis still predominates but pathological conditions typical of adult patients begin to appear as causes of peritonitis. Thus, while localized right lower quadrant pain is approached via an appendectomy incision, diffuse peritonitis is often approached via a vertical midline incision or with the periumbilical placement of the diagnostic laparoscope. Laparotomies for peritonitis secondary to trauma are best approached with a vertical midline incision to allow access to the entire abdomen.

On entering the peritoneal cavity, peritoneal fluid should be obtained for Gram stain and for aerobic, anaerobic and fungal cultures. The general strategies to control the source of infection/contamination from the gastrointestinal tract include closure, exclusion, resection with or without anastomosis and creation of a stoma. Cases in which perforation has not occurred and the infection remains contained within a viscus, for example, appendicitis or Meckel's diverticulitis, can be treated by resection alone. As in adults, primary closure or resection and anastomosis in the presence of peritonitis is generally a safe strategy for defects in the stomach and small intestine. In cases where peritoneal soilage is particularly extensive or intestinal viability is questionable, however, small bowel resection with proximal and distal enterostomies may be preferable. Because of the unique immunological and physiological considerations in neonates, it may be best to err on the conservative side in managing intestinal perforations with peritonitis. Distal small bowel perforations due to NEC are typically treated with end ileostomy, although cases of successful resection and primary anastomosis in healthy neonates have been reported [23]. For focal perforations of the distal small intestine in neonates, such as those which are the result of a complication of indomethacin therapy, exteriorization of the perforation as a diverting loop ostomy is an effective treatment option. Primary closure or anastomosis for perforations of the colon with peritonitis is not advisable due to the increased risk of anastomotic dehiscence and persisting infection. This can be attributed to many factors including the higher bacterial concentration in the colon which results in a greater degree of intraperitoneal contamination on perforation. The safest management for colonic perforations with peritonitis is exteriorization of the proximal end as an ostomy and creation of a mucous fistula or oversewing of the distal end. Exceptions to this principle, where primary closure or resection and anastomosis have been used successfully to treat colonic perforations, include penetrating trauma to the colon operated on within 12 hours of injury in the setting of minimal peritoneal contamination and iatrogenic perforation which occurs during colonoscopy in a prepared colon [21].

After controlling the source of contamination at operation, attention should be directed to reducing the bacterial inoculum and removing the substances that promote infection (adjuvants such as hemoglobin, fibrin, bile and necrotic tissue) in the hopes of preventing recurrent or persistent infection in the peritoneal cavity [3]. This can be accomplished using a combination of mechanical debridement and intraoperative peritoneal lavage. Purulent exudates should be aspirated and gently debrided and fluid loculation in the pelvis, paracolic gutters, subphrenic regions and between bowel loops should be opened and removed [2]. An attempt should also be made to remove particulate debris such as enteric contents, fecal matter or an appendicolith. The use of intraoperative mechanical lavage reduces the quantity of bacteria and rinses out adjuvant substances in the peritoneal cavity [24]. While peritoneal lavage has become standard practice during operations for peritonitis, its efficacy has not been well documented. Because the lavage fluid itself acts as an adjuvant to infection by impairing phagocytosis and leukocyte migration, it is preferred that all fluid collections be aspirated before the abdomen is closed [2]. With regard to the technique of peritoneal lavage, repeated small volume aliquots should be instilled until there are no remaining suspended particulates and the lavage fluid is clear. Temperature-controlled saline solution is typically used for irrigation with or without the addition of antiseptics and antibiotics. These additives are used to further reduce the bacterial concentration in the peritoneal cavity in the hopes of reducing infectious complications. Antiseptic agents (dilute povidine-iodine) have been shown to reduce the incidence of post-operative abscess but they have deleterious effects on white blood cell function [3]. The benefits of adding antibiotics to the irrigation solution with regard to posto-perative infection and mortality have not been statistically proven. The instillation of antibiotics into the peritoneal cavity is unlikely to be harmful, except for aminoglycosides, which can be systemically absorbed and, thus, cause toxicity [21]. One important point to remember when performing peritoneal lavage in young children is to use warmed irrigation solution to avoid hypothermia.

Intraperitoneal drains are not indicated in patients with diffuse peritonitis unless placed into a well-defined abscess cavity or used to establish a controlled fistula [3]. It is impossible to drain the entire peritoneal cavity in patients with generalized peritonitis. Morever, drains have potentially harmful effects, including erosion into the intestine and blood vessels and inhibition of normal peritoneal defense mechanisms. Wound closure in children with secondary peritonitis deviates somewhat from the principles advocated in adult patients. Fascial closure is accomplished in one or two layers depending upon the abdominal incision with either interrupted or a running suture. Whe-

re the risk of fascial dehiscence is deemed high due to severe contamination, interrupted fascial sutures may be preferred to prevent evisceration if focal fascial breakdown occurs. Whereas adult skin wounds in this setting are left open or closed by delayed primary closure of the skin and subcutaneous tissues, pediatric skin wounds can typically be closed primarily. This is usually best accomplished with widely-spaced staples or interrupted sutures which allow residual bacteria or adjuvants to drain. The mechanisms which allow these wounds to heal in children with low infection rates is not completely understood but it appears to be due in some part to the relative paucity of subcutaneous fat in pediatric abdominal wounds. Needless to say, wound surveillance is essential when managing these incisions by primary closure. Any evidence of wound infection should prompt opening of the incision, wound culture and initiation of packing changes. In children with particularly dirty wounds (for instance, with fecal peritonitis) or in adolescent patients with secondary peritonitis, the increased risk of wound infection dictates that it is more prudent to resort to delayed primary closure or secondary closure.

2. INTRA-ABDOMINAL ABSCESS

Intra-abdominal abscess formation represents the end result of the ability of peritoneal host defense mechanisms to limit and wall off infection in the peritoneal cavity [3]. From a pathophysiological standpoint, bacterial contamination of the peritoneal cavity leads to activation of the clotting cascade and production of fibrin. This fibrin then promotes adhesions between intra-abdominal structures around the source of infection, the resulting "localized" infection being an abscess. Neutrophils are present in high numbers in abscess fluid and are essential for abscess formation [21]. In addition to neutrophils, abscesses are composed of proliferating bacteria and necrotic debris. It is the persistence of this necrotic debris (devitalized tissue or residual blood) that overwhelms host mechanisms for clearance, rendering defense mechanisms inadequate to eradicate ongoing infection. While abscess formation serves a protective function in the host by containing infection and preventing the lethal effects of widely disseminated bacteremia and diffuse inflammatory activation (characteristic of peritonitis), it also perpetuates a chronic, stable infection in which bacteria are protected from phagocytosis and humorally-mediated mechanisms of destruction [25].

There are several unique aspects of intra-abdominal abscesses in the pediatric population. First, whereas prior operation has become the most common predisposing cause for intra-abdominal abscess in adults [21], appendicitis is, by far, the most common cause in children. Second, abscess formation is distinctly unusual in neonates. Newborn infants, especially the premature, demonstrate a profound lack of inflammatory response to infection and injury. This inability to form abscesses is likely related to an immaturity of the neonatal immune system, including lack of previous exposure to specific antigens [26]. An additional mechanical factor impairing localized intra-abdominal abscess formation may be the underdeveloped omentum characteristic of the neonate.

Abscesses may form in the peritoneal cavity, either within or outside of the abdominal viscera or in the retroperitoneum. Extravisceral abscesses are much more common and arise in two situations: (1) after resolution of diffuse peritonitis in which a loculated focus of infection persists and evolves into an abscess (for instance, an intra-abdominal abscess after operation for perforated appendicitis) and (2) after perforation of a viscus or an anastomotic breakdown that is successfully walled off by peritoneal defense mechanisms. Visceral abscesses in children generally occur in predisposed hosts or those suffering from an active infectious process via hematogenous or lymphatic spread of bacteria. Retroperitoneal abscesses are uncommon in children but may arise from perforation of the gastrointestinal tract (most commonly involving the retrocecal appendix) into the retroperitoneum or from hematogenous or lymphatic spread of bacteria to retroperitoneal organs [2].

2.1. Presentation

The clinical presentation of pediatric patients with intra-abdominal abscesses may range from a well-appearing child with mild abdominal pain, low grade fever and leukocytosis to one presenting with septic shock. Fever is the most common presentation, present in 75 to 95 per cent of patients, and it is typically low grade in the early course of an abscess. High spiking fever may be seen once the abscess is well established. Signs and symptoms may include ileus, diarrhea, abdominal distension, nausea and vomiting, urinary frequency and potentially a palpable abdominal mass. Abscesses in contact with the parietal peritoneum of the anterior and lateral abdominal wall usually produce localized abdominal pain, tenderness and peritoneal signs. Subphrenic, interloop, and pelvic abscesses may produce non-specific symptoms without localized clinical findings and they are more difficult to diagnose. Laboratory evaluation typically reveals leukocytosis with a left shift [21].

One group of patients that may be particularly difficult to diagnose are those patients with a post-operative intra-abdominal abscess. In this setting, the clinical presentation may be non-specific with symptoms masked by incisional pain, analgesics and possibly antibiotics. Signs of underlying abscess formation in these patients may be as subtle as: (1) failure to get well after operation or regression after an initial, apparently normal, post-operative course; (2) failure of return of bowel function; and (3) a generalized ill appearance, especially when associated with malaise and decreased activity [21].

2.2. Diagnosis

The diagnosis of intra-abdominal abscess is based on clinical suspicion and radiological confirmation. Ultrasound and CT scanning are the mainstays of radiological diagnosis and localization of intra-abdominal abscesses. Ultrasound can be done quickly, does not expose the patient to radiation and is less expensive than CT. The accuracy of ultrasonography in detecting intra-abdominal abscesses, however, is less than that achieved with CT. In addition, ultrasound can be operator-dependent and cannot penetrate intestinal gas (thus, abscesses deep in the abdomen, pelvis, or retroperitoneum may not be detected). CT can usually be performed and interpreted within a few hours and is most accurate using a combination of oral and intravenous contrast. Recent reports have shown an accuracy greater than 90 per cent when using CT to diagnose intra-abdominal abscesses [21].

The choice of utilizing ultrasound or CT scanning in a clinical setting suspicious for intra-abdominal abscess may be somewhat dependent upon the patient. If the potential site of infection can be localized clinically, ultrasound may be used to confirm clinical suspicion and to direct diagnostic aspiration of the collection. If, on the other hand, the patient appears clinically ill but the site of infection is not obvious or the ultrasound study is unsatisfactory, a CT scan can be used [2]. Both CT scanning and ultrasonography have the added advantage that if an abscess is detected and is suitably located, needle aspiration or catheter drainage of the abscess cavity can be done simultaneous to confirmation of the diagnosis [21].

2.3. Treatment

The basic principles of management of intra-abdominal abscesses include: (1) optimization of the patient's general status, (2) antibiotic administration and (3) drainage of the abscess. As previously stated, children with intra-abdominal abscesses demonstrate a wide spectrum of clinical presentations ranging from a well-appearing child to one with evidence of shock. Accordingly, the patient's initial management will be dictated by the clinical scenario. In general, these patients have some degree of intravascular volume depletion and require fluid resuscitation [3]. For ill-appearing patients, the principles of resuscitation are identical to those for patients with secondary peritonitis, that is, restoration of the patient's physiological state towards normal in order to ensure optimal tissue perfusion. As in children with peritonitis, the adequacy of resuscitation may be assessed by monitoring blood pressure, heart rate, peripheral perfusion/capillary refill and urine output. An important element in optimizing the patient's general status, particularly in those children who have been unable to tolerate feedings for several days due to nausea and vomiting or those who have been n.p.o. in the post-operative period, is nutritional support [2]. Calories may be administered either enterally (usually via a feeding tube into the stomach or small intestine) or parenterally. In the absence of an enteric fistula or evidence of bowel obstruction, the preferred method for administering nutritional supplementation is using the gut.

Microbiology of and antibiotic therapy for, intra-abdominal abscesses do not differ significantly from those of secondary bacterial peritonitis [21]. Thus, antibiotic coverage for polymicrobial flora consisting of both aerobic and anaerobic bacteria should be initiated with antibiotic combinations or single agents with appropriate broad-spectrum coverage. Antibiotics alone are unlikely to be effective in treating intra-abdominal abscesses. There are several reasons for this, including poor penetration of antibiotics into the abscess center, inactivation of antibiotics in the micro-environment of the infection (i.e., hypoxia and acidity) and lack of effectiveness of the drug against a large bacterial inoculum. Drainage of an abscess usually reverses these adverse conditions and increases the efficacy of antibiotic therapy. Intravenous antibiotic therapy can be used successfully as sole therapy for intra-abdominal abscesses in children in certain settings. Examples would include small (<2 cm) abscesses that result after operation for perforated appendicitis or in association with Crohn's disease. Antibiotic therapy is also useful in the setting of children who present with clinical suspicion of an intra-abdominal abscess after operation for complicated appendicitis but are found to have an inflammatory mass or phlegmon without frank abscess on CT scan. In this setting, antibiotic therapy will either lead to resolution of the inflammatory mass or a frank abscess will form, ultimately requiring drainage.

Drainage, either percutaneous or surgical, is the mainstay of therapy for intra-abdominal abscesses. As in adults, percutaneous drainage (PCD) of intra-abdominal collections under CT or ultrasound guidance has proved a safe and effective alternative to surgical drainage and is the preferred method of drainage in children. PCD has the advantage over operative drainage of being accomplished without general anesthesia, blood loss, visceral injury or wound complications [21]. It has been used successfully for treatment of post-operative abscesses and as a preoperative therapy for spontaneously occurring abscesses (appendiceal or Crohn's-related, for example). Initial criteria for PCD specified that the abscess should be unilocular and without enteric communication and were associated with success in more than 90 per cent of cases. As the indications for PCD have evolved and expanded, however, this technique has been applied to multilocular abscesses, abscesses with internal or enteric communications and those containing necrotic tissue or thick hematoma with predictably lower success rates. PCD with multiple catheters may be appropriate for optimal drainage of extensive or complex abscesses [27].

The management of a patient undergoing PCD requires close collaboration between radiologist and surgeon [3]. After drainage, several clinical parameters can be followed to assess the child's response to therapy. Successful drainage is typically associated with defervescence of the fever and return of the leukocyte count toward normal within 2 to 4 days. In addition, the volume of drainage in successfully treated patients steadily decreases over this time period [27].

Failure to achieve these end points suggests the presence of undrained infection and mandates repeat radiological imaging. If residual infected fluid collections or a malpo-sitioned drainage catheter is identified, in-sertion of a second catheter or relocation of the existing catheter can be undertaken. If the clinical picture fails to improve after these additional maneuvers, operative drai-nage is indicated. PCD failures usually oc-cur when the abscess contents are too thick to drain via the drainage catheter.[3]

When PCD is successful, there are several criteria that have been utilized to establish optimal timing for catheter removal. These include defervescence of fever, normaliza-tion of the leukocyte count, daily catheter output of less than 30 ml, return of appeti-te, obliteration of the cavity and healing of any communication by contrast sinography. When these criteria are met, the catheter is withdrawn in stages over a few days [27,28].

Historically, surgical drainage of intra-ab-dominal abscesses entailed a transperitone-al exploration to avoid missing small abs-cesses and leaving undrained infection within the peritoneal cavity. Improved loca-lization of intra-abdominal abscesses using ultrasound and CT scanning has greatly simplified this surgical approach [2]. When the abscess can be located accurately and the presence of multiple abscesses ruled out preoperatively, the surgeon can approach the abscess directly instead of using a com-plete laparotomy, thus potentially avoiding the risks of bleeding and enteric fistula. La-parotomy may be necessary when the abs-cesses are multiple or are located in the les-ser sac or between bowel loops. After evacuation of the abscess cavity, Penrose or soft sump drains should be left in the abs-cess cavity to effect continuing removal of purulent material and intestinal contents if an enteric fistula or leaking anastomosis is present [2,21].

The surgical approach to drainage of intra-abdominal abscesses varies depending upon the location of the collection as deter-mined by preoperative imaging. Subdiaph-ragmatic and subhepatic abscesses can be drained using posterior, anterior or lateral incisions. The abdominal wall musculature overlying the abscess is divided and dissec-tion is continued using an extraserous ap-proach down to the parietal peritoneum un-til the abscess cavity is encountered. Pelvic abscesses, which are common in children because of their association with perforated appendicitis, can be drained transrectally or transvaginally. After the abscess is palpated bulging into the lumen of the rectum or va-gina, the presence of pus is confirmed by needle aspiration and the cavity is incised, drained and Penrose drains are placed. In light of the effectiveness of this technique and the potentially difficult access to this area for percutaneous drainage, transrec-tal/transvaginal drainage should be regar-ded as first line therapy for pelvic abscesses that can be palpated via the rectum or vagi-na. Lesser sac abscesses, interloop absces-ses and pancreatic abscesses are best drai-ned using a transperitoneal approach [21].

2.4. Visceral Abscesses

HEPATIC ABSCESSES occur most commonly in children with immunodeficiencies, parti-cularly chronic granulomatous disease (CGD) in childhood. An X-linked disorder, CGD is characterized by defective killing of phagocytized bacteria by neutrophils which leads to a granulomatous as well as a sup-purative response in the host tissues which are infiltrated with large numbers of poly-morphonuclear, mononuclear cells and his-tiocytes. Abscess formation commonly oc-curs in regional nodes (usually cervical and axillary), soft tissues, lung and liver [29].

Liver abscesses in the neonatal period are usually secondary to umbilical vein catheterization [30,31]. In the preantibiotic era, these abscesses occurred following complicated appendicitis but this cause is unusual today. While liver abscesses can develop from any infectious process via hematogenous seeding, several common predisposing conditions exist. These include acute leukemia (defect of host-systemic defenses), omphalitis, sickle cell anemia, human immunodeficiency virus (HIV) infection, biliary tract operations, hepatic trauma and intestinal parasites [29]. Abscesses usually present in the right lobe of the liver as solitary cavities although multiple abscesses can occur [32]. The most common organisms cultured from hepatic abscesses are *Staphylococcus aureus*, *Streptococcus pyogenes* and *Escherichia coli*. In cryptogenic infections, anaerobic bacteria are the most likely pathogens [29].

Children with hepatic abscesses usually present with high fever, hepatosplenomegaly, right upper quadrant pain and jaundice. Associated symptoms may include abdominal distension and anorexia [33]. On initial examination, localization of the infection to the liver may not be appreciated, especially if the patient has not previously been identified as having an immune deficiency [29]. Ultrasonography and CT scan are the most useful studies to establish the diagnosis. Gallium scan and hepatic scintigram can identify abscesses as small as 2 centimeters [29].

Treatment entails prompt drainage of the abscess combined with long-term specific antibiotic therapy based on culture and sensitivity data. Percutaneous aspiration and catheter placement via ultrasound or CT-guidance is satisfactory in most cases [32]. Occasional abscesses will require surgical intervention. At operation, a transverse upper abdominal incision is made over the mass. On examining the liver, any suspicious soft areas of the liver are aspirated with a needle [34]. If pus is found, the area is walled off to minimize soiling of the peritoneal cavity and the abscess is unroofed. Necrotic tissue within the abscess cavity is debrided and surgical drains are placed. When multiple abscesses are encountered, as in CGD, as many abscesses as possible are unroofed and drained [32]. Duration of drainage is usually 2 to 3 weeks and a total antibiotic course of 4 to 6 weeks has been recommended. Microscopic and miliary (as occur from infected umbilical vein catheters) abscesses are undrainable and are treated with antibiotics alone [35].

Hepatic abscesses in children are associated with significant morbidity (recurrent abscesses, hematobilia and biliary obstruction) and mortality [32]. With effective drainage and antibiotic therapy, the mortality rates for children with hepatic abscesses are approximately 25 per cent [29,30,33].

SPLENIC ABSCESSES are uncommon in childhood and typically occur in those children that have predisposing underlying pathology. Both large solitary abscesses and smaller multiple abscesses have been reported. Solitary abscesses occur after splenic trauma or infarction due to hemoglobinopathy, while multiple abscesses are more common in immunocomprised children, especially those with leukemia. As with hepatic abscesses, splenic abscesses can develop from any infectious process via hematogenous seeding. The most common organisms cultured from splenic abscesses are *Staphylococcus*, *Streptococcus* and *Salmonella* species. *Candida* infection usually causes multiple abscesses, is more prevalent in children with leukemia and may represent a manifestation of systemic candidiasis [36].

Children with splenic abscesses present with fever and evidence of systemic sepsis. Solitary abscesses may be associated with left upper quadrant or left-sided pleuritic chest pain while multiple abscesses typically lack localizing symptoms. Splenomegaly may be present on physical examination. The diagnosis may be established by ultrasonograpy or CT scan [37].

Treatment depends upon the nature of the abscesses. For multiple abscesses, therapy is predominantly medical with administration of appropriate intravenous antibiotics. Identification of the causative organisms can be made using peripheral blood cultures (positive in 30 to 40 per cent of cases) or splenic biopsy/aspiration. Splenectomy in this setting is reserved for medical therapy failures. Solitary splenic abscesses may respond to percutaneous or operative drainage. When drainage is not felt to be safe or technically achievable, splenectomy may be necessary [37].

3. SITE-SPECIFIC INTRA-ABDOMINAL INFECTIONS

While the principles of management of peritonitis and intra-abdominal abscesses in children are similar to those in adults, the site-specific intra-abdominal infections that occur in the pediatric population are distinct in many regards. The nature of these infections varies considerably based upon the age of the patient (neonates and infants versus childhood versus adolescence) but there is considerable overlap of certain infections in more than one age group (Table 1). As previously stated, the most common pediatric intra-abdominal infections are ne-

crotizing enterocolitis (NEC) in neonates and appendicitis in childhood and adolescence.

Many of the disease entities presented in this section are intra-abdominal infections where the infectious process is contained within a diseased organ or viscus and can be eradicated by surgical resection. The remainder are intra-abdominal infections that normally respond to medical therapy. In this latter group, operative intervention may be reserved for complications of the primary diseases, medical treatment failures or definitive therapy of associated congenital diseases or anomalies.

4. THE CHILD AS A PATIENT

Children differ from adults in many ways and the evaluation of children with intra-abdominal infections must take these differences into consideration. Unlike adults, infants and young children with intra-abdominal infections are often unable to express pain or to localize complaints. The evaluation of a crying, uncooperative and ill-appearing patient in this setting can be quite challenging. Consequently, great reliance must be placed on the parents' interpretations of the child's symptoms. Details such as the onset and nature of abdominal pain as well as associated symptoms, vomiting, changes in bowel habits, feeding intolerance, lethargy and abnormal micturition, should be addressed. During questioning, special attention should be directed toward non-gastrointestinal symptoms as certain medical illnesses, especially streptococcal pharyngitis, meningitis and pneumonia, can present with apparent peritoneal findings.

The physical examination begins with observation of the child's position and move-

Table 1
Site-specific Pediatric Intra-abdominal Infections

Neonates and Infants	Childhood (Age 3-11 Years)	Adolescence
necrotizing enterocolitis	appendicitis	appendicitis
intestinal volvulus with gangrene/perforation	trauma & child abuse	pelvic inflammatory disease "adult" conditions
Hirschsprung's enterocolitis	Meckel's diverticulitis	— trauma — peptic ulcer disease
gastrointestinal perforations — meconium peritonitis — gastric perforations — intestinal perforations not related to NEC	colitis — Hirschsprung's enterocolitis — pseudomembranous colitis — diversion colitis	infectious complications of inflammatory bowel disease — fulminant colitis — toxic megacolon — peritonitis due to perforation — intra-abdominal abscess (Crohn's disease)
omphalitis & necrotizing fasciitis	acute pancreatitis	acute pancreatitis
infections of the hepatobiliary system — cholangitis — spontaneous bile duct perforation — cholelithiasis & cholecystitis — gallbladder hydrops	infections of the hepatobiliary system — cholelithiasis & cholecystitis — acute acalculous cholecystitis — gallbladder hydrops	infections of the hepatobiliary system — cholelithiasis & cholecystitis — acute acalculous cholecystitis
acute gastroenteritis	acute gastroenteritis	acute gastroenteritis
trauma & child abuse	infectious complications of inflammatory bowel disease — fulminant colitis — toxic megacolon — peritonitis due to perforation	

ment during episodes of pain to provide clues to underlying peritonitis. To optimize patient cooperation and examination reliability, the child should be kept as comfortable as possible, even if the exam has to be done in the mother's lap. If localizing symptoms have been identified, that particular area should be avoided at the start of the examination. An important part of the examination of children with abdominal pain is the digital rectal examination (i.e., to detect a pelvic abscess in a child with an acute abdomen). In females, rectal examination may allow palpation of the cervix and, when combined with bimanual palpation, uterine or adnexal masses.

Because of the frequent inability to obtain a detailed and accurate history or a reliable physical examination in infants and young children who present with potential intra-abdominal infections, laboratory testing and imaging are used more liberally than in adults to supplement clinical information. Specific lab tests and imaging studies will be outlined in subsequent sections of this chapter. Despite the use of these studies, however, a diagnosis may still remain elusive. For children in whom a diagnosis cannot be established on initial evaluation, hospitalization may be appropriate to allow observation and frequent re-evaluation (every 2 to 3 hours) with the aim of defining the nature of potential underlying pathology.

5. NEONATES AND INFANTS

The neonate is particularly susceptible to invasive infection by virtue of humoral, cellular, environmental and physiological factors and, for this reason, should be treated as a compromised host. In the term neonate, impaired host defense mechanisms are primarily related to immunological immaturity and lack of previous antigen exposure. At the extreme of prematurity, however, the neonate is not only immunologically immature but also immunologically deficient [26]. Clinically, these deficiencies are manifest as the lack of inflammatory response to infection and injury. In the premature neonate, infection is rarely resisted and abscess formation is distinctly unusual.

Limitations of humoral and cellular mechanisms of immune defense in premature neonates include quantitative and qualitative reductions in serum immunoglobulin G concentrations, absence of immunoglobulins A (IgA) and M (IgM), reduced concentrations of complement proteins, reduced antigen recognition and antibody synthesis due to altered T and B lymphocyte interactions and reduced phagocytic function. En-

vironmental factors that increase the risk of infection in premature infants requiring prolonged neonatal intensive care include prolonged use of arterial or central venous catheters, exposure to antibiotic-resistant organisms, poor skin integrity and suboptimal nutritional status [38].

From a physiological standpoint, the neonate is ill-equipped to localize or contain intra-abdominal infections or to maintain respiratory or temperature homeostasis in the setting of peritonitis. The diminutive size of the neonatal omentum limits containment of soilage from viscus perforation so that peritonitis tends to be generalized. Because the neonate is heavily reliant upon diaphragmatic ventilation, abdominal distension caused by peritonitis typically leads to ventilatory embarrassment with resulting hypercarbia and respiratory acidosis. Temperature instability in the setting of neonatal peritonitis results from immature temperature regulatory capacity, limited body fat insulation and restricted ability to utilize fat and protein as energy sources for thermogenesis [39].

5.1. Necrotizing enterocolitis (NEC)

Necrotizing enterocolitis (NEC) is the most common gastrointestinal emergency in the newborn, affecting 1 to 7.7 per cent of all NICU admissions. The overall mortality rate ranges from 20 to 40 per cent [40]. It is a syndrome with a predilection for premature or low-birth weight infants, who comprise 90 per cent of cases [41]. NEC is characterized by the clinical findings of abdominal tenderness, ileus and gastrointestinal bleeding, by the radiographic finding of pneumatosis intestinalis and by the pathological finding of crepitant necrosis of the gut [42]. he pathogenesis of NEC remains undefined but is likely multifactorial. Two principle theories regarding pathogenesis prevail, differing as to the proposed initiating events. One theory implicates perinatal insults (i.e. reduced splanchnic blood flow resulting from birth asphyxia, umbilical artery cannulation or maternal cocaine abuse) and the other presumes the presence of an infectious etiology in a vulnerable host [43]. Three essential components have been postulated, including (1) ischemic injury of the intestine, (2) bacterial colonization of the gut and (3) the presence of substrate, usually formula feedings, withint the gut lumen [44].

The most common site of involvement of NEC is the terminal ileum. In neonates with NEC, involvement of both small and large intestine (usually terminal ileum and proximal colon) is found in 44 per cent, small intestinal disease alone in 30 per cent, and colonic involvement alone in 20 per cent [42]. The disease can involve single (50 per cent of cases) or multiple segments of intestine. A fulminant form of NEC, pan-necrosis, is characterized by necrosis of at least 75 per cent of the gut and is associated with a mortality rate of nearly 100 per cent [45]. The bacteria most often associated with NEC (*Klebsiella* sp., *E. coli* and *Clostridia* sp.) are members of the normal flora of the neonatal gut, rather than pathogenic strains [46]. Blood cultures may be positive in 30 to 35 per cent of patients.

The clinical presentation of NEC may be indistinguishable from neonatal sepsis and consists of non-specific findings of physiological instability, including lethargy, temperature instability, feeding intolerance or increased gastric residuals with gavage feedings, rectal bleeding, bilious vomiting, recurrent apnea and bradycardia [43]. On physical examination, abdominal disten-

sion and tenderness are the most common findings. Erythema and edema of the abdominal wall may suggest underlying peritonitis. Palpable bowel loops, a fixed or mobile mass and crepitus may also be encountered [43]. While there are no laboratory tests specific for NEC, the findings of neutropenia, thrombocytopenia, metabolic acidosis and stool examinations which are positive for blood certainly support the diagnosis.

The diagnosis of NEC is confirmed on plain abdominal films (supine and left lateral decubitus/cross-table lateral views) with the pathognomonic finding of pneumatosis intestinalis air within the bowel wall. The intraluminal air is produced by gas-forming bacteria from fermentation of formula feedings [42]. Other radiographic findings associated with NEC include an ileus pattern with bowel distension, portal vein gas, pneumoperitoneum, ascites and persistently dilated bowel loops. The finding of portal vein gas may be associated with extensive gangrene and a high mortality rate [47]. Contrast studies of the GI tract are generally not indicated in evaluating patients with potential NEC unless the diagnosis of malrotation with midgut volvulus is entertained. In this case, a malpositioned ligament of Treitz demonstrated on upper GI would mandate emergent operative intervention.

An additional diagnostic test that has been used in infants with NEC suspected of having intestinal gangrene is paracentesis. This procedure is unnecessary in infants with suspected NEC, those with definite NEC who are improving on medical therapy or those with pneumoperitoneum, who already have an indication for operation. In the patient who does not respond to initial therapy, paracentesis may allow early detection of intestinal gangrene (prior to perforation) with a high specificity (100 per cent) and positive predictive value (97 per cent) [48]. Positive paracentesis is indicated by brown fluid or bacteria on Gram stain of the unspun fluid and mandates operative intervention.

When the diagnosis of NEC is suspected, medical therapy is begun immediately, consisting of nasogastric decompression, volume resuscitation, administration of broad-spectrum antibiotics (i.e. ampicillin, gentamicin and clindamycin or metronidazole), blood and blood product administration as needed to correct anemia or coagulopathy and serial abdominal examinations with serial abdominal radiographs (every 6 to 8 hours) to detect deterioration or the presence of pneumoperitoneum, respectively [42]. Cardiovascular and ventilatory support may also be important elements of initial therapy. Roughly one half to two-thirds of infants with NEC will recover with medical management alone. The duration of medical therapy depends upon the patient's clinical course but, in general, antibiotic therapy is continued for 7 to 10 days and feedings are restarted after 10 to 14 days of bowel rest.

Much effort has gone into defining the indications for operative intervention in NEC. Ideally, operation should be performed after the advent of intestinal gangrene but before perforation. Pneumoperitoneum is the most clear-cut indication for operation. The remaining indications for operation are recommended based upon their high specificity and positive predictive value for intestinal gangrene on retrospective review of infants treated for NEC [49]. These include positive paracentesis, portal vein gas, a fixed intestinal loop noted on X-ray, erythema of the abdominal wall and a palpable abdominal mass. Despite its potentially low

predictive value, clinical deterioration after initiation of medical therapy is regarded as an additional indication for operation.

Once operative intervention is decided on, the patient's general condition must be optimized by cardiovascular and ventilatory support as well as correction of anemia, thrombocytopenia, coagulopathy and metabolic acidosis. The general guiding principles of operation for NEC are (1) resect only perforated or frankly gangrenous bowel; (2) preserve as much intestinal length as possible; (3) make every effort to preserve the ileocecal valve and (4) leave bowel of questionable viability behind, create a stoma proximal to this bowel and be prepared to perform a second-look procedure [43].

At operation, the abdomen is opened via a transverse supraumbilical incision, peritoneal fluid is sampled for aerobic and anaerobic cultures, and the entire GI tract is examined for evidence of perforation and necrosis. The procedure performed will be dictated by the surgical pathology encountered. A single necrotic segment of bowel can be resected, and a proximal stoma and mucus fistula/Hartmann's pouch created. Alternatively, resection with primary anastomosis has been reported by a few pediatric surgeons [23]. If multiple segments of intestine are necrotic and there are intervening segments of viable small intestine that provide enough length to maintain enteral nutrition, individual necrotic segments can be excised and the remaining viable segments treated with either creation of multiple stomas or reanastomosis and proximal stoma diversion of the intestinal stream [43]. The management of NEC with pan-involvement or pan-necrosis (19 per cent of cases) is controversial. Because of the extremely high mortality in this setting, many surgeons elect to close the abdomen and forego further treatment. Others advocate high jejunostomy followed by a second-look operation 48 to 72 hours later to allow demarcation and possible resection of gangrenous segments [42]. Massive intestinal resection, leaving less that 30 cm of viable bowel, has been condemned because of the debilitating sequelae of short gut syndrome suffered by survivors.

The goals of post-operative management are (1) control of sepsis; (2) nutritional support; (3) prevention of enterostomy-induced electrolyte deficits and (4) surveillance for intestinal stricture (complication occurs in 15 to 25 per cent of survivors of acute NEC). Intravenous antibiotics are continued for 7 to 10 days. Nasogastric suction is continued until ileus has resolved and the enterostomy begins to function. Enteral feedings are usually resumed after 14 days.

In addition to laparotomy and bowel resection, surgical therapy for NEC has been undertaken using open peritoneal drainage for very low birth weight (less than 1,000 grams) infants with complicated NEC (predominantly manifest as intesinal perforation). Peritoneal drainage has been used as an adjunct to resuscitation of the critically ill infant (to decompress the abdomen, improve ventilation and release contaminated material) in preparation for later surgery [50]. Moreover, it has been used successfully as definitive therapy in this patient population in several series [51,52]. A significant number of patients (ranging from 27 to 62 per cent of cases) can be expected to make a complete recovery without further operation [53]. Laparotomy should not be delayed if the patient fails to improve within 24 hours of peritoneal drainage or if it is judged that maximum clinical improvement has been achieved with drainage alone. The procedure is performed under local anesthesia as soft Penrose drains are inserted into the iliac fossa via lower quadrant stab incisions. Broad-spectrum antibiotics are continued until all drains are removed, usually within 10 to 14 days. Nasogastric decompression is continued until return of bowel function or until patency of the GI tract is confirmed by a non-ionic upper GI series [51].

5.2. Intestinal volvulus with gangrene/perforation

Neonates and infants may suffer intestinal gangrene and perforation as a complication of intestinal volvulus. While midgut volvulus associated with malrotation is a well-described entity, intestinal volvulus can also occur in association with a Meckel's band, internal hernia or meconium ileus [54]. When this condition goes undiagnosed or untreated, intestinal strangulation ensues with eventual gangrene and perforation. In the setting of intestinal necrosis, the patient is at high risk for subsequent short bowel syndrome or death.

The classic presentation of midgut volvulus is the sudden onset of bilious emesis in a newborn and this should alert the physician to a potential surgical emergency. Findings associated with intestinal volvulus include abdominal distension, dehydration (due to vomiting and third space fluid losses) and irritability. As the intestine begins to strangulate, the infant may become lethargic and develop septic shock [55]. Hematemesis or melena are signs of mucosal ischemia. Physical examination may reveal abdominal wall erythema or peritonitis. Ventilatory embarrassment may ensue secondary to abdominal distension from peritonitis. Infants who present at this late stage are extemely difficult to diagnose because there are no localizing signs and the clinical picture is indistinguishable from sepsis.

The preoperative diagnosis of intestinal volvulus with potential gangrene or perforation may be difficult to make. While an expeditious upper GI series is essential to rule out malrotation in an infant with bilious emesis, other diagnostic studies may yield equivocal results. In the stable patient, an upper GI series may help differentiate bowel obstruction from ileus. A water-soluble contrast enema may be diagnostic and even therapeutic, in the setting of meconium ileus. In general, evidence of malrotation, viscus perforation, or intestinal obstruction on any of these studies mandates urgent operative intervention. In the patient who presents with evidence of peritonitis or clinical deterioration in the appropriate clinical setting, diagnostic studies are not indicated and all attention should be focused on stabilizing the patient in preparation for operation.

The treatment of infants with intestinal volvulus complicated by potential gangrene or perforation includes expeditious resuscitation with intravenous fluids and pressor support, as needed; correction of underlying anemia, thrombocytopenia, or coagulopathy; administration of broad-spectrum antibiotic coverage and urgent operative intervention. At operation, the intestines are eviscerated via a generous supraumbilical transverse incision. Volvulized or torsed intestine should be detorsed in hopes of restoring blood flow to the strangulated segment. For midgut volvulus, the intestine is characteristically detorsed in a counterclockwise direction. After detorsion, the intestine, regardless of how dark it may appear, should be wrapped in warm saline-soaked gauze and observed for a brief period, looking for evidence of recovery of blood flow. Short, frankly necrotic segments can

be resected with reanastomosis or stoma creation, depending upon the clinical setting. Bowel of questionable viability, especially when the majority of the small intestine is involved, may be treated with stoma creation or returned to the peritoneal cavity with planned re-exploration in 24 to 48 hours. Congenital anomalies (i.e. Meckel's band or meconium ileus) should be addressed surgically. In the case of malrotation with midgut volvulus, lysis of Ladd's bands and appendectomy should be undertaken after addressing potential intestinal compromise.

5.3. Hirschsprung's enterocolitis

Hirschsprung's disease (congenital aganglionosis of the intestine) results from arrested fetal development of the myenteric nervous system and is characterized by the absence of ganglion cells in the distal bowel (confined to the rectosigmoid colon in 75 to 80 per cent of patients). Clinically, aganglionosis results in ineffective peristalsis and manifests as partial or complete distal bowel obstruction in neonates and chronic constipation in older children.

The diagnosis of Hirschsprung's disease is based on clinical history, radiologic studies, anorectal manometrics and histologic examination of rectal biopsy specimens. Barium enema findings supporting the diagnosis include: (1) demonstration of a spasmodic distal colonic/rectal segment together with dilated proximal bowel and (2) failure to evacuate barium from the colon within 24 hours of the performance of the study [56]. Rectal biopsy is the diagnostic standard for Hirschsprung's disease. On histologic examination, the diagnosis is based upon the findings of absence of ganglion cells in the myenteric and submucosal plexuses and the presence of hypertrophied nerve trunks [57]. Using histochemical techniques, the diagnosis is established based upon the presence of increased acetylcholinesterase (AChE) content in the nerve fibers of the lamina propria and muscularis mucosa [56]. Once the diagnosis has been confirmed, one of two surgical treatment options is undertaken: (1) one-stage primary pull-through operation or (2) multi-stage approach with initial creation of a diverting colostomy and definitive pull-through when the child is 6 to 12 months old.

Roughly half of all patients with Hirschsprung's disease are diagnosed in the neonatal period, while most of the remainder are diagnosed by 2 years of age. The importance of making the diagnosis in the newborn period is underscored by the increased mortality in newborns when the diagnosis is overlooked. The typical presentation of the disease in newborns is low intestinal obstruction with or without sepsis. In the most mild cases, delayed passage of meconium (beyond 48 hours after birth) may be the only abnormality. At the other end of the spectrum is the acutely ill infant who presents with intestinal obstruction manifested by abdominal distension, bilious or feculent vomiting and failure to pass meconium.
In the most fulminant form, newborns may present with a picture of overwhelming sepsis including respiratory failure, shock, coagulopathy and temperature instability. A small number of infants may present with peritonitis from intestinal perforation [56].

Enterocolitis is the most serious complication of Hirschsprung's disease and is associated with high morbidity and mortality (25 to 30 per cent). Twenty to 58 per cent of children with Hirschsprung's disease develop enterocolitis and this may be the initial clinical presentation [58,59]. Relapses of enterocolitis can occur despite a diverting colostomy or even a definitive pull-through procedure [60]. Enterocolitis is characterized by an inflammatory and infectious process involving the colon. The pathogenesis of enterocolitis is poorly understood but stasis and bacterial overgrowth are generally believed to be involved. Proposed etiologic factors also include alterations of mucin components, increased prostaglandin E1 activity, *Clostridium difficile* infection and rotavirus infection [57]. The clinical presentation of infants with enterocolitis includes fever, abdominal distension and diarrhea which is typically explosive, malodorous and bloody. Because clinical deterioration can occur rapidly, it is important to recognize this entity and begin treatment immediately. While the physical examination of children with Hirschsprung's disease is usually non-diagnostic, the forceful decompression of gray liquid stool with rectal examination should suggest underlying enterocolitis. Treatment consists of fluid resuscitation, broad-spectrum antibiotic coverage (classic "triple" therapy, for example) and intestinal decompression, initially with rectal washouts/irrigation and, when the baby is clinically stable, with an enterostomy proximal to the aganglionic bowel segment [61]. There is no place for operative pull-through procedures in the setting of enterocolitis.

5.4. Gastrointestinal perforations

(A) Meconium peritonitis

Meconium peritonitis is an aseptic chemical and foreign-body reaction of the peritoneum to spillage of meconium from a prenatal perforation of the gastrointestinal tract. The prenatal perforation is usually caused by distal intestinal obstruction secondary to intestinal atresia or meconium ileus. Less common causes of obstruction in the fetus associated with meconium peritonitis include volvulus, internal hernia, congenital bands and intussusception. In patients without intestinal obstruction, localized mesenteric vascular insufficiency has been postulated as the etiology of perforation [62].

Three pathologic forms of meconium peritonitis have been described [63]:

(1) *Plastic.* Meconium in the peritoneal cavity induces an intense chemical reaction with subsequent formation of dense fibrous adhesions. The site of perforation is frequently sealed off by these adhesions. Calcium deposits (the result of saponification of free fatty acids) are scattered throughout.

(2) *Pseudocyst.* The intestinal perforation does not immediately seal and meconium continues to leak into the peritoneal cavity. The perforation is contained by formation of a pseudocyst, consisting of loops of intestine (which may be necrotic) and omentum surrounding the liquefied meconium. Calcium deposits line the cyst wall.

(3) *Generalized.* The intestinal perforation occurs just before birth, remains open and continues to leak meconium throughout the peritoneum, producing meconium ascites. The inflammatory reaction is less severe, and the adhesions between intestinal loops are more fibrinous. Calcium deposits may be seen throughout the peritoneum.

The most common presentations of meconium peritonitis in newborns are abdominal distension (71%) and bilious vomiting (59%). Polyhydramnios is present in the mother in 10 per cent of these patients. In less than 10 per cent of patients, meconium peritonitis is found incidentally in an asymptomatic newborn as a result of evaluation of a scrotal mass (in this case due to calcified meconium in a patent processus vaginalis) or identification of calcifications on abdominal film [62].

Meconium peritonitis is frequently detected on fetal ultrasonography. Ultrasonographic findings include polyhydramnios, acoustic shadowing from calcific foci, fetal ascites and bowel dilatation. Plain abdominal films usually reveal dilated loops of intestine and abdominal calcifications.

The indications for operative intervention in newborns with meconium peritonitis include evidence of intestinal obstruction, free intraperitoneal air, abdominal mass, cellulitis of the abdominal wall, sepsis or clinical deterioration. Infants with incidental meconium ascites or calcification in the scrotum or peritoneum who are asymptomatic and well-appearing should be carefully observed. At operation, the peritoneal cavity is carefully explored to identify and control the site of perforation, most commonly the ileum or jejunum and to address the underlying pathology (i.e. meconium ileus). All attempts should be made to preserve as much intestinal length as possible, even if this requires opening up a pseudocyst, lysing fibrous adhesions and freeing up viable bowel. Primary anastomoses can usually be performed after resection of atretic or necrotic bowel segments. Because of its high incidence in infants with meconium peritonitis, cystic fibrosis should be ruled out in all of these patients post-operatively [62].

(B) Gastric perforations

The causes of gastric perforation in neonates can be categorized as traumatic, ischemic or spontaneous. Traumatic perforations result from gastric overdistension (due to overaggressive mask resuscitation or accidental esophageal intubation with vigorous insufflation) or from puncture of the stomach during gastric intubation. Ischemic perforations occur in the setting of severe physiological stress such as extreme prematurity or birth asphyxia and sometimes accompany NEC involving the distal gastrointestinal tract. It is postulated that an initial hypoxic mucosal injury progresses to infarction of a small area of the gastric wall with subsequent perforation. It is possible that some of these lesions represent perforated stress ulcers. Spontaneous perforations generally occur in healthy neonates without obvious risk factors. One hypothesis regarding the etiology of spontaneous perforation invokes a congenital abnormality of the muscularis that causes a focal weakness prone to rupture [64].

Neonatal gastric perforation is most commonly observed between the third and fifth days of life. Clinical manifestations include abrupt onset of abdominal distension, feeding intolerance, tachycardia, lethargy and evidence of poor perfusion due to hypovolemia. Leakage of gastric contents into the peritoneal cavity will cause peritonitis, leading to third-space fluid losses and eventual respiratory compromise due, in part, to diaphragm elevation. The diagnosis is confirmed by chest x-ray or abdominal films which demonstrate massive pneumoperitoneum. Since the source of "free air" cannot be confirmed until laparotomy, the differential diagnosis includes other potential pathologies including perforated peptic ulcer, NEC and pneumoperitoneum dissecting down from the thoracic cavity/mediastinum in an infant receiving positive-pressure ventilation.

Initial treatment entails aggressive fluid resuscitation, administration of broad-spectrum antibiotics (ampicillin, gentamicin and clindamycin), careful placement of a nasogastric tube to limit further peritoneal soilage and endotracheal intubation and respiratory support as needed. At operation, the peritoneum is entered via a tranverse incision above the umbilicus. Peritoneal contents are cultured for aerobic and anaerobic bacteria and fungi. At this point, exploration is carried out to verify the site of perforation. Most gastric perforations occur along the greater curvature of the stomach [65]. In most cases, surgical management is individualized to either debridement of the perforation edges followed by a two-layer closure of the stomach or closure around a gastrostomy tube, depending upon the site of perforation [66]. Extensive gastric resections are usually not necessary. Neonatal mortality after gastric perforation is dependent upon the cause of the perforation, the presence of associated diseases, and potential delays in diagnosis and treatment and is approximately 25 per cent [65].

(C) Intestinal perforations not associated with necrotizing enterocolitis

In addition to perforations associated with NEC, premature infants, especially those weighing less than 1,000 grams, are at risk for spontaneous intestinal perforations that arise as a manifestation of underlying diseases or as a complication of treatment for diseases of prematurity. Spontaneous perforations have occurred in association with Hirschsprung's disease, meconium ileus, maternal obstetric complications, perinatal asphyxia and use of umbilical artery catheters. Perhaps best known is the association with indomethacin therapy for symptomatic patent ductus arteriosus [67,68]. Finally, intestinal perforation has also been reported with dexamethasone therapy for chronic lung disease [69].

In contrast to those resulting from NEC, spontaneous intestinal perforations are focal and demonstrate no clinical or histologic evidence of NEC or intrinsic bowel disease [70]. The most common site of perforation is the small bowel. Unlike the typical bowel flora found on culture in infants with perforation due to NEC, patients with spontaneous perforations have had cultures positive for *Candida* and/or *Staph. epidermidis* [70]. Perhaps most importantly, infants with spontaneous perforations (with patient demographics similar to those with NEC perforations) may have more favorable outcomes (reported mortality 27 versus 48 per cent) [71].

Most patients present initially with clinical findings suggestive of NEC but they do not develop the traditional clinical or radiographic findings associated with NEC. The most common finding is abdominal distension (95 per cent). Pneumoperitoneum may be present in only two-thirds of patients [72].

For distal small bowel or colon perforations, treatment is accomplished in most cases with simple exteriorization of the perforation as a stoma. Proximal small bowel perforations are probably best treated with primary closure because (1) there is minimal devitalized tissue around the focal perforation, (2) a high jejunostomy may cause severe electrolyte abnormalities and dehydration and (3) the jejunal mesentery may not stretch to the abdominal wall. When perforated appendicitis is discovered at operation in the neonate, rectal biopsies should be obtained becau-

se of potential underlying Hirschsprung's disease [73].

5.5. Omphalitis and necrotizing fasciitis

OMPHALITIS is a cellulitis of the skin and subcutaneous tissues adjacent to the umbilicus that occasionally leads to neonatal sepsis. Omphalitis is relatively uncommon because of aseptic delivery, routine umbilical care and antimicrobial therapy, with a reported incidence of approximately 2 per cent in hospital-born neonates. After birth, umbilical cords gradually become colonized with *S. aureus*, *S. epidermidis*, streptococci and, to a lesser extent, Gram-negative bacteria. Infection of the cord is necessary before sloughing and faint erythema of the skin at the base of the umbilical stump is benign. Likewise, serous or serosanguinous secretions from the cord base after separation are common [74].

Omphalitis should be suspected when more extensive erythema or inflammation is present in association with edema around the umbilical stump or when stump secretions are frankly purulent. Initial therapy with local application of bacitracin or neomycin ointment is indicated. Significant periumbilical infection or any evidence of systemic infection mandates intravenous antibiotic therapy because of possible spreading along the umbilical vein into the portal venous system. Mild cases may be treated with oral antibiotics such as erythromycin or cephalexin [74]. With severe infections, broad-spectrum antibiotics (to cover staphylococci, Gram-negative aerobic and anaerobic organisms) are warranted and, rarely, limited surgical debridement is necessary. Omphalitis may progress to peritonitis or necrotizing fasciitis of the abdominal wall [75].

NECROTIZING FASCIITIS is a rare entity in children and represents a life-threatening surgical emergency. While it is reported after local trauma and surgical procedures in older children, necrotizing fasciitis in the neonatal period is secondary to omphalitis, with a mortality rate as high as 50 per cent [76]. It is a synergistic infection that spreads rapidly along tissue planes, producing cell lysis and tissue necrosis that extends through the fascial layers. Clinical signs of necrotizing fasciitis include massive edema and induration of the abdominal wall with vibrant erythema, large fluid requirements to maintain vital signs and urine output and the "telltale" gangrenous patch of skin surrounding the umbilicus [75].

Recognition of the necrotizing infection is essential as prompt and radical surgical debridement is the infant's only hope for survival. Treatment should be initiated immediately with aggressive fluid resuscitation and administration of antibiotics to cover polymicrobial infection (typically ampicillin, gentamicin and clindamycin). Operative debridement requires sharp excision of all necrotic tissue back to a bleeding margin of viable tissue. Because the infection typically spreads along the deep fascia, it may extend along the underside of the abdominal wall between the fascia and the peritoneum. Consequently, the umbilicus should be excised completely and a limited laparotomy performed. The umbilical vessels and urachus should be divided at a site distant from the umbilicus and excised. After the initial operation, extremely close observation is necessary as evidence of clinical deterioration would suggest residual necrotic tissue and the need for further debridement. Repeat operative debridements are

required until the infection is under control [75].

5.6. Infections of the hepatobiliary system

(A) Cholangitis

Children with biliary tract obstruction (for example, due to a choledochal cyst) or dilatation (as in congenital hepatic fibrosis) are more susceptible to cholangitis. However, cholangitis in the pediatric population is most frequently observed in children who have undergone hepatic portoenterostomy for biliary atresia, occurring in 40 to 60 per cent of cases [6]. Gram-negative enteric bacteria such as *E. coli*, *Klebsiella* sp. and *Enterococcus* account for most cases but anaerobes may also be involved.

The clinical presentation includes fever, jaundice, right upper quadrant pain and, occasionally, shock. Early post-operative cholangitis (within 3 months) frequently results in the cessation of bile flow [77]. Laboratory findings include leukocytosis, hyperbilirubinemia, elevation of serum transaminases and alkaline phosphatase. Blood cultures are positive in 50 per cent of cases.

Treatment includes n.p.o. status, intravenous hydration, broad-spectrum antibiotic coverage (ampicillin, a third-generation cephalosporin and an aminoglycoside would be an appropriate regimen) and administration of choleretics such as phenobarbital, glucagon and/or steroids. Reoperation for recurrent episodes of cholangitis and to re establish bile flow may be beneficial in the patient in whom excellent bile flow has been established after portoenterostomy and then ceases abruptly. In this setting, a trial of "pulse" therapy with high-dose corticosteroids is administered before deciding upon reoperation [78].

(B) Spontaneous bile duct perforation

Although rare, spontaneous perforation of the common bile duct is second only to biliary atresia as a cause of surgically correctable jaundice in neonates. The site of perforation is typically at the junction of the common bile duct and cystic and may be due to a congenital weakness or to distal common bile duct obstruction by stones or sludge. Infants usually present between 2 and 6 weeks of age with jaundice and ascites. The disease can follow a chronic, subacute or acute course, with varying degrees of peritonitis, fever, intestinal obstruction, sepsis and even cardiorespiratory collapse. The diagnosis may be suspected at ultrasound if subhepatic fluid collections are detected but the imaging study of choice is hepatobiliary scintigraphy. The diagnosis is confirmed by extravasation of bile into the peritoneal cavity [79].

Operative intervention is undertaken to establish external drainage of the periductal area to allow healing of the perforation. An important aspect of the operation is the performance of cholangiography to rule out distal common bile duct obstruction by sludge or stones. A cholecystostomy tube should be left in cases of distal obstruction or marked ductal inflammation. Healing of the duct and the status of potential distal obstruction can be followed by cholangiography through the cholecystostomy tube [79].

5.7. Acute gastroenteritis

VIRAL GASTROENTERITIS is second only to upper respiratory infections as the most common disease observed in childhood. Rotaviruses, adenoviruses, and small round viruses (i.e. Norwalk agent) account for the majority of viral gastroenteritis in the pediatric population [80]. Rotavirus is responsible for the winter peak in childhood gastroenteritis, while the enteric adenoviruses are responsible for the summer peak [81]. Rotaviruses and adenoviruses primarily affect children 6 to 24 months of age, whereas small round viruses are usually epidemic and responsible for outbreaks of gastroenteritis in school-aged children, family contacts and adults. Symptoms of viral gastroenteritis include vomiting, diarrhea, fever and abdominal cramping and may be preceded or accompanied by other constitutional symptoms. Rapid diagnosis of rotaviruses and adenoviruses by solid-phase immunoassays are commercially available [80]. Treatment is supportive and consists of replacement of water and electrolyte losses. Oral rehydration solutions are extremely useful and are often life-saving in cases of dehydration [81]. Because enteric viruses are often spread by the fecal-oral route, adequate hand washing is important in controlling the spread of infection.

Whereas viral agents invade villus enterocytes along the entire span of the small intestine, organisms responsible for BACTERIAL GASTROENTERITIS often act on the colon. Several bacterial virulence mechanisms act specifically on the colon, causing cytotoxic injury, direct epithelial cell invasion and enteroadhesive activity [81]. The most common bacterial pathogens of the human gastrointestinal tract that cause gastroenteritis in children are *Salmonella*, *Shigella* and pathogenic strains of *E. coli*. Bacterial gastroenteritis generally results from ingestion of contaminated food or water, occurs in children under 4 years of age, presents with diarrhea and fever and requires fresh stool cultures to establish the diagnosis. Because of the risk of dehydration, prompt and appropriate replacement of fluid and electrolytes is essential.

Salmonella is the most common cause of bacterial diarrhea in children in the U.S. Because of the invasiveness of this organism, infection can result in colitis and bacteremia, especially in infants and children with impaired host immune defenses. Antibiotic treatment with ampicillin or trimethoprim-sulfamethoxazole is recommended in patients at high risk for the development of disseminated disease, those who appear septic, neonates and those with complicated cases of gastroenteritis [81]. The incidence of enteric (typhoid) fever is very rare in the absence of recent international travel.

Shigella most frequently causes a mild, self-limited diarrhea. In addition to ingestion of bacteria, the infection is spread by direct person-to-person contact and is a common cause of outbreaks of diarrhea in daycare settings. Approximately 40 per cent of children with *Shigella* infection have blood in their stools, over 50 per cent have emesis, 90 per cent have fever and 10 to 35 per cent may experience seizures due to a neurotoxin produced by the organism [82]. Treatment with trimethoprim-sulfamethoxazole is sometimes appropriate for children who are severly ill to shorten the course of disease and the period of fecal shedding of the organism [81].

Pathogenic strains of *E. coli* are important causes of diarrheal disease in children and include enteropathogenic *E. coli* (causes epidemic watery diarrhea in infants), enteroinvasive *E. coli* (related to *Shigella*; causes diarrhea with fever in all ages) and enterohemorrhagic *E. coli* (causes hemorrhagic colitis in all ages and hemolytic

uremic syndrome in children) [82]. These bacteria produce a range of symptoms from watery diarrhea to hemorrhagic colitis. Antibiotic therapy is generally not indicated except for infantile enteropathogenic *E. coli* infection, which is treated with trimethoprim-sulfamethoxazole to shorten the course of disease and to lower the risk of spread of the disease [82].

6. CHILDHOOD (AGE 3-11 YRS)

While acute gastroenteritis, Hirschsprung's enterocolitis and infections of the hepatobiliary system are common in children aged 3 to 11 years, the majority of intra-abdominal infections in this age group are due to appendicitis and trauma/child abuse. The principles of management of intra-abdominal infections resulting from pediatric trauma have been outlined above.

6.1. Appendicitis

Acute appendicitis is one of the most common pediatric intra-abdominal infections. About 1 per cent of all children younger than 15 years of age develop appendicitis, with a peak incidence between 10 and 12 years of age [83]. Children with appendicitis tend to be diagnosed at a more advanced stage of illness than adults. Because appendicitis in early childhood is uncommon, patient presentation and accurate diagnosis are frequently delayed, resulting in perforation rates reported between 20 and 50 per cent. Post-operative complications, including wound infection (1.7 per cent), bowel obstruction (1.4 per cent), intra-abdominal abscess (1.7 per cent), and enterocutaneous fistula (0.2 per cent), occur predominantly in association with perforated appendicitis [83,84].

The pathophysiology of appendicitis begins with obstruction of the lumen by fecaliths (present in 30 to 50 per cent of patients with appendicitis), lymphoid hyperplasia, foreign bodies, parasitic infections or conditions that cause increased colonic pressure and decreased motility, such as Hirschsprung's disease or meconium ileus. Continued mucous secretion by the mucosa results in increased intraluminal pressure that eventually leads to lymphatic, venous and arterial compromise. As ischemia of the appendiceal wall ensues, mucosal ulceration is followed by bacterial invasion and subsequent invasive infection of the appendix. Perforation occurs in the setting of transmural necrosis [83].

Appendicitis should be suspected in any child who presents with abdominal pain. The classic clinical presentation consisting of right lower quadrant pain, fever, anorexia, nausea and vomiting is present in less than half of children with acute appendicitis. Other symptoms may include diarrhea, constipation or urinary symptoms. The abdominal pain caused by appendicitis frequently begins in the periumbilical and epigastric regions and later shifts to the right lower quadrant. When the appendix lies in a retrocecal position, however, the classic shift of pain to the right lower quadrant may be absent because irritation of the parietal peritoneum does not occur. If symptoms have been present for more than 48 hours at presentation, the probability of perforation exceeds 70 per cent. Children with perforated appendicitis appear much "sicker" with generalized abdominal pain, high-grade fever, worsening anorexia with nausea and vomiting and dehydration.

Physical examination usually reveals focal abdominal tenderness. Rovsing's sign, referred pain in the right lower quadrant on palpation of the left lower quadrant, is a fairly specific sign for appendicitis. Evidence of peritoneal irritation may manifest with percussion tenderness, pain with internal rotation of the thigh (obturator sign), pain with hip extension (psoas sign) or involuntary guarding of the rectus muscles. Rectal examination may reveal tenderness consistent with retrocecal appendicitis or fullness associated with a pelvic abscess. Bimanual examination in postpubertal girls may help exclude pelvic inflammatory disease and ovarian pathology from the differential diagnoses. Free perforation of the appendix into the peritoneal cavity usually produces generalized peritonitis. When the perforation is "walled off" by the surrounding viscera and omentum, patients may present with a palpable mass, representing an abscess or a phlegmon.

In general, laboratory and radiographic studies do not add much to the clinical diagnosis of acute appendicitis in patients presenting with clear symptoms and physical findings. Many different laboratory tests have been used to help discriminate appendicitis from other causes of abdominal pain but none is consistently definitive [85]. The most reliable tests are the white blood cell (wbc) count and differential, as less than 5 per cent of children with appendicitis will have both a normal wbc count and differential without a left shift [83]. Perforated appendicitis is almost always associated with leukocytosis and a marked left shift. Urinalysis should be routinely performed in children with symptoms suggestive of appendicitis. The presence of leukocyte esterase, mild to moderate pyuria or hematuria may indicate underlying genitourinary tract pathology but may also be due to irritation of the bladder or ureter from an inflamed appendix.

In children whose symptoms are atypical or confusing or when faced with complicated appendicitis, radiographic studies may be helpful in establishing a diagnosis. Plain abdominal radiographs may demonstrate free air due to viscus perforation or a bowel gas pattern suggestive of obstruction secondary to a retroileal appendicitis. The finding of an appendicolith in a child with localized abdominal pain would mandate surgery for probable acute appendicitis. Ultrasound can be used to rule out pelvic or ovarian pathology as a cause of abdominal pain in girls and may be useful in diagnosing appendicitis. Ultrasonographic findings of an edematous, distended (more than 6 mm in diameter) and non-compressible appendix have been reported as accurate predictors of the presence of acute appendicitis. The use of CT scanning is probably most appropriate in evaluating atypical patients with undiagnosed intra-abdominal symptoms or in whom satisfactory ultrasound studies are not possible (i.e. for children who are obese, immunologically suppressed or neurologically impaired). In patients with suspected perforated appendicitis, CT scan may facilitate distinction of phlegmon from abscess and provide information necessary for percutaneous or transrectal abscess drainage [83].

The treatment of children with appendicitis is dictated by the severity of disease at presentation [84,86,87]. For acute (non-perforated) appendicitis, the child is promptly prepared for surgery with administration of intravenous fluids and preoperative antibiotics (a broad-spectrum single agent such as cefotetan is appropriate). Appendectomy is performed through a right lower quadrant incision. If the appendix is grossly abnormal in appearance, it should be removed and an exploration within the confines of the existing incision should be undertaken to exclude other causes of abdominal pain (such as Meckel's diverticulum, mesenteric adenitis, regional enteritis and, in females, gynecological pathology) [88]. Post-operatively, antibiotics are discontinued after one or two doses and oral intake is resumed after 12 to 24 hours.

For children with persistent right lower quadrant pain in whom the diagnosis is not clear despite a period of observation/re-examination and ancillary studies, operation is recommended due to the risk of perforation. While a standard "open" appendectomy is perfectly appropriate in this setting, consideration may be given to the use of laparoscopy, especially in postpubertal girls. The main advantage of laparoscopy is that it allows superior visualization of the peritoneal and pelvic organs when causes other than appendicitis may be the source of abdominal pain. The majority of these diseases, including appendicitis, can be treated via laparoscopy as well.

For perforated appendicitis with associated peritonitis, children are managed according to the principles outlined earlier in this chapter. After appropriate resuscitation and administration of broad-spectrum antibiotics (consisting of classic "triple-drug" therapy or combination therapy with either a third-generation cephalosporin or extended-spectrum penicillin and an aminoglycoside), appendectomy is undertaken using an incision similar to that described above. Peritoneal fluid is sampled for Gram stain, aerobic and anaerobic cultures. All debris and purulent material is removed and irrigated from the peritoneal cavity. If a localized abscess in found, this may be drained through a separate stab incision. Post-operatively, antibiotics are continued for at least 5 to 7 days until the patient is afebrile, the wbc count returns to normal and a rectal examination documents the absence of a pelvic abscess. If these criteria are not met or if the patient is ill-appearing or manifests prolonged ileus, CT scanning is used to exclude an intra-abdominal or pelvic abscess. Post-operative antibiotics may be adjusted based upon the results of intraoperative cultures, including expanding coverage if *Pseudomonas* sp. are present. Diet is advanced upon return of bowel function.

In patients with perforated appendicitis who present with a mass (abscess) and no evidence of peritonitis, conservative treatment may be appropriate. Non-operative management with percutaneous or trans-rectal/transvaginal abscess drainage and broad-spectrum antibiotic therapy followed by interval elective appendectomy after 8 weeks (to allow the inflammatory reaction to subside) is usually successful, although the patient is at risk for recurrent appendicitis.

Failure to improve with these measures (as evidenced by persistent fever or prolonged ileus) mandates earlier operation following the principles outlined above.

6.2. Meckel's diverticulitis

A Meckel's diverticulum is the most common congenital anomaly of the gastrointestinal tract, occurring in 2 per cent of the general population. It is one of several malformations that result from persistence of the embryonic vitelline or omphalomesenteric duct. Meckel's diverticulum is a true diverticulum containing all layers of the intestinal wall and is attached to the antimesenteric border of the ileum, usually within 2 feet of the ileocecal valve [89]. Up to 25 per cent of patients may have attachment of the diverticulum to the anterior ab-

dominal wall by means of a fibrous or vascular band at the umbilicus, a feature putting the child at risk for internal herniation with intestinal obstruction or volvulus [61]. The mucosa of the diverticulum may contain ectopic gastric and pancreatic mucosa in up to 25 per cent of cases. In patients who present with bleeding or perforation, peptic ulceration of adjacent ileal mucosa is responsible.

Estimates of the probability of Meckel's diverticulum causing symptoms in a patient's lifetime vary from 4 to 35 per cent with the risk diminishing substantially with increasing age. Over 60 per cent of patients who develop symptoms from this anomaly are younger that 2 years of age [83]. Based on analyses of large series of patients, the most common symptoms related to Meckel's diverticulum are: bleeding (30 to 35 per cent), intestinal obstruction (30 to 35 per cent), inflammation (20 to 25 per cent), and umbilical sinus drainage (10 per cent) [61]. The symptoms related to Meckel's diverticulum vary directly with patient age. In newborns, bowel obstruction is the most common clinical presentation. Hemorrhage is more frequent in older infants and young children, with a mean age of 2 years. Inflammation causing diverticulitis usually presents in older children [90].

Similar to the pathophysiology of appendicitis, a Meckel's diverticulum can become inflamed when the lumen is obstructed, especially when the diverticulum is long and has a narrow base. Obstruction leads to increased intraluminal pressure with decreased mucosal perfusion, tissue acidosis and bacterial invasion of the wall. Progressive distal inflammation then leads to tissue gangrene and, potentially, perforation. The role of ectopic mucosa in this process is inferred by its high incidence in resected inflamed diverticula. It is possible that the gastric or pancreatic mucosa contributes to the luminal obstruction or that gastric mucosa leads to ileal mucosal ulceration which facilitates bacterial invasion.[83] Perforation of a Meckel's diverticulum can also occur in the absence of luminal obstruction by virtue of erosion of the diverticulum wall by foreign bodies (e.g. toothpick, chicken or fish bone) [89].

The symptoms of Meckel's diverticulitis are indistinguishable from those of acute appendicitis. In fact, most patients operated on for diverticulitis have a presumptive diagnosis of acute appendicitis. Although the location of a Meckel's diverticulum within the peritoneal cavity may be somewhat variable, most present with right lower quadrant and lower midline pain and tenderness. In light of these similarities in presentation, it is imperative to search carefully for other causes of peritonitis when a non-inflamed appendix is discovered at the time of appendectomy. Perhaps because of its mobile position, a perforated Meckel's diverticulum is less likely than a perforated appendix to be walled off and, thus, may present as diffuse peritonitis [83]. In conjunction with the acute presentation of Meckel's diverticulitis, there are no laboratory or radiologic tests that are specific for this diagnosis. Pneumoperitoneum detected on abdominal plain films may suggest perforated diverticulitis.

Surgical treatment for Meckel's diverticulitis is most often accomplished using a transverse appendectomy incision which may be extended medially to allow resection of the involved ileum, if necessary [83]. Meckel's diverticulitis complicated by perforation and peritonitis requires aggressive fluid resuscitation and preoperative broad-spectrum antibiotic coverage. The extent of sur-

gical resection required for treatment of Meckel's diverticulitis depends upon several factors including the area of intestine involved in the inflammatory process and the presence of perforation and peritoneal soilage. Inflammation confined to the diverticulum, especially when perforation has not occurred, can be treated with simple diverticulectomy with transverse closure of the ileal stump to prevent luminal narrowing. Care should be taken to ligate the separate blood supply to the Meckel's diverticulum which enters the diverticulum directly from the small bowel mesentery [90]. When inflammation extends to the ileum (to a point where the ileal lumen is compromised) or when perforation is present, especially with peritoneal soilage, resection of the involved small intestine and primary end-to-end anastomosis is preferred. In patients who are hemodynamically unstable and in whom significant peritoneal soilage has occurred, a temporary enterostomy may be optimal [89].

6.3. Infections of the gall bladder and biliary system

(A) Cholelithiasis and cholecystitis

Gallstones are being recognized in children with an increasing frequency, the incidence estimated between 0.15 and 0.22 per cent.[91] The pathogenesis of cholelithiasis in children is multifactorial and differs according to age at presentation. In infants, the immaturity of both hepatic excretory function and the enterohepatic circulation lowers the threshold for stone formation when combined with other lithogenic influences (i.e. distal ileal resection for NEC, total parenteral nutrition, prolonged fasting and furosemide treatment). Cholestasis in infants can be manifest as abnormal liver function tests, biliary sludge or true chole-lithiasis. In the prepubertal child, gallsto-nes are idiopathic or related to chronic he-molysis (due to congenital hematological disorders such as sickle cell disease, here-ditary spherocytosis or thalassemia major, as well as hemolysis after open heart sur-gery and insertion of a cardiac valve), cys-tic fibrosis, ileal disease or resection, or ceftriaxone therapy. Gallstones in infants and prepubertal children are predomi-nantly pigment stones. After puberty, as in adults, stones are more likely to be choles-terol. In this age group, predisposing fac-tors include obesity, pregnancy, oral con-traceptive use and a positive family history for cholelithiasis [79].

Children can present with acute cholecysti-tis but chronic cholecystitis and cholelithia-sis are more common. Clinical presentation is strongly influenced by patient age. The presentation in infancy is often non-focal and subtle, requiring a high index of suspi-cion to make the diagnosis. Persistence of direct hyperbilirubinemia should lead to an evaluation of the biliary tract, including a search for cholelithiasis [79]. Symptoms of biliary tract disease in this age group can be severe - cholangitis, necrosis, perforation of the gallbladder, perforation of the extrahe-patic bile ducts and choledocholithiasis with obstructive jaundice have been repor-ted [92]. Younger children with gallstones may not be able to localize abdominal pain. Those children who present with re-current unexplained abdominal pain should undergo evaluation for biliary disea-se. Likewise, abdominal pain in children with chronic hemolysis or other predispo-sing conditions should raise suspicion for biliary disease [93]. Adolescent patients present in a similar fashion to adults with localized right upper quadrant pain worse-ned by fatty foods and associated with nau-

sea and vomiting. Gallstone pancreatitis or cholangitis are relatively infrequent presen-tations in children but have been reported in patients with sickle cell anemia [79].

Available tests for diagnosing cholelithiasis and cholecystitis include plain abdominal films, ultrasonagraphy and cholescinti-graphy. The value of plain films lies in the higher incidence of radiopaque stones, typi-cally pigmented, in children versus adults, reported as high as 50 per cent in patients with hemolytic disorders [94]. Ultrasono-graphy is the diagnositc modality of choice with an accuracy of approximately 96 per cent. In addition to detecting gallstones, it allows evaluation of the common hepatic and common bile ducts as well as identifying features of the gallbladder that suggest acute cholecystitis. These features include an im-pacted stone in the ampulla, associated gall bladder wall thickening or localized peri-cholecystic fluid [79]. Because of the high incidence of cholelithiasis in children with chronic hemolytic diseases, it can be very difficult to differentiate acute cholecystitis from other intra-abdominal emergencies, for example, sickle cell abdominal crisis. Cho-lescintigraphy with technetium-99m-labeled iminodiacetic acid (IDA) compounds allows assessment of the patency of the cystic duct and is the procedure of choice to diagnose acute cholecystitis. In patients with acute cholecystitis, the isotopic scan will demons-trate flow from the extrahepatic biliary sys-tem into the intestine without visualization of the gallbladder [91]. One potential draw-back of cholescintigraphy is the relatively high rate of false-positive results that have been reported in fasting patients and those receiving TPN. Although not useful in the initial evaluation of gallstones in children, CT may occasionally have value in cases complicated by choledocholithiasis or galls-tone pancreatitis [91].

Laboratory tests in patients with cholelithiasis and cholecystitis are useful to help detect potential choledocholithiasis or, rarely, gallstone pancreatitis. These test results may alter the timing of operative therapy or may mandate intraoperative cholangiography in addition to cholecystectomy. In children with acute cholecystitis, leukocytosis with a left shift is typically present. If choledocholithiasis is present, liver function tests may demonstrate elevated levels of serum bilirubin, alkaline phosphatase and gamma glutamyl transferase. Elevated serum amylase levels in the setting of cholelithiasis may be associated with gallstone pancreatitis.

The treatment of children with cholelithiasis depends upon the presence of symptoms, the age at presentation and the presence of underlying hemolytic diseases. Symptomatic or complicated cholelithiasis is treated with cholecystectomy. Unlike adults, there is little role for observation in symptomatic patients. While large series document minimal morbidity and no mortality in children treated with conventional open cholecystectomy [95], laparoscopic cholecystectomy is rapidly becoming the procedure of choice [96,97,98]. Some centers advocate routine intraoperative cholangiography, while most use cholangiography selectively in patients at high risk for choledocholithiasis (dilated common bile duct, elevated liver function tests, presence of jaundice or preoperative gallstone pancreatitis) [99,100]. If common duct stones are identified by cholangiography, treatment options include: (1) conversion to an open procedure with standard common bile duct exploration, (2) basket retrieval using a nephroureteroscope or (3) post-operative endoscopic retrograde cholangiopancreatography (ERCP) with sphincterotomy and balloon-assisted retrieval [91].

The treatment of neonates and infants who present with cholecystitis or choledocholithiasis (with or without cholangitis) requires special attention. In addition to cholecystectomy, cholecystotomy with stone removal and irrigation may be a treatment option in infants with cholecystitis or cholangitis [91]. Percutaneous puncture of the gallbladder and intrahepatic ducts with irrigation of the biliary tract to clear obstructing biliary sludge and stones has been described in infants and neonates [101]. Although spontaneous resolution has been reported, choledocholithiasis with cholestatic jaundice in infants usually requires therapeutic intervention. In this setting, ERCP and endoscopic sphincterotomy with stone removal can be used to clear the common bile duct in infants as young as 9 months of age. [102]. If gallstones remain after clearing the common bile duct, cholecystectomy should be performed. If sphincterotomy is unsuccessful or if the patient is too small for ERCP, an open procedure with irrigation of the common bile duct through the cystic duct or a transduodenal sphincterotomy may be required [91].

Treatment of children with cholelithiasis who do not have symptoms is dictated by age and associated disease. Cholelithiasis has been recognized in utero by prenatal ultrasound with spontaneous resolution occurring by one month of age [103]. Several reports have documented spontaneous resolution of asymptomatic gallstones in infants from 2 weeks to 6 months after initial discovery. For this reason, a period of careful observation is warranted in the asymptomatic infant. A trial of ursodeoxycholic acid (recommended dose is 10 to 20 mg/kg/day divided into 2 to 3 doses) may be warranted in this setting in light of its choleretic effects. Ursodeoxycholic acid has been used in cholestatic syndromes caused by parenteral nutrition [104]. Cholecystectomy is reserved for patients with persistence of gallstones for more than 6 to 12 months or for patients with radiopaque (calcified) gallstones that are unlikely to resolve [79].

In children with asymptomatic cholelithiasis secondary to chronic hemolytic disease, elective cholecystectomy has been advocated because of the likelihood of developing symptoms and subsequent complications. In children with cholelithiasis secondary to sickle cell anemia, lower complication rates have been reported in association with elective versus emergency surgery [105]. The timing of elective cholecystectomy in children with hemolytic diseases varies. While not universally accepted, early elective cholecystectomy (soon after the diagnosis is made) has been advocated for children with sickle cell anemia [106]. In children with thalassemia major, cholecystectomy is performed at the time of splenectomy when a preoperative ultrasound demonstrates concomitant cholelithiasis [107]. Similarly, in children with hereditary spherocytosis and asymptomatic cholelithiasis , cholecystectomy is performed at the time of splenectomy [91].

In older children and adolescents with asymptomatic cholelithiasis unrelated to hematologic diseases, initial management is non-operative with observation and serial ultrasound. Because these children, in comparison to adults with asymptomatic cholelithiasis, have many more years for complications to develop, a case has been made for offering these children cholecystectomy in the event of persistent or enlarged stones after 6 to 12 months of observation [79]. A more conservative approach, similar to management in adults, with continued observation until symptoms develop can also be

justified. Along this line, patients with cystic fibrosis rarely have biliary complications and should be treated non-operatively until symptoms develop [91].

Among the most important aspects of treating children with cholelithiasis are the preoperative preparation and perioperative management of patients with sickle cell anemia. Because of the risk of sickling of abnormal red blood cells which can be precipitated by a high level of hemoglobin S, among other things, preoperative transfusion to reduce the hemoglobin S level to between 30 and 40 per cent is recommended. For elective surgery, this can be accomplished using 2 to 3 transfusions (10 cc/kg) given preoperatively 2 to 3 weeks apart. An alternative technique is to use 3 partial exchange transfusions (5 cc/kg of the patient's blood is withdrawn and replaced with 10 cc/kg of washed packed red blood cells) over the 2 weeks prior to surgery. For urgent surgery, simple transfusion to a hemoglobin level of 12 g/dL or exchange transfusion through a large-bore catheter can be used. In the intraoperative and postoperative settings, it is essential to avoid hypoxia, hypothermia, hypovolemia and acidosis as these factors can precipitate sickling in this patient population [91].

(B) Acute acalculous cholecystitis

Acute acalculous cholecystitis refers to acute inflammation of the gallbladder in the absence of gallstones. It is a rare disease in children and characteristically occurs as a complication during the course of treatment of children who are severely ill based upon prior surgery, a severe burn, multisystem trauma, massive blood transfusion and various infections, including pneumonia, generalized sepsis, typhoid, salmonella, otitis media with meningitis, giardiasis and Kawasaki disease [104]. It may occur in newborns but is more common in older children. Although the exact pathogenesis of acalculous cholecystitis is not understood, bile stasis with subsequent mucosal injury and ischemia is postulated to lead to inflammation and infection in the gallbladder wall. The clinical course may be very aggressive with progression to gangrene and perforation of the gallbladder.

The presentation of acute acalculous cholecystitis is similar to calculus cholecystitis. Symptoms include fever, right upper quadrant pain, nausea, vomiting and diarrhea when the underlying infection is caused by a pathogenic intestinal organism [104]. Jaundice may occasionally be present. The mean time of onset of these symptoms has been reported between 4 and 30 days after surgery or hospitalization [108]. Physical examination reveals tenderness to palpation and muscle guarding. A right upper quadrant mass is sometimes palpable and must be distinguished from acute hydrops [104]. Laboratory abnormalities include leukocytosis, elevated liver function tests and, potentially, hyperamylasemia.

Ultrasonography is the most commonly used test to diagnose acute acalculous cholecystitis but HIDA and CT scanning can be used for confirmation in equivocal cases. The ultrasonographic criteria for making the diagnosis are: a thickened gallbladder wall (> 4mm), gallbladder distension, dependent echogenic bile sludge, pericholecystic fluid collections, subserosal edema, sloughed mucosal membrane and a sonographic "Murphy's sign" (pressure over the gallbladder by the ultrasonagraphy transducer produces tenderness and pain) [109].
The treatment for mild cases of acute acal-

culous cholecystitis is conservative with nasogastric suction, intravenous fluids, parenteral antibiotics administered according to blood culture results and serial ultrasound studies. Persistence of a right upper quadrant mass, increased gallbladder distension, or clinical deterioration constitute indications for operative intervention [104]. Although cholecystostomy (placed surgically or percutaneously via ultrasonographic guidance) is a treatment option for isolated massive distension, cholecystectomy is the procedure of choice [79].

(C) Gallbladder hydrops

Gallbladder hydrops refers to acute, massive distension of the gallbladder without wall thickening or biliary infection. The condition is characterized by the development of severe edema around the gallbladder and common bile duct and may occur in the neonatal period as well as in older children. The most common cause of hydrops is the mucocutaneous lymph node syndrome (Kawasaki disease) [79], although it has also been reported in association with scarlet fever, leptospirosis, familial Mediterranean fever, mesenteric adenitis and neonatal sepsis [104]. In hydrops associated with Kawasaki disease, the cystic duct and common bile duct are surrounded by enlarged lymph nodes.

Older infants and children with hydrops may manifest fever, a right upper quadrant mass and abdominal tenderness, whereas neonates may present with an isolated mass. The diagnosis is made by abdominal ultrasonography. Treatment is based upon the patient's clinical course, which is typically benign but can progress to gangrene and perforation. Initial management should be conservative, consisting of antibiotics for septic patients, early enteral feedings (when possible) to stimulate gallbladder contraction and emptying and serial ultrasound examinations. If gallbladder distention and pain persist, a cholecystostomy can be performed for temporary decompression. If the gallbladder wall appears gangrenous, cholecystectomy should be performed [104].

6.4. Acute pancreatitis

Acute pancreatitis is an important but uncommon cause of abdominal pain in children [110]. Unlike adult pancreatitis, which is usually related to cholelithiasis or alcohol ingestion, acute pancreatitis in the pediatric population is predominantly post-traumatic or idiopathic in origin (75 to 80 per cent of cases) [111]. Other causes of pancreatitis in children include biliary stone disease, choledochal cyst or other anatomic abnormality, cystic fibrosis, hyperlipidemia and various medications (corticosteroids, chlorothiazides, tetracycline, azathioprine, and valproic acid).

The exact pathophysiological mechanisms of pancreatitis remain unclear [112]. The injury seems to be caused by disordered release and activation of various enzymes (including trypsin, chymotrypsin, elastase, phospholipase and carboxypeptidase) that cause autodestruction of the pancreas. From a pathological standpoint, the spectrum of disease induced by this process ranges from parenchymal edema to hemorrhagic pancreatitis with gangrene and necrosis [113], although hemorrhagic and necrotizing pancreatitis are rare in children who are immunocompetent [111].

The typical clinical presentation of acute pancreatitis is abdominal pain, characteristically epigastric and constant, radiating to the midback [114]. Associated symptoms usually include fever, nausea and vomiting. Physical examination reveals abdominal distension and tenderness, at times severe enough to suggest underlying peritonitis. Approximately 5 per cent of children with severe disease may present with evidence of hypovolemic shock [113]. Measurements of serum and urinary amylase and lipase remain the most useful laboratory tests to confirm the diagnosis. Ultrasound and CT scanning are effective in detecting edema and enlargement of the pancreas, findings consistent with acute pancreatitis. While both modalities can detect pancreatic ductal dilatation, CT is particularly useful for defining the degree of parenchymal destruction and identifying areas of necrosis or abscess formation [114].

As in adults, the primary treatment of acute pancreatitis in childhood is supportive medical therapy, including intravenous hydration, bowel rest, parenteral nutrition, pain relief, nasogastric decompression (to lessen pancreatic stimulation) and careful monitoring of urine output, vital signs and laboratory parameters (electrolytes, glucose, calcium, and hemoglobin levels) [114]. As opposed to adults, in whom prophylactic antibiotics are generally not recommended, young children, especially those with severe disease, may benefit from antibiotic administration because of the risk of developing sepsis [113].

After initial stabilization of children with acute pancreatitis, early recognition of a specific cause, using CT scanning or endoscopic retrograde cholangiopancreatography (ERCP), if necessary, is important. Acute interventions may be required for such problems as ductal disruption (due to trauma), an impacted stone or a potentiating medication. Operative intervention is usually reserved for the complications of pancreatitis, including hemorrhage, necrosis, abscess, pseudocyst or ductal fistula [114].

Recurrent episodes of acute pancreatitis in children are usually associated with a specific physiological cause or anatomic abnormality. For this reason, a child with recurrent disease should be studied aggressively, including the use of ERCP, even in infants [111]. Congenital anomalies and acquired strictures of the common bile duct have been found with increasing frequency in children with recurrent pancreatitis evaluated using ERCP [113].

6.5. Colitis

(A) Pseudomembranous colitis

Pseudomembranous colitis represents one end of a wide spectrum of disease associated with *Clostridium difficile*, ranging from the mild cases of simple diarrhea without colitis to fulminant disease leading to severe diarrhea, hypovolemic shock, toxic dilatation of the colon, perforation, sepsis and death [115]. *C. difficile*-related disease develops as a result of colonization and toxin production by this organism in the colon after the normal microflora has been altered by antimicrobial therapy. Nearly all antimicrobial agents have been implicated in this disorder and the risk of development of pseudomembranous colitis appears unrelated to the dose or duration of antibiotic therapy 81. The pathogenicity of *C. difficile* is due to its production of exotoxins. Toxin A is an enterotoxin that binds to receptors on the mucosal epithelial surface, resulting in severe inflammation and fluid secretion. Toxin B is a cytotoxin that induces alterations in cell shape and causes diffuse enterocyte

cell damage [81]. Up to 70 per cent of healthy neonates are asymptomatic carriers of *C. difficile* (versus 3 per cent of healthy adults) and possess some undefined resistance to *C. difficile* colitis [116].

Pseudomembranous colitis most frequently presents with mild to moderate, watery, non-bloody diarrhea beginning 7 to 10 days after the initiation of antibiotics with associated crampy abdominal pain. The symptoms may include tenesmus, nausea, vomiting, high grade fever, chills, dehydration and occasionally hypotension. Abdominal examination may reveal abdominal distension, tenderness and guarding. Some patients present with an acute abdomen and fulminant colitis with signs of perforation or toxic megacolon, even in the absence of preceding diarrhea [81].

The diagnosis of pseudomembranous colitis is most quickly and accurately made by endoscopy with visualization of the characteristic yellow-white raised plaques scattered over mucosal surfaces [115]. In patients who present with severe abdominal pain, plain abdominal films should be obtained to detect toxic megacolon or perforation. Abdominal CT scan, usually obtained to rule out other intra-abdominal pathology, will demonstrate colonic wall thickening and inflammation. The laboratory diagnosis of *C. difficile* diarrhea depends on the identification of the organism or its toxins in the stool. Detection of toxin B by demonstration of its cytopathic effect in tissue culture is the current "gold standard" because of its high sensitivity and specificity [115].

Pediatric patients with inflammatory bowel disease or Hirschsprung's disease may be at particularly high risk for developing *C. difficile* colitis, even without an antecedent history of antibiotic use. Five to 25 per cent of patients with an apparent relapse of inflammatory bowel disease have been noted to have *C. difficile* toxin in their stool [117]. Because pseudomembranes are infrequently seen in patients with coexisting *C. difficile* infection and ulcerative colitis, it is important to assay stool samples for *C. difficile* toxin in children with inflammatory bowel disease during acute relapses [118]. Likewise, children who have undergone definitive therapy for Hirschsprung's disease appear to have an increased incidence of pseudomembranous colitis. Because the clinical picture of pseudomembranous colitis can be indistinguishable from that of Hirschsprung's enterocolitis, empiric therapy should be started while awaiting results of stool evaluation in patients who are seriously ill [81].

Treatment of pseudomembranous colitis is dictated by the severity of symptoms. For mild disease, discontinuation of antibiotic therapy, if possible, can result in complete recovery without the use of specific therapy. In more severe disease and when continued therapy with the inducing antibiotic is necessary, treatment should include oral vancomycin, 40 mg/kg/d in 3 divided doses, or metronidazole, 20 to 30 mg/kg/d in 3 divided doses, continued for 7 to 10 days. Enteral administration of these antibiotics, by rectal or stomal irrigation if the oral route is unavailable, is much more effective that intravenous administration in reaching effective intraluminal concentrations. In severely ill patients with ileus, intravenous metronidazole can achieve therapeutic fecal concentrations. Relapse after treatment occurs in 15 per cent of patients and is most often due to sporulation of *C. difficile*.[81] Treatment of a relapse is the same as initial therapy. Indications for operative therapy include perforation, toxic megacolon and refractory disease (no improvement after 7

days of aggressive medical management). Operative management ranges from decompressive colostomy to total proctocolectomy but the best results are reported with subtotal colectomy and ileostomy [119].

(B) Diversion colitis

Diversion colitis is an inflammatory process in a bypassed colorectal segment after surgical diversion of the fecal stream (i.e. for Hirshsprung's disease). Although the pathogenesis of diversion colitis is unclear, possible etiologies include an altered microflora in the bypassed segment (with decreased numbers of total bacteria and strict anaerobes) and nutritional deprivation (short-chain fatty acid/butyric acid deficiency) of the colonocytes secondary to absence of luminal nutrients [81]. The clinical presentation in symptomatic children consists of diffuse, poorly localized abdominal pain and bloody stools/rectal drainage. No correlation has been found between the severity of the colitis and the duration of diversion or age at time of diversion [81]. In children who require long-term total parenteral nutrition, diversion colitis can be a particularly difficult problem because the chronically inflamed, bypassed intestine can be a source of bacterial translocation and recurrent sepsis [120].

From the standpoint of diagnosis, it is important to distinguish diversion colitis from inflammatory changes related to the underlying disease state requiring formation of the stoma. Endoscopic findings of diversion colitis include contact irritation or bleeding, erythema and mucosal nodularity. Histological characterization consists of diffuse follicular lymphoid hyperplasia; lamina propria expansion by plasma cells, lymphocytes, and some neutrophils; cryptitis; reactive epithelium and mucin depletion. Severe cases may contain crypt abscesses, aphthous ulcers, mild architectural distortion and Paneth cell metaplasia [121].

Restoration of intestinal continuity typically leads to spontaneous resolution of diversion colitis. Successful treatment with short-chain fatty acid enemas has been reported and warrants further evaluation [122].

7. ADOLESCENCE

Intra-abdominal infections that occur during adolescence represent a mixture of disease processes that persist from childhood (i.e. appendicitis) as well as pathological entities that are more common in the adult population (i.e. peritonitis due to complicated peptic ulcer disease). These "adult" entities will not be discussed in this section because there are no specific treatment modifications for adolescents with these illnesses. Two groups of infections which characteristically occur in this age group are (1) infections of the female genital tract (specifically, pelvic inflammatory disease) and (2) infectious complications of inflammatory bowel disease. Again, appendicitis is the most common intra-abdominal infection encountered in this patient population.

7.1. Infections related to inflammatory bowel disease

Intra-abdominal infectious complications are among the indications for operative intervention in children with inflammatory bowel disease. These complications typically present as emergencies and require prompt and aggressive medical and surgical therapy to avoid significant morbidity and mortality. Fulminant colitis, toxic megacolon and peritonitis secondary to viscus perforation occur as complications of both ulcerative colitis (UC) and Crohn's disease. Intra-abdominal abscess is a complication characteristically associated with Crohn's disease only and is treated according to the principles outlined earlier in this chapter.

Severe, or fulminant, colitis is characterized by more than six bloody stools per day, abdominal tenderness, fever, weight loss, anemia, leukocytosis and hypoalbuminemia. Fifteen per cent of children with UC can present with fulminant colitis [123]. In about one-third of all patients with fulminant colitis, the fulminant attack is their first manifestation of inflammatory bowel disease [124]. Children with fulminant colitis should be treated with: (1) adequate fluid, blood and electrolyte replacement; (2) complete bowel rest; (3) broad-spectrum antibiotic coverage (metronidazole, gentamicin and ampicillin); (4) intravenous corticosteroid therapy (1 to 2 mg/kg/day of methylprednisolone); (5) nutritional support with TPN and (6) serial abdominal radiographs for surveillance. Small-intestinal tubes for decompression in patients with colonic air columns and/or increased small intestinal gas have been recommended [124]. Positive therapeutic responses may be indicated by decreased stool frequency and, on laboratory evaluation, decreasing erythrocyte sedimentation rates and C-reactive protein levels [125].

Toxic megacolon occurs in approximately 3 to 5 per cent of patients with severe colitis [126]. Although life-threatening, the mortality rate in the pediatric population is significantly lower than that reported in adults. The child usually appears febrile and toxic with abdominal distension and tenderness. Plain abdominal films demonstrate pancolonic dilatation [127]. These findings signify an emergent condition because a subsequent acute colonic perforation is common [123]. Initial therapy for toxic megacolon is as outlined above for fulminant colitis. When prompt medical therapy is instituted, subsequent surgery is not inevitable. As mentioned, nasogastric or small-intestinal tubes may be helpful to prevent progressive bowel distension.

Acute fulminant colitis should respond to medical management within the first 12 days of therapy [123]. In those children who do not respond to therapy within this time frame, there is some controversy regarding subsequent treatment options. Historically, operative therapy would be indicated in light of medical therapy failure and, in many cases, this is still true. Another option in this setting, as long as the patient in not becoming worse clinically, is administration of cyclosporine (oral dose, 4 to 8 mg/kg/day) to induce remission. Using this regimen and maintaining whole blood trough levels between 150 and 300 ng/ml, an 80 per cent remission rate in children with fulminant colitis refractory to corticosteroids has been reported [128].

The indications for operative intervention in fulminant colitis (and toxic megacolon) include: (1) failure to respond to treatment or frank deterioration in clinical condition during the first few days of intensive medical therapy, (2) continued diarrhea, abdominal tenderness or a low-grade fever after intensive medical therapy and (3) colonic perforation, increasing colonic dilatation or massive colonic bleeding [125]. Emergent colectomies for fulminant colitis require prompt preoperative fluid resuscitation, correction of anemia, continued administration of broad-spectrum antibiotics and "stress-dose" steroid replacement. Total ab-

dominal colectomy with distal closure of the retained sigmoid colon as a Hartmann pouch and creation of an ileostomy represent the procedure of choice.

Intestinal perforation occurs in 4 to 20 per cent of patients with UC who present with fulminant disease or toxic megacolon. Perforation is relatively uncommon in association with Crohn's disease (2 per cent of patients), typically occurs in the terminal ileum and is not correlated with disease activity. Perforation in patients with UC and Crohn's usually leads to rapid development of peritonitis. In a small subgroup of patients with Crohn's disease, perforation may remain contained, producing focal findings only (inflammatory mass or focal tenderness). A high index of suspicion is necessary in evaluating patients on high-dose steroids because peritoneal findings may be masked. Intestinal perforation with peritonitis is an unequivocal indication for operative intervention. When associated with UC, total abdominal colectomy with ileostomy and Hartmann's pouch is the procedure of choice [123]. For free perforations associated with Crohn's disease, operative therapy entails segmental resection of the perforated intestine and stoma creation. Initial therapy for contained perforations with Crohn's disease may include broad-spectrum antibiotics, bowel rest and TPN.

7.2. Pelvic inflammatory disease

Pelvic inflammatory disease (PID) refers to infection of the uterus, fallopian tubes and adjacent pelvic structures that is not associated with surgery or pregnancy. PID is one of the more commonly encountered causes of acute abdominal pain in the adolescent female and is the most important consequence of sexually transmitted bacterial infections [129]. The majority of infections occur via the ascending route and are polymicrobial. *Chlamydia trachomatis* and *Neisseria gonorrhoeae* are the most important causative organisms. Risk factors include young age, multiple sexual partners and an intrauterine device [129].

In the majority of cases, the onset of symptoms occurs within one week of menstruation. The classic clinical presentation is pelvic peritonitis [130]. Severe lower abdominal/suprapubic pain, usually bilateral, is the most common presenting symptom. Associated symptoms may include vaginal discharge, abnormal uterine bleeding, dysuria, dyspareunia, nausea, vomiting, fever or other constitutional symptoms [129]. In approximately 15 per cent of patients, pelvic symptoms may be associated with or indeed overshadowed by, right upper abdominal complaints secondary to PID-associated perihepatitis (Fitz-Hugh-Curtis syndrome). Findings include pleuritic right upper quadrant pain that radiates to the shoulder, liver tenderness on palpation and potential elevation of liver enzymes [130].

On physical examination, there is usually marked lower abdominal tenderness with evidence of peritoneal irritation. Pelvic exam may be remarkable for purulent discharge from the cervical os, significant adnexal and uterine tenderness on bimanual examination and exquisite cervical motion tenderness. Laboratory evaluation often reveals leukocytosis and an elevated erythrocyte sedimentation rate (ESR). White blood cells should be present in cervical secretions [130].

The diagnosis of PID should be considered in any female patient of reproductive age who has pelvic pain. Direct visualization of inflamed fallopian tubes and other pelvic structures via the laparoscope is the "gold standard" for diagnosis but is seldom practical. Consequently, the diagnosis is usually made clinically. Greater than 90 per cent of patients with PID demonstrate (1) a history of lower abdominal pain and tenderness to palpation, (2) tenderness with cervical and uterine movement and (3) adnexal tenderness. These findings, when associated with one or more of the following, fever, leukocytosis, ESR greater than 15, positive endocervical Gram stain or monoclonal-directed smear for *Chlamydia*, pelvic phlegmon/abscess or peritoneal purulence by culdocentesis or laparoscopy, have been proposed as clinical criteria for establishing the diagnosis of PID [130].

Medical management of PID is usually sufficient and consists of intravenous ceftriaxone and intravenous or oral doxycycline. Operative intervention is reserved for cases where the diagnosis is unclear or drainage of a pelvic abscess is required. The Centers for Disease Control has established the following hospitalization criteria for PID: adolescent age group, uncertainty in diagnosis (rule out appendicitis), suspected pregnancy, concurrent HIV infection, severe illness with nausea and vomiting, inability to tolerate therapy or failure to respond to therapy as an outpatient and inability to follow-up in 72 hours [131]. Close follow-up of patients is an integral part of management. Absence of clinical improvement by 24 to 48 hours after intiating therapy mandates reassessment of the diagnosis. Ultrasonography or laparoscopy should be considered to rule out an abscess. Other important aspects of therapy include removal of intrauterine devices, if present, and evaluation of the male sexual partners [129].

Tubal damage and scarring due to PID produce long-term sequelae such as recurrent disease, ectopic pregnancy (6 times more likely after PID), infertility (in 8 per cent of cases after a single episode of PID) and chronic pelvic pain (18 per cent of cases) [129]. TUBOOVARIAN ABSCESS will complicate 15 to 30 per cent of cases of PID. A unilateral or bilateral mass may be noted on bimanual examination. The diagnosis is confirmed by pelvic ultrasonography. Treatment for unruptured tuboovarian abscesses with broad-spectrum antibiotics alone is successful in 75 per cent of cases. Patients who fail to respond to antibiotic therapy require CT-guided percutaneous drainage or surgical drainage via laparotomy/laparoscopy [132]. Unilateral salpingo-oophorectomy may be required if abscess drainage and antibiotic therapy are unsuccessful [133].

8. SPECIAL CONSIDERATIONS

8.1. Intra-abdominal infections in immunocompromised patients

Depression of the humoral and cell-mediated immune function in the pediatric oncology patient and transplant patient increases the incidence of infection in these children. Opportunistic pathogens that often are indigenous to the host or commonly found in the environment are a major source of morbidity and mortality in the immunocompromised host. Susceptibility to bacterial, viral or fungal infections is directly related to the granulocytopenia associated with the type and level of immunosuppression used for chemotherapeutic regimens or antirejection therapy after organ transplantation. The incidence of bacteremia appears to be highest when the absolute neutrophil count (ANC) is less than 1,000/mm^3 [134,135]. In children with an underlying malignancy, an en-

dogenous immunosuppressive effect of the neoplasm may increase susceptibility to infection further.

One of the most challenging aspects of intra-abdominal infections in immunocompromised patients is making the diagnosis. A high index of suspicion is essential. Physical signs are inconsistently present and often difficult to elicit in this patient population. Neutropenia blunts symptomatology and allows physical signs to remain diffuse and unfocused [136]. Corticosteroids have been well-documented in their ability to mask abdominal findings [137]. The effects of chemotherapy can further confuse the picture because of blunting of the inflammatory response to intraperitoneal pathology and the background abdominal complaints (i.e. constipation, abdominal pain, nausea adynamic and ileus) that are caused by several chemotherapeutic agents. The increasing use of bone marrow transplantation in children with advanced malignancies provides another confounding element in the assessment of abdominal symptoms [136].

(A) Children with cancer

In pediatric oncology patients, an array of site-specific intra-abdominal infections may develop, including appendicitis, typhlitis, biliary tract disease, pancreatitis, pseudomembranous colitis or intestinal perforation related to malignancy (i.e. leukemic infiltrates). Of these, typhlitis or neutropenic enterocolitis, is among the most common, reported in 10 to 46 per cent of children with cancer in autopsy series [138]. Seen almost solely in children with malignancy, typhlitis occurs most often in patients with leukemia but also is seen in patients receiving chemotherapy and those with aplastic anemia or lymphoma [139].

Typhlitis refers to an inflammatory process affecting predominantly the ileocecal region and ascending colon believed to arise from chemotherapy-induced neutropenia, intestinal stasis and ischemia with resultant secondary bacterial wall invasion [136]. The clinical presentation usually includes fever, abdominal pain (equally distributed between localized right-lower-quadrant and diffuse pain), tenderness and occasional diarrhea. Less commonly, occult or gross gastrointestinal bleeding or frank sepsis may be present. The major differential diagnosis of typhlitis is appendicitis. Distinguishing these two entities can be difficult, but the distinction is critical because appendicitis mandates immediate operative intervention, whereas the treatment of typhlitis entails aggressive medical management in most cases [136].

The diagnosis of typhlitis in immunocompromised children is clinical. Laboratory studies are not particularly helpful but a complete blood count with differential should be obtained to allow calculation of the ANC. Typhlitis is characteristically uncommon with an ANC greater than 1,500. Appropriate imaging studies remain the single most important diagnostic adjunct for the immunocompromised child [136]. Plain abdominal radiographs may demonstrate free air associated with intestinal perforation or pneumatosis indicative of significant bowel wall injury. Ultrasonagraphy can be used to confirm the diagnosis and can be performed at the bedside in critically ill patients but CT scanning with bowel contrast remains the diagnostic modality of choice, especially for differentiating typhlitis from appendicitis and other potential pathological entities. In typhlitis, the CT scan often demonstrates thickening of the cecal wall with or without pneumatosis.

In the absence of peritonitis, aggressive medical therapy for typhlitis, consisting of bowel rest with nasogastric decompression, intravenous fluid resuscitation, broad-spectrum intravenous antibiotics and serial abdominal examinations, is initiated. Clinical improvement in 1 to 3 days is generally observed in patients who will respond to medical management [136]. The decision to operate on patients with typhlitis should not be taken lightly as mortality rates associated with surgical procedures in this high-risk population approaches 10 per cent [140]. Conversely, non-operative management once sepsis from an intra-abdominal source has been established carries a mortality greater than 90 per cent [141]. Objective criteria proposed to direct operative intervention for typhlitis include: (1) persistent gastrointestinal bleeding after resolution of neutropenia, thrombocytopenia and correction of clotting abnormalities; (2) free intestinal perforation; (3) clinical deterioration requiring high fluid-volume resuscitation and the use of vasopressors and (4) symptoms of a surgical process that normally would require operation in the absence of neutropenia [142]. Additional indications may include failure to improve promptly (usually in 1 to 2 days) with adequate medical therapy, persistent peritoneal findings and radiographic evidence of pneumatosis intestinalis [143]. At operation, the finding of frank necrosis or an intestinal perforation should be treated with resection of the involved bowel and creation of appropriate stomas.

(B) Infections after solid organ transplantation

Infections are a significant cause of morbidity and mortality in the pediatric patient after solid-organ transplantation. In PEDIA-

TRIC RENAL TRANSPLANTATION, trends over the past decade, including improvements in immunosuppression (with decreased reliance on steroids), a reduction in rejection episodes and an expanded donor pool (adult-to-child living-related transplants) have significantly reduced the rate of infectious complications. Intra-abdominal infectious complications in these patients have been predominantly limited to urinary tract infections, *C. difficile* colitis, and rotavirus colitis, all of which have resolved with standard therapies [134].

The overall incidence of infectious complications after PEDIATRIC LIVER TRANSPLANTATION is approximately 80 per cent, due, in part, to the preoperative severity of disease in transplant recipients and to technical difficulties resulting from previous abdominal operations [144]. The most frequent sites of infection are the wound, lung, central lines, urinary tract and operative sites of the biliary tract. Intra-abdominal bacterial infections are not as frequent now as they were in the past. Several factors have contributed to this decrease: (1) intraoperative bacterial and fungal cultures are taken of both subhepatic spaces and patients are immediately treated for any positive bacterial or fungal results; (2) intra-abdominal hematomas are surgically evacuated to remove them as a potential culture medium and (3) fungal cultures of the Roux-en-Y lumen are taken and the patient immediately treated if they are positive [145].

The spectrum of intra-abdominal infections reported after pediatric liver transplantation includes infected collections and abscesses along the cut surface of reduced-size allografts, intrahepatic abscesses (mainly due to hepatic artery stenosis or thrombosis), bowel perforations, bile leaks with infected bilomas and sepsis [146]. Of these, infected collections along the cut surface of the liver are particularly troublesome in that they may contain bacterial or fungal organisms and have been reported to occur in up to 33 per cent of reduced-size liver transplant recipients [145].

The clinical presentation of intra-abdominal infections after liver transplantation, as previously stated, may be quite subtle, consisting of no more than low grade fever, leukocytosis, prolonged ileus, failure of return of bowel function or abnormal liver function tests. Laboratory findings such as persistent metabolic acidosis and positive cultures from the abdominal drains in the first few days after transplantation may be early indications of intra-abdominal sepsis. If intra-abdominal sepsis is suspected, early reoperation has been recommended as the best method for clearly establishing the diagnosis [146]. Most infected intra-abdominal collections and abscesses are identified by ultrasound or CT scan and diagnosed by percutaneous aspiration. Percutaneous drainage may be attempted. Surgical drainage (either extraperitoneal or transperitoneal) is recommended for all fungal abscesses and for failures of percutaneous drainage [145]. The treatment of intrahepatic abscesses is determined by the vascular status of the allograft and associated bile duct abnormalities [144].

(C) Infections associated with HIV infection and AIDS

Estimates of the number of infants and children infected with the human immunodeficiency virus (HIV) in 1993 approximated 15,000 to 25,000 nationwide [147]. The ratio of HIV-infected children to those with documented acquired immunodeficiency syndrome (AIDS) is approximately 4:1. Perinatal (vertical) transmission continues to account for the overwhelming majority (greater than 90 per cent) of HIV infections in infants and children, while transmission secondary to blood transfusion and coagulation factor administration continues to decline [148]. The most significant development in the management of this illness is that perinatal transmission of HIV infection can now be avoided in as many as two thirds of cases via maternal ingestion of zidovudine (azidothymine (AZT)) during the second and third trimesters of pregnancy followed by neonatal administration of this drug for 6 weeks after delivery [149].

Advances in medical management, by improving the general health of the pediatric HIV population and delaying the onset of HIV-related symptoms and signs, have lessened the need for surgical involvement in the diagnosis and treatment of HIV-related complications in infected patients [148]. This is particularly true for intra-abdominal infections in HIV-infected children. In sharp contrast to experience in adults with AIDS, in which surgical procedures may be necessary for gastrointestinal perforation, hemorrhage, tumors or inflammatory conditions [150], surgical intervention for acute abdominal castastrophe in HIV-infected children is seldom required [151,152].

In fact, the major surgical interventions for abdominal conditions in these children are related to placement of gastric or enteric tubes for feeding and establishment of central venous access for total parenteral nutrition. Intra-abdominal infections with *Mycobacterium avium intracellulare*, cytomegalovirus, and cryptosporidiosis do occur in these children and can cause abdominal pain, diarrhea and rectal bleeding. Virtually all of these have been managed by medical therapy and supportive care [136].

With regard to the presentation of intra-abdominal infections that normally occur in the healthy pediatric population, it is believed that HIV-infected children manifest typical abdominal symptoms and signs of these acute conditions. Routine surgical treatment may be undertaken regardless of HIV status and perioperative morbidity and mortality rates are similar to those of normal children. The only caveat is that all such procedures should be performed in conjunction with broad-spectrum antibiotic coverage [136].

8.2. Short bowel syndrome and bacterial overgrowth

Short bowel syndrome is defined as malabsorption, fluid and electrolyte loss and malnutrition after massive resection of the small intestine. Infections and short bowel syndrome (SBS) are closely related with regard to etiology (i.e. NEC), complications of therapy (i.e. surgical anastomotic leak, central line infection) and their respective impacts on long-range outcome (i.e. bacterial overgrowth and nutrient absorption). Since infectious enteropathies and intra-abdominal infections are discussed above, this section will focus on the short bowel syndrome and address the role of intraluminal bacteria, their influence on nutrient absorption and their potential role in translocation across the wall of the gastrointestinal tract into the blood stream, where they may produce sepsis, central catheter seeding or even contribute to parenteral nutrition (TPN)-induced liver dysfunction.

The nutritional, medical and surgical therapies for SBS have focused on enhancement of mucosal absorption function by increasing the absorptive surface area and decreasing intraluminal transit times, thereby increasing the interval of nutrient-mucosal exposure [153]. Both the remaining small bowel length and the presence of an ileo-cecal valve have been reaffirmed as critical factors in determining which patients with SBS can eventually be weaned from TPN [154]. Recently, endoscopic and culture documentation has been used to define the role which bacterial overgrowth plays in the development of an "enteritis" as well as in the weaning from TPN [154].

Bacterial overgrowth in SBS has a multifa-ceted etiology which includes concomitant intestinal stasis, an accumulation of intralu-minal nutrients and a potential deficiency of bile flow. SBS caused by gastroschisis, NEC, bowel ischemia and long-segment Hirschsprung's disease inherently has an al-tered gut motility with secondary intralumi-nal stasis. A bowel resection with anasto-mosis may itself alter intestinal motility and promote bacterial overgrowth [155]. Addi-tionally, a focal partial bowel obstruction and even the adaptive response, with its sa-lutary compensatory increase in luminal diameter, may contribute to stasis and an ineffective cleansing peristaltic activity [156]. Malabsorbed intraluminal nutrients are available to bacterial metabolism, thus potentiating bacterial colonization as well as the production of D-lactate and its se-condary metabolic acidosis [157]. The ac-cumulation of luminal substrate may further contribute to bacterial adhesion, internali-zation and transmucosal passage, a factor contributing to enteritis [158], the potential for septicemia [159] and even the associa-ted cholestatic liver disease. The enteritis associated with SBS may have a non-infec-tious component as well [160]. Non-colitic complications of bacterial overgrowth in-clude deconjugation and rapid absorption of bile salts. These result in intraluminal de-pletion of bile salts and further impairment

of micellar solubilization and absorption of fat and fat-soluble vitamins.

Clinically bacterial overgrowth presents with an increase in bloating, cramps, diarr-hea and bloody stool output. Infectious complications including central line infec-tion or frank septicemia may be the first cli-nical signs. Several tests may be useful in diagnosing bacterial overgrowth. These in-clude quantitative small bowel aspirate cul-tures (demonstrating greater than 10^5 orga-nisms per milliliter), measurement of D-lactate production, and breath hydrogen analysis. Since translocating bacteria may be the most important pathogens in bacte-rial overgrowth, the identification of micro-organisms in gut-associated lymph node tis-sue may have the greatest clinical significance.

The treatment of bacterial overgrowth can be directed at the bacteria themselves using cyclic antibiotic administration schedules with culture-specific antimicrobials or, at ti-mes, empiric anti-anaerobic antibiotics such as metronidazole. Trophic nutrients or growth factors to enhance enterocyte as well as intestinal barrier function may be advantageous [161]. Medical and surgical therapies can be directed at intestinal dys-motility, dilatation or obstruction and their secondary luminal nutrient stasis. Finally, the incidence of parenteral nutrition cathe-ter-associated sepsis may potentially be re-duced with the use of selective bowel de-contamination [162].

REFERENCES

1. Wittman DH, Schein M, Condon RE. Mana-gement of secondary peritonitis. Ann Surg 224:10-18, 1996.

2. Rotstein O: Peritonitis and intra-abdominal abscesses. In: Wilmore DW, Cheung LY, Harken AH, Holcroft JW, Meakins JL, eds. Care of the Surgical Patient. New York: Scientific American Inc., 1992, pp 1-24.

3. Baker CC. Peritonitis and intra-abdominal abscesses. In Cameron JL, ed. Current surgical therapy, ed. 5. St. Louis: Mosby-Year Book Inc., 1995, pp 943-947.

4. Stevenson RJ. Abdominal pain unrelated to trauma. Surg Clin North Am 65(5):1181-1215, 1985.

5. McDougal WS, Izant RJ Jr, Zollinger RM Jr. Primary peritonitis in infancy and childhood. Ann Surg 181:310, 1975.

6. Molleston JP, Ziambaras T, Perlmutter DH. Liver physiology and pathophysiology. In: Oldham KT, Colombani PM, Foglia RP, eds. Surgery of infants and children: scientific principles and practice. Philadelphia: Lippincott-Raven Publishers, 1997, pp 1365-1383.

7. Bhura M, Ganger D, Jensen D. Spontaneous bacterial peritonitis: an update on evaluation, management, and prevention. Am J Med 97:169-175, 1994.

8. Yang C-Y, Liaw Y-F, Chu C-M et al. White count, pH and lactate in ascites in the diagnosis of spontaneous bacterial peritonitis. Hepatology 5:85, 1985.

9. Felisart J, Rimola A, Arroyo V et al. Cefotaxime is more effective than is ampicillin-tobramycin in cirrhotics with severe infection. Hepatology 5:457-462, 1985.

10. Fong T, Akriviadis EA, Runyon BA et al. Polymorphonuclear cell count response and duration of antibiotic therapy in spontaneous bacterial peritonitis. Hepatology 9:423-426, 1989.

11. Runyon BA, McHutchinson JG, Antillon MR et al. Short-course versus long-course antibiotic treatment of spontaneous bacterial peritonitis. Gastroenterology 100:1737-42, 1991.

12. Gines P, Rimola A, Planas R et al. Norfloxacin prevents spontaneous bacterial peritonitis recurrence in cirrhosis: results of a double-blind, placebo-controlled trial. Hepatology 12:716-724, 1990.

13. Fonkalsrud EW. Peritoneal catheter: techniques, longevity, complications. In Fine RN, ed. Chronic ambulatory peritoneal dialysis (CAPD) and chronic cycling peritoneal dialysis (CCPD) in children, Boston: Martin Nijhoff, 1987.

14. Vas SI. Peritonitis during CAPD: a mixed bag. Perit Dial Bull 1:47, 1981.

15. Peritoneal access and laparoscopic procedures. In: Rowe MI, O'Neill JA, Grosfeld JL, Fonkalsrud EW, Coran AG, eds. Essentials of pediatric surgery. St. Louis: Mosby - Year Book Inc., 1995, pp 157-164.

16. Spence PA, Mathews RE, Khanna R et al. Indications for operation where peritonitis occurs in patients on chronic ambulatory peritoneal dialysis. Surg Gynecol Obstet 161:450, 1985.

17. Bryant MS, Bremer AM, Tepas JJ et al. Abdominal complications of ventriculoperitoneal shunts. Am Surg 54 (1):50-55, 1988.

18. Ersahin Y, Mutluer S, Tekeli G. Abdominal cerebrospinal fluid pseudocysts. Child's Nerv Syst 12:755-758, 1996.

19. Gaskill SJ, Marlin AE. Pseudocysts of the abdomen associated with ventriculoperitoneal shunts: a report of twelve cases and a review of the literature. Pediatr Neurosci 15:23-27, 1989.

20. Kim HB, Raghavendran K, Kleinhaus S. Management of an abdominal cerebrospinal fluid pseudocyst using laparoscopic techniques. Surg Laparoscopy Endosc 5(2):151-154, 1995.

21. Howard RJ. Abscess and peritonitis. In: Levine BA, Copeland EM III, Howard RJ, Sugerman HJ, Warshaw AL, eds. Current practice of surgery. New York: Churchill Livingstone Inc., 1995, pp 1-45.

22. Bohnen JMA, Solomkin JS, Dellinger EP et al. Guidelines for clinical care: anti-infective agents for intra-abdominal infection: a Surgical Infection Society policy statement. Arch Surg 127:83-89, 1992.

23. Ade-ajayi N, Kiely E, Drake D et al. Resection and primary anastomosis in necrotizing enterocolitis. J R Soc Med 89:385-388, 1996.

24. Hau T, Ahrenholz DH, Simmons RL. Secondary bacterial peritonitis: the biologic basis of treatment. Curr Prob Surg 16:1, 1979.

25. Magnuson DK, Rice CL. Intra-abdominal infection and sepsis following trauma. In: Fonkalsrud EW, Krummel TM, eds. Infections and immunologic disorders in pediatric surgery. Philadelphia: W. B. Saunders Company, 1993, pp 239-261.

26. Flake AW. Ontogeny of fetal immunity. In: Fonkalsrud EW, Krummel TM, eds. Infections and immunologic disorders in pediatric surgery. Philadelphia: W. B. Saunders Company, 1993, pp 239-261.

27. van Sonnenberg E, D'Agostino HB, Casola G et al. Percutaneous abscess drainage: current concepts. Radiology 181(3):617-626, 1991.

28. Brolin RE, Flancbaum L, Ercoli FR et al. Limitations of percutaneous catheter drainage of abdominal abscesses. Surg Gynecol Obstet 173:203-210, 1991.

29. Hepatocellular disorders. In: Rowe MI, O' Neill JA, Grosfeld JL, Fonkalsrud EW, Coran AG, eds. Essentials of pediatric surgery. St. Louis: Mosby - Year Book Inc., 1995, pp 619-624.

30. Lazarchick J, de Souza N, Nichols D et al. Pyogenic liver abscess. Mayo Clin Proc 48:349, 1973.

31. Tariq A, Rudolph N, Levin F. Solitary hepatic abscess in a newborn infant: a sequelae of umbilical vein catheterization and infusion of hypertonic glucose solution. Clin Pediatr 16:577, 1977.

32. Breuer CK, Vacanti JP. Surgical liver disease. In: Oldham KT, Colombani PM, Foglia RP, eds. Surgery of infants and children: scientific principles and practice. Philadelphia: Lippincott-Raven Publishers, 1997, pp 1385-1394.

33. Harrington E, Bleicher M. Cryptogenic hepatic abscess in two immunocomprised children. J Pediatr Surg 15:660, 1980.

34. Baum ES, Raffensperger JG. Liver tumors. In: Raffensperger JG, ed. Swenson's pediatric surgery, ed. 5. Norwalk: Appleton and Lange, 1990, pp 371-381.

35. Kays DW. Pediatric liver cysts and abscesses. Semin Pediatr Surg 2(1):107-114, 1992.

36. Keidl CM, Chusid MJ. Splenic abscesses in childhood. Pediatr Infect Dis J 8:368, 1989.

37. Mollitt DL, Dokler ML. Spleen. In: Oldham KT, Colombani PM, Foglia RP, eds. Surgery of infants and children: scientific principles and practice. Philadelphia: Lippincott-Raven Publishers, 1997, pp 1425-1436.

38. Dawson JG, August AM, Cole FS. The neonate: complications of premature infants. In: Oldham KT, Colombani PM, Foglia RP, eds. Surgery of infants and children: scientific principles and practice. Philadelphia: Lippincott-Raven Publishers, 1997, pp 65-72.

39. Martin JB. Peritonitis in the newborn - current concepts. Pediatr Clin North Am 32(5):1181-1201, 1985.

40. Holman RC, Stehr-Green JK, Zelasky MT. Necrotizing enterocolitis mortality in the United States. Am J Publ Health 79:987, 1989.

41. Kliegman RM, Fanaroff AA. Necrotizing enterocolitis. N Engl J Med 310:1093, 1984.

42. Kosloske AM. Necrotizing enterocolitis. In: Oldham KT, Colombani PM, Foglia RP, eds. Surgery of infants and children: scientific principles and practice. Philadelphia: Lippincott-Raven Publishers, 1997, pp 1201-1213.

43. Albanese CT, Rowe MI. Necrotizing enterocolitis. Semin Pediatr Surg 4(4):200-206, 1995.

44. Santulli TV, Schullinger JN, Heird WC et al. Acute necrotizing enterocolitis in infancy: a review of 64 cases. Pediatrics 55:376, 1975.

45. Ballance WA, Dahms BB, Shenker N et al. Pathology of neonatal necrotizing enterocolitis: a ten-year experience. J Pediatr 117:506-513, 1990.

46. Kosloske AM, Ulrich JA. A bacteriologic basis for the clinical presentation of necrotizing enterocolitis. J Pediatr Surg 15:558, 1980.

47. Kosloske AM, Musemeche CA, Ball WS Jr et al. Necrotizing enterocolitis: value of radiographic findings to predict outcome. AJR 151:771, 1988.

48. Kosloske AM, Lilly JR. Paracentesis and lavage for diagnosis of intestinal gangrene in neonatal necrotizing enterocolitis. J Pediatr Surg 13:315-320, 1978.

49. Kosloske AM. Indications for operation in necrotizing enterocolitis revisited. J Pediatr Surg 29(5):663-666, 1994.

50. Cheu HW, Sukarochana K, Lloyd DA. Peritoneal drainage for necrotizing enterocolitis. J Pediatr Surg 23(6):557-561, 1988.

51. Morgan LJ, Schochat SJ, Hartman GE. Peritoneal drainage as primary management of perforated NEC in the very low birth weight infant. J Pediatr Surg 29(2):310-315, 1994.

52. Azarow KS, Ein SH, Shandling B et al. Laparotomy or drain for perforated necrotizing enterocolitis: who gets what and why? Pediatr Surg Int 12:137-139, 1997.

53. Ein SH, Shandling B, Wesson D et al. A 13-year experience with peritoneal drainage under local anesthesia for necrotizing enterocolitis perforation. J Pediatr Surg 25:1034-1037, 1990.

54. Agrons GA, Corse WR, Markowitz RI et al. Gastrointestinal manifestations of cystic fibrosis: radiologic-pathologic correlation. Radiographics 16(4):871-893, 1996.

55. Warner BW. Malrotation. In: Oldham KT, Colombani PM, Foglia RP, eds. Surgery of infants and children: scientific principles and practice. Philadelphia: Lippincott-Raven Publishers, 1997, pp 1229-1240.

56. Hirschsprung's disease. In: Rowe MI, O' Neill JA, Grosfeld JL, Fonkalsrud EW, Coran AG, eds. Essentials of pediatric surgery. St. Louis: Mosby - Year Book Inc., 1995, pp 586-595.

57. Puri P. Hirschsprung disease. In: Oldham KT, Colombani PM, Foglia RP, eds. Surgery of infants and children: scientific principles and practice. Philadelphia: Lippincott-Raven Publishers, 1997, pp 1277-1299.

58. Nixon HH. Hirschsprung's disease in newborn. In: Hosschneider AM, ed. Hirschsprung's disease. Stuttgart: Hippokrates Verlag, 1982, p 103.

59. Surana R, Quinn FMJ, Puri P. Evaluation of risk factors in the development of enterocolitis complicating Hirschsprung's disease. Pediatr Surg Int 9:234, 1994.

60. Fujimoto T, Puri P. Persistence of enterocolitis following diversion of faecal stream in Hirschsprung's disease: a study of mucosal defense mechanisms. Pediatr Surg Int 3:141, 1988.

61. Oldham KT. The pediatric abdomen: gastrointestinal disorders. In: Greenfield LJ, Mulholland MW, Oldham KT, Zelenock GB, eds. Surgery: scientific principles and practice. Philadelphia: J. B. Lippincott Company, 1993, pp 1838-1882.

62. Tibboel D, Molenaar JC. Meconium peritonitis: a retrospective, prognostic analysis of 69 patients. Z Kinderchir 39:25-28, 1984.

63. Lorimer WS, Ellis DH. Meconium peritonitis. Surgery 60:470, 1966.

64. Holgerson LO. The etiology of spontaneous gastric perforation of the newborn: a re-evaluation. J Pediatr Surg 16:608, 1981.

65. Rosser SB, Clark CH, Elechi EN. Spontaneous neonatal gastric perforation. J Pediatr Surg 17:390, 1982.

66. Other conditions of the upper gastrointestinal tract. In: Rowe MI, O' Neill JA, Grosfeld JL, Fonkalsrud EW, Coran AG, eds. Essentials of pediatric surgery. St. Louis: Mosby - Year Book Inc., 1995, pp 501-507.

67. Scholz TD, McGuinness GA. Localized intestinal perforation following intravenous indomethacin for patent ductus arteriosus. J Pediatr Gastroenterol Nutr 7(5):773-775, 1988.

68. Kuhl G, Wille L, Bolkenius M et al. Intestinal perforation associated with indomethacin treatment in premature infants. Eur J Pediatr 143(3):213-216, 1985.

69. McDonnell M, Evans N. Upper and lower gastrointestinal complications with dexamethasone despite H2 antagonists. J Paediatr Child Health 31(2):152-154, 1995.

70. Mintz AC, Applebaum H. Focal gastrointestinal perforations not associated with necrotizing enterocolitis in very low birth weight neonates. J Pediatr Surg 28(6):857-860, 1993.

71. Grosfeld JL, Molinari F, Chaet M et al. Gastrointestinal perforation and peritonitis in infants and children: experience with 179 cases over ten years. Surgery 120(4):650-655, 1996.

72. Hsiao PH, Chou YH, Tsou YK et al. Gastrointestinal perforation in infants: cases unrelated to necrotizing enterocolitis. Acta Paediatr Sin 34(6):429-435, 1993.

73. Stringer MD, Drake DP. Hirschsprung's disease presenting as neonatal gastrointestinal perforation. Br J Surg 78(2):188-189, 1991.

74. Cushing A. Omphalitis: a review. Pediatr Infect Dis 4:282, 1985.

75. Kosloske AM. Sepsis and infection in the neonate. In: Fonkalsrud EW, Krummel TM, eds. Infections and immunologic disorders in pediatric surgery. Philadelphia: W. B. Saunders Company, 1993, pp 131-144.

76. Sawin RS, Schaller RT, Tapper D et al. Early recognition of neonatal abdominal wall necrotizing fasciitis. Am J Surg 167:481-484, 1994.

77. Ohi R, Ibrahim M. Biliary atresia. Semin Pediatr Surg 1(2):115-124, 1992.

78. Kobayashi A, Utsunomiya T, Ohbe T et al. Ascending cholangitis following hepatic portoenterostomy for biliary atresia. J Pediatr 99:656, 1981.

79. Flake AW. Disorders of the gallbladder and biliary tract. In: Oldham KT, Colombani PM, Foglia RP, eds. Surgery of infants and children: scientific principles and practice. Philadelphia: Lippincott-Raven Publishers, 1997, pp 1405-1414.

80. Offit PA. Viral gastroenteritis. In: Rudolph AM, Hoffman JIE, Rudolph CD, eds. Rudolph's pediatrics, ed. 20. Stamford: Appleton and Lange, 1996, pp 642-644.

81. Katz AL. Colon. In: Oldham KT, Colombani PM, Foglia RP, eds. Surgery of infants and children: scientific principles and practice. Philadelphia: Lippincott-Raven Publishers, 1997, p 1319.

82. Pickering LK. Salmonella, Shigella, and enteric E. coli infections. In: Rudolph AM, Hoffman JIE, Rudolph CD, eds. Rudolph's pediatrics, ed. 20. Stamford: Appleton and Lange, 1996, pp 592-601.

83. Sawin RS. Appendix and Meckel diverticulum. In: Oldham KT, Colombani PM, Foglia RP, eds. Surgery of infants and children: scientific principles and practice. Philadelphia: Lippincott-Raven Publishers, 1997, pp 1215-1228.

84. Neilson IR, Laberge JM, Nguyen LT et al. Appendicitis in children: current therapeutic recommendations. J Pediatr Surg 25:1113, 1990.

85. Hoffman J, Rasmussen OO. Aids in the diagnosis of acute appendicitis. Br J Surg 76:774, 1989.

86. Samuelson S, Reyes HM. Management of perforated appendicitis in children revisited. Arch Surg 122:691, 1987.

87. Lund DP, Murphy EP. Management of perforated appendicitis in children: a decade of aggressive treatment. J Pediatr Surg 29:1130, 1994.

88. Lau WY, Fan ST, Yiu TF et al. Negative findings at appendectomy. Am J Surg 148:375, 1984.

89. Meckel's diverticulum. In: Rowe MI, O' Neill JA, Grosfeld JL, Fonkalsrud EW, Coran AG, eds. Essentials of pediatric surgery. St. Louis: Mosby - Year Book Inc., 1995, pp 515-519.

90. St-Vil D, Brandt ML, Panic S et al. Meckel's diverticulum in children: a 20 year review. J Pediatr Surg 26:1289, 1991.

91. Rescorla FJ, Grosfeld JL. Cholecystitis and cholelithiasis in children. Semin Pediatr Surg 1(2):98-106, 1992.

92. Man DWK, Spitz L. Choledocholithiasis in infancy. J Pediatr Surg 20:65-68, 1985.

93. Reif S, Sloven DG, Lebenthal E. Gallstones in children. Am J Dis Child 145:105-298, 1991.

94. Stephens CG, Scott RB. Cholelithiasis in sickle cell anemia. Arch Intern Med 140:648-651, 1980.

95. Holcomb GW Jr, O' Neill JA Jr, Holcomb GW III et al. Cholecystitis, cholelithiasis, and common duct stenosis in children and adolescents. Ann Surg 191:626-635, 1980.

96. Sigman HH, Laberge JM, Croitoru D et al. Laparoscopic cholecystectomy: a treatment option for gallbladder disease in children. J Pediatr Surg 26:1181-1183, 1991.

97. Newman KD, Marmon LM, Attorri R et al. Laparoscopic cholecystectomy in pediatric patients. J Pediatr Surg 26:1184-1185, 1991.

98. Holcomb GW, Olsen DO, Sharp KW. Laparoscopic cholecystectomy in the pediatric patient. J Pediatr Surg 26:1186-1190, 1991.

99. Sackier JM, Berei G, Phillips E et al. The role of cholangiography in laparoscopic cholecystectomy. Arch Surg 126:1021-1026, 1991.

100. Gregg RO. The case for selective cholangiography. Am J Surg 155:540-545, 1988.

101. Pariente D, Bernard O, Gauthier F et al. Radiological treatment of common bile duct lithiasis in infancy. Pediatr Radiol 19:104-107, 1989.

102. Jonas A, Yahar J, Fradkin A et al. Choledocholithiasis in infants: diagnostic and therapeutic problems. J Pediatr Gastroenterol Nutr 11:513-517, 1990.

103. Beretsky I, Lankin DH. Diagnosis of fetal cholelithiasis using real-time high-resolution imaging employing digital detection. J Ultrasound Med 2:381-383, 1983.

104. Gallbladder diseae. In: Rowe MI, O' Neill JA, Grosfeld JL, Fonkalsrud EW, Coran AG, eds. Essentials of pediatric surgery. St. Louis: Mosby - Year Book Inc., 1995, pp 656-662.

105. Stephens CG, Scott RB. Cholelithiasis in sickle cell anemia. Arch Intern Med 140:648-651, 1980.

106. Alexander-Reindorf C, Nwaneri RU, Worrell RG. The significance of gallstones in children with sickle cell anemia. J Natl Med Assoc 82:645-650, 1990.

107. Chandrcharoensis-Wilde C, Chairoongruang S, Jitnuson P el at. Gallstones in thalassemia. Birth Defects 23:263-267, 1988.

108. Tsakayannis DE, Kozakewich HP, Lillehei CW. Acalculous cholecystitis in children. J Pediatr Surg 31(1):127-130, 1996.

109. Babb RR. Acute acalculous cholecystitis: a review. J Clin Gastroenterol 15(3):238-241, 1992.

110. Weizman Z, Durie PR. Acute pancreatitis in childhood. J Pediatr 113:24, 1988.

111. Coran AG. The pediatric pancreas. In: Greenfield LJ, Mulholland MW, Oldham KT, Zelenock GB, eds. Surgery: scientific principles and practice. Philadelphia: J. B. Lippincott Company, 1993, pp 1898-1899.

112. Marshall JB. Acute pancreatitis. Arch Intern Med 153:1185, 1993.

113. Disorders of the pancreas. In: Rowe MI, O' Neill JA, Grosfeld JL, Fonkalsrud EW, Coran AG, eds. Essentials of pediatric surgery. St. Louis: Mosby - Year Book Inc., 1995, pp 663-667.

114. Lillehei C. Pancreas. In: Oldham KT, Colombani PM, Foglia RP, eds. Surgery of infants and children: scientific principles and practice. Philadelphia: Lippincott-Raven Publishers, 1997, pp 1417-1419.

115. Devenyi AG. Antibiotic-induced colitis. Semin Pediatr Surg 4(4):215-220, 1995.

116. Larson HE, Barclay FE, Honour P et al. Epidemiology of Clostridium difficile in infants. J Infect Dis 146:727-733, 1982.

117. Greenfield C, Ramirez JRA, Pounder RE et al. Clostridium difficile and inflammatory bowel disease. Gut 24:713-717, 1983.

118. Trnka YU, Lamont JT. Association of Clostridium difficile toxin with symptomatic relapse of chronic inflammatory bowel disease. Gastroenterology 80:693-696, 1981.

119. Bradley SJ, Weaver DW, Maxwell NP et al. Surgical management of pseudomembranous colitis. Am Surg 54:329-332, 1988.

120. Ordein JJ, DiLorezzo C, Flores A et al. Diversion colitis in children with severe gastrointestinal motility disorder. Am J Gastroenterol 87:88, 1992.

121. Hague S, Eisen RN, West AB. The morphologic features of diversion colitis: studies of a pediatric population with no other disease of the intestinal mucosa. Hum Pathol 24(2):211-219, 1993.

122. Hague S, West AB. Diversion colitis - 20 years a-growing. J Clin Gastroenterol 15(4):281-283, 1992.

123. Dudgeon DL. Ulcerative colitis. In: Oldham KT, Colombani PM, Foglia RP, eds. Surgery of infants and children: scientific principles and practice. Philadelphia: Lippincott-Raven Publishers, 1997, pp 1301-1311.

124. Present DH. Fulminant colitis. Semin Gastrointest Dis 2(2):107-114, 1991.

125. Travis SPL, Farrant JM, Ricketts C. Predicting outcome in severe ulcerative colitis. Gut 38(6):905-910, 1996.

126. Ament ME, Vargas JH. Medical therapy for ulcerative colitis in childhood. Semin Pediatr Surg 3(1):28-32, 1994.

127. Hofley PM, Piccoli DA. Inflammatory bowel disease in childhood. Med Clin North Am 78(6):1281-1302, 1994.

128. Treem WR, Cohen J, Davis PM et al. Cyclosporine for the treatment of fulminant ulcerative colitis in children. Immediate response, long-term results, and impact on surgery. Dis Colon Rectum 38(5):474-479, 1995.

129. McCormack WM. Pelvic inflammatory disease. N Engl J Med 330(2):115-119, 1994.

130. Mollitt DL, Dokler ML. The teenage girl. Semin Pediatr Surg 6(2):100-104, 1997.

131. Adkins ES. Female genital tract. In: Oldham KT, Colombani PM, Foglia RP, eds. Surgery of infants and children: scientific principles and practice. Philadelphia: Lippincott-Raven Publishers, 1997, pp 1559-1575.

132. Hurt WG, Soper DE. Female genital tract. In: Greenfield LJ, Mulholland MW, Oldham KT, Zelenock GB, eds. Surgery: scientific principles and practice. Philadelphia: J. B. Lippincott Company, 1993, pp 2005-2018.

133. Wiesenfeld HC, Sweet RL. Progress in the management of tuboovarian abscesses. Clin Obstet Gynecol 36(2):433-444, 1993.

134. Gilbert JC, Vacanti JP. Infection and immunosuppression in children with cancer or organ transplants. In: Fonkalsrud EW, Krummel TM, eds. Infections and immunologic disorders in pediatric surgery. Philadelphia: W. B. Saunders Company, 1993, pp 219-238.

135. Albano EA, Pizzo PA. Infectious complications in childhood acute leukemias. Pediatr Clin North Am 35:873-901, 1988.

136. Bensard DD, Haase GM. Special consideration for the neurologically and immunologically impaired child. Semin Pediatr Surg 6(2):92-99, 1997.

137. Remine S, McIlrath D. Bowel perforation in steroid-treated patients. Ann Surg 192:581-586, 1980.

138. Kunkel JM, Rosenthal D. Management of the ileocecal syndrome, neutropenic enterocolitis. Dis Colon Rectum 29:196-199, 1986.

139. Foglia RP. Surgical considerations in the immunocompromised patient. In: Fonkalsrud EW, Krummel TM, eds. Infections and immunologic disorders in pediatric surgery. Philadelphia: W. B. Saunders Company, 1993, pp 119-129.

140. Rice M, Cordy-Udy C, Little K et al. Surgical complications in acute leukemia in childhood: a 20-year experience. Med Pediatr Oncol 20:32-37, 1992.

141. Skibber J, Matter G, Pizzo P et al. Right lower quadrant pain in young patients with leukemia. Surgical perspective. Ann Surg 711-716, 1987.

142. Shamberger R, Weinstein H, Delorey M et al. The medical and surgical management of typhlitis in children with acute nonlymphocytic (myelogenous) leukemia. Cancer 57:603-609, 1986.

143. Silliman CC, Haase GM, Strain JD et al. Indications for surgical intervention for gastrointestinal emergencies in children receiving chemotherapy. Cancer 74:203-216, 1994.

144. Ryckman FC, Fisher RA, Pedersen SH et al. Liver transplantation in children. Semin Pediatr Surg 1(2):162-172, 1992.

145. Andrews W. Liver. In: Oldham KT, Colombani PM, Foglia RP, eds. Surgery of infants and children: scientific principles and practice. Philadelphia: Lippincott-Raven Publishers, 1997, pp 721-738.

146. Bilik R, Yellen M, Superina RA. Surgical complications in children after liver transplantation. J Pediatr Surg 27(11):1371-1375, 1992.

147. Centers for Disease Control and Prevention. HIV/AIDS surveillance report. Atlanta: Centers for Disease Control and Prevention, February 1993, pp 1-23.

148. Cooper A. Human immunodeficiency virus and acquired immunodeficiency syndrome: recent developments and their implications for pediatric surgeons. Semin Pediatr Surg 4(4):252-261, 1995.

149. Connor EM, Sperling RS, Gelber R et al. Reduction of maternal-infant transmission of human immunodeficiency virus type 1 with zidovudine treatment. N Engl J Med 331:1173-1180, 1994.

150. LaRaja R, Rothenberg R, Odom J et al. The incidence of intra-abdominal surgery in acquired immunodeficiency syndrome: a statistical review of 904 patients. Surgery 105:175-179, 1989.

151. Beaver B, Hill J, Vachon D et al. Surgical intervention in children with human immunodeficiency virus infection. J Pediatr Surg 25:79-84, 1990.

152. Dolgin SE, Larsen JG, et al. CMV enteritis causing hemorrhage and obstruction in an infant with AIDS. J Pediatr Surg 25:696-698, 1990.

153. Ziegler MM. Short bowel syndrome: remedial features that influence outcome and the duration of parenteral nutrition. J Pediatr 1997, in press.

154. Kaufman SS, Loseke CA, Lupo et al. Influence of bacterial overgrowth and intestinal inflammation on duration of parenteral nutrition in children with short bowel syndrome. J Pediatr 1997, in press.

155. Hocking MP, Carlson RG, Courington, KR et al. Altered motility and bacterial flora after functional end-to-end anastomosis. Surgery 108:384-392, 1990.

156. Debas HT, Mulvihill SJ. Neuroendocrine design of the gut. Am J Surg 161:243-249, 1991.

157. Perlmutter DH, Boyle JT, Campos JM et al.

D-lactic acidosis in children: an unusual metabolic complication of small bowel resection. J Pediatr 102:234-238, 1983.

158. Go LL, Ford HR, Watkins SC et al. Quantitative and morphologic analysis of bacterial translocation in neonates. Arch Surg 129:1184-1190, 1994.

159. Pierro A, van Saene HKF, Donnell SC et al. Microbial translocation in neonates and infants receiving long-term parenteral nutrition. Arch Surg 131:176-179, 1996.

160. Taylor SF, Sondheimer JM, Sokol RJ et al. Non-infectious colitis associated with short gut syndrome in infants. J Pediatr 119:24-28, 1991.

161. Byrne TA, Persinger RL, Young LS et al. A new treatment for patients with short bowel syndrome, growth hormone, glutamine, and a modified diet. Ann Surg 222:243-255, 1995.

162. Kurkubasche AG, Smith SD, Rowe MI. Catheter sepsis in short bowel syndrome. Arch Surg 127:21-25, 1992.

Pelvic Inflammatory Disease

William J. Ledger, MD

1. INTRODUCTION

This attempt to write a chapter on pelvic inflammatory disease faces two obstacles. The first is definition. Currently, the term pelvic inflammatory disease (PID) is applied to a diverse group of patients with very different types of clinical pathophysiology. The next problem is structure. Attempts to categorize clinical pathophysiology in a textbook may not mimic nature.

Pelvic inflammatory disease (PID) encompasses all infection disorders of the upper genital tract (i.e. the uterus, fallopian tubes and ovaries) of non-pregnant women. Most of these infections are the result of sexual activity but a few cases follow operative manipulations of the genital tract. The overriding problem in physician understanding reflects the varied presentations of disease. The clinical range is very great. Infected women may not feel sick enough to seek medical attention. In one study by Cates et al. 238 of 283 white women with tubal infertility (84%) did not have a history of pelvic inflammatory disease [1]. The authors called this group "atypical pelvic inflammatory disease" but I prefer the term silent pelvic inflammatory disease, because these women represent the majority of the patients I see with (PID). I am not comfortable

applying a term that means not typical, not characteristic or abnormal to the largest single subgroup of patients with this disease. There is controversy about the designation of silent with reference to PID. In a recent study of infertile women found to have adhesions or distal tubal occlusion at laparoscopy, only 11 of 36 (30.6%) had a history of PID [2]. Utilizing a preoperative questionnaire, 29 of 36 (80.6%) had a history of lower abdominal pain [2]. In the author's eyes, this puts in doubt the terminology silent PID. I am not convinced. These women neither sought medical attention nor were they aware they had PID. In contrast to this large group of women with absent or negligible symptomatology, there are many seriously ill women in whom there is no doubt in the physician's mind about the diagnosis. One group encompasses a category of patients with what I call Emergency Room PID. These urban poor young women present on an emergent basis with fever, obvious purulent material exuding from the cervix and serious pain with any movement of the uterus or palpation of the tubes at the time of pelvic examination. Soper has documented the clinical and laboratory findings of this population with a prospective laparoscopic study [3]. The most striking correlation in his evaluation was the frequency with which *Neisseria gonorrhea* was recovered. It was isolated in 25 of 36 patients (69.4%). In addition to this population of seriously ill women, there is another group of women with an obvious pelvic infection. These are the critically ill women who present with an acute abdomen, the result of the intra-abdominal rupture of a tubo-ovarian abscess [4]. This is a wide variety of presentations. Clearly, there is no single category of clinical symptomatology that defines the designation, PID. The term covers a range of patients from asymptomatic women to those who are close to death.

The other problem in my presentation of this subject resides with the very nature of medical textbook writing. As a result of a background in biology that over-emphasizes classification, physician writers generally take a huge bank of clinical, laboratory and therapeutic data and categorize these findings into specific designations. Diseases become graded as mild, moderate or severe; bacterial isolates represent colonization or pathogens; therapeutic responses are called a cure, improvement or failure. In many ways, medical texts resemble the neat rows of saplings seen in a nursery [5]. To me, each row could represent a chapter in this text devoted to infection or a chapter heading in any medical text. In my mind's eye, row three could be pelvic inflammatory disease with each individual tree representing such categories for discussion as signs and symptoms, physical findings, laboratory findings, theories of pathophysiology, preventive measures and treatment options. This is a form of writing with which doctors are comfortable. Habit has made this type of presentation logical and understandable. Unfortunately, our comfort level with this standard medical writing form may not equate with reality. For individual practitioners, with a responsibility to care for this wide variety of pa-

tients, this textbook picture of ordered clarity, often bears no relationship to the clinical muddle of the individual patient seen in the office or the hospital with PID. In many patients, the presenting signs and symptoms can be absent or confusing. The physical examination finding of pain may not conform to any scale. Microbiology laboratory results may be confusing or absent. Sometimes this is the result of the absence of reliable scientific data in the literature. More often, the commercial microbiology laboratory or the hospital microbiology laboratory is not equipped to provide the depth of information that has been achieved in research microbiology laboratories that publish studies on pelvic infection. This certainly has been my experience. The isolation of anaerobes from clinical specimens became commonplace when I established an anaerobic laboratory at the Los Angeles County-University of Southern California Medical Center. The prior use of the term, a "sterile abscess", applied to a tubo-ovarian abscess was not an event that occurred by chance. It represented the best clinical logic at that time, which unfortunately was based upon laboratory reports associated with inadequate or unavailable anaerobic isolation techniques[6]. Two examples specifically illustrate microbiology laboratory shortcomings. A 1962 study of tubo-ovarian abscesses, had no anaerobic bacterial isolates and there was no bacterial growth reported in 52 of 67 cases (77.6%) [7]. Another study of tubo-ovarian abscesses published in 1969, also had no anaerobic isolates and reported no growth in 53 of 121 cases (43.8%) [8]. In the 1960's, clinical logic, based upon this type of faulty laboratory investigation, confused the true microbiological nature of pelvic abscesses. Incomplete or inaccurate information always has this outcome as a possibility. In preparing this chapter, I acknowledge the difficulty of accurately labeling the various aspects of this diverse clinical problem. Categorization is the basis for the ordered presentation of materials in this chapter on PID but it relies upon my own personal decisions and judgments based upon current data that may not withstand the harsh light of future science. What follows is my best bet on the nature of PID in the world today.

2. HISTORICAL REVIEW

A dominant theme for anyone reviewing the topic of pelvic inflammatory disease is the changing nature of the disease. The clinical presentations change, the therapeutic outcomes differ and the prognosis varies from decade to decade. To me, there is a constant underlying current of change. In any one time frame, the most serious problems of infection are recognized. These stimulate laboratory and clinical research studies, done to determine the nature of the problems. New diagnostic and treatment strategies are devised. To the credit of the medical investigators in the past, these new interventions usually work. Unfortunately, over and over again, a new previously unrecognized clinical problem emerges. The process of laboratory and clinical investigation begins again with a focus on a new problem. Let me cite a few examples.

With the introduction of antibiotics into clinical practice in the mid-1940's, physicians first focused their attention on seriously ill women who had pelvic inflammatory disease. These represented the most vexing serious problems in gynecology. Two categories of patients received most of the medical attention in the interval 1945-1965. Efforts at understanding led to improvements in care.

There was a group of acutely ill women who presented regularly to the emergency rooms of urban hospitals in this post-World War II era. The issue that commanded physician attention was the severity of this, the patient's first pelvic illness. These sexually active young women were febrile and they had obvious lower abdominal pain at the time of the general physician examination. The pelvic examination findings were striking. Purulent material was issuing from the cervix and these women had acute pain when the pelvic organs were manipulated. The clinical diagnosis of PID was never in doubt. To care for these women, the investigators focused on two unknowns. First, what was the organism involved? Careful microbiologic evaluations demonstrated in the over-riding majority of cases that the pathogen was *Neisseria gonorrhea*. This changed clinical practice. The heightened awareness of the significance of this pathogen was followed by modifications in physician behavior so that this organism could be isolated in the clinical microbiology laboratory. The sterile swab in a sterile tube would no longer suffice as a specimen collection technique. These fragile organisms in the laboratory with the then routine collections system required new strategies. New transport tubes with liquid media present to maintain the viability of the gonococci were introduced. These changes in technique markedly increased the yield of positive cultures for *Neisseria gonorrhea* on gynecology services. A clinical need had been recognized and met. The next focus was therapy. Fortunately, early on, *Neisseria gonorrhea* was very susceptible to the antibiotics available, such as penicillin and tetracycline. For clinicians in these early years of antibiotic prescriptions, antibiotics represented a magic bullet and there was little concern about resistance. The immediate outcome was obvious. A serious clinical problem had been recognized and a diagnostic and treatment regimen had been established that markedly shortened the clinical course of the disease. Even today, acute PID is still with us [3] but the prognosis for these women is excellent. Nearly all of them respond to medical therapy and over 80% of these woman remain fertile after treatment has been completed [9].

In these early years of antibiotic experience, another group of patients commanded physician attention. These were critically ill women with recurrent pelvic infections who had developed a pelvic abscess. This was a frustrating infectious disease entity. There was physician confusion about the pathophysiology of these abscesses and this limited therapeutic strategies. The absence of good anaerobic isolation techniques in the laboratory led most gynecologists to postulate the concept of a "sterile" abscess [7]. These mistaken microbiologic assumptions, plus the clinical observations that the then prescribed antibiotics did not achieve a cure, led to the option of more aggressive operative interventions. Physician frustration with the then available medical treatment is apparent in the paper by Anderson and Bucklew [7]. They noted seven patients who ruptured a tubo-ovarian abscess while under medical treatment and close observation in the hospital. Despite what seemed then to be appropriate antibiotic therapy, these women with a serious medical problem, the unruptured pelvic abscess, had their disease progress to a life threatening medical condition, the intraperitoneal rupture of pelvic abscess. When this rupture occurred, a medical emergency existed. If operative intervention was delayed because the diagnosis was missed these women could have died [4,10]. The therapeutic emphasis was on the immediate diagnosis of a ruptured tube-ovarian abscess followed by operative removal of all pelvic organs combined with vigorous lavage of the peritoneal cavity. Academic gynecology had a macho pride in the operative skills needed to do this difficult pelvic organ extirpation and in conferences the gynecological surgical advocates would intone that an abscess can only be cured by the scalpel, not by antibiotics. The short-term outcomes of this aggressive operative approach were beneficial. Lives were saved. The patients were cured of their infections and they survived. Yet, this clinical care strategy was disquieting. Physicians mused, "There ought to be a better way". Long-term concerns remained. This operative strategy castrated these young women and eliminated any future hope of a pregnancy. Defenders of the operative status noted that with the tubal damage from the infection, in these women, future concerns about a pregnancy seemed a misplaced priority.

Frustration with this therapeutic status quo led to important studies in the mid sixties and the 1970's. It was apparent to observant clinicians then, that there were large gaps between published clinical observation and their personal evaluation of patients. Some of the dogma in that era had such incantations as the "sterile abscess" or the observation of a typical E. coli odor when an abscess was drained. For the questioning physician, the problem with the former was that these patients had clinical evidence of sepsis and a gram stain of the purulent material from these abscesses showed myriads of bacteria. These were not "sterile" abscesses. The problem with the latter was the awareness that *Escherichia coli* had no odor in the laboratory. The then inadequate microbiology techniques isolated only the aerobes in these mixed infections. The breakthrough occurred when improved laboratory technology resulted in an increased ability to isolate anaerobes from the purulent material in these abscesses. This technology became part of the hospital microbiology procedures and the view of pelvic infections broadened. Also two new observations were made. These abscesses were not sterile. Instead anaerobes were the dominant organisms recovered. In addition it became obvious that the commonly isolated Gram negative anaerobes, particularly *Bacteroides fragilis* were not susceptible to the antibiotics that were the standard treatment for women with serious pelvic infections. The statement that only a scalpel can cure an abscess is probably true in an environment when the antibiotics given are not effective against the pathogen. Into this therapeutic void, new antibiotics were introduced specifically because of their activity against these Gram negative anaerobes. In the mid-1960's and early '70's, these included clindamycin [11], cefoxitin [12] and metronidazole [13]. Their early use in patients with serious pelvic infections dramatically changed the universe of pelvic infections seen by gynecologists. Fewer pelvic abscesses were seen and the ruptured tubo-ovarian abscess became a rarity. This expanded knowledge about anaerobes dramatically improved medical antibiotic options and decreased the numbers of patients with a pelvic abscess, who required operative intervention.

This 1965-1980 era was also important for a shift in physician focus. It marked the first published awareness of a subtle presentation of pelvic inflammatory disease. Prior to this time, the overriding physician focus was patients with obvious pelvic inflammatory disease. The criteria for a diagnosis of pelvic infection was a standard that emphasized obvious signs. (See Table 1) [14] Patients with a pelvic infection were presumed to have pain, fever, adnexal swelling

Table 1
1960's Criteria for the Diagnosis of Pelvic Inflammatory Disease

1. Acute Pelvic Pain.

2. Oral temperature above 38°C.

3. Bilateral tender adnexal swelling or masses.

4. Elevated white blood cell count and/or elevated erythrocyte sedimentation rate.

or masses and a high white blood cell count or an elevated sedimentation rate. Physicians touting this rigid set of criteria justified it as a way to avoid the indiscriminate use of antibiotics for a patient with pelvic pain. As strategies for the successful medical treatment of acute symptomatic pelvic inflammatory disease worked, it became obvious to astute clinician observers that more subtle presentations of this disease existed. An early published study to demonstrate the inaccuracies of the traditional diagnostic criteria was reported by Westrom et al. in 1969 [15]. Gynecologists were shocked with the results of this study. If true, it meant that they were guilty of clinical diagnostic errors in a substantial number of patients. In this Swedish study, all women with a clinical diagnosis of pelvic inflammatory disease were subjected to immediate laparoscopy before antibiotics were begun. The clinical diagnosis of infection was much less accurate than assumed, only 65% of those thought to have pelvic inflammatory disease actually had this confirmed by laparoscopy. In addition, the study demonstrated that the clinical criteria for making a diagnosis of pelvic inflammatory disease were much less sensitive than had been assumed. (See Table 2) [15] Pelvic pain did not distinguish those with laparos-

Table 2
Clinical and Laboratory findings in laparoscopy proven
Pelvic Inflammatory Disease

Clinical Sign	Laparoscopy Results	
	PID patients (%)	Normal patients (%)
1. Acute Pelvic Pain.	94%	94%
2. Oral temperature above 38°C.	41.4%	19.6%
3. Tender adnexal swelling or mass.	49.4%	24.5%
4. Elevated sedimentation rate.	75.9%	52.7%

copic evidence of PID from those free of infection. In this study, just over 40% of the patients with PID were febrile and fewer than half had pelvic swelling or a mass on pelvic examination. Although over 75% had an elevated sedimentation rate, more than half of those women with no evidence of an infection had an elevated sedimentation rate as well. This was both a seminal as well as a disturbing study. It meant that the traditional clinical and laboratory criteria for making a diagnosis (See Table 1) were not sensitive enough to be relied upon. Too few patients with pelvic inflammatory disease would be detected. One response to these observations has been to broaden the criteria for the diagnosis of infection [16,17]. (See Tables 3 & 4). There are pluses and minuses with this empirical approach. It will increase the number of women with pelvic inflammatory disease who will be detected with minimal symptomatology. However, the downside is that there is no scientific basis for this new diagnostic menu. In my eyes, these new criteria have no more scientific basis than the four criteria shown in Table 1.

There were other evidences of a milder form of pelvic inflammatory disease in this same era. A study from the United States in

1975 delineated another subtle form of PID [18]. Many patients seen in an urban emergency room and not suspected by physicians on clinical grounds to have PID were found to be endocervical culture positive for *Neisseria gonorrhea*. Their presenting complaints were vaginal discharge, urinary urgency and frequency and abnormal uterine bleeding. (See Table 5) [18] This was another published suggestion that the clinical diagnosis of PID was not as obvious as we had assumed in the past. This study should heighten physician awareness of the subtleties of the early clinical presentation of pelvic inflammatory disease in the young sexually active patient. A new vaginal discharge, cystitis symptoms, or abnormal uterine bleeding in the absence of any demonstrable pelvic pathology should increase the physician's suspicion of pelvic infection.

In the 1980's, a major breakthrough in our understanding of "silent" pelvic inflammatory disease came with the discovery that *Chlamydia trachomatis* could be isolated from these patients [19,20]. This was an important discovery. A possible role for *Chlamydia trachomatis* in the pathophysiology of PID had not been recognized before this because the standard culture techniques

Table 3
Criteria for the diagnosis of acute PID (without laparoscopy)

A. Three of the following signs or symptoms must be present.

1. Lower abdominal pain and tenderness, with or without

2. Cervical motion tenderness

3. Adnexal tenderness

B. In addition, one or more of the following conditions must be present.

1. Fever equal to or greater than 38°C.

2. White blood cell count equal to or greater than 10,000/cu.mm.

3. Inflammatory pelvic mass documented by clinical examination or sonogram or both.

4. Culdocentesis reveals white blood cells and bacteria on gram stain of peritoneal fluid

5. Gram-negative intracellular diplococci found on gram stain of material from cervix.

---

then employed, would not isolate this organism. Both culture [19,20] and antibody studies [21,22] showed the role of Chlamydia in patients with tubal damage sequelae of infection and as a causative factor in women with tubal damage who had an ectopic pregnancy. This new awareness of the importance of *Chlamydia trachomatis* changed diagnostic and antibiotic strategies. Cell culture techniques used in research laboratories, were not adapted by clinical laboratories because of their complexity and expense. Monoclonal antibody testing [23], DNA probes [24] and Polymerase Chain Reaction (PCR) testing [25] were introduced to enable clinicians to more easily detect this organism. These identification techniques became established standards of practice but there were problems. There were difficulties with the sensitivity and specificity of both the fluorescent antibody testing and the DNA probes. This meant that some infected women would not be detected and some test positive patients

would not be infected. Obviously, a false positive test result for an organism acquired by sexual contact poses serious problems for the patient and physician. The sensitivity and specificity of the PCR makes it the current test of choice. There were treatment problems. Two of the popular antibiotics in the treatment of PID, cefoxitin and metronidazole, both effective against anaerobes, had no activity against Chlamydia. One study showed the continued isolation of *Chlamydia trachomatis* in PID patients who were clinically cured with cefoxitin [26]. New antibiotic combinations were employed using tetracycline, erythromycin and clindamycin as agents effective against Chlamydia.

Another modification in the presentation of pelvic inflammatory disease occurred in the 1980's. There was an increase in the number of penicillin resistant *Neisseria gonorrhea* isolates, particularly in urban centers [27]. Penicillin, the old mainstay of therapy

Table 4
Criteria for the diagnosis of PID

MINIMUM CRITERIA

Presence of all three:

1. Lower abdominal tenderness

2. Adnexal tenderness, and

3. Cervical motion tenderness

ADDITIONAL CRITERIA

ROUTINE

1. Oral temperature > 38.3°C

2. Abnormal cervical or vaginal discharge

3. Elevated sedimentation rate

4. Elevated C-reactive protein

5. Laboratory confirmation of cervical infection with Neisseria gonorrhea or Chlamydia trachomatis

ELABORATE

1. Histopathological evidence of endometritis on endometrial biopsy

2. Tubo-ovarian abscess on sonography or other radiological tests

3. Laparoscopic abnormalities consistent with PID

---

was replaced by a variety of cephalosporins or a combination of clindamycin and aminoglycosides.

Also, in the 1980's, another new variant of pelvic inflammatory disease was seen. The most rapidly increasing segment of HIV positive patients are women who have acquired the disease through heterosexual sex [28]. In this expanding population, pelvic infections can be more serious and less amenable to treatment [29]. A protracted clinical response to antibiotics should be a stimulus for the physician to order HIV antibody testing.

3. DIAGNOSIS OF ACUTE PELVIC INFLAMMATORY DISEASE

There has been a remarkable change in the criteria for the diagnosis of acute pelvic inflammatory disease in the past 30 years. In the early 1960's, there were rigid criteria for the diagnosis of pelvic inflammatory disease. (See Table 1) [14] A subsequent laparoscopic study by Jacobson et al. published in 1969 demonstrated that these established requirements for the diagnosis of PID were not sensitive enough (See Table 2) [15] The Jacobson study caused a revision in thinking about PID but retrospective criticism of the criteria noted in Table 1, has to take into account some of the underlying concerns of the clinical decision makers of that era. Prior to the Jacobson publication, they had been unaware of the existence of a silent form of PID. This was justified. There were major clinical problems with pelvic infections that captured all of their attentions. In urban academic centers, PID was too frequently a life threatening problem that was not responsive to the antibiotic strategies then in vogue. Operative intervention with the removal of reproductive organs was the standard rather than the exception. These seriously ill women commanded the attention of academic gynecologists. There was another important reason for the reliance upon the academic dogma presented in Table 1 [14]. Pelvic pain could be caused by conditions other than PID; a tubal pregnancy or torsion of the adnexa to name just two. Diagnostic techniques were much less

Table 5
Neisseria gonorrhea culture results by diagnostic category in the emergency room

Diagnostic Category	Number positive	Number negative	Total	% Positive
1. Pelvic Inflammatory Disease or Bartholin's abscess.	42	9	51	82.4%
2. Abnormal uterine bleeding.	7	9	16	43.8%
3. Urinary tract symptoms.	10	25	35	28.6%
4. Cervicitis or Vaginitis.	6	17	23	26.1%
5. Other Patients	8	129	137	5.8%

sophisticated. The tests for the presence of chorionic gonadotrophin required high levels of the hormone to be positive, ultrasound had not yet been introduced into clinical practice and laparoscopy was just beginning to be employed by American physicians. In this milieu of diagnostic uncertainty, there was a concern that antibiotics might be given to women without infection, delaying their eventual actual diagnosis and appropriate operative intervention.

The result of the seminal study by Jacobson, et al. [15] was a realization that a milder clinical form of PID existed. This has elicited a number of responses. The first has been to ease the clinical and laboratory criteria for diagnosis. This has taken a variety of forms. One was the 1984 publication by a group of American gynecologists with new revised guidelines for the diagnosis of pelvic inflammatory disease. (See Table 3) [16]. Utilizing these new criteria, more women with PID would be correctly diagnosed as having an infection and would be treated with antibiotics. The standards for the diagnosis of PID have been relaxed even more in the most recent Center for Disease Control (CDC) Guidelines for the tre-

atment of PID. (See Table 4) [17]. There are some good aspects of these less rigid criteria for diagnosis. They require new physician awareness of the frequency of silent PID and their employment by practicing physicians should result in more women receiving antibiotics than in the past. Despite this, I have major reservations about this approach. The first is the lack of any scientific support for the criteria now in place. There have been no large prospective studies to demonstrate the significance of each of the criteria in these guidelines. Does lower abdominal pain have the same sensitivity and specificity as adnexal pain? No large prospective studies have been carried out to confirm or deny this. My other problem with this diagnostic strategy is related to the target population. It is aimed at physicians rather than patients. All of these new diagnostic formulas require a patient to seek medical care. This frequently does not occur for a number of reasons. They may not have symptoms that they judge serious enough to seek medical attention. This was documented in the aforementioned Cates study [1]. Alternatively, the symptoms may not be serious enough for the woman to either seek or receive medical attention [2]. In setting up educational programs for physicians to increase their awareness of "silent" PID, we have overlooked some of the needs of sexually active young women. In the United States, the current reality for most sexually active urban poor young women is that they do not seek medical care until they are pregnant or have symptomatic Emergency Room PID. Our current medical care system does not provide preventive care for these women. Difficulty in achieving access to care is not limited to the urban poor. Every private gynecologist's office that I have encountered has a "gatekeeper." This person will make it difficult for anyone with minimal symptoms to be seen. What is the answer?

There has to be a shift in strategy on two broad fronts. There needs to be a new focus for physicians and their patients.

Physicians need to concentrate on new diagnostic techniques that identify a larger number of women with "silent" PID. Too often in the past, we have stressed either physical findings or invasive techniques to make the diagnosis. There was and continues to be an emphasis upon pelvic examination findings [16,17]. To confirm the diagnosis over the years there have been proponents for culdocentesis [30], endometrial biopsy [31] and laparoscopy [32]. All can be helpful but all are invasive. For the woman in an outpatient setting who has undergone endometrial biopsy or culdocentesis, they are painful. For the woman who has laparoscopy, anesthesia is required. I have never understood the American disregard of the findings of Westrom et al. [33] He has stated that he has never seen a patient with laparoscopic proven PID who did not have an abundance of white cells on the vaginal smear. This is a simple, non-invasive test, that can be done within minutes by the gynecologist. Westrom's observa-

tions indicate it is a very sensitive test [33] and this was confirmed by a recent study where it was more sensitive than the white blood cell count, sedimentation rate and the C-Reactive protein [34]. Obviously, it is not specific for white cells can be seen in the vagina of a woman with a cervicitis. Despite this, this diagnostic test should be part of the physician's diagnostic armamentarium. I for one, am surprised that it is not included in CDC guidelines.

A more significant future focus should be on new and improved microbiological techniques that will increase our ability to diagnose and then to treat "silent" PID.

An emphasis upon *Chlamydia trachomatis* is important because of the major role it has in the etiology of "silent" PID. This silent clinical presentation is accounted for by the interesting human host response to this organism. *Chlamydia trachomatis* evokes a different response than we are accustomed to seeing with bacterial infections. It is an obligate intracellular organism. If you add *Chlamydia trachomatis* to a tissue culture, there is mutual symbiosis. Both bacteria and the tissue culture cells survive without any damage to either. *Chlamydia trachomatis* survives and there is no visual damage to the cells [35]. What happens when this same organism is introduced into the human host? Why does tissue damage occur? There are some clues that suggest an auto-immune mechanism. In monkeys, a single exposure to *Chlamydia trachomatis* caused transient inflammation but repeated inoculations resulted in permanent tubal damage and occlusion [36]. Work by Steve Witkin suggests a pathway for this response. A surface *Chlamydia trachomatis* antigen and a heat shock protein, have a remarkably similar parallel amino acid sequence homology with the surface heat shock protein present in normal fallopian tube and endometrial epithelium [37]. The human host response to exposure to the heat shock protein of Chlamydia is to produce antibodies. With subsequent exposure, these antibodies activate a lymphocyte response to the heat shock protein. Unfortunately, because of the similarities to the heat shock protein of normal tissue, the lymphocytes attack this tissue as well. This probably accounts for the clinically silent situations that we encounter in which tissue damage occurs [1]. This cell mediated response is rarely seen in women with a cervicitis, while it is commonly seen in those women who have had more than one episode of salpingitis [37,38]. There is an important take home clinical lesson here. Early detection and effective treatment of *Chlamydia trachomatis* infections should be beneficial to women. To achieve this, better microbiological techniques need to be employed and new strategies in self-care should be presented to women. One recent study suggested vaginal specimens collected by patients and subjected to PCR testing were nearly as sensitive as those obtained by health care workers doing a pelvic examination [39]. Self-testing avoids an office visit. This is done now in pregnancy testing. Clearly, this is a future option for the diagnosis of infection.

There have been long delays in effective microbiological techniques to detect the presence of *Chlamydia trachomatis* in women. Because it is an obligate intracellular organism, it could not be isolated with ordinary culture techniques and media used by physicians. Early on, detection of this organism depended upon the use of tissue culture techniques [19,20]. This was a major problem. Clinical laboratories were either unwilling or unable to put together the resources to provide this as a standardized service. In this void, there was evidence of

clinicians grasping at straws. Some early emphasis was on the detection of Chlamydia by the simple cytologic examination of a gram stained endocervical smear [40]. Although this is a sensitive test, it is not specific. A major breakthrough occurred with the introduction of alternative laboratory techniques. These included DNA probe testing [24] or fluorescent antibody testing [23]. These had great appeal to clinicians and directors of laboratories. For the clinician, it meant that testing for *Chlamydia trachomatis* could be done. For laboratory directors, these tests could be performed, with much less complexity or expense than the then "gold standard," the tissue culture. There were problems. Their sensitivity and specificity were less than the tissue culture standards. This gave clinicians two concerns. The lack of sensitivity meant that some patients with a *Chlamydia trachomatis* infection would not be detected. The lack of specificity meant that some women who were test positive did not have a *Chlamydia trachomatis* infection. A false positive test for a sexually transmitted disease is a source of unnecessary angst for young couples.

4. TREATMENT OF ACUTE PELVIC INFLAMMATORY DISEASE

There is ample evidence from a number of studies that soft tissue pelvic infections often have more than one bacterial species involved in the infection. In these patients, physicians will find a wide range of isolates, including at times, *Neisseria gonorrhea*, *Chlamydia trachomatis*, Gram positive and negative aerobes and anaerobes. With such a variety, it is apparent that broad spectrum antibiotic regimens should be employed.

The best antibiotic treatment for patients with acute pelvic inflammatory disease is not clear at the present time. There are a host of reasons for this uncertainty. It is clear in discussing the protean nature of acute PID that there is a wide range of patient presentations with this disease. Patients with Emergency Room PID are obviously sicker, more easily recognized and more easily confirmed to have PID than those with "silent" PID, in whom the diagnosis is difficult and in many cases will be suspect in retrospect. Prospective studies evaluating modes of treatment are few and far between and they suffer from a number of shortcomings. There can be patient selection bias, that is the urban poor black population is over-represented [3] and does not fit the universe of the population with PID [1]. There is a more serious problem in the analysis of treatment results. Nearly all of the studies published to date have looked at short term outcomes alone. These are important observations. Physicians want to know if the patients get better clinically or if they fail treatment as measured by a need to switch antibiotics or the necessity for operative care in the rare instances in which pelvic abscess formation developed. This data was used by clinicians in order to anticipate the expected immediate outcome of therapy. For example, one pooled analysis of several reports showed the best immediate result when the antibiotic regimen had good anaerobic coverage [41]. There are shortcomings to these studies. The clinical evaluation can be flawed. A study by Sweet et al. had patients with PID who were thought to be clinically cured with cefoxin. A culture at the time of the post-treatment examination was still culture positive for *Chlamydia trachomatis* in a few of these patients [26]. This observation highlights the inaccuracy of some clinical evaluations. In addition to these concerns about immediate treatment outcome, physicians should also be knowledgeable about the long term outcomes of therapy. How many of these patients "successfully" treated with anti-

biotics have tubal damage sufficient to cause infertility or are debilitated with persistent pelvic pain? Observations made in the past demonstrated the frequency of tubal infertility after antibiotic treatment of acute pelvic inflammatory disease [9,42]. Unfortunately, there has been a limited focus on these outcomes, based upon initial antibiotic treatment choices. The data base is very limited. One evaluation of 608 women showed no difference in the incidence of tubal occlusion following treatment with four different antibiotic regimens, chloramphenicol alone, penicillin and streptomycin, ampicillin alone and doxycycline alone [43]. Oviously, none of these regimens are currently employed. The caveat for the reader should be that many of the currently used treatment regimens are based upon both a limited data base and the best judgment of clinician investigators. Whether these current treatment pronouncements will withstand the test of time is unknown.

The first important question of therapeutic strategy revolves around the question of the site of treatment. Should these women be routinely admitted to the hospital or should they be treated as outpatients? There are many experts, myself included, who believe all of these patients are best served by admission to hospital. This flies in the face of clinical logic, i.e. why admit a patient who is minimally ill for treatment when it can be provided on an outpatient basis? Also, in the United States, there are pressures from patient funding agencies, such as private insurance companies, to direct such treatment to an outpatient setting. In defense of this stand, based upon economics, there again, are no prospective studies comparing inpatient and outpatient treatment in women with similar types of pelvic infection. The CDC has developed a set of guidelines to try to help guide physicians in

Table 6
Hospitalization for patients with PID is especially recommended
when the following criteria are met

1. The diagnosis is uncertain and surgical emergencies such as appendicitis and ectopic pregnancy cannot be excluded.

2. Pelvic abscess is suspected.

3. The patient is pregnant.

4. The patient is an adolescent (among adolescents, compliance with therapy is unpredictable).

5. The patient has HIV infection.

6. Severe illness or nausea and vomiting preclude outpatient management.

7. The patient is unable to follow or tolerate an outpatient regimen.

8. The patient has failed to respond clinically to outpatient therapy.

9. Clinical follow-up within 72 hours of starting antibiotic treatment cannot be arranged.

the selection of patients for admission. (See Table 6.) [17] These are logical and helpful but have not been subjected to any scientific prospective study to test their validity.

Currently in the United States, the majority of patients with acute PID are managed as outpatients. The physician's decision about the site of treatment is usually dictated by the clinical evaluation of the severity of the infection. Generally, patients with mild symptoms or those that are culture positive and asymptomatic are treated as outpatients. In the United States, the CDC recommends two antibiotic strategies. See Table 7 [17]. Regimen A combines a single antibiotic dosage plus oral doxycycline for 14 days. There are many positive aspects to this approach. It provides excellent coverage against *Neisseria gonorrhea* and *Chlamydia trachomatis*. A single intramuscular injection plus doxycycline is an easily tolerated treatment schedule for a patient. Compliance should be high. My criticism of this regimen is that it provides an inadequate length of treatment of infections caused by Gram negative anaerobes. As a result, on occasion I have had women admitted to the New York Hospital who developed a pelvic abscess despite this treatment. The second regimen appeals to me more because of my views about the importance of anaerobes. Ofloxacin effectively covers both *Neisseria gonorrhea* and *Chlamydia trachomatis*. The two-week regimen with either clindamycin or metronidazole provides much better anaerobic coverage than regimen A. There are difficulties with this regimen. Patients will not tolerate it as well as regimen A and they can develop diarrhea and pseudomembranous enterocolitis while taking clindamycin [44]. Also they need to be cautioned to inform their medical care provider if they develop diarrhea and to discontinue the antibiotic if they have five or more loose bowel movements in one day. Oral metronidazole for 14 days can be a difficult regimen for patients to tolerate. They should be warned to avoid alcohol and alerted to the fact that they can have many uncomfortable gastrointestinal symptoms while taking this drug and an occasional patient

Table 7
CDC Recommended Outpatient Treatment of PID

Regimen A.

   1. Cefoxitin two grams IM plus oral probenecid 1.0 gram in a single dose concurrently, or

   2. Ceftriaxone 250 mg IM, or

   3. Other third-generation cephalosporins, i.e.

      Ceftizoxime or

      Cefotaxime

PLUS

   Doxycycline 100 mg, two times a day for 14 days

Regimen B

   Oflaxicin 400 mg, orally two times a day for 14 days

PLUS

   1. Clindamycin 450 mg orally four times a day for 14 days or

   2. Metronidazole 500 mg orally two times a day for 14 days

can develop a peripheral neuropathy [45]. With both outpatient-antibiotic treatment schedules, the sexual partners of these patients should be treated as well.

Patients who are thought clinically to be more seriously ill are treated as inpatients. This is an individual physician judgment and varies from service to service. The inpatient regimens recommended by the CDC are listed in Table 8 [17]. Regimen A has been widely used. It is a very appealing regimen because of the excellent coverage of *Neisseria gonorrhea*, *Chlamydia trachomatis*, and Gram negative anaerobic bacteria. In addition, these antibiotics are usually well tolerated by patients. Regimen B is also popular because it has been widely used by American obstetrician-gynecologists for many years. Although neither clindamycin

nor gentamicin alone have great effect against *Neisseria gonorrhea* in the laboratory, they are effective in combination in eliminating this organism from the patient treated. I have never had a *Neisseria gonorrhea* culture positive patient remain culture positive after treatment with this combination. Both clindamycin and gentamicin pose difficulties for the gynecologist. There is the potential for gastrointestinal ill effects with clindamycin. With gentamicin, standard dosing schedules in young women can produce sub-optimal serum antibiotic levels in more than a third of patients [46]. Peak and trough levels of gentamicin are indicated in the patient who fails to initially respond to treatment. The alternative regimens have been less well studied but they seem to be effective and offer the clinician a wide range of therapeutic possibilities. All

Table 8
CDC Recommended Inpatient Treatment of PID

Regimen A.

Cefoxitin two grams IV every six hours or Cefotetan two grams every 12 hours.

PLUS

Doxycycline 100 mg IV or orally every 12 hours.

Regimen B.

Clindamycin 900 mg IV every eight hours

PLUS

Gentamicin loading dose IV or IM (two mg/kg of body weight) followed by maintenance dose (1.5 mg/kg) every eight hours

Alternative Inpatient Regimens

1. Ampicillin/sulbactam plus doxycycline

OR

2. Intravenous ofloxacin plus either clindamycin or metronidazole

of these antibiotic combinations require close patient observation. Some patients will not be able to tolerate the antibiotic schedule. Some patients will continue to spike temperatures and require modification of the initial antibiotic combination or operative intervention. The care of all inpatients should include outpatient antibiotic treatment of their sexual partners as well.

There is an unresolved question in the treatment of PID in which *Chlamydia trachomatis* is one of the species of bacteria involved in the infection. The therapeutic assumption in the past was that the treatment regimen, either outpatient or inpatient, eliminated *Chlamydia trachomatis*. This has been called into question by several clinical studies. *Chlamydia trachomatis* DNA and antigens were detected in biopsy

tissues of the fimbrial and peritubal adhesions by *in situ* hybridization or immunoperoxidase stain, suggesting a persistent infection in these women after antibiotic therapy [46]. Dr. Henry-Suchet has made similar observations in Paris [48]. Is this persistent infection or biological markers of killed *Chlamydia trachomatis* organisms? I favor the former. These findings have been a stimulus to prolong the length of antibiotic treatment for *Chlamydia trachomatis* PID. The benefits or dangers of such a strategy need to be subjected to clinical testing.

5. DIAGNOSIS OF PELVIC ABSCESS

There are two presentations of patients with PID who develop a pelvic abscess. There are those patients who when seen by the physician for the first time have a pelvic abscess present. In most cases, these women give a protracted history of not feeling well, even though they have not availed themselves of medical care. The other group of patients with a pelvic abscess are those women who have had prior antibiotic treatment and have failed to respond. Initially, they had no abscesses but upon re-evaluation are found to have a pelvic abscess.

The diagnosis of a pelvic abscess is usually suspected on clinical grounds. This category of infection fits our model of a bacterial infection. These patients feel ill, they are febrile, have an elevated white count and a tender mass can usually be palpated on pelvic examination. This is the clinical situation in which imaging techniques are a tremendous aid to the clinician. The delineation of a pelvic mass is difficult when solely dependent upon pelvic examination findings. Every clinician in my age group who has practiced before ultrasonography became an integral part of clinical practice remembers a laparotomy for the huge pelvic mass, greater than 10 cm. in diameter, which on operative exploration was found to be a much smaller inflamed enlarged tube, surrounded by adhesions with adherent bowel and omentum. Confirmation of a suspected pelvic mass is possible with imaging techniques. The most popular mode of diagnostic imaging for American gynecologists is ultrasonography. This is a highly sensitive technique to determine the presence of a fluid filled, adnexal structure [49]. An experienced gynecological ultrasonographer can accurately differentiate tubal and ovarian masses. CT can be used to better determine if the fluid filled mass is sterile. CT is more accurate than sonography with good anatomic resolution and is not opera-

tor-dependent [49]. It has been used to carry percutaneous drainage of these pelvic abscesses, eliminating in most cases the necessity for an operation [50]. It has the disadvantage of radiation exposure and expense.

6. TREATMENT OF A PELVIC ABSCESS

A physician responsible for a patient, suspected of having a pelvic abscess, should obtain all information that could be helpful in the care of the patient. There are some sub-categories of infection that will require different treatment strategies. If a patient with a pelvic abscess has an intrauterine device (IUD) in place or has recently had one removed, a major etiologic concern for the physician should be *Actinomycosis Israeli* [51]. This anaerobic organism is susceptible to penicillin and clindamycin but a long course of treatment, i.e. months, will be required to achieve a cure [51]. Tubo-ovarian abscesses in post-menopausal women are uncommon [52,53] but they dictate new diagnostic concerns. In addition to the clinician's legitimate focus upon the immediate concern, the pelvic abscess, some of these women can have other diseases including diverticulitis of the colon or a malignancy, either pelvic or gastrointestinal. An ordered diagnostic workup for these possibilities is indicated in the total care of this population. Finally, HIV antibody testing can be very helpful in determining prognoses in these women. There is good evidence that these women are more likely to have a pelvic abscess and more often require operative care, because they fail to respond to antibiotic treatment [29].

There have been remarkable changes in the therapeutic strategies for women suspected of having a pelvic abscess in the past three decades. In the past, gynecological treatment was based upon operative intervention and the dogma was that a pelvic abscess could only be treated surgically, not medically. One very good clinical review of tubo-ovarian abscesses published in 1969 mentions antibiotics only as adjunctive treatment to the more significant operative intervention [54]. In another review of the care of patients with a tubo-ovarian abscess from 1970-1974, only 10% were cured with medical management alone [55]. This former dependence upon an operative approach for initial therapy has been superseded by medical therapies. Today, in nearly every patient with a pelvic abscess, the initial course of therapy is systemic antibiotics. The exception is the acutely ill patient with generalized point and rebound tenderness, hypoactive bowel sounds and tachycardia. This should make the physician suspect the intraperitoneal rupture of a tubo-ovarian abscess [4,10]. If rupture is suspected, immediate operative intervention is indicated. Fortunately, these operative emergencies are rare events in the 1990's. Nearly all of the patients suspected of having a pelvic abscess are now treated with antibiotics. This change in strategy was dictated by two important observations. The importance of anaerobes, particularly Gram negative anaerobes, in abscess formation was noted in an animal model [56] and in the human [57]. *Bacteroides fragilis*, a Gram negative anaerobe, seemed particularly important [57]. New antibiotic strategies were employed, directed at those Gram negative anaerobes, and it became apparent to clinicians that women with pelvic abscesses could be cured medically.

For patients with a suspected unruptured tubo-ovarian abscess, antibiotic treatment is the first line of therapy. This should be ad-

ministered as parenteral antibiotics given to the patient within the hospital. These abscesses are mixed bacteria species infections but the importance of Gram negative anaerobes in their formation cannot be overstated. Combination antibiotic treatment is usually employed and one part of this combination should be an antibiotic effective against Gram negative anaerobic bacteria. There are limited clinical series to compare results but one study of patients with tubo-ovarian abscesses had a higher medical cure rate when clindamycin was used in comparison to regimens in which it had not been prescribed [50]. These differences were statistically significant ($p<0.01$). In addition to clindamycin, there are a variety of antibiotic agents introduced into clinical practice in the last 20 years that have good activity against Gram negative anaerobes. These include certain cephalosporins, penicillins, penicillins with a beta lactamase inhibitor, imipenem, ofloxacin and metronidazole. Personally, I favor metronidazole as one arm of therapy in the patient with a pelvic abscess, although there are no prospective studies to show its superiority. It is bactericidal, and there has not been the development of resistance to it by Gram negative anaerobic bacteria. However, it must be used in combination with other antibiotics. I prefer an aminoglycoside to cover Gram negative aerobes and penicillin for gram positive aerobes and anaerobes.

Despite the use of other antibiotics, some patients will not respond to medical treatment. When this occurs, there are a variety of treatment options for the clinician. One popular form of operative intervention is colpotomy drainage of a pelvic abscess [59]. This procedure is possible when the abscess expands and presses into the posterior cul-de-sac of the vagina. The procedure has the advantage of being easy to perform with little intraoperative stress or morbidity for the patient. The simplicity of the procedure should not blind physicians to its shortcomings. In one series of 65 patients published in the 1970's, approximately a third of the patients required another operation before they were finally cured [59]. The cases in this report were collected from 1968 to 1973, before there was a heightened awareness of the importance of using antibiotics effective against Gram negative anaerobes. With that adjunctive help, the subsequent reoperation rate might have been lower. More serious post-operative complications can be seen. A report published in 1982 of operative experience with colpotomy in Mississippi and South Africa from 1961 to 1976 documented diffuse peritoneal sepsis in 18 of 298 patients (6%) [60]. This report emphasizes close post-operative evaluation of these patients, although no details of the antibiotics used in this series was given. Colpotomy is done infrequently on most services in the 1990's. The early use of effective antibacterial agents against Gram negative anaerobes may have diminished the progression of pelvic abscesses in patients receiving medical treatment to a size where operative drainage is easily done. Alternatively, there has been increased enthusiasm for alternate methods of abscess reduction. These include transabdominal percutaneous aspiration guided by CT scanning [50]. I have been impressed in my contacts with different hospital services that the frequency this intervention is used depends upon both the enthusiasm and the skills of the interventional radiologists at that institution. There are other options. Dr. Henry-Suchet et al. have championed the use of intra-abdominal aspiration of tubo-ovarian abscesses with a laparoscope [61]. This is a viable alternative to either colpotomy or laparotomy and has been successfully employed by other investigators [62,63]. When this approach is successful, it preserves pelvic reproductive organs and gives the patient the opportunity for a further pregnancy. The immediate post-operative recovery time is shorter than after a laparotomy. Despite all of these alternative treatments, some women will come to laparotomy for the care of their pelvic abscess. The guidelines for operative care at the time of laparotomy have remarkably changed in the past three decades. Historically, this intervention required removal of all pelvic organs for a cure [4,10]. This is no longer true for a variety of reasons. With effective antibiotics available against Gram negative anaerobes, infected pelvic tissue can be preserved and a cure achieved medically. There is a growing awareness that in many instances of pelvic abscess the findings were unilateral, not bilateral. This is particularly true in women with PID who have an intrauterine device in place [64]. Obviously, the uninvolved adnexa would not require operative removal. Finally, the acceleration of assisted reproductive technology means that a woman can achieve a subsequent pregnancy with donor eggs if only a uterus is left behind and *in vitro* fertilization can be employed if an ovary and a uterus remain. These are powerful influences for a more conservative operative approach. The most serious operative problem in an infected patient is the ruptured tubo-ovarian abscess. Even here, operative criteria have changed. In the past, the treatment of choice was a total abdominal hysterectomy and bilateral salpino-oophorectomy [4,10]. More recent experience indicates that partial removal of adnexa, with uterine preservation and peritoneal lavage, accompanied by broad spectrum antibiotic coverage is effective in the majority of cases [65]. Anyone choosing a strategy of partial pelvic tissue extirpation must be aware and alert the patient to the possibility that a second operation may be required.

7. POST-OPERATIVE PELVIC INFECTIONS

Physicians caring for women will also see some patients who develop a pelvic infection after a gynecological operation. These complications make up a much smaller number of incidents than the universe of patients with community acquired pelvic inflammatory disease.

The most frequent infection in this category is the pelvic infection following termination of a pregnancy. Preoperative risk factors have been identified. Those women who are asymptomatic but culture positive for *Neisseria gonorrhea* [66] and *Chlamydia trachomatis* [67] are much more likely to have a post termination infection. Fortunately, most patients respond rapidly to antibiotics and one study showed a consistently low number of degree hours of fever when this patient category was evaluated [68]. There is a smaller group of patients where the problem of infection can be much more serious. If there is pelvic tissue damage as a result of the termination, some of these patients can have a complicated post-operative course with hospitalization required for parenteral antibiotic treatment. In some cases, an operation is indicated for the drainage or removal of an abscess [69]. These are rare events in the 1990's. Pre-operative screening for *Neisseria gonorrhea* and *Chlamydia trachomatis* is done on most services; prophylactic antibiotics are employed for coverage of this procedure and the legalization of pregnancy termination in the United States allows the procedure to be done early in the pregnancy. All of these

events have contributed to the low incidence of pelvic infection following this operative procedure.

The other common sources of pelvic infection following an operation are the adnexal abscesses following hysterectomy [71]. This was seen more often following vaginal hysterectomy as compared to abdominal hysterectomy. These abscesses were different from the tubo-ovarian abscesses in community acquired PID, for ovarian abscesses were commonly seen in which the endosalpinx was not involved [72]. This was a complication most frequently encountered in premenopausal women undergoing vaginal hysterectomy in which the protective capsule of the ovary was breached with post-operative ovulation. These abscesses were serious post-operative problems and usually required operative removal of the infected adnexa. Fortunately, these clinical problems are rarely seen in the 1990's. There was a dramatic drop in incidence when prophylactic antibiotics for vaginal hysterectomy were shown to be effective [73]. Another post-operative infection problem seen, is the vaginal cuff infection following hysterectomy. These infections usually respond to systemic antibiotics but occasionally, operative drainage of the vaginal cuff is needed for a cure.

REFERENCES

1. Cates, W. Jr., Joesoef, M.B., & Goldman, M.R.: Atypical pelvic inflammatory disease: can we identify clinical predictors? Am. J. Obstet. Gynecol. 1993; 169: 341-346.

2. Wolner-Hanssen, P.: Silent Pelvic Inflammatory Disease: is it overstated? Obstet. Gynecol. 1995; 86: 321-325.

3. Soper, D.E., Brockwell, N.J., & Dalton, H.P.: Microbial etiology of urban emergency de-

partment acute salpingitis. Am. J. Obstet. Gynecol. 1992; 167: 648-652.

4. Vermeeren, J., & TeLinde, R.W.: Intra-abdominal rupture of pelvic abscesses. Am. J. Obstet. Gynecol. 1954; 68: 402-409.

5. Ledger, W.J.: Chronic vaginitis. Inf. Dis. in Clin. Prac. 1993; 2: 60-64.

6. McNamara, M.T. & Mead, P.B.: Diagnosis and management of the pelvic abscess. J. Reprod. Med. 1976; 17: 299-304.

7. Anderson, G.V. & Bucklew, W.B.: Abdominal surgery and tubo-ovarian abscesses. West. J. Surg., Obstet. and Gynec. 1962; 70: 67-70.

8. Mickal, A. & Sellmann, A.H.: Management of tubo-ovarian abscess. Clin. Obstet. Gynecol. 1969; 12: 252-264.

9. Svensson, L., Mardh, P-A., & Westrom, L.: Infertility after acute salpingitis with special reference to *Chlamydia trachomatis*. Fertil. Steril. 1983; 40:322-329.

10. Collins, C.G., Nix, F.G., & Cerha, H.: Ruptured tubo-ovarian abscess. Am. J. Obstet. Gynecol. 1956; 72: 820-829.

11. Ledger, W.J., Kriewall, T.J., Sweet, R.L., & Fekety, F.R. Jr.: The use of parenteral clindamycin in the treatment of obstetric-gynecologic patients with severe infections: a comparison of a clindamycin-kanamycin combination with penicillin-kanamycin. Obstet. Gynecol. 1974; 43: 490-497.

12. Sweet, R.L., & Ledger, W.J.: Cefoxitin: single-agent treatment of mixed aerobic-anaerobic pelvic infections. Obstet. Gynecol. 1979; 54: 193-198.

13. Platt, L.D., Yonekura, M.L. & Ledger, W.J.: The role of anaerobic bacteria in post partum endomyometritis. Am. J. Obstet. Gynecol. 1979; 135: 814-817.

14. Ledger, W.J.: Infection in the Female. 2nd edition. Philadelphia; Lea & Febiger. 1986.

15. Jacobson, L., & Westrom, L.: Objectivized diagnosis of acute pelvic inflammatory disease. Diagnostic and prognostic value of rou-

tine laparoscopy. Am. J. Obstet. Gynecol. 1969; 105: 1088-1098.

16. Hager, W.D., Eschenbach, D.A., Spence, M.R. , & Sweet, R.L.: Criteria for diagnosis and grading of salpingitis. J. Obstet. Gynecol. 1983;61:113-114.

17. Centers for Disease Control.: 1993 Sexually Transmitted Diseases. Treatment guidelines. 1993; 42:1-102.

18. Curran, J.W., Rendtorff, R.C., Chandler, R.W., Wiser, W.L., & Robinson, H.: Female gonorrhea. Its relation to abnormal uterine bleeding, urinary tract symptoms, and cervicitis. Obstet. Gynecol. 1975; 45: 195-198.

19. Mardh, P-A., Ripa, T., Svensson, L., & Westrom, L.: *Chlamydia trachomatis* infection in patients with acute salpingitis. N. Engl. J. Med. 1977;296:1377-.1379.

20. Shepard, M.K., & Jones, R.B.: Recovery of *Chlamydia trachomatis* from endometrial and fallopian tube biopsies in women with infertility of tubal origin. Fertil. Steril 1989; 52:232-238.

21. Brunham, R.C., Maclean, I.W., Binns, B., & Peeling, R.W.: *Chlamydia trachomatis*: Its role in tubal infertility. J. Inf. Dis. 1985;152:1275-1282.

22. Hartford, S.L., Silva, P.D., di Zerega, G.S., & Yonekura, M.L.: Serologic evidence of prior chlamydial infection in patients with tubal ectopic pregnancy and contralateral tubal disease. Fertil. Steril. 1987; 47:118-121.

23. Livengood, C.H. III, Schmitt, J.W., Addison, W.A., Wrenn, J.W., & Magruder-Habib, K.: Direct fluorescent antibody testing for endocervical *Chlamydia trachomatis*: factors affecting accuracy. Obstet. Gynecol. 1988; 72:803-809.

24. Hosein, I.K., Kaunitz, A.M., & Craft, S.J.: Detection of cervical *Chlamydia trachomatis* and *Neisseria gonorrhea* with deoxyribonucleic acid probe assays in obstetric patients. Am. J. Obstet. Gynecol. 1992; 167:588-591.

25. Witkin, S.S., Jeremias, J., Toth, M., & Ledger, W.J.: Detection of *Chlamydia trachomatis* by the polymerase chain reaction in the cervices of women with acute salpingitis. Am. J. Obstet. Gynecol. 1993;168:1438-1442.

26. Sweet, R.L., Schachter, J., and Robbie, M.O.: Failure of B-Lactam antibiotics to eradicate *Chlamydia trachomatis* in the endometrium despite apparent clinical cure of acute salpingitis. JAMA 1983;250:2641-2645.

27. Handsfield, H.H., Sandstrom, E.G., Knapp, J.S., Perine, P.L., Whittington, W.L., Sayers, D.E., & Holmes, K.K.: Epidemiology of penicillinase-producing *Neisseria gonorrhea* infections: analysis by autotyping and serogrouping. N. Engl. J. Med. 1982;306:950-954.

28. Quinn, T.C., Zacarias, F.R., & St. John, R.K.: AIDS in the Americas: an emerging public health crisis. N. Engl. J. Med. 1989;320:1005-1007.

29. Kamenga, M.C., DeCock, K.M., St. Louis, M.E., Toure, C.K., Zakaria, S., N'gbichi, J.M., Ghys, P.D., Holmes, K.K., Eschenbach, D.A., Gayle, H.D., & Kreiss, J.K.: The impact of human immunodeficiency virus infection on pelvic inflammatory disease: a case control study in Abidjan, Ivory Coast. Am. J. Obstet. Gynecol. 1995;172:919-925.

30. Monif, G.R., Welkos, S.L., Baer, H., & Thopson, R.J.: Cul-de-sac isolates from patients with endometritis-salpingitis-peritinitis and gonococcal endocervicitis. Am. J. Obstet. Gynecol. 1976;126:158-161.

31. Paavonen, J., Aine, R., Teisala, K., Heinonen, P.K., & Punnonen, R.: Comparison of endometrial biopsy and peritoneal fluid cytologic testing with laparoscopy in the diagnosis of acute pelvic inflammatory disease. Am. J. Obstet. Gynecol. 1985;151:645-650.

32. Chaparro, M.V., Ghosh, A., Nashed, A., & Poliak, A.: Laparoscopy for the confirmation and prognostic evaluation of pelvic inflammatory disease. Int. J. Gyn. Obstet. 1978;15:307-309.

33. Westrom, L.: Clinical manifestations and diagnosis of pelvic inflammatory disease. J. Reprod. Med. 1983;28:703-708.

34. Peipert, J.F., Boardman, L., Hogan, J.W., Sung, J. & Mayer, K.H.: Laboratory evaluation of acute upper genital tract infection. Obstet. Gynecol. 1996; 87: 730-736.

35. Hutchinson, G.R., Taylor-Robinson, D., & Dourmashkin, R.R.: Growth and effect of chlamydiae in human and bovine oviduct organ cultures. Brit. J. Ven. Dis. 1979; 55:194-202.

36. Patton, D.L., Kuo, C-C., Wang, S-P., & Halbert, S.A.: Distal tubal obstruction induced by repeated *Chlamydia trachomatis* salpingeal infections in pig-tailed macaques. J. Inf. Dis. 1987; 155:1292-1299.

37. Witkin, S.S., Jeremias, J., Toth, M., & Ledger, W.J.: Proliferative response to conserved epitopes of the *Chlamydia trachomatis* and human 60-Kilodalton heat shock proteins by lymphocytes from women with salpingitis. Am. J. Obstet. Gynecol. 1994; 171:455-460.

38. Witkin, S.S., Jeremias, J., Toth, M., & Ledger, W.J.: Cell-mediated immune response to the recombinant 57-kDa heat-shock protein of *Chlamydia trachomatis* in women with salpingitis. J. Inf. Dis. 1993; 167:1379-1383.

39. Wiesenfeld, H.C., Heine, R.P., Rideout, A., Macio, I., DiBiasi, F. & Sweet, R.L.: The vaginal introitis: A novel site for *Chlamydia trachomatis* testing in women. Am. J. Obstet. Gynecol. 1996; 174: 1542-1546.

40. Moscicki, B., Shafer, M-A., Millstein, S.G., Irwin, C.E. Jr., & Schachter, J.: The use and limitation of endocervical Gram stains and mucopurulent cervicitis as predictors for *Chlamydia trachomatis* in female adolescents. Am. J. Obstet. Gynecol. 1987; 157:65-71.

41. Dodson, M.G.: Antibiotic regimens for treating acute pelvic inflammatory disease. J. Repro. Med. 1994; 39:285-296.

42. Westrom, L.: Effect of acute pelvic inflammatory disease on fertility.: Am. J. Obstet. Gynecol. 1975; 121:707-713.

43. Westrom, L., Iosif, S., Svensson, L., & Mardh, P-A.: Infertility after acute salpingitis: results of treatment with different antibiotics. Curr. Ther. Res. 1979; 26:752-759.

44. Bartlett, J.G., Chang, T.W., Gurwith, M., Gorbach, S.L., & Onderdonk, A.B.: Antibiotic associated pseudomembranous colitis due to toxin producing Clostridia. N. Eng. J. Med. 1978;298:531-534. .

45. Bartlett, J.G.: Metronidazole. Johns Hop. Med. J. 1981;149:89-92.

46. Zaske, D.E., Cipolle, R.J., Strate, R.J. & Dickes, W.F.: Increased gentamicin dosage requirements: rapid elimination in 249 gynecology patients. Am. J. Obstet. Gynecol. 1981; 139:896-900.

47. Patton, D.L., Askienazy-Elbha, M., Henry-Suchet, J.,Campbell, L.A., Cappucio, A., Tannous, W., Wang, S-P., & Kuo, C-C.: Detection of *Chlamydia trachomatis* in fallopian tube tissue in women with post-infectious tubal infertility. Am. J. Obstet. Gynecol. 1994;171:95-101.

48. Henry-Suchet, J., Catalan, F., Loffredo, V., Serfaty, D., Siboulet, A., Perol, Y., Sanson, M.J., Debache, C., Pigeau, F., Coppin, R., deBrux, J., & Poynard, T: Microbiology of specimens obtained by laparoscopy from controls and from patients with pelvic inflammatory disease or infertility with tubal obstruction. *Chlamydia trachomatis* and *Ureaplasma urealyticum* Am. J. Obstet. Gynecol. 1980;138:1022-1025.

49. Montgomery, R.S., & Wilson, S.E.: Intraabdominal abscesses: image-guided diagnosis and therapy. Clin. Inf. Dis. 1996; 23:28-36.

50. Tyrrel, R.T., Murphy, F.B., and Bernardino, M.E.: Tubo-ovarian abscesses: CT-guided percutaneous drainage. Rad. 1990;175:87-89.

51. Burkman, R., Schlesselman, S., McCaffrey, L., Gupta, P.K., & Spence, M.: The relationship of genital tract actinomycetes and the development of pelvic inflammatory disease. Am. J. Obstet. Gynecol. 1982;143:585-589.

52. Heaton, F.C., & Ledger, W.J.: Postmenopausal tubo-ovarian abscess. Obstet. Gynecol. 1976;47:90-94.

53. Hoffman, M., Molpus, K., Roberts, W.S., Lyman, G.H., & Cavanaugh, D.: Tubo-ovarian abscess in postmenopausal women. J. Reprod. Med. 1990; 35:525-528.

54. Mickel, A., & Sellmann, A.H.: Management of tubo-ovarian abscess. Clin. Obstet. Gynecol. 1969; 12:252-264.

55. Hager, W.D.: Follow-up of patients with tubo-ovarian abscesses in association with salpingitis. Obstet. Gynecol. 1983;61:680-684.

56. Bartlett, J.G., Louie, T.J., Gorbach, S.L., & Onderdonk, A.B.: Therapeutic efficacy of 29 antimicrobial regimens in experimental interabdominal sepsis. Rev. Inf. Dis. 1981; 3:535-542.

57. Ledger, W.J.: Anaerobic infections. Am. J. Obstet. Gynecol. 1975; 123:111-118.

58. Landers, D.V., & Sweet, R.L.: Tubo-ovarian abscess: contemporary approach to management. Rev. Inf. Dis. 1983; 5:876-884.

59. Rubenstein, P.R., Mishell, D.R. Jr., & Ledger, W.J.: Colpotomy drainage of pelvic abscess. Obstet. Gynecol. 1976; 48:142-145.

60. Rivlin, M.E., Golan, A., & Darling, M.R.: Diffuse-peritoneal sepsis associated with colpotomy drainage of pelvic abscess. J. Reprod. Med. 1982; 27:406-410.

61. Henry-Suchet, J., Soler, A., & Loffredo, V.: Laparoscopic treatment of tubo-ovarian abscesses. J. Reprod. Med. 1984; 29:579-582.

62. Reich, H., & McGlynn, F.: Laparoscopic treatment of tubo-ovarian and pelvic abscess. J. Reprod. Med. 1987; 32:747-752.

63. Teisala, K., Heinonen, P., & Punnonen, R.: Laparoscopic diagnosis and treatment of

acute pyosalpinx. J. Reprod. Med. 1990; 35:19-21.

64. Golde, S.H., Israel, R., & Ledger, W.J.: Unilateral tubo-ovarian abscess: a distinct entity. Am. J. Obstet. Gynecol. 1977; 127:807-810.

65. Rivlin, M.E., & Hunt, J.A.: Ruptured tubo-ovarian abscess: Is hysterectomy necessary? Obstet. Gynecol. 1977; 50:518-522

66. Burkman, R.T., Tonascia, J.A., Atienza, M.F., & King T.M.: Untreated endocervical gonorrhea and endometritis following elective abortion. Am. J. Obstet. Gynecol. 1976; 126:648-651.

67. Moller, B.R., Ahrons, S., Laurin, J., & Mardh, P-A.: Pelvic infection after elective abortion associated with *Chlamydia trachomatis*. Obstet. Gynecol. 1982; 59:210-213.

68. Ledger, W.J., Moore, D.E., Lowensohn, R.J., & Gee, C.L.: A fever index evaluation of chloramphenicol or clindamycin in patients with serious pelvic infection. Obstet. Gynecol. 1977; 50:523-530.

69. Ledger, W.J., Gassner, C.B., & Gee, C.: Operative care of infection in Obstetrics-Gynecology. J. Reprod. Med. 1974; 13:128-133.

70. Sonne-Holm, S., Heisterberg, L., Hebjorin, S., Pyring-Anderson, K., Anderson, J.T., & Hejl, B.L.: Prophylactic antibiotic in first trimester abortions: a clinical controlled trial. Am. J. Obstet. Gynecol. 1981; 139:693-696.

71. Ledger, W.J., Campbell, C., Taylor, P., & Willson, J.R.: Adnexal abscess as a late complication of pelvic operations. Surg. Gynecol. Obstet. 1969; 129:973-978.

72. Ledger, W.J., Campbell, C., & Willson, J.R.: Post-operative adnexal infections. Obstet. Gynecol. 1968; 31:83-89.

73. Ledger, W.J., Sweet, R.L., & Headington, J.T.: Prophylactic cephaloridine in the prevention of post-operative pelvic infection in premenopausal women undergoing vaginal hysterectomy. Am. J. Obstet. Gynecol. 1973; 115:766-774.

Intra-Abdominal Infections Originated from Tropical Surgical Diseases

Ricardo Vitor Cohen, MD, PhD- FACS and
Frederico Aun, MD, PhD- FACS

Infectious and parasitic diseases are endemic in tropical and subtropical areas of the world. The number of individuals with such illnesses is staggering and it is fair to state that a substantial percentage of the world population is affected by one or more of them.

Many "Tropical Surgical Diseases" often lead to situations amenable only to surgical treatment, whelher urgent or elective. Those problems are no longer merely limited to the tropics and the Third World. Migratory movements due to famine, economic hardship, war, –or even tourism–, pose an additional challenge. Nowadays, it is conceivable that a physician in Europe or North America may have to deal with surgical problems not frequently found in these parts of the world and information regarding the surgical treatment of infectious and parasitic diseases of the tropics is often incomplete or unavailable in standard textbooks of surgery [1].

There are some tropical affections that may have their clinical course complicated, leading to intra-abdominal infections (IAI) and

urgent clinical/surgical approach. This chapter will gather those diseases, pediatric and adult, making an overview of the clinical picture, diagnosis and management of each situation.

1. MOST COMMON PEDIATRIC TROPICAL AFFECTIONS THAT GENERATE IAI.

1.1. Ascaris lumbricoides infestation

Massive *Ascaris lumbricoides* infestation in children may result in significant morbidity and mortality. IAI may be generated from some complications following some mechanisms [2]:

a) Mechanical obstruction

Worms can obstruct the intestinal lumen. An intestinal segment " packed " with Ascaris becomes heavier and may twist around its vascular pedicle causing a volvulus with posterior intestinal necrosis and

Figure 1
Plain abdominal film showing small intestinal distension and radiopaque images corresponding to the ' bolus of ascaris "
(arrow)

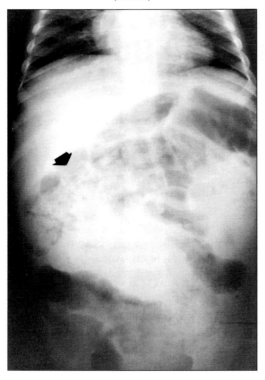

b) Inflammation

Toxic products secreted by Ascaris or resulting from decomposition of dead worms cause intense mucosal inflammation and muscular spasm. Progression of the process associated to intestinal distension and compression by the worms, can lead to intestinal necrosis (Figure 2). In this case, surgical specimens may show bowel necrosis without apparent mechanical strangulation or vascular compromise.

c) Perforation

Ascaris can perforate through bile ducts, intestinal wall, appendix, Meckel's diverticulum or gallbladder - wherever there is severe inflammation and necrosis.

It is interesting to note that those infectious surgical situations usually lead to severe diffuse peritonitis and high morbidity and mortality rates, as the children bearing those conditions are of a low socio-economic level and have poor nutritional status [3].

Clinical manifestations of ascariasis vary. A well-nourished individual can tolerate a

diffuse peritonitis if unrecognized initially (Figure 1).

Fever, spicy food and some drugs are believed to promote Ascaris migration. The main complications when treating an eventual ascaridiasis are cholangitis and pancreatitis secondary to bilio-pancreatic tree obstruction, leading to a typical clinical picture of inflammatory acute abdomen and appendicitis. In busy emergency rooms in the Third World,an incidence of 7.2% of acute appendicitis due to ascaridial luminal obstruction, has been reported.

Figure 2
Intraoperative view of necrotic intestinal segment due to massive infestation of *Ascaris*

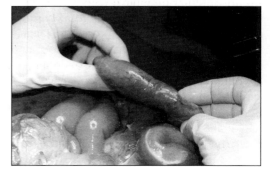

mild infestation with few significant symptoms. Adult Ascaris in the intestines produce few or no symptoms. Chronic infestation in children causes malnutrition, failure to thrive, anemia and poor general health. Massive infestation causes intestinal obstruction, usually in the terminal ileum, manifested by colicky abdominal pain, distension and bilious vomiting. Initially diarrhea may be present as well as non-specific gastrointestinal symptoms like periumbilical pain, nausea and anorexia. The worms are frequently eliminated in these situations in vomitus or stools. Ascaridial elimination through vomiting may occur in chronically infected children or secondary to other causes of acute abdomen like intussusception or appendicitis. These conditions must be ruled out before treatment for ascaridial intestinal obstruction. An abdominal mass consisting of the ascaris " bolus " can be occasionally palpated. Granulomatous peritonitis is a rare complication in chronic ascariasis with symptoms simulating tuberculous peritonitis, lymphoma or Crohn's disease. It is caused by chronic granulomatous reaction of the peritoneum to worms or eggs that perforate into the peritoneal cavity.

As obstruction progresses, abdominal tenderness and guarding appear as well as systemic findings of intestinal necrosis/perforation. Care of malnourished children with Ascaris obstruction must be prompt. Intense dehydration and Gram negative sepsis usually develop under these conditions. Biliary and pancreatic obstruction are characterized by the clinical findings of cholangitis, pancreatitis and cholestasis (Table 1).

Biliary and pancreatic complications can happen simultaneously, since the parasite obstructs the ampulla of Vater and both biliary and pancreatic ducts. In cases of biliary obstruction, hepatic abscesses can originate from ascending cholangitis. These abscesses are either large and solitary or small and multiple and they may rupture to the cavity or erode the diaphragm causing a secondary thoracic empyema. A disintegrated, fractured worm inside the bile ducts causes inflammation of ductal mucosa acting as a predisposing factor to strictures and stone's formation. This entity is known as Chinese biliary syndrome [3,4]. Hepatic involvement also can be due to chronic granulomatous process elicited by a response to larvae, eggs or the adult worm. Hepatic granulomata presents as a tender hepatomegaly and diagnosis is made by liver biopsy. Its chronic course may lead to portal hypertension and splenomegaly.

The treatment of partial or complete uncomplicated obstruction is initially conservative and consists of nasogastric tube insertion, fluid replacement, broad-spectrum antibiotics when sepsis or biliary involvement is thought and analgesia. After initial resuscitation, piperazine-citrate is given through the nasogastric tube (75 mg/Kg), in order to paralyze worms and mineral oil (40-60 ml initially) to help their elimination

Table 1
Signs and symptoms of bilio-pancreatic ascariasis

Epigastric and right upper quadrant pain	100%
Hepatomegaly	100%
Vomiting	80%
Fever, chills	68%
Jaundice	13%
Hemobilia	3%

From: Pinus J.Surgical complications of ascariasis. Progr Pediat Surg 1982, 15:79-86.

by peristalsis. During treatment, physical examination must be repeated in order to identify early signs of perforation, necrosis and/or peritonitis. Anti-helminthic drugs are not recommended, as they promote hypermotility and favor worm migration to bile and pancreatic ducts. Surgical management is warranted for: (1) refractory intestinal obstruction; (2) deterioration of clinical status; (3) signs of necrosis/peritonitis and (4) hematochezia. During the operation, the surgeon tries to free the bolus and gently milk it down toward the large bowel and sometimes an enterotomy must be performed for worm removal. Necrotic bowel must be resected and primary anastomosis attempted unless severe peritonitis is present or the patient is in systemic critical conditions. In such cases a double-barreled enterostomy is performed.

Uncomplicated biliary ascariasis is also treated conservatively. The question about the administration route of anthelmintic drugs is controversial, either systemically or into the biliary tree. Decomposed worms can elicit intense inflammation and act as a nidus for calculus formation. The live worm usually migrates spontaneously out of the biliary system. Bilio-pancreatic ascariasis must be regularly followed by ultrasound to assess the efficacy of treatment and to identify livers abscess formation. ERCP is effective in identifying and removing Ascaris from biliary and pancreatic ducts (Figure 3). Should it fail, formal surgical exploration of the biliary tree is indicated. Hepatic abscesses can be drained percutaneously, with ultrasound or CT guidance, or surgically. Gram-negative antimicrobial coverage is initiated empirically and is guided by Gram stain and culture. Pancreatitis is treated conservatively with oral fasting, nasogastric decompression, H_2 blockers, analgesics and eventually parenteral nutrition.

Figure 3
ERCP showing *Ascaris* in the left hepatic duct

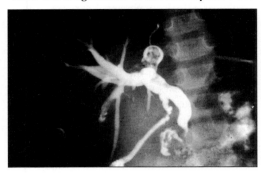

1.2. Intestinal Angiostrongyliasis

Acute abdomen secondary to angiostrongyliasis is rare and it is found mainly in Central and South America. Intestinal granulomatous or necrotic lesions can occur secondary to an intense inflammatory reaction against the worm (*Angiostrongilous costarricences*), its larvae or eggs. The parasite also produces an intense necrotizing vasculitis with thrombus formation leading to ischemia and/or necrosis of intestinal segments[5].

Diagnosis is usually presumptive as identification of the parasite on stool examination is not possible since the worm remains firmly fastened the intestinal wall. It can only be confirmed by the observation of eggs, larvae or adult worms on histopathological examination of surgical specimens (Figure 4). The clinical diagnosis will present the classic findings of an acute abdomen. Laboratorial findings are non-specific, with only mild eosinophilia. Unfortunately, identification of the parasite on stool examination is not possible, since the worm remains entrapped inside the intestinal wall. Serological tests are non-conclusive.

Figure 4
***A. costarricencis* inside a vessel
at the intestinal submucosa -HE stain - x 120**

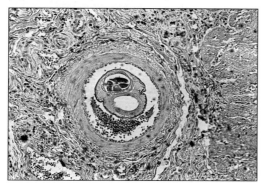

So far, no drug has been demonstrated to be effective against *Angiostrongylus costarricensis*. Thiabendazole has been employed prior or after surgery but the results are uneven. Surgical management will focus on intestinal resections and the treatment of eventual associated peritonitis. Th postoperative period must be closely followed, as progression of intestinal necrosis due to autogenous reinfestation in adjacent areas to the resected segment may occur and reoperation might be required [6,7].

1.3. Toxic colitis following amebiasis

It is estimated that about 10% of the world's population is infected with *Entamoeba histolytica*. What used to be an exclusive public health concern of tropical zones has now taken on worldwide proportions, mainly due to immigration to developed countries.

Amebic dysentery may have potentially lethal complications, especially if early diagnosis is not made and adequate treatment initiated. Perforation and peritonitis are the most common complications observed in children and carry a high mortality rate. Shock, electrolyte and acid-base disorders are frequent and increase the severity of the infection. The other complication that can generate IAI is liver abscess secondary to massive intestinal infestation and portal dissemination. It can be drained percutaneously or laparoscopically and laparotomy is indicated when perforation occurs with secondary peritonitis [8].

Regarding intestinal complications, surgical therapy is straightforward and consists of laparotomy with resection of the compromised intestinal segment. In case of diffuse colic lesions associated to poor systemic status, total colectomy is preferred to partial resections. Lower rates of recurrence and better outcome are more frequently observed with this radical approach. Ostomies are preferred to primary anastomosis.

2. MOST COMMON TROPICAL AFFECTIONS THAT GENERATE IAI. (ADULT)

2.1. Chagasic Megacolon

In 1921 Carlos Chagas described a disease caused by a parasite, entirely based on clinical and epidemiological observation. This disease, named after him, causes myocarditis and significant motility disorders in the digestive tract. Because of its wide prevalence, distribution and severity of its effects, Chagas' disease is considered one of the most urgent public health problems in Latin America [9].

Chagas' disease has been reported from the southern United States to southern Argentina and Chile. The incidence of cardiac and gastrointestinal (GI) manifestations varies throughout Latin America. This is probably due to different strains of the *Trypanosoma cruzii*. In countries north of the Equator, the GI form has never been described and in South American countries other than Brazil, there is a very low incidence of this form compared to the cardiac one. Almost 8% of the population in Latin America is supposed to be infected by the parasite yet have no clinical manifestations. The majority of the patients have cardiac manifestations and only 7%-18% have GI symptoms. The incidence of Chagas' disease is predominant in males (3:2). The age distribution of chagasic megacolon in Brazil is around 4% under 20 years old, 88% from 20-60 and 8% over 60 [10].

The infection is transmitted by a hematophagous insect of the Triatomidae family. While sucking the host's blood, the insect produces feces containing *Trypanosoma cruzii*.

The clinical manifestations of Chagas' disease in the digestive tract are caused by the destruction of neural cells of intramural plexi of Meissner and Auerbach. The destruction mechanism is mediated by neurotoxins and inflammatory reactions produced by the trypanosoma. In the colon, motility disorders occur and they are especially marked in distal segments, mainly in the rectum. Achalasia of the internal anal sphincter contributes to defecation impairment [11].

Diagnosis is made through history and mainly collecting epidemiological data. In the acute form, the parasite can be detected in the blood. In the chronic form, the Machado-Guerreiro test, carried out by hemagglutination or immunofluorescence, is positive in 80%-90% of patients and demonstrates previous infection by the parasite.

The two main complications of chagasic megacolon are fecaloma and sigmoid volvulus. Fecaloma occurs in severely obstipated patients. Sigmoid volvulus develops when this segment becomes extremely elongated and mobile. The bowel rotates around its mesentery from 90° to 320°. With minor torsion (90°-180°), also called " incomplete torsion ", there are usually no ischemic complications and the patient can endure this condition for several days. With major torsion, called " complete torsion ", the likehood of ischemia increases. In these cases, perforation with fecal peritonitis is followed by high mortality. Pain, abdominal distension and obstipation are the clinical signs and symptoms of the uncomplicated form. When abdominal tenderness appears, the complicated form is suspected. Another not-so-frequent complication that may lead to IAI is ischemic colitis. It carries a very high mortality rate as diagnosis is usually delayed [12].

Plain abdominal films, when volvulus is suspected, may show marked left lower quadrant bowel dilatation (Figures 5 and 6) and pneumoperitoneum may be present. Iodine contrast may be employed to perform a rectal enema and the "candle's flame " sign indicates sigmoid torsion.

With sigmoid volvulus, the first procedure to be attempted is bowel distortion with rigid or flexible sigmoidoscopy, as there is mainly air or liquid stools within the proximal bowel. A rectal tube may be left inside the colon, above the torsion point to prevent recurrence. When ischemic complications are suspected, laparotomy and bowel resection are indicated. A Hartmann's procedure or a decompressive colostomy is performed and the patient remains in the hospital after volvulus' treatment for the definitive surgical approach. The operations that could prevent further complications of megacolon can be

Figure 5 and Figure 6
Plain abdominal films. Sigmoid volvulus

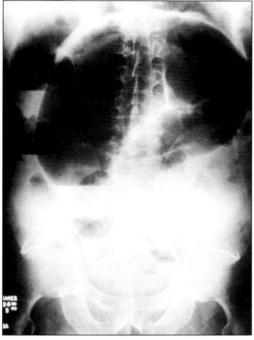
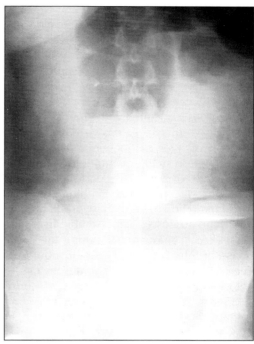

divided into 2 major groups : abdominal and abdomino-perineal procedures. The abdominal operations are sigmoidectomy, rectosigmoidectomy and hemicolectomy and the abdomino-perineal are the endoanal pull-through resection with delayed colorectal anastomosis [13], endoanal pull-through resection with delayed colo-anal anastomosis [14] and the Duhamel-Haddad operation [15,16]. The description, advantages and disadvantages of each operation are beyond the scope of this chapter.

2.2. Amebic liver abscess

Amebiasis has a worldwide distribution with the highest incidence observed in sub-

tropical/tropical areas with poor sanitary conditions. Human carriers that eliminate *Entamoeba histolytica* in their stools are the primary source of infection. In its cystic form, the parasite survives outside the human body, reaching the digestive tract by ingestion of contaminated food or water. The cysts are resistant to gastric acid and are digested by pancreatic enzymes releasing invasive trophozoites. The trophozoites live and multiplicate in the large bowel lumen, especially in the cecum, migrate to distal colon and change into round or oval cysts passed in the feces. The parasite can live in the bowel lumen without tissue invasion. yet trophozoites generally invade the colonic mucosa, where superficial may be seen. From the mucosa they enter mesenteric venules or lymphaticus and are carried to the liver via portal circulation.

The most common site of extraintestinal colonization is the liver [17]. Massive embolization of parasites or ameba's multiplication can lead to venular obstruction or thrombosis with infarction of liver parenchyma cells. The coalescence of the necrotic areas associated with ameba-induced cytolysis results in extensive cavitary destruction of liver parenchyma. The lesions produced are single or multiple and of variable size. Occasionally parasites pass through hepatic sinusoids reaching the systemic circulation where they produce lung and brain abscesses [18]. Amebic liver abscesses (ALA) may appear during the acute phase of intestinal amebiasis or months or even years later. Sometimes abscesses develop in patients who never have had prior symptoms. The abscess is usually large and solitary, most of the time located in the right liver lobe, often in a superior and anterior position just below the diaphragm. It consists of a large, central necrotic liquefied area with thick chocolate-brown pus. Histologically, degenerated hepatocits, white blood cells are found. During early stages of amebic hepatitis, ameba are found most frequently in the focal area of necrosis and as the process develops into abscess formation, protozoa are found in the bordering tissue or in the abscess' wall [19].

Young men are more commonly affected than women (9:1). Patients bearing ALA are younger than those with pyogenic lesions. Patients usually live or come from an endemic area. The onset is gradual. The earliest and most common manifestations are pain and right upper quadrant tenderness. Amebic dysentery is present in only 10 % of patients and in an autopsy study of patients with ALA, 27% had colonic lesions. Fever is low, intermittent or even absent, unless secondary infection is present. Nausea, vomiting, anorexia and weight loss occur but are non-specific. Jaundice is unusual and is mild if present [20,21].

Diagnosis may be supported by subsidiary examinations. Leukocytosis is found in 70% of patients. Serum alkaline phosphatase is about twice the normal value; elevated serum bilirubin is rare and low serum albumin and elevated globulin with normal total protein values are found. *Entamoeba histolytica* is isolated from abscesses in about 20% of cases; ameba are more likely to be detected in the peripheral margin or the abscess wall. The protozoa can be isolated in stool in 15%-47% of cases. Pitt [22] reported ameba in the stools of 66% of patients with amebic hepatitis and 47% of those with ALA. Many serological tests are available and they have an accuracy of 95%. The enzyme linked immunosorbent assay (ELISA) technique is sensitive to the *E. Histolytica* antibody from serum and abscess aspirate.

Chest films may show an elevated right diaphragm or pleural effusion. Ultrasound is accurate in 80%-90% of cases of hepatic abscess and guides needle aspiration but findings are not ALA specific. Abul-Khair [23] suggest that ALA have a thin wall with internal echoes less dense than surrounding tissue (Figure 7). Computed tomography is very sensitive , with accuracy ranging from 90% to 95%, demonstrating lesions as small as 0.5cm. Percutaneous aspiration for the diagnosis of ALA should be reserved for patients with suspected abscess and negative serology.

Adams and MacLeod [21] reviewed 2074 patients with amebic liver abscess (ALA); 9.6% were uncomplicated. In contrast to

Figure 7
Ultrasonography showing a liver amebic abscess with a thin wall and internal echoes (debris)

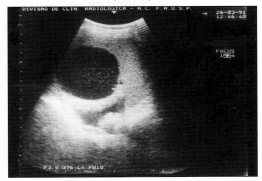

pyogenic liver abscess, ALA tends to rupture, reflecting the thin band of granulation tissue surrounding the abscess, in comparison to the fibrous wall in pyogenic cases. The most common sites of rupture are into the peritoneal cavity and the pleura but also rupture to the retroperitoneum, biliary tract and bowel loops can occur. Secondary bacterial infection occurs in about 20% of the patients and is suspected if prostration, fever and a rise in white blood cells is present. In those cases, the pus in the abscess becomes grayish-yellow or green.

The treatment of amebic abscess includes amebicidal agents, aspiration and percutaneous drainage and surgical conventional drainage [24]. Medical treatment with antiamebic agents, as nitroimidazoles such has in, part replaced surgical drainage. The use of metronidazole[25], 750 mg three times/24 hs for 10 days is highly effective and is the treatment of choice for ALA. Failures are uncommon and may be related to persistence of intestinal disease, inadequate drug absorption or resistance. Other drugs such as chloroquine, used alone or in com-

bination with emetine or dihydroemetine, are also effective to treat amebiasis. Advances in treatment modalities has decreased mortality from 81% in 1956 to 3.9% in 1974. Medical management is usually effective and should always be the first step in the management of ALA. Invasive measures are reserved for patients with complications such as free cavity rupture or secondary bacterial infection.

Percutaneous drainage (PD) under ultrasound guidance can provide diagnostic aspiration and avoid surgical treatment. PD is being frequently used for the treatment of pyogenic liver abscess but this approach is not very effective for ALA management because the abscess content is usually thick, making adequate drainage difficult and secondary bacterial superinfection may happen. Surgical treatment is required in up to 10% of cases and is reserved for complications such as rupture or imminent rupture. Surgical drainage is also required in abscesses in locations inaccessible to needle puncture and after an unsuccessful trial of medical or combined medical and percutaneous drainage therapy. When diagnosis is difficult or diagnostic facilities are poor, the rate of surgical treatment is greater. The decision of an invasive approach is based on the physician's experience. Filice [24] suggests ultrasound-guided drainage with intralesion injection of nitroimidazole. The disease resolves more promptly with fewer relapses and less residual hepatic scarring when compared to open surgical drainage and medical associated treatment. It is emphasized that combined therapy should be used in patients with abscesses exceeding 5-6cm in diameter. The time required for the abscess cavity to resolve after treatment depends on its size and can vary from 10 days to a year. The mortality rate for the treatment of ALA is about 4%, and when secondary infection is present is as high as 20%. The prognosis depends on the organism's virulence and host defense, the number of liver lesions, presence of secondary infection and the type of therapy employed.

2.3. Primary Intrahepatic Lithiasis

Primary intrahepatic lithiasis (IHL), also known as hepatolithiasis or recurrent pyogenic cholangitis, is a rare disease in the western world but is frequent in eastern Asia, with unknown etiology [26].

The etiology and pathophysiology of IHL are not completely understood. Poor sanitation and nutrition seem to predispose to the development of the disease. Clinical and experimental data suggest that intestinal bacteria pass through the portal system to the liver by translocation through mucosal lesions caused by chronical parasitic intestinal disease, a characteristic of developing countries. Some worms, as *Ascaris lumbricoides and Clonorchis sinensis,* may cause inflammatory lesions in the biliary tract and act as a nidus for stone formation [27,28]. The association of biliary stasis and infection are determinant factors in lithogenesis. Bacterial infection is very common, mainly by *E. Coli, Klebsiella sp. and Streptococcus fecalis.* Anaerobes are found in 30% of the cases and *Clostridium* and *Bacteroides* are the most frequent.

Stones occur most commonly in both hepatic lobes and if there is unilateral involvement, the left lobe is more frequently affected. Stones in the extra-hepatic bile duct and gallbladder are found in 50% and 33% of cases, respectively. Biliary stasis associated to infection can lead to biliary strictures or abscess formation in one-third of the patients. Repeated episodes of cholangitis

characterize the disease. It can lead to destruction of liver parenchyma and atrophy of the affected part of the liver. In severe cases, secondary biliary cirrhosis can be found [29,30].

The peak of incidence of the disease is in the third decade of life, earlier than in patients bearing cholelithiasis. Males and females are equally affected. Cholangitis is almost a constant in patients with IHL. Charcot's triad is present in 60% of patients. Symptoms vary from mild abdominal pain to severe septic shock and mental confusion. On physical examination the liver is enlarged and the right upper quadrant is tender. Scars of previous biliary surgery are observed in 30%-50% of patients. In chronic and severe disease, signs of liver failure can be found secondary to biliary cirrhosis.

Laboratory data demonstrate leukocytosis, abnormal liver function tests`as elevated bilirubin, alkaline phosphatase and gamma-glutamil-transpeptidase, confirming the obstructive nature of jaundice. If a stone is present in the distal portion of the common bile duct, serum amylase may be as well elevated. Stool examination for parasites should always be performed. Blood cultures are positive in up to 50% of cases. Ultrasonography in expert hands can detect over 90% of intrahepatic stones but it cannot be employed for the diagnosis of strictures. Computed tomography is less sensitive than ultrasound but is useful to detect livers atrophy and intrahepatic stones location (Figure 8). CT is also helpful in demonstrating hepatic abscesses and for guidance of percutaneous drainage. Percutaneous (PTC) or endoscopic (ERCP) cholangiography, provides the most accurate diagnosis including location and shape of stones (Figure 9) and strictures' evaluation. The choice of either PTC or ERCP depends

Figure 8
Computed tomography demonstrating stones in the right liver lobe

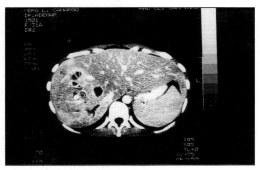

Figure 9
Cholangiography disclosing bilateral intrahepatic stones

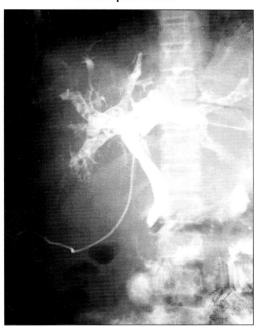

on experience and sometimes both can be used in association to assure that the entire biliary tree is visualized. PTC and ERCP may also have therapeutic value by providing an access for drainage of the infected bile ducts in patients with severe infection waiting definitive treatment.

Treatment of primary intrahepatic lithiasis is essentially surgical and the goal is to decompress the biliary tree, control the infection and clear the stones. Broad spectrum antibiotics must be given at the time of diagnosis and, when cultures are available, should be the bacterias targeted. Recently, several operative procedures have been proposed for biliary drainage (bilioenteric anastomoses or papillotomy), hepatic resection and a combination of both.

Treatment should be individualized for each patient, according to stone location, presence of extrahepatic stones, presence of biliary strictures, liver atrophy or unremovable stones. Hepatic resection is recommended for patients in whom the involved segment or livers lobe, which includes biliary strictures and stones, can be completely removed (Figure 10). It is in-

dicated in cases of associate atrophy of livers parenchyma. This approach, used for localized disease, leads to good results in 80%-100% of cases. The mortality rate in specialized reference centers for liver resection is less than 4%,

For patients with bilateral disease, biliary drainage procedures such as hepatojejunal Roux-en-Y anastomosis or papillosphincterotomy are recommended. When stones are found in both major lobes,biliary drainage procedures with stone clearance and biliary decompression provide good results in 50-70% of patients. The incidence of stone recurrence is high, ranging from 16% to 50%. Auxiliary procedures as postoperative cholangioscopy and lithotripsy for residual or recurrent stones, have improved long-term

Figure 10
Left hepatectomy. Left liver lobe with intrahepatic calculi

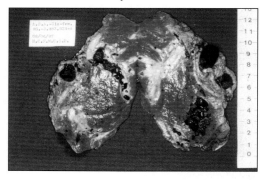

results. Complete stone clearance with surgical treatment and complementary methods is possible in 80-90 % of the cases [31,32,33,34].

2.4. Hydatid liver cyst

The hydatid liver cyst is a cyclozoonotic infection that affects humans and other animals and it is caused by *Taenia echinococcus* in its larval cystic stage. The adult form of *Echinococcus granulosus* inhabits the first portion of the small bowel of the definitive host, household dogs and wild canines. It is fixed by its scolex to the bowel's villi. The larvae can be found in herbivorous animals and in humans. In humans, one or several bags of liquid, fixed in the liver in almost 60% of cases, comprises the hydatid liver cyst [35].

The disease is endemic in southern Brazil, Uruguay and Argentina. It is also reported in Central Europe, Northern and Southern Africa, Australia, New Zealand and in lower rates in Saudi Arabia, Siberia, Northern China, Japan and Philippines.

The hydatid liquid is sterile and uncolored, with a density of 1007 to 1015. It contains small amounts of albumin, urea, glucose, uric acid, creatinine, chloride, sulphate, sodium phosphate and traces of other salts and is slightly alkaline. Host immunoglobulin have been found in some cysts, however the mechanism of entrance remains unknown, Hydatid liver cysts, when large my have a long course, becoming hydatidoses. In the liver they compress the parenchyma, sometimes even the whole left or right hepatic lobe, causing severe hepatic lesions as well as serious hemodynamic disorders. Cysts located in the cortical regions have less significant vascular and biliary effects. Left lobe cysts rarely cause biliary or vascular complications, unlike those of the right lobe. The cysts may be under high pressure, causing the proligerous membrane to rupture into biliary ducts with hydatid obstruction of the main biliary tree and jaundice. With suprahepatic venous compression, Budd-Chiari syndrome has been reported [36].

Most of the clinical manifestations have a long course of evolution. The hydatid liver cyst is usually asymptomatic for a long time. It elicits no, or only a weak immune response and requires continuous surveillance after the diagnosis is done through imaging methods, such as ultrasonography and/or CAT scan. Complication rate decreases with close follow-up. Complications include cyst rupture into the biliary tract, liver abscess, bronchial fistula, rupture to free peritoneal cavity, cystic wall calcification that may predispose to a cystic-digestive tract fistula and compression of biliary ducts and suprahepatic and portal veins. The diagnosis of " hydatid peritonitis " is difficult to make, as the hydatid liquid is sterile and clinical manifestations arise after any possible bacterial secondary infection [37].

The overall mortality, according to most authors, ranges between 3% and 8%, while morbidity is 15%-35% [35,37].

When discussing subsidiary elements for diagnosis, the main laboratory tools are electrophoresis, ELISA and hemagglutination. The specificity of electrophoresis is high and ELISA is very sensitive.

Conventional radiological methods can demonstrate liver enlargement, pleural reaction, air level inside the cysts and calcified rings (Figure 11).

Ultrasonography and computed tomography determine the number, location, cyst volume and anatomical relations of the cyst and the vascular and biliary structures (Figure 12).

Figure 11
Plain film showing a drained hydatid liver cyst without biliary communication

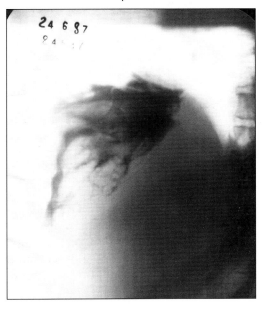

Figure 12
Computed tomography showing a right liver's lobe hydatid cyst

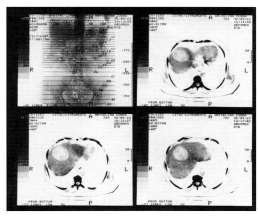

The treatment of hydatidosis is basically surgical. However, the use of imidazole components has been successful. Mebendazole was first introduced in 1977 with good results. It may be indicated by: 1) patients with multiple cysts; 2) complicated forms; 3) pre- or post-operatively ; 4) significant surgical risks. The recommended duration of treatment is 6 months. Recently, other drugs have been used to treat hydatidosis, such as praziquantel, albendazole and fluobendazole. The maximum dose of mebendazole is 300 mg/Kg/day. Medical treatment is contraindicated in pregnancy and in children under 2 years old. Clinical and laboratorial follow-up during treatment should include hematological, hepatic, renal and cardiac monitoring.

Although the management of hydatidosis is basically surgical, techniques vary. Operative risk is high; in the first operation mortality is 2%-8 %. The approach must be conservative, bearing a variety of therapeutic procedures with the same goals: to eliminate the parasite, to enucleate or resect cysts,

Figure 13
Completed pericystectomy

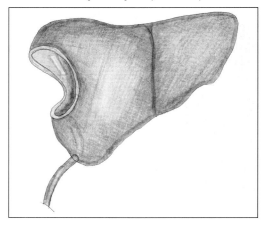

Figure 14
Pericystic resection

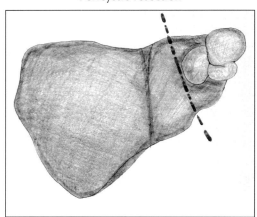

to treat the remaining cavity and assure biliary patency and function. Abdominal exploration must be conducted with care and should be supplemented by intraoperative echography to elucidate the exact number of cysts and their anatomical relation to biliary and vascular landmarks. In order to protect the abdominal cavity, several solutions may be employed as formol 2%, saline 30% and ethanol. However, H_2O_2, silver nitrate 0.5% and cetrimide can be safely employed to avoid peritoneal dissemination during the cyst's manipulation. The surgical options include total pericystectomy and liver resections (Figures 13 and 14). More conservative methods include percutaneous cyst's drainage, internal drainage (cyst-biliary/cyst-jejunal anastomosis) and drainage of the residual cavity [36,37,38].

Hydatid liver disease is usually asymptomatic for a long time. It elicits its no or weak immune response and requires continuous surveillance. Complication rate decreased with imaging monitoring and close follow-up. Complications include cyst rupture into the biliary tract, to the peritoneal cavity, cyst wall calcification that may predispose to cyst-digestive tract fistula and compression of the extrahepatic biliary tree and suprahepatic and portal veins. Complications are also related to liver parenchymal compromise. Mortality ranges between 3% and 8% and morbidity is 15%-35% [39].

2.5. Acute pancreatitis due to Ascaris lumbricoides

Parasitic pancreatitis accounts for less than 1% of the causes of acute pancreatitis.

Ascaris lumbricoides is a common intestinal parasite in tropical and temperate regions and biliary ascariasis is a well-known complication caused by this roundworm [40].

The clinical manifestations are similar to any acute pancreatitis, mild or severe but when marked eosinophilia (greater than

Figure 15
Worm's extrusion through duodenal papilla

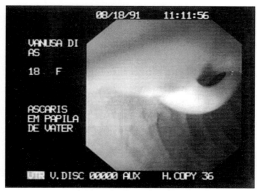

Figure 16
Ascaris' entrapment with a polypectomy loop

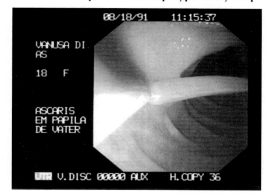

15%) is found, a parasitic etiology should always be considered. Advances in diagnosis have probably contributed to an increased number of reported cases. Several types of imaging modalities, such as ultrasonography, computed tomography (CAT scan) and particularly endoscopic retrograde cholangiopancreatography (ERCP), have all been employed to confirm diagnosis. Some authors have reported that ultrasonography demonstrates the characteristic morphology of worms in patients with biliary/pancreatic ascaridiasis, however, the role of ultrasonography is still controversial [41]. Ultrasonography and CAT scan can be used to even detect complications but ERCP is important for intervention as well as diagnosis [42,43]. Definitive diagnosis can be made by visualization of the worm in the duodenal lumen should penetration into pancreatic or biliary tree be incomplete. Moreover, endoscopic removal can be performed in several ways with forceps or polypectomy loops (Figures 15 and 16) [42]. The indications for ERCP following successful removal of the nematode is subject to debate. If doubts remain regarding removal of the entire worm, endoscopy is mandatory but it should not be employed if removal is com-

plete and recovery is uneventful. If patient's clinical conditions deteriorate or evidence of cholangitis appear, open surgery is indicated, with nematode removal through the common bile duct and T-tube insertion. There is a relatively common situation when the surgeon makes the diagnosis intraoperatively during intraoperative cholangiography in elective cholecystectomies. The worm emerges through the cystic duct stump and the best option is to remove the nematode by choledochotomy followed by T-tube insertion. Patients who recover may expect good long-term results unless they become reinfested [44].

2.6. Typhoid fever

Typhoid fever is an acute infectious systemic disease caused by *Salmonella typhi*. It appears worldwide; however it is endemic in some areas of Asia, the Middle East, the Eastern Europe, and in Central and South America.Incidence is higher in areas where there is rapid population growth, increased urbanization, limited water supply and overburdened health care systems [45].

Typhoid fever (TF) continues to be a global health problem. Approximately 12.5 million cases occur per year with an incidence of 0.5% of the world population. Seven million cases are estimated to occur annually in South and East Asia alone. Other areas with high incidence include Africa and Latin America. In the United States, significant progress has been made in the eradication of *Salmonella typhi*; 35,994 cases were reported in 1920 and 493 in 1991[46,47]. This result is related to improved food hygiene and water treatment. Transmission by contaminated food or water is responsible for most of the recent epidemics.

The incubation period after ingestion of *Salmonella typhi* varies from 5 to 21 days depending on the inoculum ingested and the health of the patient; 10.38% are constipated at onset. Some patients, most commonly those in certain geographic areas, AIDS patients and children under 1 year, will have diarrhea at onset. The mean duration of diarrhea is 6 days. Some non-specific symptoms, such as chills, sore throat, headache, anorexia, dizziness and muscular pain are often present and may be the initial complaint before the onset of fever. The ' typhoid state " described as psychosis and confusion, can occur in 5%-10% of patients. Seizures may even happen. Consequently, a lumbar puncture must be carried out to rule out meningitis. The pathophysiology of CNS features is unknown and may relate to cytokine release from macrophages infected with the Gram-negative bacteria [48].

Physical examination usually reveals a severely ill patient. The pulse may be relatively slow in spite of fever intensity. Around 30% of patients have rose spots which are usually quite subtle and frequently fade to small maculae that seem like minor, resolving skin hemorrhages. Also rales and cervical lymphadenopathy are noted. Abdominal examination usually reveals pain upon deep palpation and increased peristalsis. Half of patients present hepatosplenomegaly and about 3% may have cholangitis. Pancreatitis, although rare, has been described. After the fourth week of infection , without antibiotics, 90% of patients recover from the acute illness. However weakness, weight loss and debilitation may persist for months. In contrast, after proper treatment, fever usually passes in 3-5 days.

Laboratory confirmation of the diagnosis may be done in 2 ways : culture or serology. A definitive diagnosis can be made by hemoculture, which is more likely to be positive during the septic period. Stool cultures are positive during the early phase of the disease, although the greater chance of a positive finding occurs during the third week of infection. This test is of extreme value in identifying chronic carriers who are continuously or intermittently positive. *Salmonella* can be isolated from other sources such as rose spots, mononuclear blood cell-platelet fraction, bronchial fluid, gastrointestinal secretions and bile [49]. Many serological tests, including the classical Widal reaction, are not sensitive, reliable or rapid enough for daily clinical use [50]. Additional findings include leukopenia, mildly elevated bilirubin, elevation in transaminase and alkaline phosphatasis. Urinalysis frequently reveals proteinuria, pyuria and casts. Coagulation abnormalities compatible with intravascular coagulation are common but rarely clinically significant. Plain chest films reveal infiltrates in 2%-11% of the cases. In patients with diarrhea, a methylene blue stain of fresh stools may reveal mononuclear cells. Plain abdominal films are important when intestinal perforation is suspected.

There are many options for the treatment of typhoid fever [51]: quinolone, chloramphenicol, trimethropim-sulfamethoxazol (TMP/SMX) and ß lactams. Since *S. typhi* from many areas of the world (Central America, Southeast Asia, India, Pakistan, the Middle East and Africa) are resistant to chloramphenicol, ampicillin and TMP/SMX, a patient's recent travel history must be considered before initial antimicrobial therapy. Since its introduction in 1948, chloramphenicol has been the drug of choice for typhoid fever therapy , reducing mortality and period of fever. Nevertheless, drug resistance, high relapse rate and high rate of chronic carrier state diminish the value of that drug. Quinolones have theoretical advantages over other antibiotics, as they reduce the incidence of chronic carriers and relapse rate. Quinolones, however, cannot be given to children and pregnant women because of the potential cartilage damage. For multi resistant organisms or empiric treatment, parenteral third generation cephalosporin, particularly ceftriaxone, appears to be the initial agent of choice for children. For oral therapy of sensitive organisms, chloramphenicol and TMP/SMX seem equivalent for chronic or initial therapy. Glucocorticoid in severe typhoid fever with evidence of altered mental status (delirium, obtundation, stupor, coma or shock) has been advocated, with reduction of mortality rate.

The use of oral live vaccine Ty21 is recommended for travelers to high-risk areas because of its low frequency of side effects [52]. Children under 6, immuno supressed individuals and those under antibiotics should not receive it. The protection given by the vaccine in endemic population ranges from 6% to 43% following administration of three doses on alternate days. None of the available vaccines have demonstra-

ted enough efficacy for travelers to broadly recommend their use.

As in all septic diseases, typhoid fever can be associated with complications in any organ. Many of the complications in untreated patients occur during the second to fourth weeks of infection. Intestinal hemorrhage and perforation are the most feared and frequent complications. Focal infections, such as pericarditis, endocarditis, osteomyelitis, cholecystitis, orchitis and splenic (7.3%) and liver abscess may occur. Intestinal perforation occurs in 3% of patients. Lymphoid hyperplasia in the ileocecal area followed by sloughing, ulceration and necrosis with subsequent intestinal hemorrhage and perforation, are typical complications in the small intestine. Rarely perforation occurs in the colon or proximal bowel segments. With antimicrobial therapy these complications have a rate of less than 3%. Some patients appear to improve only to later develop a high fever and increased abdominal pain. Absence of pneumoperitoneum on plain films or leukocytosis are not enough criteria to exclude the diagnosis of typhoid visceral perforation , wich is better based on accurate clinical examination. Early surgery after prompt and adequate resuscitation is lifesaving. Perforation classically occurs on the antimesenteric border of the terminal ileum. During laparotomy, excision of ulcer's margins and primary suture/stapling of the ileum is simple and effective. Resection is advisable if three or more perforations are present. Right hemicolectomy is justified only in patients with cecal perforation. Peritoneal lavage with warm saline and drainage of established abscesses must be part of the procedure.

The underlying problem in typhoid fever can only be solved by public hygiene measures such as provision of clean water and people's basic sanitary education. With

such easy and simple precautions, the incidence and, therefore, treatment and/or
complication rate could improve [53,54].

2.7. Peritoneal tuberculosis

Tuberculosis is one of the main causes of
peritoneal disease. It is observed with greater frequency as the incidence of tuberculosis (TBC) increases, especially in association with AIDS [55].

In fact, peritoneal compromise secondary to
TBC carries a very low rate of associated
bacterial infection, thus it is not an important cause of IAI but its incidence in Middle
East and Africa is increasing. The same phenomenon is happening in developed countries, such as the United States and Western
Europe as migratory and immigratory movements are day by day increasing, paralleled
by AIDS increased incidence. Medical treatment is based on antiTBC drugs with relatively good results [56].

The complications of peritoneal TBC are rare; they include intestinal obstruction and
eventually digestive tract fistulae. They are
usually resolved with conservative treatment and do not require surgery. Mortality
from TBC peritonitis in treated patients is
about 5%, and is considerably higher in
malnourished, alcoholic and elder patients
[57,58,59].

2.8. Intestinal tuberculosis

Primary tuberculosis of the intestine, caused by the ingestion of *Mycobacterium bovis* is rare. Secondary intestinal TBC caused
by *Mycobacterium tuberculosis* is increasing in incidence, mainly due to emigration
from endemic areas to developed countries

and secondary to a higher prevalence of
HIV infection [60].

The distal ileum is the most common site of
the disease. The intestinal form is usually
secondary to a pulmonary focus and has
two forms: **ulcerative** with caseous submucosal lesions responsible for free peritoneal
perforation and visceral fistulas and **hypertrophic** tuberculous enteritis that usually
provokes an inflammatory reaction in Pa-
yer's patches and leads to obstruction of the
compromised segment.

Non-specific symptoms related to TBC are
usually present. Hypertrophic form is cha-
ractherized by signs and symptoms of intestinal obstruction. In the ulcerative form,
crampy, diffuse abdominal pain and diarrhea are common features. Perforation to the
peritoneal cavity may happen in 25% and
during laparotomy, diagnosis of intestinal
TBC may be difficult as it is not easy to rule
out Crohn's disease and right colon cancer.

When perforation associated to fecal peritonitis occurs, right hemicolectomy is usually
required. Reoperations are not rare, as patients bear poor clinical and nutritional status. In a series of 29 ileal perforations secondary to intestinal TBC operated at the
Emergency Service of the University of Sao
Paulo, 65% of all were reoperated to drain
intra-abdominal abscesses and mortality rate was about 30%. Anastomotic complications were present in 20% of cases. Tuber-
culostatic agents, broad spectrum
antibiotics and parenteral nutrition are the
mainstay of post-operative care [61,62].

2.9. Intestinal Paracoccidioidomycosis

Paracoccidioidomycosis is a granulomatous disease, first described by Lutz in

1908. It is caused by a dimorphic fungus, the *Paracoccidioides brasiliensis*, which leads to a progressive and chronic illness characterized by primary pulmonary infection that disseminates by lymphatic or hematogenic routes to other organs, such as the brain, intestine, spleen, pancreas and bones, among others.

The fungal agent is found in Central and South America, from Mexico to Argentina, although is uncommon in Chile [63].

The disease presents in 4 distinct forms, according to both clinical and immunological criteria [64,65] ; a) the **localized** form is rare. There are no changes in serum proteins and low level of complement-fixing antibodies. In the so-called primary type, the oral mucosa or the lungs are involved. The delayed hypersensivity skin reaction (paracoccidiodoioidine) is always positive in this form. b) the **acute or septicemic** form follows the primary infection or recrudescence of pre-existing localized or disseminated chronic disease. It presents as a systemic disease and is responsible for most of the fatal cases. It progresses rapidly and leads to marked cachexia. There is an increase of levels of alpha-1, alpha- 2 and gammaglobulins. Precipitation tests are strongly positive and the serum levels of complement-fixing antibodies are elevated. c) the **chronic disseminated** form is the most common, corresponding to 90% of cases. The evolution of the disease is insidious and is characterized by skin, mucosal and variable degrees of visceral involvement. It tends to be restricted to the lymphaticus. The most frequent form of presentation is the lymphatic-tegumental-visceral. Pulmonary involvement occurs in 90 % of the cases, almost without any symptoms, and diagnosis is based only on chest films. d) The **chronic disseminated**

form occurs in 14.5% of all patients and in 45% of the necropsy cases. It is typical in the second and third decades of life and symptoms are non-specific. The clinical manifestations are lymphnode enlargement, abdominal pain, weight loss, spleen enlargement, ascites and jaundice, plus mucosal-skin lesions. Jaundice is usually secondary to extrinsic compression of the biliary tree from enlarged lymph nodes but less frequently it may be caused by a mycotic granuloma in bile duct mucosa. Diarrhea or dysentery often assume similar characteristics to those in ulcerative colitis. Patients may present with marked protein and fat loss, as severe malabsorption. Constipation or cramps are due to stenosis of the small and/or large intestine, or to extrinsic compression by enlarged abdominal lymph nodes. Diagnosis is based on careful history, direct examination of secretions from fistulized nodes, pulmonary mucus, bronchial lavage, material from lesions or intestinal mucosa, with either an unstained specimen or with a specimen stained with Giemsa. Chest films should be done routinely, since pulmonary symptoms are non-specific.The lack of findings does not exclude paracoccidioidomycosis, especially the acute form. The radiological appearance is variable, ranging from gross to small nodules, pneumonia or cavities. Also calcifications, pleural thickness and fibrosis are frequent features.

Serum specific antibodies and skin tests are extremely helpful in diagnosis, prognosis and treatment. They may identify infected patients who are asymptomatic, although they are negative in the acute form [66].

Small bowel involvement can be evaluated by barium studies. Some features can be appreciated as rapid transit, stenotic areas and/or irregular mucosa, usually in the ter-

Figure 17
Epithelioid granuloma with fungi.
Typical lesion. (Gomori 100x)

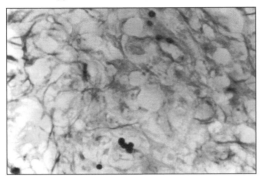

Figure 18
Large ulcerated lesions.
Transmural compromise

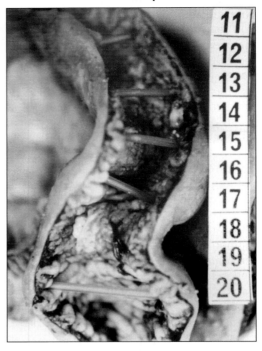

minal ileum which resembles findings seen in intestinal tuberculosis and Crohn's disease. The colon may be studied by either barium enema or colonoscopy. Barium enema may show reduced colon luminal area , simulating neoplastic lesions, extrinsic compression or intra-abdominal calcifications. Large masses, usually located in the right colon can also be detected. However, colonoscopy is considered a better diagnostic procedure since the mucosa can actually be visualized. Moreover, colonoscopy biopsies can be taken and can confirm the etiological diagnosis (Figure 17) as the disease may simulate ulcerative colitis, intestinal tuberculosis, Crohn's disease and cancer.

Drugs used to treat paracoccidioidomycosis are sulfa derivates, azoles and amphotericin B. with Ketoconazole being the main drug. In spite of short-term good clinical results, ketoconazole therapy is usually maintained for 18-24 months. Very severe cases are managed with amphotericin B until a total dose of 1.5-2,5 g is achieved. Occasionally, resistance to amphotericin B may develop; concomitant administration of rifampicin, 600 mg/day may be indicated.

Surgical treatment is restricted to the complications secondary to abdominal lymph node enlargement or intestinal involvement. When large masses are present and CAT scan- guided needle biopsy cannot be performed to confirm diagnosis, laparotomy may be necessary. Other indications for an operative approach are treatment of bowel's (Figure 18) or common bile duct extrinsic compression, lavage of the peritoneal cavity to wash out purulent material from lymph nodes and bowel's obstruction. Intestinal perforation - usually involving the terminal ileum or colon - occurs due to deep mucosal ulceration. Segmental resection is usually the procedure of choice. When surgery is undertaken, regardless of the extension of the disease in the abdomen, specific drug therapy should be promptly initiated, since intestinal involvement is just a part of a systemic disease [67,68,69].

REFERENCES

1. Lacaz CS- Tropical pathology and medical geography. In Cohen RV; Aun F- Tropical Surgery, pg. 1-3. Karger-Landes Systems, 1997, Basel, Switzerland

2. Pinus J. Surgical complications of Ascariasis. Progr Pediatr Surg 1982;15:79-86.

3. Chen D,Li X.-Forty-two patients with acute ascaris pancreatitis in China. J Gastroenterol 1994;29(5);676-78.

4. Ochoa B-Surgical complications of ascariasis. World J Surg 1991;152: 222-27.

5. Morera P.-Life,history and redescription of *Angyostrongilus costaricenses* . Am J Trop Med Hyg 1973;22:613-621.

6. Frontal JK.- *Angyostrongilus costaricenses* infection. In: Branford C;Connors D-Pathology of tropical and extraordinary diseases. Washington,DC. The Armed Forces Institute of Pathology 1976;2(1):452-54.

7. Maksoud Filho JG, Rocha RF- Abdominal complications of intestinal angiostrongyliasis. In Cohen RV; Aun F- Tropical Surgery, pg. 115-17. Karger-Landes Systems, 1997, Basel, Switzerland.

8. Reed SL.-Amebiasis: an update Clin Infect Dis 1992;14:385-93

9. Wendel S,Brener Z,Camargo NE,Rassi A-Chagas' disease: Its impact on transfusion and clinical medicine. São Paulo, Biomedical Institute, Univ. Of São Paulo, ISBT,1992.

10. Branford C;Connors D-Pathology of tropical and extraordinary diseases. Washington, DC. The Armed Forces Institute of Pathology 1976;2(1):323-34.

11. Zapata MT,McGreevy , Mardsen PD-American trypanosomiasis.In Hunter GW-Tropical Medicine. Pg. 628-37, WB Saunders, Philadelphia USA, 1991.

12. Cutait DE,Cutait R-Surgery of chagasic megacolon. World J Surg 1991;15:188-97.

13. Cutait DE, Figliolini FJ- A new method of colorectal anastomosis in abdominoperineal resection. Dis Colon Rect 1961;4:335-42.

14. Simonsen O, Habr A, Gazal P-Retossigmoidectomia endoanal com ressecção da mucosa retal(English abstract). Rev Paul Med 1960;57:116-20.

15. Duhamel B. Une nouvelle operation pour le mégacolon congenital. Press Med 1956;64:2249-2250.

16. Haddad J, Raia A, Corre-Neto A-Abaixamento coloretal com colostomia perineal no megacolon chagásico. Operação de Duhamel modificada (Engl abst) Rev Ass Med Bras 1965;11:83-88.

17. Donovan AJ,Yellin AE,Ralls PW- Hepatic abscess World J Surg 1991;15:162-169.

18. Hai AA,Singh A,Mittal VK,Karan GC- Amoebic liver abscess. Int Surg 1991;76:81-83.

19. Conter RL,Pitt HA,Tompkins RK, Longmire WP- Differentiation of pyogenic from amebic hepatic abscess. Surg Gynecol Obstet 1986; 162:114-119.

20. Crane PS,Lee YT,Seel DJ- Experience in the treatment of 200 patients with amebic abscess of the liver in Korea. Am J Surg 1972; 123:332-37.

21. Adams EB, Mc Leod IN- Invasive amebiasis. Amebic liver abscess and its complications. Medicine 1977; 56: 325-334.

22. Pitt HA- Surgical management of hepatic abscess. World J Surg 1990;14:498-504.

23. Abul-Khair MH, Kenawi MM, Korashi EEA-Ultrasonography and amebic liver abscess. Ann Surg 1981; 193:221-28.

24. Filice C, Di Pierri G, Strosselli M,Brunetti E;Scotti-Foglieni C- Outcome of hepatic

amebic abscess managed with 3 different therapeutic strategies.

25. Powell SJ, MacLeod IN, Wilmot AJ- Metronidazole in amebic dysentery and amebic liver abscess. Lancet 1996; 2:1329-1333.

26. Bove P, Ramos de Oliveira M, Speranzini M- Intrahepatic lithiasis. Gastroenterology 1963;44:251-256.

27. Vachell HR, Stevens WM- Case of intrahepatic calculi. Br Med J 1906;1:434-36.

28. Chen HH,Zhang WH,Wang SS,Carvana JA- Twenty-two years experience with the diagnosis and treatment of intrahepatic calculi Surg Gynecol Obst 1984;159:519-24

29. Nakayama F,Koga A-Hepatolithiasis: present status. World J Surg 1984;8:9-14.

30. Wong J- Recurrent pypgenic cholangitis. In: Schwartz SI, Ellis H- Maingot's Abdominal Operations pg. 908-917, New York, Appleton-Century-Crofts, 1984.

31. Chijiwa K,Kameoka N,Yamazaki T,Nochiro H,Nakano K- Hepatic resection for hepatolithiasis. Long term results. J Am Coll Surg 1995;180:43-48.

32. Choi TK,Wong J- Current management of intrahepatic stones. World J Surg 1990; 14:487-491.

33. Choi TK, Wong J, Ong GB- The surgical management of primary hepatic lithiasis. Br J Surg 1982,69:86-90.

34. Machado MCC,Herman P, Bachela T, Pugliese V, Pinotti HW- Primary intrahepatic lithiasis. Surgical treatment of a rare western's world disease. HPB surgery 1995; 9(1):102-103.

35. Edelweiss EL,Hidatidose. In-Diagnostico e tratamento das doenças infecciosas e parasitárias.pg. 334-342. Ed. Guanabara, Rio de Janeiro, Brazil, 1978.

36. Pinto C, Almeida JL- Hidatidose Humana no Brasil. Arch Int Hidat 1941;5:143-155.

37. Rohner A-Traitment du KHF. Ann Chir 1988; 42:635-38.

38. Bellakhdar A,Iamhamedi A,Neijar M-Irrigation-lavage de la cavite residuelle de KHF. J Chir 1987; 124:189-91.

39. Karkow F, Amendola D- Hydatid liver cyst. Abdominal complications of intestinal angiostrongyliasis. In Cohen RV; Aun F- Tropical Surgery, pg. 225-234. Karger-Landes Systems, 1997, Basel, Switzerland.

40. Capallo D, Gongaware R. Biliary ascariasis. South med J 1984; 77(9):1201-02.

41. Kamath P, Joseph DC, Ramkumar C. Biliary ascariasis: Ultrasonography, ERCP and biliary drainage. Gastroenterology 1986;91: 730-32.

42. Cohen RV,Pereira PR, Tozzi FL,Hashiba K, Maruta L-Acute pancreatitis due to *Ascaris lumbricoides* . Postgrad Gen Surg 1993;5(4):185-86.

43. Lee MJR, Choi TC, Wong J- ERCP after acute pancreatitis. Surg Gynecol Obst 1986; 163: 354-56.

44. Philips RD, Yung HY- Surgical helminthiasis of the biliary tract. Ann Surg 1960; 152(2): 905-10.

45. Edelman R, Levine MM,- Summary of an international workshop on typhoid fever. Rev Infect Dis 1986; 8: 329-49.

46. Waterman SH, Juarez G, Carr SJ- *Salmonella arizona* infections latins associated with rattlesnake folk medicine. Am J Public Health 1990; 80: 286-89.

47. Committee on Salmonella, Division of Biology and Agriculture of the National Research Council. An evaluation of the Salmonella problem. National Academy of Science. Washington DC, USA, 1969.

48. Budd W- Typhoid fever: Its nature, spread and prevention. Longmans Publishers, London, 1973.

49 Gilman RH, Terminel M,Hernandez-Mendoza P- Relative efficacy of blood, urine, rectal swab, bone-marrow and red spots culture for recovery of Salmonella in typhoid fever. Lancet 1975;1:1211-23.

50. Isomaki O,Vuento R, Granfors K- Serological diagnosis of Salmonella infections by immunological assay. Lancet 1989; 6: 1411-14.

51. Nguyen VS- Typhus perforations in the tropics. A report of 83 observations. J Chir (Paris) 1994: 131(2): 90-95.

52. Benavente L, Gotuzzo E, Guerra J- Diagnosis of typhoid fever using a string capsule device. Trans R Soc Trop Med Hyg 1984; 78: 564-65.

53. Vineeta G, Sanjeev KG, Vijay KS, Saroj G- Perforated typhoid enteritis in children. Postgrad Med J 1994; 70:19-22.

54. Kizilcan F, Tanyel FC, Buyukpamukçu A.- Complications of typhoid fever requiring laparotomy during childhood. J Ped Surg 1993; 28:1490-93.

55. Ganga UR, Schaffer L- Tuberculous peritonitis; a case report and review of literature. S D J Med 1992;45(10)287-89.

56. Ihekwaba FN- Abdominal tuberculosis ; a study of 881 cases. J R Coll Surg Edinb 1993; 38(5):293-95.

57. Ahmed ME, Hassan MA- Abdominal tuberculosis. Ann R Coll Surg Engl 1994; 76(2):75-9.

58. Al Quorain AA, Satti MB; Al Gindan YM, Al Ghassab GA, Al Freihi HM - Tuberculous peritonitis. Hepatogastroenterology 1991; 38(1):37-40.

59. Gotzinger RP, Michalik-Himmelmann R, Koop I - Peritoneal tuberculosis. Also current in Germany. Radiologe 1993; 33(6):372-75.

60. Harries AD- Tuberculosis and AIDS in developing countries. Lancet 1990; 335:387-90.

61. Rieder HL - Tuberculosis in the United States. JAMA 1989; 262: 385-88.

62. Cohen RV- Intestinal tuberculosis. In Cohen RV; Aun F- Tropical Surgery, pg. 251-52. Karger-Landes Systems, 1997, Basel, Switzerland.

63. Perea VD, Gallegos MM, Hurtado JMC, herrera JV, Aspicuelca FA - Blastomicosis sudamericana. Presentacion de caso com compromisso extenso y primitivo del colon. Acta Méd Peru 1974; 3:117-21.

64. Sodré LA, Cerrutti H- Retite blastomitótica. Bol Soc Med Cir São Paulo 1930; 14: 167-76.

65. Olivaira E - Blastomicose do reto. An Paul Med Cir 1950; 83: 113-21.

66. Veronesi R, Del Negro G, Albuquerque FJ, Soares JCM- Blastomicose retal primitiva. Rev Hosp Clin Fac Med Univ S Paulo 1954; 9: 327-36.

67. Fonseca LC, Mignone C - Paracoccidioidomicose do intestino delgado. Aspectos clinicos e radiológicos de 125 casos. Rev Hosp Clin Fac Med Univ S Paulo 1976; 31:199-207.

68. Martinez R, Meneghelli UG, Dantas RO, Fiorillo AM - O comprometimento intestinal na blastomicose sul americana. Rev Ass Med Bras 1979; 25:31-34.

69. Arantes Pereira A - A paracoccidioidomicose gastro-entérica. Estudo radiológico. Thesis - Univ. Of Rio de Janeiro, Brazil, 1983.

Index

Abdominal compartment syndrome, *154, 159*
Acute appendicitis, *313*
Acute cholangitis, *212, 217, 331, 319*
    Recurrent pyogenic cholangitis, *374*
Acute Cholecystitis, *209, 318*
    Acalculous cholecystitis, *210, 261, 320*
    Calculous cholecystitis, *210, 319*
    Emphysematous cholecystitis, *211*
    Pericholecystic abscess, *211*
Acute fluid collections, *222*
Acute fulminant colitis, *326*
Acute pancreatitis, *322*
Acute pseudocysts, *223*
Adenovirus, *275, 312*
Adverse drug effects, *130*
AIDS in pediatric patients, *274*
AIDS-appendicitis, *270*
AIDS-associated "cholangiopathy", *261, 262*
AIDS-related gastritis, *269*
AIDS-related lymphoma, *273, 274*
AIDS-related non-Hodgkin lymphoma, *272*
Amebic dysentery, *369*
Amebicidal agents, *373*
Aminoglycoside, *125, 127*
Aminoglycoside peak levels, *131*
Amphotericin B, *186, 384*
Anabolic "flow" phase, *112*
Anaerobic bacteria, *122, 123*
Anti-enterococcal agents, *182*
Anit-helminthic drugs, *368*
Anti-Pseudomonal therapy, *137*
Antibiotic Therapy, *200, 297*
    β-lactamase inhibitor, *132, 135*
    Carbapenems, *125, 135, 184*
    Combination therapy, *73*
    Duration, *137, 291*
    Fourth generation cephalosporins, *132*
    In biliary tract infections, *215*
    In hepatic abscesses, *200*
    In PID, *351*

    In SBP, *93*
    In secondary peritonitis, *120*
    In tertiary peritonitis, *179*
    Monotherapy, *135*
    Quinolones, *381*
    Short-course treatment, *83*
    SIS recomendations, *132*
    Third generation cephalosporins, *82, 135, 286*
    Triple drug therapy, *291, 307*
Antibiotic-resistan pathogens, *135*
Antienterococcal coverage, *139, 182*
Antifungal therapy, *137, 184*
Antiseptics, *107, 294*
APACHE II, *99, 111, 124, 225*
Artificial Burr, *166*
Ascaris lumbricoides, *365, 374, 378*
Atlanta Classification System, *219, 220*
Aztreonam, *127*
β-lactamase inhibitor, *132, 135*
Bacteremias, *249*
Bacterial gastroenteritis, *312*
Bacterial overgrowth, *332*
Bacteroides fragilis, *122, 357*
Biliary pancreatitis, *219*
Bilio-pancreatic ascariasis, *367*
Budd-Chari syndrome, *376*
Candida albicans, *89, 276*
Candida glabrata, *186*
Candida krusei, *186*
Carbapenems, *135*
Carbenicillin, *134*
Carboxypenicillins, *184*
Catabolic "ebb" phase, *112*
Cefonicid, *132*
Ceforanide, *132*
Cephalopthin, *107, 124*
Cephazolin, *107*
Ciprofloxacin, *139*
Clinafloxacin, *183*

Clindamycin, *124, 125, 353*
Clinical trials, *124, 125*
Clonorchis sinensis, *374*
Clostridium difficile, 268, 303, 307, 323
Colpotomy drainage of a pelvic abscess, *357*
Continuous ambulatory peritoneal dialysis
(CAPD), *87*
Contrast-enhanced CT scans, *227*
Covered Abdominostomy (COLA), *157*
Crohn´s disease, *326*
Cryptosporidium, *262, 265, 268, 275, 276*
CSF pseudocysts, *288*
Culture of the peritoneal fluid, *102*
Cullens´sign, *225*
Cytokine plasma levels, *54*
Cytomegaloviral cholecystitis, *265, 266*
Chagasic Megacolon, *369*
Chinese biliary syndrome, *367*
Chlamydia trachomatis, 327, 346, 347, 350
Chloramphenicol, *127, 183, 381*
Cholangiopancreatography (ERCP), *322*
Cholecystectomy, *216*
Chronic granulomatous disease (CGD), *298*
D-xylose absorption test, *275*
Damage control laparotomies, *103*
Design of clinical trials, *65*
Diagnosis of intra-abdominal infection, *31*
    Liver abscesses, *197*
    Non-directed relaparotomy, *33*
    Non-therapeutic laparotomy, *33*
    Peritoneal tap, *34*
    Radionuclide clolescintigraphy, *37, 214*
    Splenic abscesses, *207*
Diarrehal gastrointestinal infections, *275*
Diversion colitis, *324*
Drug approval process, *68*
Echinoccocus granulosus, *376*
Endoscopic retrograde cholangio-
pancreatography (ERCP), *215, 227*
Entamoeba histolytica, 369, 371
Enterobacter cloacae, 184
Enterobacter spp, 180, 184
Enterococcus faecalis, 138
Enterococcus faecium, 138, 183
Escherichia coli, 285, 299
Ethizip, *160*
Familial Mediterranean fever, *321*
Fecaliths, *314*
Fitz-Hugh-Curtis syndrome, *327*
Fluconazole, *186*
Flucytosine, *186*
Fluoroquinolones, *139, 183*
Fosfomycin, *183*
Ganciclovir, *267*

Ganglion cells, *306*
Gastric ulcer with perforation, *103*
Gastrointestinal tuberculosis, *264*
Genetic factors, *56*
    HLA-DR6 serotype, *57*
    Homozygous TNFB2, *57*
Giardia lamblia, 275
Granulomatous peritonitis, *367*
Grey-Turner sign, *225*
Guidelines
    CDC for treatment of PID, *354, 355*
    Criteria for PCD, *297*
    Diagnosis of PID, *348, 349*
    IDSA / FDA for clinical trials, *66*
    Nutritional support, *113*
    SIS, *135*
    STAR, indications, *171*
Hartmann´s pouch, *304, 326*
Hereditary spherocytosis, *318*
Hirschsprung´s enterocolitis, *306*
HIV-infected children, *331*
Human inmunodeficiency virus (HIV)
    Infection, *299*
Human Peritoneal Macrophages, *1*
Human Peritoneal Mesothelial Cells
    (HPMC), *2*
Hydatid liver cyst, *376*
"Hydatid peritonitis", *376*
Hypobaric Wound shield, *162*
Imidazole components, *377*
Imipenem, *125, 184*
Infected pancreatic necrosis, *221*
Infectious proctitis, *268*
Inflammatory bowel disease, *325*
"Intention to treat" analysis, *71*
Intestinal Angiostrongyliasis, *368*
Intestinal Paracoccidioidomycosis, *382*
Intestinal perforation, *381*
Intra-abdominal abscess, *97, 111, 138, 294, 295*
    Percutaneous drainage, *112*
    Post-operative, *296*
    Surgical drainage, *112, 204, 298*
Intracolonic bypass devices, *105*
Intraoperative cholangiography, *217*
Intraperitoneal drains, *294*
Itraconazole, *186*
Kanamycin, *124*
Kaposis sarcoma, *271*
Kawasaki disease, *321*
Ketaconazole, *384*
Klebsiella, 303
Laparoscopic cholecystectomy, *39, 216, 319*
Laparoscopy, *34, 292, 327*
Laparostomy, *110*

Liver abscesses
    Amebic, *201, 371, 372*
    Crytogenic, *196*
    ERCP, *198*
    Pyogenic, *193, 205, 298*
Machado-Guerreiro test, *370*
Marlex mesh, *106, 160, 162*
Meckel´s diverticulitis, *293, 316, 317, 366*
Meconium peritonitis, *290, 307, 308*
Meropenem, *184*
Methicillin-resistant staphylococci, *184*
Metronidazole, *107, 125, 357*
Microbial flora of the gastrointestinal tract, *13*
Midgut volvulus, *305, 306*
Monomicrobial peritonitis, *185*
Multi-drug resistant organisms, *127*
Multiple organ dysfunction syndrome
   (MODS), *45, 99*
Mycobacterium aivum intracellulare
   (MAI), *263, 275, 276, 331*
Mycobacterium aivum complex (MAC), *276*
Mycobacterium bovis, 382
Necrosectomy, *231, 232*
Necrotizing enterocolitis (NEC), *302*
Necrotizing fasciitis, *311*
Neisseria gonorrhoeae, 327, 343
Neonatal gastric perforation, *309*
Nitrofurantoin, *183*
Non-surgical causes of peritonitis, *101*
Norwald agent, *312*
Omphalitis, *310*
Open Abdominostomy (OPA), *157*
Oral vancomycin, *324*
Pancreatic abscess, *224*
Paracoccidioides brasiliensis, 383
Pediatric liver transplantation, *330*
Pediatric renal transplantation, *329*
Pelvic inflammatory disease
   (PID), *326, 341, 346*
Percutaneous drainage, *232, 297, 373*
    CT-guided, *202*
    Cholecystectomy, *217*
    Failure, *203*
    Intra-abdominal abscesses, *112*
    Liver abscesses, *201*
    Splenic abscesses, *209*
    Transhepatic, *215*
Percutaneous transhepatic cholangiography, *215*
Perforated appendicitis, *315*
Perforated sigmoid diverticulitis, *103*
Perihepatic fluid collection, *250*
Peritoneal Inflammatory Response, *5*
    Ascitic fluid, *77*
    Failure, *46*

    Fibrinolitic activity, *7*
    Modulation, *49, 52*
    Neutrophil influx, *7*
    Protein concentration, *285*
    Trans-diaphragmatic absortion, *5*
Peritoneal lavage, *106, 293*
    Diagnostic, *33*
    Intra-operative, *106, 293*
    Post-operative, *109*
Peritoneal tuberculosis, *382*
Peritoneal-associated Lymphoid Tissue (PALT), *3*
PID-associated perihepatitis, *327*
Piperacillin-tazobactam, *134, 183*
Pieprazine-citrate, *367*
Planned relaparotomy (PR), *158*
Pneumatosis intestinalis, 267, 290
Polymyxins, *132*
Post-operative pelvic infections, *359*
Predictors of SBP, *85*
Primary anastomosis of the colon, *104*
Primary Intrahepatic Lithiasis, *374*
Primary peritonitis, *87, 284*
Prophylaxis SBP, *85*
    Cirrhotic patients with gastrointestinal
      hemorrhage, *85*
    Long-term intestinal decontamination, *85*
Pseudo-Whipple disease, *264*
Pseudomembranous colitis, *268, 323, 328*
Pseudomonas aeruginosa, *183*
Quinolones, *381*
Radionuclide scanning, *214*
Regulation of normal microbial ecology, *17*
Risk factors
    Candidal infection, *185*
    CAPD, *87*
    Ventriculoperitoneal shunt infection, *90*
Rotaviruses, *312*
S. pneumoniae, 285
Scores for monitoring peritonitis, *52, 99*
    APACHE I, *52*
    APACHE II, *99, 124*
    APACHE III, *53*
    Legal-score, *53*
    Mannheim Peritonitis Index, *52, 99*
    MOF-score, *53*
    Peritonitis Index Altona, *52, 99*
    Sepsis Severity Score, *53*
    SOFA-score, *53*
Second-look operation, *305*
Secondary Peritonitis, *97, 289*
Selective decontamination of the digestive
   tract (SDD), *229*
Short bowel syndrome (SBS), *331*
Sickle cell anemia, *320*

Sigmoid volvulus, *370*
Small bowel perforation, *103*
Sparfloxacin, *183*
Splenectomy, *209, 300*
Splenic abscess, *206, 299*
Spontaneous bacterial peritonitis, *77, 269, 285*
Spontaneous bile duct perforation, *312*
Spontaneous intestinal perforations, *310*
Staged abdominal repair (STAR), *158, 171*
Standard operative management, *155*
Staphylococcus aureus, 88, 90, 283, 310
Staphylococcus epidermidis, 88, 103, 180, 310
Streptococcus viridans, 90, 287, 310
Streptococcus fecalis, 374
Streptococcus pneumoniae, 285
Streptococcus pyogenes, 299
Stress hormone response, *112*
Sulbactam, *135*
Systemic inflammatory response syndrome
    (SIRS), *52, 97, 225*
Tazobactam, *135*
Temporary closing devices, *105*

Tertiary peritonitis, *143, 179, 181*
Tetracyclines, *183*
Thalassemia major, *318, 320*
Thiabendazole, *369*
Ticarcillin, *134*
Tobramycin, *127*
Toxic megacolon, *325*
Toxin B, *323*
Translocation, *222, 247, 251*
Tripsinogen activation peptides, *220*
Trypanosoma cruzii, *370*
Tubo-ovarian abscess, *328, 342, 357*
Typhlitis, *268, 328, 329*
Typhoid fever, *379*
Ulcerative colitis, *324*
Uncomplicated biliary ascariasis, *368*
Ureidopenicillins, *184*
Ursodeoxycholic acid, *319*
Vancomycin, *88*
Ventriculoperitoneal (VP) shunt infection, *89, 288*
Viral gastroenteritis, *312*
Visceral abscesses, *295*